DRUG GUIDE FOR PSYCHIATRIC NURSING

DRUG GUIDE FOR PSYCHIATRIC NURSING

SECOND EDITION

Mary C. Townsend, RN, MN
Advanced Registered Nurse Practitioner
Clinical Nurse Specialist
Psychiatric/Mental Health Nursing

Private Practice
Affiliated Psychiatric Services
Wichita, Kansas

In consultation with:

Donna J. Schroeder, PharmD
Director of Drug Information Analysis Service
Assistant Clinical Professor
School of Pharmacy
University of California
San Francisco, California

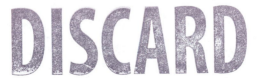

 F. A. DAVIS COMPANY • Philadelphia

F. A. Davis Company
1915 Arch Street
Philadelphia, PA 19103

Printed in the United States of America

Last digit indicates print number: 10 9 8 7 6 5 4 3 2 1

As new scientific information becomes available through basic and clinical research, recommended treatments and drug therapies undergo changes. The author(s) and publisher have done everything possible to make this book accurate, up to date, and in accord with accepted standards at the time of publication. The authors, editors, and publisher are not responsible for errors or omissions or for consequences from application of the book, and make no warranty, expressed or implied, in regard to the contents of the book. Any practice described in this book should be applied by the reader in accordance with professional standards of care used in regard to the unique circumstances that may apply in each situation. The reader is advised always to check product information (package inserts) for changes and new information regarding dose and contraindications before administering any drug. Caution is especially urged when using new or infrequently ordered drugs.

Library of Congress Cataloging-in-Publication Data
Townsend, Mary C., 1941–
    Drug guide for psychiatric nursing / Mary C. Townsend, in consultation with Donna J. Schroeder.—Ed. 2.
        p.   cm.
    Includes bibliographical references and index.
    ISBN 0-8036-8584-X (alk. paper) :
    1. Psychotropic drugs—Handbooks, manuals, etc.
2. Psychopharmacology—Handbooks, manuals, etc. 3. Psychiatric nursing—Handbooks, manuals, etc. I. Schroeder, Donna J.
II. Title.
    [DNLM: 1. Psychiatric Nursing—handbooks. 2. Psychotropic Drugs--handbooks. 3. Psychotropic Drugs—nurses' instruction. QV 39 T749d 1995]
    RM315.T68 1995
    616.89'18—dc20
    DNLM/DLC
    for Library of Congress   94-24449

This Book is Dedicated:

To Virginia Farley French, whose input into the first edition of this text is still highly visible, and who is one of the most courageous individuals I have ever known.

MCT

Acknowledgments

My special thanks and appreciation:

To Joanne DaCunha for guidance and editorial assistance throughout this project.

To the individuals who read and critiqued the manuscript, providing valuable input into the final product.

To Donna Schroeder, who critically reviewed each monograph, and so graciously responded each time I needed assistance.

And to my family, for always being there, and for continuing to believe in me.

MCT

Consultants

James Beach, RPN, BA
Program Supervisor
Wascana Institute
Regina, Saskatchewan, Canada

Marjorie F. Bendik, DNSc, (candidate, RN)
Associate Professor of Nursing
Pt. Loma Nazarene College
San Diego, California

Suellen M. Bryan, RN, BS, MEd
Psychiatric Nursing Instructor
Beebe School of Nursing
Lewes, Delaware

Barbara T. D'Silva, BS, PharmD
Pharmacist
The William W. Backus Hospital
Norwich, Connecticut

Rita Hunt, RN, MS
Instructor
Methodist Hospital
School of Nursing
Lubbock, Texas

Mary Elizabeth Martucci, RN, PhD
Associate Professor Emerita
Former Nursing Department Chair
Saint Mary's College
Notre Dame, Indiana

Gene D. Morse, PharmD
Assistant Professor of Pharmacy
Erie County Medical Center
State University of New York at Buffalo
Buffalo, New York

J. LaRue Pope, RN, MS
Psychiatric Nursing Education Director
Atascadero State Hospital
Atascadero, California

Katy Reynolds, RN, MSN
Professor of Nursing
Long Beach City College
Associate Degree Nursing Program
Long Beach, California

Ann G. Ross, MN, ARNP, CS
Professor of Nursing
Shoreline Community College
Seattle, Washington

Ross A. Stewart, RPN, RN, MHSc
Director
Department of Psychiatric Nursing
Douglas College
New Westminster, British Columbia, Canada

Kathleen L. Talbott, RN, MSN
Assistant Professor
West Texas State University
Canyon, Texas

Reg Arthur Williams, PhD, RN, FAAN
Associate Professor
University of Michigan
School of Nursing
Ann Arbor, Michigan

Table of Contents

Introduction

PHARMACOLOGY: ADJUNCT PSYCHOTHERAPY

What sort of behavior warrants the label of "mental illness"?[1] Horwitz has suggested a strong cultural influence in the application of this label. Behaviors considered indicative of mental illness in one society may not necessarily be considered as such in another. Standards by which behaviors are measured include:

1. The degree to which the behavior conforms to societal norms
2. The ability of an observer to comprehend the behavior (or the motivation behind the behavior)

Historically, reaction to and treatment of the mentally ill ranged from benign involvement to intervention some would consider inhumane. Mentally ill individuals were feared due to common beliefs associating them with demons or the supernatural. They were looked upon as loathsome and often were mistreated.

Beginning in the late 18th century, a type of "moral reform" in the treatment of the mentally ill began to occur. This resulted in the establishment of community and state hospitals concerned with the needs of the mentally ill. Considered a breakthrough in the humanization of care, these institutions, however well intentioned, fostered the concept of custodial care. Patients were assured the provision of food and shelter but had little or no hope of change for the future. As they became increasingly dependent upon the institution to fill their needs, the likelihood of their return to the family or community diminished.

The early part of the 20th century saw the advent of the somatic therapies in psychiatry. Mentally ill individuals were treated with insulin shock therapy, wet sheet packs, ice baths, electroconvulsive therapy, and psychosurgery. Before 1950, no important chemical agents existed in psychiatric practice except sedatives and amphetamines, which had limited use due to their toxicity and addicting effects.[2] Since the 1950s, the development of psychopharmacology has expanded to include widespread use of antipsychotic, antidepressant, and antianxiety medications. Research into how these drugs work has provided an understanding of the etiology of many psychiatric disorders.

Psychotropic medications are not intended to "cure" mental illness. Most physicians who prescribe these medications for their patients use them as an adjunct to individual or group psychotherapy. Although the contribution of these drugs to psychiatric care cannot be minimized, it must be emphasized that psychotropic medications relieve physical and/or behavioral symptoms. They do not resolve any underlying condition or emotional problems that may exist.

---

[1]Horwitz, AV: The Social Control of Mental Illness. Academic Press, New York, 1982, pp. 14–30.

[2]Burgess, AW: Psychiatric Nursing in the Hospital and the Community, ed 4. Prentice-Hall, Englewood Cliffs, NJ, 1985, p. 755.

Nurses must understand the legal implications associated with administration of psychotropic medications. Laws differ from state to state, but most adhere to the patient's right to refuse treatment. Exceptions exist in emergency situations when it has been determined that patients are likely to harm themselves or others.

It is important for nurses to be familiar with the psychotropic medications being administered. This text is designed to provide the information needed to administer medications in a safe manner and to provide a framework of the nursing process for delivery of care. Common psychotropic medications are included, as well as other medications that have implications in psychiatry. Each medication monograph includes GENERIC and TRADE NAMES, CONTROLLED SUBSTANCE and PREGNANCY CATEGORIES, CLASSIFICATION, MECHANISM OF ACTION, INDICATIONS, CONTRAINDICATIONS AND PRECAUTIONS, PHARMACOKINETICS, ADVERSE REACTIONS AND SIDE EFFECTS, INTERACTIONS, ROUTE AND DOSAGE, and PHARMACODYNAMICS sections. In addition, application of the nursing process as it relates specifically to each medication is discussed. This includes assessment data necessary for safe administration, NANDA-accepted nursing diagnoses with potential or actual relevance to administration of the medication, nursing actions important in the implementation of drug administration (including a section on patient/family education), and evaluation of patient response to the medication regimen.

This integration of psychopharmacology with nursing process will provide the nurse with a useful, quick, and up-to-date reference for systematic and accurate administration of medications commonly used in psychiatry.

How to Use Drug Guide for Psychiatric Nursing*

The purpose of DRUG GUIDE FOR PSYCHIATRIC NURSING is to provide readily accessible, easy-to-understand information on the most commonly prescribed drugs for use in psychiatric/mental health clinical settings. The sections below describe the organization of the book and the information provided for each drug.

SPECIAL DOSING CONSIDERATIONS

In many clinical situations, the average dosing range can be inappropriate. This section presents general guidelines for situations in which special dosing considerations must be made to ensure optimum therapeutic outcome.

CLASSIFICATIONS

Brief summaries of the various drug classifications are provided, along with a list of drugs contained in each classification and the page numbers on which the individual drug monographs may be found.

DRUG MONOGRAPHS

The following information appears for each drug:

Generic/Trade Name: The generic name appears first, followed by the pronunciation key (in parentheses). Next is an alphabetical listing of popular trade names. Canadian trade names appear in brackets. If the generic name is not known to the reader, he or she may refer to the Comprehensive Index. It contains entries both for trade names and generic names, as well as for classifications, and is designed to provide this information quickly and easily.

Classification(s): The classification of a drug by its most common use in psychiatric/mental health nursing is listed first, followed by other classification(s) for which the drug is used. For example, amantadine (Symmetrel) is classified first as an antiparkinsonian agent for its primary use in psychiatry and secondly as an antiviral agent. Refer to the Classification section, which provides brief summaries of the classifications contained within the book, lists the drugs included in each classification, and identifies the page numbers on which the drugs can be found.

Controlled Substance Category: If a drug is a controlled substance, the category under which it has been scheduled in terms of abuse potential is listed. This information alerts the reader to observe necessary regulations when handling these drugs. As a further aid, an explanation of controlled substance categories is contained in Appendix A. The appendix describes the five categories and lists

---

*Adapted from Deglin, JH and Vallerand, AH: Davis's Drug Guide for Nurses, ed 4. FA Davis, Philadelphia, 1994.

the drugs included in this book under each category, along with the page numbers on which they appear.

Pregnancy Category: The Food and Drug Administration (FDA) has established five categories to which a drug may be assigned, based on documentation of risk to the fetus balanced against potential benefits to the patient. If a drug has been assigned, its category is listed. The reader may refer to the Key to FDA Pregnancy Control Categories in Appendix B for an explanation of these ratings, along with a list of the drugs included in this book within each category and the page numbers on which they appear.

Action: This section contains a concise description of how a drug is known or believed to act in producing the desired therapeutic effect.

Indications: The indications for use of the drug as commonly prescribed in psychiatry are listed. Those indications not approved by the FDA are listed as "Investigational Uses," or "Unlabeled Uses."

Pharmacokinetics: This section describes what happens to a drug following administration. It includes information on absorption, distribution, metabolism, excretion, and half-life (the amount of time for drug levels to decrease by 50%). Such information is useful because, for example, if only a small fraction of a drug is absorbed when administered orally (diminished bioavailability), the oral dose must be much larger than the parenteral dose.

Following absorption, drugs are distributed, sometimes selectively, to various body tissues and fluids. These factors become important in choosing one drug over another, as in avoiding drugs that cross the placenta in pregnancy or concentrate in breast milk during lactation. If drugs are extensively metabolized in the liver, patients with severe liver disease may require a reduction in dosage. If the kidney is the major organ of elimination, dosage adjustment may be necessary in cases of renal impairment. Premature infants, neonates, and persons over age 60 have diminished renal excretory and hepatic metabolic capacities, and so may require dosage adjustments.

The half-life of a drug is useful to know in planning effective regimens, since it correlates roughly with the duration of action. Half-lives given are based on patients with normal renal and hepatic functions. Conditions that may alter the half-life are noted.

Contraindications and Precautions: Situations in which use of the drug should be avoided or alternatives strongly considered are listed as contraindications. In general, most drugs are contraindicated in pregnancy or lactation unless the potential benefits outweigh the possible risks to the mother, fetus, or neonate (e.g., anticonvulsants). Absolute contraindication—that is, situations in which the drug in question should be avoided completely—are introduced by the heading "Contraindicated in." Relative contraindications, in which certain clinical situations may allow the cautious use of a drug, are introduced by the heading "Use Cautiously in." The contraindications and precautions section includes disease states or clinical situations in which drug use involves particular risks or in which dosage modification may be necessary.

Adverse Reactions and Side Effects: This information is organized using a systems approach. Although it is not possible to include all reported reactions, an effort has been made to include all major side effects. Life-threatening adverse reactions or side effects are capitalized. The problems encountered most commonly are underlined.

The following abbreviations are used to designate affected systems: CNS, central nervous system; CV, cardiovascular; DERM, dermatologic; EENT, eye, ear, nose, and throat; ENDO, endocrinologic; GI, gastrointestinal; GU, genitourinary; HEMAT, hematologic; METAB/NUTRIT, metabolic, nutritional; MS, musculoskeletal; NEURO, neurologic; OCULAR, eye/vision; PSYCH, psychiatric; RESP, respiratory; SPECIAL SENSES, vision, hearing, touch, taste, smell; OTHER or MISC, miscellaneous reactions not otherwise listed.

Interactions: As the number of medications a patient receives increases, so does the likelihood of drug interaction. The most clinically important interactions are explained under the headings "Drug-Drug" and "Drug-Food."

Route and Dosage: The usual routes of administration relating to psychiatric/mental health are listed, as well as recommended dosages for adults and children (including specific age groups when necessary). Dosage units are listed using the terminology in which they are most commonly prescribed. Dosage intervals are also presented in the manner in which they usually are ordered. This section also includes routes and dosages of drugs with investigational uses that have implications for psychiatry.

Pharmacodynamics: This information is provided so that the drug's onset of action, peak effect, and duration of action can be anticipated and considered in planning dosage schedules. The pharmacodynamics of all routes of administration are tabulated for easy comparison.

Nursing Implications: This section has been developed to help the nurse apply the nursing process to pharmacotherapeutics. It is divided into subsections consistent with the steps of the nursing process, providing the nurse with a systematic framework for the provision of medication therapy.

ASSESSMENT

This subsection includes parameters for patient history, lab tests, and physical and behavioral data that should be assessed prior to and during drug therapy. Separate headings for "Lab Test Alterations," "Withdrawal (signs and symptoms)," "Withdrawal Management," "Toxicity and Overdose" (therapeutic serum drug levels and signs and symptoms of intoxication or overdose), and "Overdose Management" are also included, when appropriate.

POTENTIAL NURSING DIAGNOSES

Nursing diagnoses approved through the Eleventh National Conference of the North American Nursing Diagnosis Association (NANDA) are used. Those diagnoses that may be identified for a patient receiving the medication are listed, along with possible etiological ("related to") factors.

PLAN/IMPLEMENTATION

Specific guidelines for medication administration are discussed in this subsection. Information is further specified according to whether it is general or related specifically to PO, IM, or IV administration. These subsections describe actions appropriate for administration regardless of route (e.g., take vital signs prior to administration) as well as actions specific to PO administration (e.g., may be taken with food; may crush tablet or empty capsule), IM administration (e.g., do not mix with any other solution in syringe; administer deep into large muscle mass), and IV administration (e.g., administer at rate of 5 mg or fraction thereof over 1 minute).

PATIENT/FAMILY EDUCATION

This section includes material that should be taught to patients receiving a specific medication or to family members/caregivers who may be administering or assisting with the administration of the medication. Most commonly reported side effects, details of administration, and follow-up requirements are presented. Although most of the pertinent information is included, the nurse should also refer to the "Adverse Reactions and Side Effects" and "Interactions" sections for additional data to complete the patient teaching plan.

EVALUATION

Measurable objectives for determination of the therapeutic effectiveness of a medication are provided.

APPENDICES

The following appendices are intended to provide additional reference information:

Appendix A: Controlled Substance Categories
Appendix B: Key to FDA Preganacy Control Categories
Appendix C: Measurement Conversion Table
Appendix D: Dietary Guidelines for Food Sources
Appendix E: Common Street Names of Drugs
Appendix F: Alphabetical Listing of NANDA Nursing Diagnoses
Appendix G: Classification of NANDA Nursing Diagnoses by Doenges'/Moorhouse's Diagnostic Divisions
Appendix H: Classification of NANDA Nursing Diagnoses by Gordon's Functional Health Patterns

BIBLIOGRAPHY

COMPREHENSIVE INDEX

An alphabetical listing consisting of generic names, trade names (in capital letters), and classifications (in italics) is included.

Alpha-Adrenergic Blocking Agents

General Action and Information: Alpha-adrenergic blocking agents non-competitively block alpha-adrenergic receptors, inhibiting the normal excitatory responses to epinephrine and norepinephrine. Receptors primarily affected are located in vascular smooth muscle and exocrine glands.

General Use: Used in situations of adrenergic (sympathetic) excess, such as pheochromocytoma or hypertensive crises associated with excessive sympathomimetic amines (the result of interaction between MAO inhibitors and tyramine-containing foods).

Contraindications: Hypersensitivity; conditions in which a precipitous fall in blood pressure could be dangerous.

Precautions: Cardiovascular effects may be severe and may require intervention and supportive treatment. Use cautiously in patients with a history of peptic ulcer.

Interactions: Any drugs that stimulate alpha-adrenergic receptors will be antagonized. Alpha- and beta-adrenergic amines in combination with alpha-adrenergic blockers will result in exaggerated hypotension and arrhythmias.

ALPHA-ADRENERGIC BLOCKERS INCLUDED IN THIS DRUG GUIDE

phentolamine, 330

Anesthetics

General Action and Information: The ultrashort-acting barbiturate anesthetics depress the central nervous system by inhibiting impulse conduction in the ascending reticular activating system. They produce anesthesia and muscle relaxation (except methohexital) but do not possess analgesic properties.

General Use: Used to induce a hypnotic state; as anesthesia for short procedures (minor surgery or electroconvulsive therapy) with minimal painful stimuli; and as supplementation of other anesthetics in longer procedures.

Contraindications: Hypersensitivity; latent or manifest porphyria; absence of suitable veins for IV administration; status asthmaticus.

Precautions: Use cautiously in patients with severe cardiovascular disease; hypotension or shock; conditions in which hypnotic effects may be prolonged or potentiated; increased intracranial pressure; asthma, myasthenia gravis; debilitation; impaired function of respiratory, circulatory, renal, hepatic, or endocrine systems.

---

*Adapted from Deglin, JH and Vallerand, AH: Davis's Drug Guide for Nurses, ed. 4. FA Davis, Philadelphia, 1994.

Interactions: Additive CNS and respiratory depression with other CNS depressants. Orthostatic hypotension when administered with furosemide.

ANESTHETICS INCLUDED IN THIS DRUG GUIDE

methohexital, 258
thiamylal, 396
thiopental, 399

Antianxiety Agents

General Action and Information: Antianxiety agents cause generalized CNS depression. They may produce tolerance with chronic use and have the potential for psychological or physical dependence.

General Use: Used to treat anxiety disorders and for the temporary relief of anxiety symptoms.

Contraindications: Hypersensitivity. Should not be used in combination with other CNS depressants, in narrow-angle glaucoma, in comatose patients, or in patients with uncontrolled pain. Avoid use during pregnancy or lactation.

Precautions: Use cautiously in elderly and debilitated patients, patients with hepatic or renal dysfunction, individuals with a history of drug abuse/addiction, and depressed or suicidal patients. Should not be discontinued abruptly following prolonged use.

Interactions: Increased effects with alcohol, barbiturates, narcotics, antipsychotics, antidepressants, antihistamines, neuromuscular blocking agents, cimetidine, disulfiram. Decreased effects with cigarette smoking and caffeine.

ANTIANXIETY AGENTS INCLUDED IN THIS DRUG GUIDE

alprazolam, 31
buspirone, 81
chlordiazepoxide, 96
chlormezanone, 100
clorazepate, 121
diazepam, 136

halazepam, 195
hydroxyzine, 203
lorazepam, 222
meprobamate, 243
oxazepam, 283
prazepam, 340

Anticholinergics

General Action and Information: Inhibits the muscarinic actions of acetylcholine at postganglionic parasympathetic neuroeffector sites, including smooth muscle, secretory glands, and sites within the central nervous system. Specific anticholinergic responses are dose-related.

General Uses: Used as a preoperative or pre-procedural (including electroconvulsive therapy) medication to decrease secretions and block cardiac vagal inhibitory reflexes. Also used in the control of symptoms of parkinsonism.

Contraindications: Hypersensitivity; narrow-angle glaucoma; tachycardia; unstable cardiovascular status in acute hemorrhage; myocardial ischemia; paralytic ileus; myasthenia gravis.

Precautions: Use cautiously in patients with GI or GU pathophysiology; elderly, debilitated, and pediatric patients; and those with chronic renal, hepatic, pulmonary, or cardiac disease.

Interactions: Increased anticholinergic effects with antihistamines, procainamide, quinidine, antipsychotics, antiparkinsonian agents, buclizine, meperidine, orphenadrine, benzodiazepines, tricyclic antidepressants, MAO inhibitors. Decreased therapeutic effects of anticholinergics with guanethidine, histamine, reserpine. Increased effects of sympathomimetics, nitrofurantoin, thiazide diuretics with anticholinergics. Decreased effects of cholinesterase inhibitors, metoclopramide with anticholinergics.

ANTICHOLINERGICS INCLUDED IN THIS DRUG GUIDE

atropine sulfate, 56
glycopyrrolate, 192
scopolamine, 373

Anticonvulsants

General Action and Information: Anticonvulsants include a variety of agents, all of which are capable of depressing abnormal neuronal discharges in the CNS that may result in seizures. They work by preventing the spread of seizure activity, depressing the motor cortex, raising the seizure threshold, or altering the levels of neurotransmitters, depending on the drug group (see individual drugs).

General Uses: Used in the control of absence (petit mal), psychomotor, simple partial, partial with complex symptomatology, akinetic, myoclonic, mixed, and tonic-clonic (grand mal) seizures, and in the treatment of status epilepticus. See individual drugs for specific uses.

Contraindications: Hypersensitivity.

Precautions: Use cautiously in patients with severe hepatic or renal dysfunction; dosage adjustment may be required. Choose agents carefully in pregnant and lactating women. Should not be discontinued abruptly.

Interactions: Barbiturates stimulate the metabolism of other drugs that are metabolized by the liver, decreasing their effectiveness. Hydantoins are highly protein bound and may displace or be displaced by other highly protein-bound drugs. For more specific interactions, see individual drugs. Many drugs are capable of lowering the seizure threshold and may decrease the effectiveness of anticonvulsants. These drugs include tricyclic antidepressants and phenothiazines.

ANTICONVULSANTS INCLUDED IN THIS DRUG GUIDE

barbiturates
mephobarbital, 239
phenobarbital, 320

benzodiazepines
clonazepam, 118
clorazepate, 121
diazepam (IV), 136

hydantoins
ethotoin, 169
mephenytoin, 236
phenytoin, 332

succinimides
ethosuximide, 166
methsuximide, 260
phensuximide, 324

oxazolidinediones
paramethadione, 289
trimethadione, 436

other
acetazolamide, 24
carbamazepine, 86
felbamate, 172
paraldehyde, 286
phenacemide, 307
primidone, 343

Antidepressants

General Action and Information: Antidepressant activity most likely is due to prevention of the reuptake of dopamine, norepinephrine, and/or serotonin by presynaptic neurons, resulting in the accumulation of these neurotransmitters. They also possess significant anticholinergic and sedative properties, which explains many of their side effects.

General Uses: Used in the treatment of major depression, bipolar disorder, and dysthymic disorder, often in conjunction with psychotherapy. Other uses include treatment of depression accompanied by anxiety (doxepin), childhood enuresis (imipramine), and obsessive-compulsive disorder (sertraline).

Contraindications: Hypersensitivity; acute recovery phase following myocardial infarction; angle-closure glaucoma; pregnancy, and lactation.

Precautions: Use cautiously in elderly or debilitated patients; in patients with hepatic, renal, or cardiac insufficiency; benign prostatic hypertrophy; psychotic patients; and in children. Dosage requires slow titration; onset of therapeutic response may be 2–4 weeks. May decrease seizure threshold.

Interactions: Tricyclic antidepressants may cause hyperpyretic crisis, hypertensive crisis, severe seizures, and tachycardia when used with MAO inhibitors. May prevent therapeutic response to some antihypertensives (clonidine, guanethidine). Additive CNS depression with other CNS depressants. Additive sympathomimetic and anticholinergic effects with other drugs possessing these same properties. Hypertensive crisis may result with concurrent use of MAO inhibitors and amphetamines, methyldopa, levodopa, dopamine, epinephrine, norepinephrine, reserpine, vasoconstrictors, or ingestion of tyramine-containing foods (see Appendix D). Hypertension or hypotension, coma, convulsions, and death may occur with meperidine or other narcotic analgesics when used with MAO inhibitors. Additive hypotension may result with concurrent use of antihypertensives or spinal anesthesia and MAO inhibitors. Additive hypoglycemia may result with concurrent use of insulin or oral hypoglycemic agents and MAO inhibitors.

ANTIDEPRESSANTS INCLUDED IN THIS DRUG GUIDE

amitriptyline, 38
amoxapine, 45
bupropion, 78
clomipramine, 114
desipramine, 128
doxepin, 151
fluoxetine, 178
imipramine, 206
isocarboxazid, 210
maprotiline, 229

nortriptyline, 276
paroxetine, 291
phenelzine, 313
protriptyline, 366
sertraline, 381
tranylcypromine, 412
trazodone, 416
trimipramine, 439
venlafaxine, 445

Antimanic Agents

General Action and Information: Alters sodium metabolism within nerve and muscle cells and enhances the reuptake of biogenic amines in the brain, lowering levels in the body and resulting in decreased hyperactivity. May block development of sensitive dopamine receptors in the CNS of manic patients. Has both antimanic and antidepressant properties.

General Use: Used in the prevention and treatment of manic episodes associated with bipolar disorder. May also be effective for depression associated with bipolar disorder. Normalization of symptoms is achieved within 1–3 weeks.

Contraindications: Hypersensitivity; severe cardiovascular or renal disease; severe dehydration; sodium depletion; brain damage; pregnancy and lactation.

Precautions: Use cautiously in elderly patients; thyroid disorders; diabetes mellitus; urinary retention; patients with a history of seizure disorder; children (safety not established).

Interactions: May prolong neuromuscular blockage. Encephalopathic syndrome may occur with haloperidol. Diuretics, methyldopa, probenecid, indomethacin, and other nonsteroidal anti-inflammatory agents may increase the risk of toxicity. Aminophylline, phenothiazines, sodium bicarbonate, and sodium chloride may hasten excretion, leading to decreased effect. Lithium may decrease the effectiveness of phenothiazines. Hypothyroid effects may be additive with potassium iodide.

ANTIMANIC AGENTS INCLUDED IN THIS DRUG GUIDE

lithium carbonate, 218
lithium citrate, 218

Antimigraine Agents

General Action and Information: Binds to specific vascular serotonin receptor sites, resulting in vasoconstriction of the basilar artery and in the vasculature of the isolated dura mater.

General Use: Used in the treatment of acute migraine attacks, with or without aura.

Contraindications: IV use; ischemic heart disease; Prinzmetal's angina; uncontrolled hypertension; concomitantly with basilar or hemiplegic migraine.

Precautions: Postmenopausal women; males over 40; patients at risk for coronary artery disease; impaired heptaic or renal function; pregnancy, lactation, and children.

Interactions: Prolonged vasospastic reactions with ergot-containing drugs. Avoid use of either drug within 24 hours of each other, as effects may be additive.

ANTIMIGRAINE AGENTS INCLUDED IN THIS DRUG GUIDE

sumatriptan, 387

Antiparkinsonian Agents

General Action and Information: Drugs used in the treatment of the parkinsonian syndrome and other dyskinesias are aimed at restoring the natural balance of two major neurotransmitters in the CNS: acetylcholine and dopamine. The imbalance is a deficiency in dopamine that results in excessive cholinergic activity. Drugs used are either anticholinergics (benzotropine, trihexyphenidyl) or dopaminergic agonists (amantadine, bromocriptine, levodopa).

General Use: Used in the treatment of parkinsonism of various causes, including degenerative, toxic, infective, neoplastic, or drug-induced.

Contraindications: Hypersensitivity. Anticholinergics should be avoided in patients with angle-closure glaucoma; pyloric, duodenal, or bladder-neck obstructions; prostatic hypertrophy; myasthenia gravis.

Precautions: Use cautiously in patients with hepatic, renal, or cardiac insufficiency; elderly and debilitated patients; those with tendency toward urinary retention, or exposed to high environmental temperatures.

Interactions: Pyridoxine, MAO inhibitors, benzodiazepines, phenytoin, phenothiazines, and haloperidol may antagonize the effects of levodopa.

ANTIPARKINSONIAN AGENTS INCLUDED IN THIS DRUG GUIDE

amantadine, 34
benztropine, 63
biperiden, 70
bromocriptine, 74
carbidopa/levodopa, 90
diphenhydramine, 144

ethopropazine, 162
levodopa, 214
orphenadrine, 280
procyclidine, 352
trihexyphenidyl, 432

Antipsychotics

General Action and Information: Antipsychotics block dopamine receptors in the brain and alter dopamine release and turnover. Peripheral effects include anticholinergic properties and alpha-adrenergic blockade. Commonly used groups include the phenothiazines (chlorpromazine, thioridazine, fluphenazine); thioxanthenes (thiothixene); butyrophenones (haloperidol); dibenzoxazepines (loxapine); tricyclic dibenzodiazepine derivatives (clozapine); and dihydroindolones (molindone). Differences occur in the level of anticholinergic effects, sedation, and extrapyramidal reactions produced, and drug selection is based on capacity to decrease psychotic symptoms with a minimum of these effects.

General Use: Used in the treatment of acute and chronic psychoses, particularly when accompanied by increased psychomotor activity. Selected agents are used as antiemetics (chlorpromazine, perphenazine, prochlorperazine); in the treatment of intractable hiccoughs (chlorpromazine, perphenazine); and for the control of tics and vocal utterances in Tourette's disorder (haloperidol, pimozide).

Contraindications: Hypersensitivity (cross-sensitivity may exist among phenothiazines). Should not be used when CNS depression is evident; when blood dyscrasias exist; in Parkinson's disease; or in liver, renal, or cardiac insufficiency. Safety in pregnancy and lactation has not been established.

Precautions: Use cautiously in elderly, severely ill, or debilitated patients; diabetics; patients with respiratory insufficiency, prostatic hypertrophy, or intestinal obstruction. May lower seizure threshold. Individuals should avoid exposure to extremes in temperature while taking antipsychotic medication.

Interactions: Additive hypotensive effects with beta-adrenergic blocking agents (propanolol, metoprolol). Antacids and antidiarrheals may decrease absorption. Barbiturates may increase metabolism and decrease effectiveness. Additive CNS depression with other CNS depressants, including alcohol, antihistamines, antidepressants, sedative-hypnotics.

ANTIPSYCHOTICS INCLUDED IN THIS DRUG GUIDE

benzisoxazole derivatives
risperidone, 369

butyrophenones
droperidol, 155
haloperidol, 198
pimozide, 336

dibenzoxazepines
loxapine, 225

dihydroindolones
molindone, 268

thioxanthenes
chlorprothixene, 109
thiothixene, 407

phenothiazines
acetophenazine, 26
chlorpromazine, 102
fluphenazine, 181
mesoridazine, 245
perphenazine, 301
prochlorperazine, 346
promazine, 355
thioridazine, 402
trifluoperazine, 422
triflupromazine, 427

tricyclic dibenzodiazepine derivatives
clozapine, 124

Beta-Adrenergic Blocking Agents

General Action and Information: Beta-adrenergic blocking agents compete with beta-adrenergic agonists for beta-receptor sites. They may inhibit beta-1 receptors (located chiefly in cardiac muscle) or beta-2 receptors (located chiefly in the bronchial and vascular musculature), or both, thereby inhibiting the chronotropic, inotropic, and vasodilator responses to beta-adrenergic stimulation.

General Uses: Used in the treatment of hypertension, angina pectoris, cardiac arrhythmias, myocardial infarction, pheochromocytoma, and as a prophylactic for migraine headaches. Used investigationally for recurrent GI bleeding in cirrhotic patients, in schizophrenia, essential tremors (e.g., those induced by lithium carbonate and other psychotropic drugs), tardive dyskinesia, and acute panic symptoms.

Contraindications: Hypersensitivity to beta-adrenergic blocking agents; congestive heart failure; acute bronchospasm; severe COPD; sinus bradycardia; heart block; cardiogenic shock.

Precautions: Use cautiously in diabetes mellitus; patients prone to hypoglycemia; myasthenia gravis; Wolff-Parkinson-White syndrome; thyrotoxicosis; impaired hepatic or renal function; patients undergoing major surgery. Beta-adrenergic blockers should not be discontinued abruptly, particularly in patients with cardiovascular disease.

Interactions: May cause additive myocardial depression and bradycardia when used with other agents having this effect (e.g., digitalis, glycosides, IV phenytoin, IV verapamil). May antagonize the therapeutic effect of bronchodilators. Hypoglycemic effects of insulin and oral hypoglycemics may be prolonged. Effects of beta-adrenergic blockers are increased with chlorpromazine, cimetidine, oral contraceptives, furosemide, and hydralazine; effects are decreased with barbiturates, rifampin, and thyroid hormones.

BETA-ADRENERGIC BLOCKING AGENTS INCLUDED IN THIS DRUG GUIDE

propranolol, 361

Calcium Channel Blocking Agents

General Action and Information: Calcium channel blockers inhibit movement of calcium ions across the membrane of myocardial and vascular smooth muscle cells, resulting in inhibition of muscle contraction, vasoconstriction, and cardiac conduction. The mechanism of action of verapamil in the treatment of bipolar disorder is unknown.

General Uses: Used in the treatment of angina pectoris, essential hypertension, supraventricular tachyarrhythmias. Investigational uses include bipolar disorder and migraine headache.

Contraindications: Hypersensitivity to calcium channel blockers; bradycardia; hypotension; second and third degree heart block; and uncompensated congestive heart failure. Safe use in pregnancy and lactation has not been established.

Precautions: Use cautiously in patients with Duchenne's muscular dystrophy, increased intracranial pressure, impaired hepatic or renal function, and in elderly or debilitated patients.

Interactions: Additive depression of myocardial contractility and AV conduction when used with beta-adrenergic blockers. Effects may be decreased with rifampin, calcium salts, and vitamin D, and increased with cimetidine. Effects may be increased or decreased when given with other highly protein-bound drugs such as warfarin, oral hypoglycemics, hydantoins, sulfonamides, salicylates. Interaction of verapamil with cardiac glycosides may increase serum digitoxin/digoxin levels and result in toxicity.

CALCIUM CHANNEL BLOCKING AGENTS INCLUDED IN THIS DRUG GUIDE

Central Nervous System Stimulants

General Action and Information: CNS stimulants increase levels of neurotransmitters in the CNS. They produce CNS and respiratory stimulation, dilated pupils, increased motor activity and mental alertness, diminished sense of fatigue, and brighter spirits.

General Use: Used in the management of narcolepsy and attention deficit disorder with hyperactivity in children. Also used as adjunctive therapy to caloric restriction in the treatment of exogenous obesity.

Contraindications: Hypersensitivity to sympathomimetic amines. Should not be used in advanced arteriosclerosis, symptomatic cardiovascular disease, hypertension, hyperthyroidism, glaucoma, agitated or hyperexcitability states, in patients with a history of drug abuse, during or within 14 days of receiving therapy with MAO inhibitors, in children under 3 years of age, and in pregnancy.

Precautions: Use cautiously in lactation; psychotic children; Tourette's disorder; patients with anorexia or insomnia; elderly, debilitated, or asthenic patients; and patients with a history of suicidal or homicidal tendencies. Prolonged use may result in physical or psychological dependence.

Interactions: Use with or within 14 days following administration of MAO inhibitors may result in hypertensive crisis, headache, hyperpyrexia, intracranial hemorrhage, bradycardia. Insulin requirements may be altered with CNS stimulants. Urine alkalinizers decrease excretion, enhancing the effects of amphetamines; urine acidifiers increase excretion, decreasing the effects. May result in decreased effects of both drugs when administered with phenothiazines.

CENTRAL NERVOUS SYSTEM STIMULANTS INCLUDED IN THIS DRUG GUIDE

amphetamine sulfate, 49
benzphetamine, 60
dextroamphetamine sulfate, 132
diethylpropion, 140
fenfluramine, 175
mazindol, 233

methamphetamine, 254
methylphenidate, 263
pemoline, 294
phendimetrazine, 310
phenmetrazine, 317
phentermine, 326

Cholinergics

General Action and Information: Cholinergics intensify and prolong the action of acetylcholine by either mimicking its effects at cholinergic receptor sites (bethanechol) or preventing the breakdown of acetylcholine by inhibiting cholinesterase activity. Effects include increased GI secretions, motility, and muscle tone; bladder contraction; and increased skeletal muscle tone.

General Uses: Used to treat postoperative and postpartum nonobstructive urinary retention, neurogenic atony of the urinary bladder with retention, and urinary retention associated with use of certain drugs, such as antidepressants and antipsychotics. Also used in the diagnosis and treatment of myasthenia gravis, and as an antidote for nondepolarizing neuromuscular blocking agents. Tacrine is used to improve cognition and functional autonomy in mild to moderate dementia of the Alzheimer type.

Contraindications: Hypersensitivity. Avoid use in patients with possible obstructions or lesions of the GI or GU tract; following recent GI or bladder surgery; when there is questionable strength or integrity of the GI or bladder wall. Safe use in children and during pregnancy and lactation has not been established.

Precautions: Use with extreme caution in patients with a history of asthma, peptic ulcer disease, cardiovascular disease, epilepsy, or hyperthyroidism. Atropine should be available to treat excessive dosage.

Interactions: Additive cholinergic effects with other cholinergic drugs. Use with ganglionic blocking agents (mecamylamine, trimethaphan) may result in severe hypotension. Do not use with depolarizing neuromuscular blocking agents, such as succinylcholine and decamethonium (depolarizing action is prolonged).

CHOLINERGICS INCLUDED IN THIS DRUG GUIDE

bethanechol, 67
neostigmine, 272
tacrine, 390

Neuromuscular Blocking Agents (Depolarizing)

General Action and Information: Produces skeletal muscle relaxation of ultrashort duration by combining with cholinergic receptors of the motor endplate, resulting in depolarization of the muscle membrane. This is observed as muscle fasciculations, followed by a flaccid paralysis.

General Use: Used as an adjunct to general anesthesia to facilitate endotracheal intubation and to induce skeletal muscle relaxation during surgery or mechanical ventilation. Also used to reduce the intensity of muscle contractions of pharmacologically or electrically induced convulsions (e.g., electroconvulsive therapy).

Contraindications: Hypersensitivity. Should not be used in disorders of plasma pseudocholinesterase; patients with a personal or familial history of malignant hyperthermia; myopathies associated with elevated creatine phosphokinase (CPK) values; acute narrow-angle glaucoma; penetrating eye injuries. Safe use during pregnancy and lactation has not been established.

Precautions: Use cautiously in patients undergoing delivery by cesarean section; patients with cardiovascular, hepatic, pulmonary, metabolic, or renal disorders; patients with severe burns, electrolyte imbalance, hyperkalemia; degenerative or dystrophic neuromuscular disease; spinal cord injury; eye surgery.

Interactions: Prolonged neuromuscular blocking action may occur when administered concomitantly with any of the following drugs: phenelzine, promazine, oxytocin, gentamycin, kanamycin, neomycin, streptomycin, quinidine, beta-adrenergic blocking agents, procainamide, lidocaine, trimethaphan, lithium carbonate, furosemide, magnesium sulfate, quinine, chloroquine, acetylcholine, anticholinesterases, procaine-type local anesthetics, isoflurane.

DEPOLARIZING NEUROMUSCULAR BLOCKING AGENTS INCLUDED IN THIS DRUG GUIDE

succinylcholine, 384

Sedative-Hypnotics

General Action and Information: Sedative-hypnotics cause generalized CNS depression. They may produce tolerance with chronic use and have the potential for psychological or physical dependence.

General Uses: Used in the short-term management of various anxiety states and to treat insomnia. Selected agents are used as anticonvulsants and preoperative sedatives (phenobarbital, pentobarbital, secobarbital) and to reduce anxiety associated with drug withdrawal (chloral hydrate).

Contraindications: Hypersensitivity. Should not be used in comatose patients or in those with pre-existing CNS depression. Should not be used in patients with uncontrolled pain. Avoid use during pregnancy or lactation.

Precautions: Use cautiously in patients with hepatic dysfunction or severe renal impairment. Use with caution in patients who may be suicidal or who may have been addicted to drugs previously. Hypnotic use should be short term. Elderly patients may be more sensitive to CNS depressant effects, and dosage reduction may be required.

Interactions: Additive CNS depression with alcohol, antihistamines, antidepressants, phenothiazines, or any other CNS depressants. Barbiturates induce hepatic drug-metabolizing enzymes and can decrease the effectiveness of drugs metabolized by the liver. Should not be used with MAO inhibitors.

SEDATIVE-HYPNOTICS INCLUDED IN THIS DRUG GUIDE

amobarbital, 42
aprobarbital, 54
butabarbital, 83
chloral hydrate, 94
ethchlorvynol, 158
ethinamate, 160
flurazepam, 187
glutethimide, 189

methyprylon, 266
pentobarbital, 298
phenobarbital, 320
secobarbital, 377
temazepam, 394
triazolam, 419
zolpidem, 452

Special Dosing Considerations*

For almost every drug there is an average dosing range. In some situations, however, this average range can become either toxic or ineffective. The purpose of this section is to describe situations in which special dosing considerations must be evaluated in order to ensure a successful therapeutic outcome. The guidelines presented here are general but should lead to a finer appreciation of individual dosing parameters. When these clinical situations are encountered, dosage for the drugs ordered should be reviewed, and necessary adjustments made.

THE PEDIATRIC PATIENT

The most obvious reason for adjusting dosages in pediatric patients is smaller body size. Many drug dosages for this population are given on a mg/kg body weight basis, or even more specifically, on the basis of body surface area.

The neonate and the premature infant require drug dosage adjustments in addition to those made on the basis of size. With this population, absorption following oral administration may be incomplete or altered, due to changes in gastric pH or GI motility; distribution may be altered due to varying amounts of total body water; and metabolism and excretion may be delayed because liver and kidney function have not yet matured. Hepatic and renal function maturation as well as weight changes may necessitate frequent dosage adjustments during the course of therapy. Dosages for the premature infant or neonate may have to be readjusted to reflect improved drug handling, within even a period of several days.

In addition to the evaluation of pharmacokinetic variables, other nursing considerations should be assessed. The route of administration chosen for pediatric patients often reflects the seriousness of the illness. The nurse should consider the child's developmental level and ability to understand the situation. Medications that must be administered intravenously or by intramuscular injection may seem frightening to a young child or cause undue concern to the parents. The nurse should allay these fears by educating the parents and comforting the child. As with any age group, intramuscular or subcutaneous injection sites should be carefully selected to prevent any possibility of nerve or tissue damage.

THE GERIATRIC PATIENT

The pharmacokinetic behavior of drugs changes considerably in patients over the age of 60. Drug absorption may be delayed secondary to diminished GI motility (resulting from age or other drugs) or passive congestion of abdominal blood

---

*Adapted from Deglin, JH and Vallerand, AH: Davis's Drug Guide for Nurses, ed 4. FA Davis, Philadelphia, 1994.

19

vessels (as seen in congestive heart failure). Distribution of the drug may be altered due to low levels of plasma proteins, particularly in malnourished patients. Because plasma proteins are decreased, a larger proportion of free or unbound drug will result in an increase in drug action. This may cause the patient to exhibit toxicity while receiving a standard dose of a drug. Drug metabolism by the liver and excretion by the kidneys are both slowed as part of the aging process and may cause prolonged and exaggerated drug action. Body composition also changes with age. There is an increase in fatty tissue and a decrease in skeletal muscle and total body water. Height and weight also usually decrease. A dosage of medication that was acceptable for the robust 50-year-old patient may be excessive in the same patient 20 years later.

An additional concern is that many elderly patients are already receiving numerous drugs. With increasing numbers of drugs being used, there is greater risk of one drug negating, potentiating, or otherwise altering the effects of another drug (drug-drug interaction). In general, doses of most medications should be decreased in the geriatric population.

Dosing regimens should be kept simple in this patient population since many of these patients are taking multiple drugs. Doses should be scheduled so that the patient's day is not interrupted numerous times to take medications. The use of fixed-dose combination drugs may help to simplify dosing regimens. However, some of these combinations are more expensive than the individual components.

In explaining medication regimens to elderly patients, bear in mind that hearing deficits are common in this age group. Patients may find it embarrassing to disclose this information, and full compliance may be hindered.

THE OBSTETRICAL PATIENT

During pregnancy, both the mother and the fetus must be considered. The placenta, once thought to be a protective barrier, is simply a membrane that is capable of protecting the fetus from only extremely large molecules. The placenta may transfer drugs to the fetus by both passive and active processes. The fetus is particularly vulnerable during two of the three stages of pregnancy: the first trimester and the last trimester.

Many drugs have been categorized by the FDA according to potential risk to the fetus weighed against benefit to the mother. Refer to Appendix B for a key to the definitions of these categories.

The possibility of medications altering sperm quality and quantity in potential fathers is also becoming an area of increasing concern. These considerations should be explained to patients who are trying to conceive.

During the first trimester, the vital organs of the fetus are being formed. Ingestion of drugs that cause harm (potential teratogens) during this stage of pregnancy may lead to fetal malformation or miscarriage. Unfortunately, this is the time when a woman is least likely to know that she is pregnant. Therefore, it is wise to inform all patients of childbearing age of this potential harm to an unborn child.

In the third trimester, the major concern is that drugs administered to the mother and transferred to the fetus may not be safely metabolized and excreted by the fetus. This is especially true of drugs administered near term. After the infant is delivered, he or she no longer has the placenta available to help with drug excretion. If drugs administered before delivery are allowed to accumulate, toxicity may result.

There are situations in which, for the sake of the mother's health and to protect the fetus, drug administration is required throughout pregnancy. Two examples of this are the epileptic patient and the hypertensive patient. In these circumstances, the safest drug in the lowest effective dose is chosen. Because of changes in the behavior of drugs that may occur throughout pregnancy, dosage adjustments may be required during the progression of pregnancy and after delivery.

A special situation related to the drug behavior of women during pregnancy is that of the mother who abuses drugs. Infants born to mothers addicted to alcohol, sedatives (including benzodiazepines), heroin, or cocaine may be of low birth weight, may experience drug withdrawal after birth, and may display developmental delays and/or behavior disorders. A careful history should alert the nurse to these possibilities.

KIDNEY DISEASE

The kidneys are the major organs of drug elimination. Some drugs are excreted only after being metabolized or biotransformed by the liver. Others may be eliminated by the kidneys unchanged. The premature infant has immature renal function. Elderly patients have an age-related decrease in renal function. To make dosage adjustments for patients with renal dysfunction, one must know the degree of renal impairment in the individual patient, and the percentage of drug that is eliminated by the kidneys. The degree of renal function can be quantitated by laboratory testing, most commonly by using the creatinine clearance value. The percentage of each drug excreted by the kidneys can be determined from references on pharmacokinetics. In addition, the dosage frequently can be optimized by measuring blood levels of the drug in the individual patient and making any further necessary changes.

LIVER DISEASE

The liver is the major organ for the metabolism of drugs. For most drugs, this is an inactivation step. Most inactive metabolites are subsequently excreted by the kidneys. The conversion process usually changes the drug from a relatively lipid- or fat-soluble compound to a more water-soluble substance. Liver function is not as easily quantified as renal function; therefore it is difficult to predict the correct dosage for a patient with liver dysfunction based on laboratory tests alone. In addition, it appears that only a minimal level of liver function may be required for complete drug metabolism.

A patient who is severely jaundiced or has very low serum proteins (particularly albumin) may be expected to have some problems metabolizing drugs. Chronic alcoholic patients are at risk for developing this type of problem. In advanced liver disease, drug absorption may be impaired secondary to portal vascular congestion. Drugs that require the liver for activation should also be avoided in patients with severely compromised liver function.

CONGESTIVE HEART FAILURE

Patients with clinical congestive heart failure also require dosage modifications. In these patients, drug absorption may be impaired due to passive congestion of blood vessels feeding the GI tract. This same passive congestion slows drug delivery to the liver and delays metabolism. In addition, renal function may be compromised, leading to delayed elimination and prolonged drug action. Many patients who have congestive heart failure are already in a special dosing category because of their age. Dosages of drugs that are mainly metabolized by the liver or mainly excreted by the kidneys should be decreased in patients with apparent congestive heart failure.

BODY SIZE

In most situations, drug dosing is based on total body weight. Some drugs selectively penetrate fatty tissues. If the drug is known to not penetrate fatty tissues and the patient is obese, dosage should be determined by ideal body weight or estimated lean body mass. These quantities may be determined from tables of desirable weights or may be estimated using formulas for lean body mass when the patient's height and weight are known. If this type of adjustment is not made, considerable toxicity may result.

DELIVERY TO SITES OF ACTION

To have a successful therapeutic outcome, a drug must reach its intended site of action. Under the most desirable of conditions, a drug may have only a minimal effect on other tissues or body systems. An example is topical drugs for skin conditions that are only minimally absorbed systemically. Sometimes unusual routes of administrtion must be used to guarantee the presence of a drug at the intended site of response. In some cases, local absorption may not occur, and therefore the desired systemic effect will not occur. In patients with shock or poor tissue perfusion due to other causes, drugs may not be absorbed into systemic circulation from subcutaneous sites. When considering the route of administration, remember where the drug is intended to have its primary action. To achieve its maximal effect, it must be delivered to its intended site of action.

DRUG INTERACTIONS

The presence of other drugs may necessitate dosage adjustments. Drugs that are highly bound to plasma proteins may be displaced by other highly protein-bound drugs. When this phenomenon occurs, the drug that has been displaced exhibits an increase in its activity, since it is the free, or unbound, drug that is active.

Some agents decrease the ability of the liver to metabolize other drugs. Drugs that can have this effect include cimetidine and chloramphenicol. Concurrently administered drugs that are highly metabolized by the liver may therefore need to be administered in decreased dosages. Other agents, such as phenobarbital, other barbiturates, and rifampin, are capable of stimulating (inducing) the liver to metabolize drugs more rapidly, requiring larger doses to be administered.

Drugs that significantly alter urine pH can affect excretion of other drugs for which the excretory process is pH-dependent. Alkalinizing the urine will hasten the excretion of acidic drugs. Acidification of the urine will enhance reabsorption of acidic drugs, prolonging and enhancing drug action. Drugs that acidify the urine will hasten the excretion of alkaline drugs. An example of this is administering sodium bicarbonate in cases of aspirin overdose. Alkalinizing the urine promotes renal excretion of aspirin.

DOSAGE FORMS

The nurse will frequently encounter problems that relate to the dosage form itself. Some medications may not be commercially available in liquid or chewable dosage forms. The pharmacist may have to compound such dosage forms for an individual patient. It may be necessary to disguise the taste or appearance of a medication in food or a beverage so that a patient will fully comply with a given regimen. Finally, some dosage forms, such as aerosol inhalers, may not be suitable for very young patients because their use requires cooperation beyond the patient's developmental level.

Before altering dosage forms (crushing tablets or opening capsules), check to be sure that the effect of the drug won't be altered by doing so. In general, extended- or prolonged-release dosage forms should not be crushed, nor should capsules containing beads of medication be opened. Altering these dosage forms may shorten and intensify their intended action. Enteric-coated tablets, which may appear to be sugar-coated or candy-coated, also should not be crushed. This coating is designed to protect the stomach from irritating effects of the drugs. Crushing them will expose the stomach lining to these agents and increase GI irritation. If a dosage form must be crushed, it should be ingested right away. A glass of water should be taken prior to administration of powders or crushed tablets to wet the esophagus and prevent the material from sticking to upper GI mucosal surfaces.

ENVIRONMENTAL FACTORS

Cigarette smoke can induce liver enzymes to metabolize drugs more rapidly. Patients who smoke may need larger doses of liver-metabolized drugs to compensate for this. Patients who are passively exposed to cigarette smoke may also exhibit otherwise unexplained needs for larger doses of medications.

NUTRITIONAL FACTORS

Certain foods can alter the dosing requirement for some medications. For example, foods that are high in pyridoxine (vitamin B_6) can negate the antiparkinsonian effect of levodopa. (This can be counteracted with coadministration of carbidopa.) The absorption of some medications is facilitated if they are taken on an empty stomach. Foods that alter urine pH may affect the excretion patterns of medications, thereby enhancing or diminishing their effectiveness. There are no general guidelines for nutritional factors. It is prudent to check whether or not these problems exist (or if they could explain therapeutic failures) and to make any necessary dosage adjustments.

SUMMARY

The average dosing range for drugs is intended for an average patient. However, every patient is an individual with specific drug-tolerance capabilities. Taking into account these special dosing considerations allows the planning of an individualized drug regimen that is more likely to result in a desired therapeutic outcome while minimizing the risk of toxicity to the patient.

ACETAZOLAMIDE

(a-set-a-zole'a-mide)
Diamox

Classification(s):
Anticonvulsant; Diuretic; Carbonic anhydrase inhibitor
Pregnancy Category C

INDICATIONS

♦ Absence (petit mal) seizures ♦ Tonic-clonic (grand mal) seizures ♦ Focal seizures ♦ Also useful in women whose seizures appear to be related to menstruation.

ACTION

♦ Mechanism of anticonvulsant action not fully understood ♦ Inhibits the enzyme carbonic anhydrase, which in the central nervous system appears to result in a retarding of abnormal, paroxysmal, excessive discharge from the neurons.

PHARMACOKINETICS

Absorption: Readily absorbed from GI tract.
Distribution: Widely distributed. Crosses blood–brain and placental barriers; excretion in breast milk unknown.
Metabolism and Excretion: Not metabolized; excreted by the kidneys unchanged.
Half-Life: 2.4–5.8 hours.

CONTRAINDICATIONS AND PRECAUTIONS

Contraindicated in: ♦ Hypersensitivity to sulfonamides ♦ Renal, hepatic, or adrenocortical insufficiency ♦ Hypokalemia ♦ Hyponatremia ♦ Electrolyte imbalance ♦ Severe pulmonary obstructive disease ♦ Long-term use in patients with chronic noncongestive angle-closure glaucoma.
Use Cautiously in: ♦ Patients with di-

abetes mellitus ♦ Digitalized patients ♦ Patients receiving high-dose salicylate therapy ♦ Pregnancy and lactation (safety not established).

ADVERSE REACTIONS AND SIDE EFFECTS*

CNS: <u>drowsiness</u>, ataxia, dizziness, confusion, headache, weakness, tremor, tinnitus, depression, sedation, malaise, irritability, vertigo, paresthesia, SEIZURE.
Derm: <u>skin rashes</u>, urticaria, pruritus, hirsutism, photosensitivity, pain at IM injection site.
GI: <u>nausea/vomiting</u>, <u>anorexia</u>, constipation, melena, diarrhea, dry mouth, excessive thirst.
GU: hematuria, glycosuria, <u>urinary frequency</u>, renal colic, renal calculi, polyuria, alkaline urine, <u>hypokalemia</u>, dysuria, crystalluria.
Hemat: BONE MARROW DEPRESSION, THROMBOCYTOPENIA, LEUKOPENIA, HEMOLYTIC ANEMIA, AGRANULOCYTOSIS, APLASTIC ANEMIA.
Other: exacerbation of gout, transient myopia, metabolic acidosis, jaundice, fever, hypernea, cyanosis.

INTERACTIONS

Drug-Drug: ♦ **Amphetamines; ephedrine; tricyclic antidepressants; quinidine; procainamide:** increased or prolonged effects of these drugs ♦ **Salicylates:** possible salicylate or acetazolamide toxicity ♦ **Corticosteroids; ACTH; amphotericin B; most diuretics:** increased risk of hypokalemia ♦ **Lithium:** increased lithium excretion ♦ **Phenytoin; primidone:**increased calcium excretion (risk of osteomalacia) ♦ **Digitalis:** drug-induced hypokalemia may sensitize patient to digitalis toxicity ♦ **Oral hypoglycemics; insulin:** decreased hypoglycemic effects ♦ **Methenamine:** decreased effectiveness of methenamine.

*Underlines indicate most frequent; CAPITALS indicate life-threatening.

ROUTE AND DOSAGE

Absence (petit mal), Tonic-Clonic (grand mal), and Focal Seizures

♦ **PO (Adults and Children):** 3–30 mg/kg/day in divided doses. Optimal range: 375–1000 mg/day. When given in combination with other anticonvulsants, the starting dose is 250 mg once daily.
♦ **IM/IV (Adults and Children):** 8–30 mg/kg/day in divided doses.

PHARMACODYNAMICS

Route	Onset	Peak	Duration
PO	1–1.5 hr	1–3 hr	8–12 hr
PO (SR)	2 hr	8–12 hr	18–24 hr
IM	UK	UK	UK
IV	2 min	≤15 min	4–5 hr

NURSING IMPLICATIONS

Assessment

♦ Assess baseline vital signs.
♦ Assess and record extent and characteristics of seizure activity.
♦ Assess for suicidal ideation (depression may be an adverse reaction to acetazolamide therapy).
♦ Assess for signs of hypokalemia: • fatigue • malaise • weakness • postural hypotension • tachycardia • muscle cramps • vomiting • impaired thought processes.
♦ Assess for signs of blood dyscrasias: • sore throat • fever • malaise • unusual bleeding • easy bruising.
♦ Assess history of allergies, sensitivity to this drug and to sulfonamides.
♦ Assess for presence of adverse reactions or side effects.
♦ Assess date of last menses (possible pregnancy); use of contraceptives.
♦ Assess if currently breast-feeding a child.
♦ Assess current and past alcohol and drug consumption.
♦ Assess operation of automobile and/or other dangerous machinery.
♦ Assess patient/family knowledge about illness and need for medication.

♦ In collaboration with physician, assess CBC and liver function tests in patients on long-term therapy.
♦ **Lab Test Alterations:** False-positive urine protein determinations.
◊ Depression of iodine uptake by thyroid in patients with altered thyroid function.
♦ **Toxicity and Overdose:** Long-term or high-dosage therapy may result in metabolic acidosis. Symptoms include: • headache • lethargy • weakness • nausea/vomiting • abdominal pain • diarrhea • dyspnea.
♦ **Management of Acidosis:** Monitor vital signs.
◊ Monitor electrolytes.
◊ Administration of sodium bicarbonate is usually successful in reversing acidosis.

Potential Nursing Diagnoses

♦ High risk for injury related to seizures.
♦ High risk for fluid volume deficit related to medication-induced diuresis.
♦ High risk for self-directed violence related to depressed mood.
♦ Activity intolerance, high risk for, related to acetazolamide side effects of: • drowsiness • dizziness • ataxia • weakness • confusion.
♦ Knowledge deficit related to medication regimen.

Plan/Implementation

♦ **General Info:** Monitor vital signs before beginning therapy/and at regular intervals (bid or tid) throughout therapy.
◊ Encourage increase in fluid intake, if condition permits, to prevent kidney stone formation.
◊ Ensure patient is protected from injury. Supervise and assist with ambulation if dizziness and drowsiness are problems. Pad siderails and headboard for patient who experiences seizures.
◊ Frequently monitor lab results of serum electrolytes, blood glucose, pH, CBC, BUN, and creatinine.

○ Store medication at controlled room temperatures between 15° and 30°C (59°–86°F). Protect from heat and moisture.

♦ **PO:** Give with food to minimize GI upset.

○ Tablets may be crushed and mixed with soft food for patient who has difficulty swallowing.

○ Sustained-release form of the drug is not recommended as an anticonvulsant.

♦ **IM:** Due to high alkaline pH (~9.2) of the the the solution, IM administration is extremely painful and not the preferred parenteral mode. It is not commonly used.

♦ **IV:** Each 500 mg should be diluted in 5 mL of sterile water for injection.

○ Administer direct IV at rate of 500 mg or less over at least 1 minute, or add to IV fluids to be given over 4–8 hours.

○ Use of reconstituted solutions within 24 hours is recommended to prevent contamination.

Patient/Family Education

♦ Do not drive or operate dangerous machinery until individual response has been determined. Drowsiness and dizziness can occur.

♦ Epileptic patient should not stop taking the drug abruptly. Could precipitate seizures or even status epilepticus.

♦ May take drug with food if GI upset occurs.

♦ Nofity physician immediately if any of the following symptoms occur: • sore throat • fever • malaise • weakness • persistent nausea • vomiting • diarrhea • unusual bleeding • easy bruising • fast heart beat • leg cramps • disorientation.

♦ Carry card or other identification at all times describing condition and medications being taken.

♦ To protect patient during a tonic-clonic (grand mal) seizure, do not restrain. Padding (towels, blankets, pillows) may be used to prevent bumping against hard objects. When convulsion has subsided, turn patient on side to allow secretions to drain, preventing aspiration. Keep records of occurrence, characteristics, and duration of seizures, so that accurate reports may be given to physician for providing assistance in stabilization and control of seizures. If patient has difficulty breathing or continues to experience subsequent seizures, family should call for emergency assistance immediately.

♦ Be aware of risks of taking acetazolamide during pregnancy. Safe use during pregnancy and lactation has not been established. It is known that acetazolamide crosses the placental barrier, so fetus could experience adverse effects of the drug. Notify physician immediately if pregnancy occurs, is suspected, or is planned.

♦ Be aware of possible side effects. Refer to written materials furnished by healthcare providers regarding correct method of self-administration.

Evaluation

♦ Patient demonstrates stabilization of seizure activity with regular administration of acetazolamide.

♦ Patient verbalizes understanding of side effects and regimen required for prudent self-administration of acetazolamide.

ACETOPHENAZINE

(a-set-oh-fen′a-zeen)
Tindal

Classification(s):
Antipsychotic; Neuroleptic; Phenothiazine
Pregnancy Category C

INDICATIONS

♦ Symptomatic management of psychotic disorders.

ACTION

♦ The exact mechanism of antipsychotic action is not fully understood but probably is related to antidopaminergic effects ♦ Antipsychotics may block postsynaptic dopamine receptors in the basal ganglia, hypothalamus, limbic system, brain stem, and medulla ♦ Antipsychotic effects also appear to be related to inhibition of dopamine-mediated neurotransmission at the synapses ♦ Antipsychotic effects may also result from the drug's alpha-adrenergic blocking, muscarinic blocking, and adrenergic activity, as well as its effects on other amines (such as GABA) or peptides.

PHARMACOKINETICS

Absorption: Generally well absorbed, but may be erratic and variable.
Distribution: Widely distributed. Highly lipophilic, accumulating in brain, lungs, and other tissues with high blood supply. Highly protein bound. Crosses placental barrier. Enters breast milk.
Metabolism and Excretion: Metabolized by the liver and kidneys. Excreted through kidneys and enterohepatic circulation. Active metabolites accumulate and are stored in fatty tissue over a prolonged period of time and may be detected in urine up to 3–6 months following discontinuation of the drug.
Half-Life: Not well established.

CONTRAINDICATIONS AND PRECAUTIONS

Contraindicated in: ♦ Hypersensitivity to this drug, other phenothiazines ♦ Comatose or severely CNS-depressed patients ♦ Presence of large amounts of CNS depressants ♦ Bone marrow depression ♦ Blood dyscrasias ♦ Subcortical brain damage ♦ Parkinson's disease ♦ Liver, renal, and/or cardiac insufficiency ♦ Severe hypotension or hypertension ♦ Safe use in children and during pregnancy and lactation not established.
Use Cautiously in: ♦ Patients with history of seizures ♦ Respiratory (i.e., infection, COPD), renal, hepatic, thyroid (i.e., thyrotoxicosis), or cardiovascular (i.e., mitral insufficiency, angina pectoris) disorders ♦ Prostatic hypertrophy ♦ Glaucoma ♦ Diabetes ♦ Elderly and debilitated patients ♦ Patients exposed to high or low environmental temperatures or to organophosphate insecticides ♦ Hypocalcemia ♦ Patients with history of severe reactions to insulin or ECT.

ADVERSE REACTIONS AND SIDE EFFECTS*

CNS: sedation, headache, seizures, insomnia, dizziness, exacerbation of psychotic symptoms, extrapyramidal symptoms (pseudoparkinsonism, akathisia, akinesia, dystonia, oculogyric crisis), tardive dyskinesia, fatigue, cerebral edema, ataxia, blurred vision, NEUROLEPTIC MALIGNANT SYNDROME, restlessness, anxiety, depression, hyperthermia, hypothermia.
CV: hypotension, orthostatic hypotension, hypertension, tachycardia, bradycardia, CARDIAC ARREST, ECG changes, ARRHYTHMIAS, PULMONARY EDEMA, CIRCULATORY COLLAPSE.
Derm: skin rashes, urticaria, petechiae, seborrhea, photosensitivity, eczema, erythema, hyperpigmentation, contact dermatitis, EXFOLIATIVE DERMATITIS (rare).
Endo: galactorrhea, gynecomastia (men), changes in libido, impotence, hyperglycemia, hypoglycemia, amenorrhea, retrograde ejaculation, weight gain, high or prolonged glucose tolerance curves.
GI: dry mouth, nausea, vomiting, increased appetite and weight gain, anorexia, dyspepsia, constipation, diarrhea, jaundice, polydipsia, PARALYTIC ILEUS.
GU: urinary retention, frequency, incontinence, bladder paralysis, polyuria, enuresis, priapism.

---

*Underlines indicate most frequent; CAPITALS indicate life-threatening.

Hemat: AGRANULOCYTOSIS, LEUKOPENIA, ANEMIA, THROMBOCYTOPENIA, PANCYTOPENIA. **Ocular:** lens deposition. **Resp:** LARYNGEAL EDEMA, LARYNGOSPASM, BRONCHOSPASM, SUPPRESSION OF COUGH REFLEX. **Other:** decreased sweating.

INTERACTIONS

Drug-Drug: ♦ **CNS depressants (including alcohol, barbiturates, narcotics, anesthetics and other sedative drugs):** additive CNS depressant effects ♦ **Anticholinergic agents (e.g., atropine):** additive anticholinergic effects; decreased antipsychotic effects ♦ **Barbiturate anesthetics:** increased incidence of excitatory effects and hypotension ♦ **Barbiturates:** possible decreased effects of phenothiazines ♦ **Metyrosine:** potentiation of extrapyramidal side effects ♦ **Levodopa:** decreased efficacy of levodopa ♦ **Quinidine:** additive cardiac depressive effects ♦ **Magnesium- or aluminum-containing antidiarrheal mixtures; antacids:** reduced phenothiazine absorption effectiveness ♦ **Guanethidine:** decreased antihypertensive action ♦ **Lithium:** decreased plasma levels and effect of antipsychotic drug; severe neurotoxicity reported ♦ **Epinephrine:** reversal of usual pressor action of epinephrine, resulting in decreased blood pressure and tachycardia ♦ **Bromocriptine:** impairment of prolactin-suppressing action ♦ **Angiotensin converting enzyme (ACE) inhibitors:** increased effects of ACE inhibitors ♦ **Phenytoin:** decreased phenytoin metabolism; increased risk of toxicity ♦ **Polypeptide antibiotics:** possible neuromuscular respiratory depression ♦ **Metrizamide:** seizures ♦ **Cimetidine:** decreased effect of phenothiazines ♦ **Clonidine:** possibility of severe hypotension ♦ **Piperazine:** increased seizure potential.

Drug-Food: ♦ **Caffeine-containing beverages (e.g., coffee, tea, colas):** counteraction of antipsychotic effect.

ROUTE AND DOSAGE

Psychotic Disorders

♦ **PO (Adults):** 20 mg tid. In patients who have difficulty sleeping, take last tablet 1 hour before retiring. Total daily dosage range is 40–80 mg. **Hospitalized Patients:** Optimum dosage is 80–120 mg/day in divided doses. Certain hospitalized patients with severe schizophrenia have received doses as high as 400–600 mg/day.

PHARMACODYNAMICS

Route	Onset*	Peak†	Duration‡
PO	30–60 min	2–4 hr	4–6 hr

*Full clinical effects may not be observed for 4–8 weeks.

†Steady-state plasma levels are achieved in approximately 4–7 days.

‡Drug may be detected in urine for 3–6 months after last dose.

NURSING IMPLICATIONS

Assessment

♦ Assess mental status daily. Assess mood: • appearance • thought and communication patterns • level of interest in the environment and in activities • level of anxiety or agitation • presence of hallucinations or delusions • suspiciousness • interactions with others • ability to carry out activities of daily living.

♦ Assess for symptoms of blood dyscrasias: • sore throat • fever • malaise • unusual bleeding • easy bruising.

♦ Assess for extrapyramidal symptoms: • pseudoparkinsonism (tremors, shuffling gait, drooling, rigidity) • akinesia (muscular weakness) • akathisia (continuous restlessness and fidgeting) • dystonia (involuntary muscular movements of face, arms, legs, and neck) • oculogyric crisis (uncontrolled rolling back of the eyes) • tardive dyskinesia (bizarre facial and tongue movements, stiff neck, difficulty swallowing).

- Assess for symptoms of neuroleptic malignant syndrome: • hyperpyrexia up to 107°F • elevated pulse • increased or decreased blood pressure • severe parkinsonian muscle rigidity • elevated creatinine phosphokinase blood levels • elevated white blood count • altered mental status (including catatonic signs or agitation) • acute renal failure • varying levels of consciousness (including stupor and coma) • pallor • diaphoresis • tachycardia • arrhythmias • rhabdomyolysis.
- Assess vital signs, weight. Record baseline values for comparison.
- Assess history of allergies, sensitivity to this drug or other phenothiazines.
- Assess for signs and symptoms of cholestatic jaundice: • abdominal pain • nausea • rash • fever • yellow skin • flu-like symptoms • abnormal lab (eosinophilia • bile in urine • increased serum transaminases • bilirubin • alkaline phosphotase).
- Assess date of last menses (possible pregnancy); use of contraceptives.
- Assess if currently breast-feeding a child.
- Assess current and past alcohol and drug consumption.
- Assess for operation of automobile and/or other dangerous machinery.
- Assess for presence of adverse reactions or side effects.
- Assess patient/family knowledge about illness and need for medication.
- In collaboration with physician, assess CBC and liver function tests and ophthalmological exams in patients on long-term therapy.
- **Lab Test Alterations:**
  ◇ Increased serum alkaline phosphatase, transaminases, bilirubin.
  ◇ Increase in protein-bound iodine.
  ◇ False-positive urine pregnancy test, possibly caused by drug metabolite which discolors the urine (less likely to occur when serum test is used).
  ◇ Increased urinary glucose.

◇ Decreased urinary estrogen, progestin, and gonadotropin.
◇ Increased plasma cholesterol level.
◇ Increased serum prolactin.
- **Withdrawal:** Assess for symptoms of abrupt withdrawal from long-term therapy: • gastritis • nausea • vomiting • dizziness • headache • tachycardia • insomnia • tremulousness • sweating.
- **Toxicity and Overdose:** No correlation has been established between blood level and therapeutic effect.
◇ Assess for symptoms of overdose: • CNS depression, from heavy sedation to deep sleep to coma • hypotension • confusion • excitement • extrapyramidal symptoms • agitation • restlessness • convulsions • fever • autonomic reactions • ECG changes • cardiac arrhythmias • tachycardia • hypothermia • tremor • seizures • cyanosis.
- **Overdose Management:** Ensure maintenance of open airway.
◇ Gastric lavage.
◇ Do not induce emesis (nuchal rigidity may result in aspiration of vomitus).
◇ Give antiparkinsonian drugs or diphenhydramine to counteract extrapyramidal symptoms.
◇ IV fluids or administration of a vasoconstrictor to maintain adequate blood pressure. **Note:** Epinephrine is not recommended due to interaction with phenothiazines, which causes further drop in blood pressure.
◇ IV phenytoin for ventricular arrhythmias.
◇ Phenobarbital or diazepam to control convulsions or hyperactivity.
◇ Dialysis does not appear to be a useful intervention.

Potential Nursing Diagnoses

- High risk for violence directed at others related to mistrust and panic anxiety.
- High risk for injury related to acetophenazine's side effects of sedation,

dizziness, ataxia, weakness, lowered seizure threshold; abrupt withdrawal after prolonged use; overdose.

♦ Sensory-perceptual alteration related to panic anxiety, evidenced by hallucinations.

♦ Altered thought processes related to panic anxiety, evidenced by delusional thinking.

♦ Social isolation related to inability to trust others.

♦ Activity intolerance, high risk for, related to acetophenazine's side effects of: ● drowsiness ● dizziness ● ataxia ● weakness.

♦ Noncompliance with medication regimen related to suspiciousness and mistrust of others.

♦ Knowledge deficit related to medication regimen.

Plan/Implementation

♦ Monitor vital signs before beginning therapy and at regular intervals (bid or tid) throughout therapy. Take BP lying and standing to monitor for possible hypotensive reaction. Elderly are particularly susceptible. Dosage adjustment may be required.

♦ Ensure that patient who is ambulatory is protected from sun when spending time outdoors.

♦ Weigh patient 2–3 times a week, at same time of day, on same scale, if possible. A rapid weight gain or evidence of edema should be reported to physician immediately. Record I&O.

♦ Ensure that patient is protected from injury. Provide supervision and assistance when ambulating if dizziness and drowsiness are problems. Pad siderails and headboard for patient who experiences seizures.

♦ Give hard candy, gum, or frequent sips of water if dry mouth is a problem.

♦ Store medication at controlled temperatures between 15° and 30°C (59°–86°F). Protect from heat and moisture.

♦ Administer oral medication with food to minimize GI upset.

♦ Ensure patient swallows tablet and does not "cheek" to avoid medication or hoard for later use.

♦ Crush tablet and mix with food or fluid for patient who has difficulty swallowing.

Patient/Family Education

♦ Use caution when driving or operating dangerous machinery. Drowsiness and dizziness can occur.

♦ Do not stop taking the drug abruptly. To do so might produce withdrawal symptoms, such as nausea, vomiting, gastritis, headache, tachycardia, insomnia, tremulousness.

♦ Use sunscreens and wear protective clothing when spending time outdoors. Skin is more susceptible to sunburn.

♦ Report occurrence of any of the following symptoms to physician immediately: sore throat, fever, malaise, unusual bleeding, easy bruising, persistent nausea/vomiting, severe headache, rapid heart rate, difficulty urinating, muscle twitching, tremors, darkly colored urine, pale stools, yellow skin or eyes, muscular incoordination, skin rash.

♦ Drug may turn urine pink or reddish-brown in color. This is not significant nor is it harmful.

♦ Rise slowly from a sitting or lying position to prevent a sudden drop in blood pressure.

♦ If dry mouth is a problem, take frequent sips of water, chew sugarless gum, or suck on hard candy. Good oral care (frequent brushing, flossing) is very important.

♦ Consult physician regarding smoking while on acetophenazine therapy. Smoking increases metabolism of acetophenazine, requiring adjustment in dosage to achieve therapeutic effect.

♦ Dress warmly in cold weather and avoid extended exposure to very high or low temperatures. Body temperature is harder to maintain with this medication.

* Do not drink alcohol while on acetophenazine therapy. These drugs potentiate each other's effects.

* Do not consume other medications (including over-the-counter meds) without physician's approval. Many medications contain substances that interact with acetophenazine in a way that may be harmful.

* Be aware of possible risks of taking acetophenazine during pregnancy. Safe use during pregnancy and lactation has not been established. Acetophenazine readily crosses the placental barrier, so fetus could experience adverse effects of the drug. Inform physician immediately if pregnancy occurs, is suspected, or is planned.

* Be aware of side effects of acetophenazine. Refer to written materials furnished by healthcare providers for safe self-administration.

* Continue to take medication, even if feeling well and as though it is not needed. Symptoms may return if medication is discontinued.

* Carry card or other identification at all times describing medications being taken.

Evaluation

* Patient demonstrates a subsiding/resolution of the symptoms for which acetophenazine was prescribed (panic anxiety, altered thought processes, altered perceptions).

* Patient verbalizes understanding of side effects and regimen required for prudent self-administration of acetophenazine.

ALPRAZOLAM

(al-pray'zoe-lam)
Xanax

Classification(s):
Antianxiety; Benzodiazepine;
Skeletal muscle relaxant;
Anticonvulsant
Schedule C IV
Pregnancy Category D

INDICATIONS

* Anxiety disorders * Temporary relief of anxiety symptoms * Anxiety associated with depression. **Investigational Uses:** * Panic disorder. Efficacy for periods greater than 4 months has not been evaluated.

ACTION

* Depresses subcortical levels of the CNS, particularly the limbic system and reticular formation * May potentiate the effects of the powerful inhibitory neurotransmitter gamma-aminobutyric acid (GABA) in the brain, thereby producing a calmative effect * All levels of CNS depression can be effected, from mild sedation to hypnosis to coma.

PHARMACOKINETICS

Absorption: Rapid absorption from the GI tract.
Distribution: Is widely distributed. Crosses blood–brain and placental barriers; excreted in breast milk.
Metabolism and Excretion: Metabolized by the liver; produces inactive metabolites that are rapidly excreted for the most part by the kidneys.
Half-Life: 12–15 hours.

CONTRAINDICATIONS AND PRECAUTIONS

Contraindicated in: * Hypersensitivity to the drug * Combination with other CNS depressants * Pregnancy and lactation *

Narrow-angle glaucoma ✦ Children under 18.

Use Cautiously in: ✦ Elderly and debilitated patients ✦ Patients with hepatic or renal dysfunction ✦ Individuals with a history of drug abuse/addiction ✦ Depressed/suicidal patients.

ADVERSE REACTIONS AND SIDE EFFECTS*

CNS: <u>drowsiness</u>, <u>fatigue</u>, <u>ataxia</u>, <u>dizziness</u>, confusion, headache, syncope, paradoxical excitement, blurred vision.
CV: tachycardia, orthostatic hypotension, ECG changes.
Derm: rash, dermatitis, itching.
Endo: gynecomastia, galactorrhea.
GI: dry mouth, nausea/vomiting, diarrhea, constipation, anorexia.
GU: urinary retention, incontinence, irregular menses, libidinal changes.
Other: tolerance, physical and psychological dependence.

INTERACTIONS

Drug-Drug: ✦ **Other CNS depressants (including alcohol, barbiturates, narcotics), antipsychotics, antidepressants, antihistamines, anticonvulsants:** additive CNS depression ✦ **Cimetidine:** increased effects of alprazolam ✦ **Oral contraceptives:** increased or decreased effects of alprazolam ✦ **Cigarette smoking and caffeine:** decreased effects of alprazolam ✦ **Neuromuscular blocking agents:** increased respiratory depression ✦ **Digoxin:** reduced excretion of digoxin; increased potential for toxicity ✦ **Disulfiram:** decreased clearance of alprazolam ✦ **Rifampin, valproic acid:** decreased effects of alprazolam ✦ **Levodopa:** decreased effects of levodopa.

ROUTE AND DOSAGE

Anxiety; Anxiety Disorders; Anxiety Associated with Depression

✦ **PO (Adults):** 0.25–0.5 mg tid; total dose not to exceed 4 mg/day in divided doses.
✦ **PO (Geriatric or Debilitated Patients):** Initial dose 0.25 mg bid–tid

Panic Disorder

✦ **PO (Adults):** Range 1.0–10 mg/day. Usual dosage 3–6 mg/day. Start at 0.25–0.5 mg/day in 2–3 divided doses; slowly increase over several weeks.

PHARMACODYNAMICS

Route	Onset	Peak	Duration
PO	30–60 min	0.7–1.6 hr	*

*Varies with individual age, disease state, number of doses.

NURSING IMPLICATIONS

Assessment

✦ Assess level of anxiety. Symptoms include: • restlessness • pacing • insomnia • inability to concentrate • increased heart rate • increased respiration • elevated blood pressure • confusion • tremors • rapid speech.
✦ Assess for suicidal ideation. (CNS depressants may aggravate symptoms in depressed patients.)
✦ Assess history of allergies, sensitivity to this drug or to other benzodiazepines.
✦ Assess history of glaucoma.
✦ Assess date of last menses (possible pregnancy); use of contraceptives.
✦ Assess if currently breast-feeding a child.
✦ Assess current and past alcohol and drug consumption.
✦ Assess operation of automobile and/or other dangerous machinery.
✦ Assess for presence of adverse reactions or side effects.
✦ Assess patient/family knowledge about illness and need for medication.
✦ In collaboration with physician, assess CBC and liver function tests in patients on long-term therapy.
✦ **Lab Test Alterations:** Abnormal renal function tests.

*<u>Underlines</u> indicate most frequent; CAPITALS indicate life-threatening.

♦ **Withdrawal:** Assess for symptoms of withdrawal: • depression • insomnia • increased anxiety • abdominal and muscle cramps • tremors • vomiting • sweating • convulsions • delirium.

♦ **Withdrawal Management:** Monitor vital signs.

◊ Place in quiet room with low stimuli.

◊ Institute seizure precautions.

◊ A long-acting barbiturate, such as phenobarbital, may be ordered to suppress withdrawal symptoms.

◊ Phenytoin may be ordered to prevent seizures.

◊ Some physicians may order oxazepam, as needed, for objective withdrawal symptoms, gradually decreasing the dosage until the drug is discontinued.

♦ **Toxicity and Overdose:** Assess for symptoms of intoxication: • euphoria • relaxation • drowsiness • slurred speech • disorientation • mood lability • incoordination • unsteady gait • disinhibition of sexual and aggressive impulses • judgment and/or memory impairment.

◊ Assess for symptoms of overdose: • shallow respiration • cold and clammy skin • hypotension • dilated pupils • weak and rapid pulse • hypnosis • coma. Death is possible.

♦ **Overdose Management:** Ensure maintenance of adequate airway.

◊ Monitor vital signs.

◊ Vomiting should be induced if patient is conscious.

◊ Gastric lavage in unconscious patient.

◊ Administer IV fluids as ordered.

◊ Physician may also order flumazenil, a benzodiazepine antagonist.

Potential Nursing Diagnoses

♦ High risk for injury related to seizures; panic anxiety; abrupt withdrawal from long-term alprazolam use; effects of alprazolam intoxication or overdose.

♦ High risk for self-directed violence related to depressed mood.

♦ Anxiety (specify level) related to threats to physical integrity and/or self-concept.

♦ Activity intolerance, high risk for, related to alprazolam's side effects of lethargy, drowsiness, dizziness, muscular weakness.

♦ Knowledge deficit related to medication regimen.

Plan/Implementation

♦ Monitor vital signs before beginning therapy and at regular intervals (two times a day) throughout therapy.

♦ Ensure patient practices good mouth care. Offer hard, sugarless candy; gum; frequent sips of water for dry mouth.

♦ Ensure patient is protected from injury. Supervise and assist with ambulation if dizziness and muscular weakness are problems. Pad siderails and headboard for patient who experiences seizures.

♦ To minimize nausea, give medication with food or milk.

♦ If patient has difficulty swallowing tablet, it may be crushed and mixed with food or fluid.

♦ Ensure tablet has been swallowed and not "cheeked" to avoid medication or to hoard for later use.

♦ Store medication at controlled room temperatures of 15°–30°C (59°–86°F).

Patient/Family Education

♦ Do not drive or operate dangerous machinery. Drowsiness and dizziness can occur.

♦ Do not stop taking the drug abruptly. Can result in serious withdrawal symptoms.

♦ Do not consume other CNS depressants (including alcohol).

♦ Do not take nonprescription medication without approval from physician.

♦ Be aware of risks of taking alprazolam during pregnancy (congenital malformations have been associated with use during first trimester). Notify physi-

cian of desirability to discontinue drug if pregnancy is suspected or planned.
- Report any of the following symptoms to nurse or physician immediately: • excessive drowsiness or dizziness • palpitations • severe nausea/vomiting • skin rash • difficulty urinating • increased agitation.
- Be aware of potential side effects. Refer to written materials furnished by healthcare providers regarding correct method of self-administration.
- Carry card or piece of paper at all times stating names of medications being taken.

Evaluation
- Patient demonstrates a subsiding/resolution of the symptoms for which alprazolam was prescribed (anxiety symptoms, anxiety disorder, anxiety associated with depression).
- Patient verbalizes understanding of side effects and regimen required for prudent self-administration of alprazolam.

AMANTADINE

(a-man'ta-deen)
Symmetrel

Classification(s):
Antiparkinsonian agent; Antiviral agent
Pregnancy Category C

INDICATIONS
- Treatment of symptoms associated with idiopathic, postencephalitic, or arteriosclerotic parkinsonism, or symptomatic parkinsonism following injury to the nervous system by carbon monoxide intoxication • Control of drug-induced extrapyramidal reactions • Prophylaxis and symptomatic treatment of influenza A viral infections.

ACTION
- Not completely understood • Thought to relieve symptoms of parkinsonism by potentiating the release of dopamine within the CNS • Antiviral action may be related to prevention of viral penetration of host cell or blockage of the transfer of viral nucleic acid into the host cell.

PHARMACOKINETICS
Absorption: Well absorbed following oral administration.
Distribution: Is widely distributed. Crosses blood–brain and placental barriers; excreted in saliva, nasal secretions, and breast milk.
Metabolism and Excretion: Minimal metabolism by the liver; excreted by the kidneys unchanged.
Half-Life: 9–37 hours (average 24 hours).

CONTRAINDICATIONS AND PRECAUTIONS
Contraindicated in: • Hypersensitivity to the drug • Safe use in pregnancy, lactation, and in children under 1 year not established.
Use Cautiously in: • Patients with a history of seizures • Hepatic or renal impairment • Uncontrolled psychiatric disturbances • History of congestive heart failure or peripheral edema • Recurrent eczematoid dermatitis • Elderly and debilitated patients • Orthostatic hypotension • Concomitant use of CNS stimulating drugs.

ADVERSE REACTIONS AND SIDE EFFECTS*
CNS: <u>confusion</u>, <u>anxiety</u>, <u>irritability</u>, <u>ataxia</u>, <u>dizziness</u>, <u>difficulty concentrating</u>, headache, fatigue, insomnia, weakness, slurred speech, visual disturbances, seizures, oculogyric episodes, psychosis, nervousness.

---

*<u>Underlines</u> indicate most frequent; CAPITALS indicate life-threatening.

CV: CONGESTIVE HEART FAILURE, orthostatic hypotension, peripheral edema.
Derm: skin rash, eczematoid dermatitis, livedo reticularis (skin mottling), photosensitivity.
GI: anorexia, nausea, vomiting, constipation, dry mouth.
GU: urinary retention, increased frequency of urination.
Hemat: LEUKOPENIA, NEUTROPENIA.
Resp: dyspnea.
Psych: depression, psychosis, hallucinations.

INTERACTIONS

Drug-Drug: ♦ **Anticholinergic drugs:** additive anticholinergic effects ♦ **CNS stimulants:** increased CNS stimulation ♦ **Thiazide-type diuretics; triamterene:** possible decreased urinary excretion of amantadine with increased potential for toxicity ♦ **Note:** Amantadine does not interfere with antibody response to influenza vaccine and may be given concomitantly.

ROUTE AND DOSAGE

Parkinsonism; Drug-Induced Extrapyramidal Symptoms

♦ **PO (Adults):** 100 mg bid when used alone. For patients with serious associated medical illnesses or those receiving high doses of other antiparkinsonian drugs, the initial dosage is 100 mg daily for 1 to several weeks. Dosage may then be increased to 100 mg bid, if necessary. If response is not achieved at 200 mg/day, dosage may be increased up to 400 mg/day in divided doses, under close medical supervision.

Prophylaxis and Symptomatic Treatment of Viral Influenza A

♦ **PO (Adults 13–64):** 100 mg bid or 200 mg as single daily dose.
♦ **PO (Children 10–12):** 100 mg bid.
♦ **PO (Children under 10):** 4.4–8.8 mg/kg/day given in one or two doses (not to exceed 150 mg/day).

Patients with Renal Impairment

Dose is based on individual creatinine clearance, as follows:

Creatinine Clearance	Dose
≥80	100 mg bid
60–79	200 mg/100 mg on alt. days
40–59	100 mg qd
30–39	200 mg twice weekly
20–29	100 mg three times weekly
10–19	200 mg/100 mg alternating every 7 days

PHARMACODYNAMICS

Route	Onset	Peak	Duration
PO	4–48 hr*	1–4 hr	12–24 hr

*Time required to achieve maximal therapeutic response: 2 weeks.

NURSING IMPLICATIONS

Assessment

♦ Assess for symptoms of Parkinson's disease: ● tremors ● muscular weakness and rigidity ● drooling ● shuffling gait ● disturbances of posture and equilibrium ● flat affect ● monotone speech.
♦ Assess for extrapyramidal symptoms: ● pseudoparkinsonism (tremors, shuffling gait, drooling, rigidity) ● akinesia (muscular weakness) ● akathisia (continuous restlessness and fidgeting) ● dystonia (involuntary muscular movements of face, arms, legs, and neck) ● oculogyric crisis (uncontrolled rolling back of the eyes) ● tardive dyskinesia (bizarre facial and tongue movements, stiff neck, difficulty swallowing). **Note:** Amantadine is not effective in alleviating symptoms of tardive dyskinesia.
♦ Assess vital signs, weight. Record baseline values for comparison.
♦ Assess history of allergies, sensitivity to this drug.
♦ Assess date of last menses (possible pregnancy); use of contraceptives.
♦ Assess for symptoms of blood dyscrasias: ● sore throat ● fever ● malaise.

♦ Assess for symptoms of mental changes: • psychosis • hallucinations • delusions • paranoid ideations • depression with or without suicidal tendencies.

♦ Assess if currently breast-feeding a child.

♦ Assess current and past alcohol and drug consumption.

♦ Assess for operation of automobile and/or other dangerous machinery.

♦ Assess for presence of adverse reactions or side effects.

♦ Assess level of knowledge about illness and need for medication.

♦ In collaboration with physician, assess CBC, hepatic and renal function tests in patients on long-term therapy.

♦ **Withdrawal:** Assess for symptoms of abrupt withdrawal: parkinsonian crisis (rapid decomposition of condition) with severe akinesia, rigidity, tremor.

♦ **Toxicity and Overdose:** Neurotoxicity has been associated with plasma concentrations greater than 1.5 mcg/mL.

◊ Assess for symptoms of toxicity/overdose: • nausea • vomiting • anorexia • hyperexcitability • tremors • ataxia • blurred vision • lethargy • depression • slurred speech • convulsions • urinary retention • acute toxic psychosis • arrhythmias • hypotension.

♦ **Overdose Management:** Initiate immediate induction of emesis or gastric lavage.

◊ Maintain adequate airway.

◊ Monitor vital signs.

◊ Monitor electrolytes.

◊ Monitor urine pH and urinary output.

◊ Cardiac monitor.

◊ Force fluids (IV if necessary).

◊ Physician may elect to administer physostigmine salicylate to treat CNS toxicity.

◊ Administer urinary acidifier to promote drug elimination.

◊ Sedatives, anticonvulsants, antiarrhythmics, and vasopressors may be administered as required.

◊ Only minimal amount of amantadine is removed by hemodialysis.

Potential Nursing Diagnoses

♦ High risk for injury related to symptoms of Parkinson's disease or side effects of amantadine (dizziness, weakness, confusion).

♦ High risk for self-directed violence related to side effects of depressed mood with suicidal ideations.

♦ Sensory-perceptual alteration related to side effects of amantadine, evidenced by hallucinations.

♦ Altered thought processes related to side effects of amantadine, evidenced by confusion, difficulty concentrating.

♦ Social isolation related to embarrassment by symptoms of Parkinson's disease.

♦ Activity intolerance, high risk for, related to amantadine side effects of dizziness, ataxia, weakness, confusion, fatigue.

♦ Knowledge deficit related to medication regimen.

Plan/Implementation

♦ Monitor vital signs tid. Notify physician of significant elevations, arrhythmias, or changes in respiratory rate or rhythm.

♦ Weigh patient 2–3 times a week, at same time of day, on same scale, if possible. A rapid weight gain or evidence of edema should be reported to physician immediately. Record I&O.

♦ Ensure that patient is protected from injury. Provide supervision and assistance when ambulating if dizziness and ataxia are problems. Patient should change positions slowly to minimize effects of orthostatic hypotension.

♦ Give hard candy, gum, or frequent sips of water if dry mouth is a problem, or treat with saliva substitute.

♦ Ensure patient swallows capsule and

does not "cheek" to avoid medication or to hoard for later use.

♦ May administer with food to minimize gastric upset.

♦ May empty contents of capsule and mix with food or fluid for patient who has difficulty swallowing, or use the syrup form.

♦ Monitor vital signs before beginning therapy and at regular intervals (bid or tid) throughout therapy. Take BP lying and standing to monitor for possible hypotensive reaction. Elderly are particularly susceptible. Dosage adjustment may be required.

♦ Store medication at controlled room temperatures between 15° and 30°C (59°–86°F). Protect from heat and freezing.

♦ For influenza prophylaxis, start medication in anticipation of contact or as soon as possible after exposure. Continue for 10 days, or up to 90 days in the event of repeated or unknown exposures.

♦ For treatment of influenza symptoms, start medication as soon as possible after onset of symptoms and continue for 24–48 hours after symptoms disappear.

Patient/Family Education

♦ May take with food if GI upset occurs.

♦ Use caution when driving or operating dangerous machinery. Dizziness and confusion can occur.

♦ Do not stop taking the drug abruptly. To do so might produce withdrawal symptoms, such as muscle rigidity, weakness, tremors.

♦ Report occurrence of any of the following symptoms to physician immediately: swelling in the extremities, difficulty urinating, shortness of breath, persistent nausea and vomiting, significant weight gain, mental disturbances, dizziness or lightheadedness.

♦ Rise slowly from a sitting or lying position to prevent a sudden drop in blood pressure.

♦ If insomnia becomes a problem, take last dose earlier in the evening (e.g., with evening meal).

♦ If dry mouth is a problem, take frequent sips of water, chew sugarless gum, or suck on hard candy. Good oral care (frequent brushing, flossing) is very important.

♦ Do not consume other medications (including over-the-counter meds) without physician's approval. Many medications contain substances that interact with amantadine in a way that may be harmful.

♦ Be aware of possible risks of taking amantadine during pregnancy. Safe use during pregnancy and lactation has not been established. It is thought that amantadine crosses the placental barrier; if so, fetus could experience adverse effects of the drug. Inform physician immediately if pregnancy occurs, is suspected, or is planned. Use is not recommended in nursing mothers.

♦ Be aware of side effects of amantadine. Refer to written materials furnished by healthcare providers for safe self-administration.

♦ Continue to take medication, even if feeling well and as though it is not needed. Symptoms may return if medication is discontinued.

♦ Carry card or other identification at all times describing medications being taken.

Evaluation

♦ Patient demonstrates a subsiding of the symptoms for which amantadine was prescribed (symptoms of parkinsonism, drug-induced extrapyramidal symptoms, influenza A).

♦ Patient verbalizes understanding of side effects and regimen required for prudent self-admnistration of amantadine.

AMITRIPTYLINE

(a-mee-trip′ti-leen)
Amitril, Elavil, Endep, {Levate, Meravil, Novotriptyn}

Classification:
Tricyclic antidepressant
Pregnancy Category C

INDICATIONS

✦ Major depression with melancholia or psychotic symptoms ✦ Depression associated with organic disease, alcoholism, schizophrenia, or mental retardation ✦ Depressive phase of bipolar disorder. **Investigational Uses:** ✦ Chronic pain ✦ Cluster, migraine, and tension headaches.

ACTION

✦ Exact mechanism unclear ✦ Blocks reuptake of the neurotransmitters norepinephrine and serotonin, increasing their concentration at the synapse and correcting the deficit that is thought to contribute to the melancholy mood of the depressed person.

PHARMACOKINETICS

Absorption: Readily absorbed from the GI tract following oral administration.
Distribution: Is widely distributed. Crosses blood–brain and placental barriers. Enters breast milk.
Metabolism and Excretion: Metabolized by the liver. Excreted in urine; small amount excreted in feces.
Half-Life: 10–50 hours.

CONTRAINDICATIONS AND PRECAUTIONS

Contraindicated in: ✦ Hypersensitivity to this drug or other tricyclic antidepressants ✦ Concomitant use with MAO inhibitors ✦ Acute recovery period following myocardial infarction ✦ Untreated angle-closure glaucoma ✦ Children under age 12 ✦ Pregnancy and lactation (safety not established).
Use Cautiously in: ✦ Patients with a history of seizures ✦ Urinary retention ✦ Benign prostatic hypertrophy ✦ Glaucoma ✦ Cardiovascular disorders ✦ Respiratory difficulties ✦ Hepatic or renal insufficiency ✦ Psychotic patients ✦ Elderly and debilitated patients.

ADVERSE REACTIONS AND SIDE EFFECTS*

CNS: drowsiness, dizziness, weakness, headache, fatigue, confusion, lethargy, memory deficits, disturbed concentration, tremors, ataxia, tinnitus, extrapyramidal symptoms, paresthesias of extremities, lowered seizure threshold, blurred vision, agitation, excitement, restlessness, insomnia, exacerbation of psychosis, shift to manic behavior.
CV: orthostatic hypotension, tachycardia and other arrhythmias, hypertension, MYOCARDIAL INFARCTION, HEART BLOCK, CONGESTIVE HEART FAILURE, ECG CHANGES, syncope, CARDIOVASCULAR COLLAPSE.
Derm: skin rash, urticaria, photosensitivity, erythema, petechiae.
GI: dry mouth, constipation, nausea, vomiting, anorexia, diarrhea, abdominal cramps, adynamic ileus, esophageal reflux, stomatitis, black tongue.
GU: urinary retention, gynecomastia (males), testicular swelling, menstrual irregularity, breast engorgement and galactorrhea (females), changes in libido, impotence, delayed micturation.
Hemat: AGRANULOCYTOSIS, THROMBOCYTOPENIA, LEUKOPENIA, eosinophilia, purpura.
Hepat: jaundice, hepatitis.
Other: weight gain, nasal congestion, alopecia, hypothermia, peripheral neuropathy.

INTERACTIONS

Drug-Drug: ✦ **MAO inhibitors:** hyperpyretic crisis, hypertensive crisis, severe

{} = Only available in Canada.
*Underlines indicate most frequent; CAPITALS indicate life-threatening.

seizures, tachycardia, death ✦ **Guaneth-idine; clonidine; (possibly) guanabenz:** decreased effects of these medications ✦ **Cimetidine:** increased amitriptyline serum levels ✦ **Amphetamines; sympathomimetics:** increased hypertensive and cardiac effects of these drugs ✦ **CNS depressants (including alcohol, barbiturates, benzodiazeines):** potentiation of CNS effects ✦ **Thyroid medications:** tachycardia; arrhythmias ✦ **Methylphenidate; phenothiazines; haloperidol:** increased serum amitriptyline levels ✦ **Ethchlorvynol:** transient delirium ✦ **Quinidine; procainamide; disopyramide:** potentiates adverse cardiovascular effects of amitriptyline ✦ **Oral contraceptives:** decreased effects of amitriptyline ✦ **Smoking:** increases amitriptyline metabolism ✦ **Disulfiram:** decreases amitriptyline metabolism ✦ **Levodopa; phenylbutazone:** delayed or decreased absorption of these drugs ✦ **Warfarin:** increased prothrombin time ✦ **Dicumarol:** increased plasma dicumarol concentrations.

ROUTE AND DOSAGE

Depression

- **PO (Hospitalized Adults):** Initial dose: 100 mg/day in divided doses or as a single bedtime dose. Gradually increase to 200 mg/day. Some patients may require as much as 300 mg/day. Total daily dose may be administered once a day, preferably at bedtime.
- **PO (Outpatient Adults):** Initial dose: 75 mg/day. Gradually increase to 150 mg/day. Maximum daily dose: 200 mg/day. Total daily dose may be administered once a day at bedtime.
- **PO (Adolescents, Geriatrics):** Initial dose: 10 mg tid and 20 mg at bedtime.
- **IM (Adults):** 20–30 mg qid. Used only when initiating therapy with patients who are unable or unwilling to use the oral medication. (Switch to oral form as soon as possible.)

- **PO (Maintenance, Adults):** Reduce dose as possible, usually to 50–100 mg/day but sometimes as low as 25–40 mg/day.

Chronic Pain

- **PO (Adults):** 75–150 mg/day.

Prevention of Cluster, Migraine, and Tension Headaches

- **PO (Adults):** 25 mg at bedtime; may be increased by 25 mg at weekly intervals until maximum of 150 mg/day is reached. In most patients, 50–75 mg/day. Allow 6-week trial before concluding drug is ineffective.

PHARMACODYNAMICS

Route	Onset	Peak	Duration
PO, IM	2–4 wk	2–12 hr	weeks*

*Allow up to 2 weeks following cessation of therapy for complete drug elimination.

NURSING IMPLICATIONS

Assessment

- Assess for suicidal ideation, plan, means. Assess for sudden lifts in mood, which could indicate patient's decision to commit suicide.
- Assess mental status daily: • mood • appearance • thought and communication patterns • level of interest in the environment and in activities • suicidal ideation. Improvement in these behavior patterns and level of energy should be expected within 2–4 weeks following initiation of therapy.
- Assess for symptoms of blood dyscrasias: sore throat, fever, malaise, unusual bleeding, easy bruising.
- Assess vital signs, weight.
- Assess history of allergies, sensitivity to this drug or other tricyclic antidepressants.
- Assess for history of glaucoma.
- Assess date of last menses (possible pregnancy); use of contraceptives.
- Assess if currently breast-feeding a child.
- Assess current and past alcohol and drug consumption.

♦ Assess for operation of automobile and/or other dangerous machinery.

♦ Assess for presence of adverse reactions or side effects.

♦ Assess patient/family knowledge about illness and need for medication.

♦ In collaboration with physician, assess CBC and liver function tests in patients on long-term therapy.

♦ **Lab Test Alterations:** Increased serum bilirubin, alkaline phosphatase, transaminase, and glucose.

◊ Decreased urinary 5-hydroxyindoleacetic acid (HIAA) and vanillylmandelic acid (VMA) excretion.

♦ **Withdrawal:** Assess for symptoms of abrupt withdrawal from long-term therapy: • nausea • headache • vertigo • malaise • insomnia • nightmares.

♦ **Toxicity and Overdose:** Range of therapeutic serum concentration is 150–300 ng/mL.

◊ Assess for symptoms of overdose: • confusion • agitation • irritability • hallucinations • seizures • flushing • dry mouth • dilated pupils • delirium • hyperpyrexia • hypotension or hypertension • coma • tachycardia • arrhythmias • respiratory depression • cardiac arrest • renal failure • shock • congestive heart failure • acid-base disturbances.

♦ **Overdose Management:** Monitor vital signs and ECG.

◊ Ensure adequate airway.

◊ Induce emesis or initiate gastric lavage.

◊ Administer activated charcoal to minimize absorption.

◊ Physician may prescribe IV physostigmine (given cautiously) to reverse anticholinergic effects.

◊ Administer sodium bicarbonate, vasopressors, phenytoin, propranolol, or lidocaine for cardiovascular effects.

◊ Administer IV diazepam for seizures.

Potential Nursing Diagnosis

♦ High risk for self-directed violence related to depressed mood.

♦ High risk for injury related to amitriptyline side effects of sedation, dizziness, ataxia, weakness, confusion, lowered seizure threshold; abrupt withdrawal after prolonged use; overdose.

♦ Social isolation related to depressed mood.

♦ Activity intolerance, high risk for, related to amitriptyline side effects of drowsiness, dizziness, ataxia, weakness, confusion.

♦ Knowledge deficit related to medication regimen.

Plan/Implementation

♦ **General Info:** Monitor vital signs before beginning therapy and at regular intervals (bid or tid) throughout therapy. Take BP lying and standing in patients experiencing orthostatic hypotension (elderly are particularly susceptible). Contact physician if tachycardia/arrhythmias are noted.

◊ Ensure that patient who is ambulatory is protected from sun when spending time outdoors.

◊ Weigh patient 2–3 times a week, at same time of day, on same scale, if possible. Rapid weight gain or evidence of edema should be reported to physician immediately. Record I&O.

◊ Ensure that patient is protected from injury. Provide supervision and assistance when ambulating if dizziness and drowsiness are problems. Pad siderails and headboard for patient who experiences seizures.

◊ Give hard candy, gum, or frequent sips of water if dry mouth is a problem.

♦ **PO:** Administer oral medication with food to minimize GI upset.

◊ Ensure patient swallows tablet and does not "cheek" to avoid medication or to hoard for later use.

◊ Crush tablet and mix with food or fluid for patient who has difficulty swallowing.

◊ Store tablets in a well-closed container. Avoid storage at temperatures above 40°C (104°F). In addition, 10-mg tablets must be protected from light and stored in a well-closed, light-resistant container.

♦ **IM:** Administer IM only if patient is unwilling or unable to use oral medication.

◊ Do not administer parenteral solution IV.

◊ Protect amitriptyline injection from freezing and avoid storage above 40°C (104°F).

◊ Replace with oral maintenance therapy as soon as possible.

Patient/Family Education

♦ Therapeutic effect may not be seen for as long as 4 weeks. If no improvement is noted after this time, physician may prescribe a different medication. Continue to take medication even though symptoms have not subsided.

♦ Use caution when driving or operating dangerous machinery. Drowsiness and dizziness can occur. If these side effects become persistent or interfere with daily activities, report to physician. Dosage adjustment may be necessary.

♦ Do not abruptly stop taking the drug. To do so might produce withdrawal symptoms, such as nausea, vertigo, insomnia, headache, malaise, nightmares.

♦ Use sunscreens and wear protective clothing when spending time outdoors. Skin may be sensitive to sunburn.

♦ Report occurrence of any of the following symptoms to physician immediately: sore throat, fever, malaise, unusual bleeding, easy bruising, persistent nausea/vomiting, severe headache, rapid heart rate, difficulty urinating.

♦ Rise slowly from a sitting or lying position to prevent a sudden drop in blood pressure.

♦ If dry mouth is a problem, take frequent sips of water, chew sugarless gum, or suck on hard candy. Good oral care (frequent brushing, flossing) is very important.

♦ Avoid smoking while on amitriptyline therapy. Smoking increases metabolism of amitriptyline, requiring adjustment in dosage to achieve therapeutic effect.

♦ Do not drink alcohol while on amitriptyline therapy. These drugs potentiate each other's effects.

♦ Do not consume other medications (including over-the-counter meds) without physician's approval. Many medications contain substances that, in combination with tricyclics, could precipitate a life-threatening hypertensive crisis.

♦ Be aware of possible risks of taking amitriptyline during pregnancy. Safe use during pregnancy and lactation has not been established. It is known that amitriptyline readily crosses the placental barrier, so fetus could experience adverse effects of the drug. Inform physician immediately if pregnancy occurs, is suspected, or is planned.

♦ Be aware of side effects of amitriptyline. Refer to written materials furnished by healthcare providers for safe self-administration.

♦ Carry card or other identification at all times describing medications being taken.

Evaluation

♦ Patient demonstrates a subsiding/resolution of the symptoms for which amitriptyline was prescribed (depressed mood, suicidal ideation, chronic pain, headaches).

♦ Patient verbalizes understanding of side effects and regimen required for prudent self-administration of amitriptyline.

AMOBARBITAL

(am-oh-bar'bi-tal)
Amytal

Classification(s)
Sedative-hypnotic; Anticonvulsant;
Barbiturate; CNS depressant
Schedule C II
Pregnancy Category D

INDICATIONS

♦ Moderate anxiety states ♦ Insomnia
♦ Seizure disorders ♦ Status epilepticus
♦ Preanesthetic sedative.

ACTION

♦ Depresses the central nervous system ♦
Interferes with transmission through the
reticular formation, which is concerned
with arousal ♦ Action on neurotransmitters is not well defined ♦ All levels of CNS
depression can occur, from mild sedation to hypnosis to coma to death.

PHARMACOKINETICS

Absorption: Readily absorbed following
oral administration.
Distribution: Rapidly and widely distributed. Crosses blood–brain and placental barriers; excreted in breast milk.
Metabolism and Excretion: Metabolized by the liver and excreted by the
kidneys as inactive metabolites.
Half-Life: 16–40 hours.

CONTRAINDICATIONS AND PRECAUTIONS

Contraindicated in: ♦ Hypersensitivity
to the drug ♦ Severe hepatic, renal, cardiac, or respiratory disease ♦ Individuals
with a history of drug dependence ♦ Porphyria.
Use Cautiously in: ♦ Elderly and debilitated patients ♦ Patients with hepatic,
renal, cardiac, or respiratory dysfunction
♦ Depressed/suicidal patients ♦ Patients

with ammonia intoxication ♦ Pregnancy
and lactation ♦ Drug-dependent person-
alities.

ADVERSE REACTIONS AND SIDE EFFECTS*

CNS: drowsiness, headache, lethargy,
dizziness, mental depression, ataxia, re-
sidual sedation ("hangover"), confusion,
paradoxical excitement and/or euphoria.
CV: hypotension, bradycardia.
Derm: skin rashes, urticaria, dermatitis
(may precede potentially fatal reactions);
redness and pain at IM injection site,
phlebitis at IV site.
GI: nausea/vomiting, diarrhea/constipa-
tion, epigastric pain.
Hemat: AGRANULOCYTOSIS, THROMBOCYTO-
PENIA.
Resp: hypoventilation, apnea, RESPIR-
ATORY DEPRESSION, LARYNGOSPASM, BRONCHO-
SPASM.
Other: tolerance, physical and psycho-
logical dependence.

INTERACTIONS

Drug-Drug: ♦ **Other CNS depressants**
(including alcohol, benzodiaze-
pines, antihistamines, opiates): additive CNS depression ♦ **Chloramphen-**
icol, MAO inhibitors, valproic acid,
cimetidine, disulfiram: increased effects of amobarbital ♦ **Phenytoin:** increased or decreased effects of either
drug (close monitoring of serum levels
to control seizure activity) ♦ **Oral con-**
traceptives: decreased effectiveness of
oral contraceptives ♦ **Oral anticoagu-**
lants: decreased anticoagulant effects ♦
Corticosteroids, digitoxin, doxycy-
cline: decreased effects of these drugs ♦
Furosemide: orthostatic hypotension
♦ **Griseofulvin:** decreased griseofulvin
levels.
Drug-Food: ♦ **Vitamin D:** increased vitamin D metabolism; possible deficiency
♦ **Folic acid:** decreased absorption of
folic acid; possible deficiency.

*Underlines indicate most frequent; CAPITALS indicate life-threatening.

ROUTE AND DOSAGE
Anxiety
- **PO (Adults):** 15–120 mg bid–qid (usual dose 30–50 mg bid or tid).
- **PO (Children):** 2 mg/kg daily, in four equally divided doses.

Insomnia
(Limit use to 2 weeks.)
- **PO (Adults):** 65–200 mg at bedtime.
- **IM (Adults):** 65–200 mg at bedtime.
- **IM (Children):** 2–3 mg/kg at bedtime.

Anticonvulsant
- **IM (Adults):** 65–500 mg (maximum IM dose: 500 mg).
- **IV (Adults):** 65–500 mg (maximum IV dose, 1 g).

Preanesthetic Sedation
- **PO, IM (Adults):** 200 mg 1–2 hours before surgery.

PHARMACODYNAMICS

Route	Onset	Peak	Duration
PO	30–60 min	6 hr	8–10 hr
IM	10–30 min	20–60 min	3–6 hr
IV	5 min	30 min	3–6 hr

NURSING IMPLICATIONS
Assessment
- Assess sleep patterns. Keep records for adequate baseline data before initiation of therapy.
- Assess occurrence, characteristics, and duration of seizure activity.
- Assess for suicidal ideation in depressed patients.
- Assess history of allergies, sensitivity to this drug or to other barbiturates.
- Assess date of last menses (possible pregnancy), use of contraceptives.
- Assess if currently breast-feeding a child.
- Assess current and past alcohol and drug consumption.
- Assess for operation of automobile and/or other dangerous machinery.
- Assess for presence of adverse reactions or side effects.
- Assess patient's and family's response to diagnosis of seizure disorder.
- Assess patient/family knowledge about illness and need for medication.
- In collaboration with physician, assess CBC and renal and liver function tests in patients on prolonged amobarbital therapy.
- **Lab Test Alterations:** May increase values of bromsulphalein (BSP) retention and protein-bound iodine (PBI).
  ◇ Elevation of blood ammonia.
- **Withdrawal:** Assess for symptoms of withdrawal: • anxiety • tremors • insomnia • nausea/vomiting • weakness • diaphoresis • orthostatic hypotension • delirium • convulsions.
- **Withdrawal Management:** Monitor vital signs.
  ◇ Place in quiet room with low stimuli.
  ◇ Institute seizure precautions.
  ◇ A long-acting barbiturate, such as phenobarbital, may be ordered to suppress withdrawal symptoms.
  ◇ Phenytoin may be ordered to prevent seizures.
  ◇ Some physicians may order oxazepam, as needed, for objective withdrawal symptoms, gradually decreasing the dosage until the drug is discontinued.
- **Toxicity and Overdose:** Assess for symptoms of intoxication: • confusion • drowsiness • dyspnea • slurred speech • staggering.
  ◇ Assess for symptoms of overdose: • CNS and respiratory depression • hypoventilation • hypothermia • hypotension • oliguria • tachycardia • coma.
  ◇ May progress to respiratory arrest, circulatory collapse, and death.
- **Overdose Management:** Monitor vital signs.
  ◇ Ensure maintenance of airway.
  ◇ Induce vomiting (in conscious patient).
  ◇ Initiate gastric lavage (in unconscious patient).

◇ Administer activated charcoal to minimize absorption of drug.

◇ For severe intoxication, forced diuresis or hemodialysis may be used.

Potential Nursing Diagnoses

◆ Ineffective breathing pattern related to side effects of hypoventilation and respiratory depression.

◆ High risk for injury related to seizures; abrupt withdrawal from long-term use; decreased mental alertness caused by side effect of residual sedation; side effects of dizziness and ataxia; effects of overdose.

◆ High risk for self-directed violence related to depressed mood.

◆ Sleep pattern disturbance related to situational crises, physical condition, severe level of anxiety.

◆ Activity intolerance, high risk for, related to side effects of residual sedation, drowsiness, dizziness.

◆ Knowledge deficit related to medication regimen.

Plan/Implementation

◆ **General Information:** Monitor vital signs before beginning therapy, at regular intervals (bid) throughout therapy, every 3–5 minutes during IV administration and every 10 minutes for 30 minutes following IM administration.

◇ Ensure that patient is protected from injury. Supervise and assist with ambulation if dizziness and drowsiness are problems. Ensure that patient avoids participation in any activity that requires mental alertness (including smoking). Raise siderails, and instruct patient to remain in bed following administration.

◇ Store medication at controlled room temperatures between 15° and 30°C (59°–86°F). Protect from heat and freezing.

◆ **PO:** To minimize nausea, medication may be given with food or milk. However, rate of absorption is increased if taken on an empty stomach.

◇ Ensure that tablet or capsule has been swallowed and not "cheeked" to avoid medication or to hoard for later use.

◇ Crush tablet or empty capsule, and mix with food or fluid for patient who has difficulty swallowing.

◆ **IM:** Dilute with sterile water for injection. Do not shake to mix. Do not use if solution is not clear or if precipitate is visible. Use within 30 minutes of preparation.

◇ Administer deep into large muscle mass to minimize subcutaneous tissue irritation/necrosis. Use Z-track method.

◇ Volume of injection should not exceed 5 mL at any one site.

◇ Maximum IM dose should not exceed 500 mg.

◇ Aspirate carefully before injecting drug. Inadvertent arterial injection can result in pain, tissue necrosis, gangrene.

◇ Patient should remain in bed with siderails up and be observed closely for at least 3 hours following IM administration. Monitor vital signs every 15–30 minutes during this time.

◆ **IV:** Prepare IV solution immediately prior to administration. Dilute with sterile water for injection. Do not shake to mix. Do not use if solution is not clear or if precipitate is visible. Use within 30 minutes of preparation.

◇ Solution is irritating. Extravasation may result in tissue necrosis. Stop infusion immediately if patient complains of pain. Inadvertent arterial injection may result in gangrene.

◇ Administer IV solution at no more than 100 mg/min for adults, 60 mg/min for children. Observe closely for potential depression of vital signs.

◇ Patient should be recumbent during IV administration and should remain in bed with siderails up for at least 3 hours following IV administration. Observe closely and monitor vital signs every 5 minutes for first 30 minutes, then every 15–30 minutes for 3 hours.

◇ Ensure availability of artificial ventilation and resuscitation equipment.

Patient/Family Education

♦ Use caution in driving or operating dangerous machinery. Drowsiness and dizziness can occur.

♦ Do not stop taking the drug abruptly. Can produce serious (even life-threatening) withdrawal symptoms. If you forget a dose, take it as close as possible to prescribed time. If it is already close to time for next dose, wait until then; do not double the dose at the next prescribed time.

♦ Do not consume other CNS depressants (including alcohol).

♦ Be aware of how to protect patient during a seizure: Do not restrain, but do protect from injury. Padding (towels, blankets, pillows) may be used to prevent bumping against hard objects. When convulsion has subsided, turn patient on side to allow secretions to drain and to prevent aspiration. Be sure to keep records of occurrence, characteristics, and duration of seizures, so that accurate reports may be given to physician for providing assistance in stabilization and control of seizures. If patient has difficulty breathing or continues to experience subsequent seizures, call for emergency assistance immediately.

♦ Be aware of the risks of taking barbiturates during pregnancy. Congenital malformations have been associated with use during the first trimester. Also, evidence of withdrawal symptoms has been observed in neonates born to mothers who had ingested barbiturates regularly during the last trimester of pregnancy. Notify physician if pregnancy is suspected or planned.

♦ Because barbiturates decrease the effectiveness of oral contraceptives, use alternative methods of birth control during amobarbital therapy.

♦ Be aware of potential side effects. Refer to written materials furnished by healthcare providers regarding correct method of self-administration.

♦ Report symptoms of sore throat, fever, malaise, severe headache, conjunctivitis, rhinitis, urethritis, balanitis, easy bruising, petechiae, epistaxis to physician immediately.

♦ Carry card or other identification at all times stating names of medications being taken.

Evaluation

♦ Patient demonstrates a subsiding/resolution of the symptoms for which amobarbital was prescribed (seizures, sleep disturbances, anxiety).

♦ Patient verbalizes understanding of side effects and regimen required for prudent self-administration of amobarbital.

AMOXAPINE

(a-mox′a-peen)
Asendin

Classification(s):
Tricyclic antidepressant
Pregnancy Category C

INDICATIONS

♦ Major depression with melancholia or psychotic symptoms ♦ Depression associated with organic disease and alcoholism ♦ Depressive phase of bipolar disorder ♦ Psychoneurotic anxiety ♦ Mixed symptoms of anxiety and depression.

ACTION

♦ Exact mechanism of action unclear ♦ Blocks reuptake of the neurotransmitters norepinephrine and serotonin, increasing their concentration at the synapse and correcting the deficit that is thought to contribute to the melancholy mood of the depressed person ♦ May also decrease response to dopamine by blocking dopaminergic receptors.

PHARMACOKINETICS

Absorption: Readily and almost completely absorbed from the GI tract following oral administration.

Distribution: Is widely distributed. Crosses blood–brain and placental barriers. Enters breast milk.

Metabolism and Excretion: Metabolized by the liver. Excreted in urine and feces.

Half-Life: Approximately 8 hours. 8-hydroxyamoxapine (major active metabolite) 30 hours.

CONTRAINDICATIONS AND PRECAUTIONS

Contraindicated in: ◆ Hypersensitivity to this drug or other tricyclic antidepressants ◆ Concomitant use with MAO inhibitors ◆ Acute recovery period following myocardial infarction ◆ Untreated angle-closure glaucoma ◆ Patients with tendency for urinary retention ◆ Safety in children under age 16 and in pregnancy and lactation not established.

Use Cautiously in: ◆ Patients with history of seizures ◆ Benign prostatic hypertrophy ◆ Cardiovascular disorders ◆ Respiratory difficulties ◆ Hepatic or renal insufficiency ◆ Psychotic patients ◆ Elderly and debilitated patients.

ADVERSE REACTIONS AND SIDE EFFECTS*

CNS: <u>drowsiness</u>, <u>dizziness</u>, weakness, headache, fatigue, confusion, lethargy, memory deficits, disturbed concentration, tremors, ataxia, tinnitus, extrapyramidal symptoms, paresthesias of extremities, lowered seizure threshold, blurred vision, agitation, excitement, restlessness, insomnia, exacerbation of psychosis, shift to manic behavior.

CV: <u>orthostatic hypotension</u>, <u>tachycardia</u> and other arrhythmias, hypertension, MYOCARDIAL INFARCTION, HEART BLOCK, CONGESTIVE HEART FAILURE, <u>ECG changes</u>, syncope, CARDIOVASCULAR COLLAPSE.

Derm: skin rash, urticaria, photosensitivity, erythema, petechiae.

GI: <u>dry mouth</u>, <u>constipation</u>, nausea, vomiting, anorexia, diarrhea, abdominal cramps, adynamic ileus, esophageal reflux, stomatitis, black tongue.

GU: <u>urinary retention</u>, gynecomastia (males), testicular swelling, menstrual irregularity, breast engorgement and galactorrhea (females), changes in libido, impotence, delayed micturation.

Hemat: AGRANULOCYTOSIS, THROMBOCYTOPENIA, LEUKOPENIA, eosinophilia, purpura.

Hepat: jaundice, hepatitis.

Other: weight gain, nasal congestion, alopecia, hypothermia, peripheral neuropathy.

INTERACTIONS

Drug-Drug ◆ **MAO inhibitors:** hyperpyretic crisis, hypertensive crisis, severe seizures, tachycardia, death ◆ **Guanethidine, clonidine, (possibly) guanabenz:** decreased effects of these medications ◆ **Cimetidine:** increased amoxapine serum levels ◆ **Amphetamines, sympathomimetics:** increased hypertensive and cardiac effects of these drugs ◆ **CNS depressants (including alcohol, barbiturates, benzodiazepines):** potentiation of CNS effects ◆ **Thyroid medications:** tachycardia, arrhythmias ◆ **Methylphenidate, phenothiazines, haloperidol:** increased serum amoxapine levels ◆ **Ethchlorvynol:** transient delirium ◆ **Quinidine, procainamide, disopyramide:** potentiation of adverse cardiovascular effects of amoxapine ◆ **Oral contraceptives:** decreased effects of amoxapine ◆ **Smoking:** increased amoxapine metabolism ◆ **Disulfiram:** decreased amoxapine metabolism ◆ **Levodopa, phenylbutazone:** delayed or decreased absorption of these drugs ◆

---

*Underlines indicate most frequent; CAPITALS indicate life-threatening.

Dicumarol: increased plasma dicumarol concentrations.

ROUTE AND DOSAGE
Anxiety/Depression
- **PO (Adults and Children Over 16):** Initially, 50 mg bid or tid. Increase dosage to 100 mg bid or tid by end of first week. Increase above 300 mg/day (maximum 400 mg/day outpatient or 600 mg/day hospitalized patient) only if 300 mg/day has been ineffective for at least 2 weeks. Once desired effect has been achieved, may be given in single bedtime dose (not to exceed 300 mg). If total daily dosage exceeds 300 mg, give in divided doses.
- **PO (Geriatrics):** Initially, 25 mg bid or tid. Dose may be increased by end of first week to 50 mg bid or tid. 100–150 mg/day is usually adequate, but some patients may require up to 300 mg/day.
- **PO (Maintenance):** Reduce to lowest possible dose required to achieve relief of symptoms.

PHARMACODYNAMICS

Route	Onset	Peak	Duration
PO	2–4 wk	90 min	weeks*

*Allow up to 2 weeks following cessation of therapy for complete drug elimination.

NURSING IMPLICATIONS
Assessment
- Assess mental status daily: • mood • appearance • thought and communication patterns • level of interest in the environment and in activities • suicidal ideation. Improvement in these behavior patterns and level of energy should be expected within 2–4 weeks following initiation of therapy.
- Assess for suicidal ideation, plan, means. Assess for sudden lifts in mood, which could indicate patient's decision to commit suicide.
- Assess level of anxiety. Symptoms include: • restlessness • pacing • insomnia • inability to concentrate • increased heart rate • increased respiration • elevated blood pressure • confusion • tremors • rapid speech.
- Assess for symptoms of blood dyscrasias: • sore throat • fever • malaise • unusual bleeding • easy bruising.
- Assess vital signs, weight.
- Assess history of allergies, sensitivity to this drug or to other tricyclic antidepressants.
- Assess for history of glaucoma.
- Assess date of last menses (possible pregnancy), use of contraceptives.
- Assess if currently breast-feeding a child.
- Assess current and past alcohol and drug consumption.
- Assess for operation of automobile and/or other dangerous machinery.
- Assess for presence of adverse reactions or side effects.
- Assess patient/family knowledge about illness and need for medication.
- In collaboration with physician, assess CBC and liver function tests in patients on long-term therapy.
- **Lab Test Alterations:** Increased serum bilirubin, alkaline phosphatase, transaminase, and glucose.
- ◇ Decreased urinary 5-hydroxyindoleacetic acid (HIAA) and vanillylmandelic acid (VMA) excretion.
- **Withdrawal:** Assess for symptoms of abrupt withdrawal from long-term therapy: • nausea • headache • vertigo • malaise • insomnia • nightmares.
- **Toxicity and Overdose:** Range of therapeutic serum concentration not well substantiated.
- ◇ Assess for symptoms of overdose: • confusion • agitation • irritability • hallucinations • seizures • flushing • dry mouth • dilated pupils • delirium • hyperpyrexia • hypotension or hypertension • coma • tachycardia • arrhythmias • respiratory depression • cardiac arrest • renal failure • shock

- congestive heart failure • acid-base disturbances.
♦ **Overdose Management:** Monitor vital signs and ECG.
◊ Ensure adequate airway.
◊ Induce emesis or initiate gastric lavage.
◊ Administer activated charcoal to minimize absorption.
◊ Physician may prescribe IV physostigmine (given cautiously) to reverse anticholinergic effects.
◊ May administer sodium bicarbonate, vasopressors, propranolol, or lidocaine for cardiovascular effects.
◊ Administer IV diazepam or phenytoin for seizures.

Potential Nursing Diagnosis

♦ High risk for self-directed violence related to depressed mood.
♦ High risk for injury related to amoxapine side effects of sedation: • dizziness • ataxia • weakness • confusion • lowered seizure threshold • abrupt withdrawal after prolonged use • overdose.
♦ Anxiety (moderate to severe) related to threat to physical integrity or self-concept.
♦ Social isolation related to depressed mood.
♦ Activity intolerance, high risk for, related to amoxapine side effects of: • drowsiness • dizziness • ataxia • weakness • confusion.
♦ Knowledge deficit related to medication regimen.

Plan/Implementation

♦ Monitor vital signs before beginning therapy and at regular intervals (bid or tid) throughout therapy. Take BP lying and standing in patients experiencing orthostatic hypotension (elderly are particularly susceptible). Contact physician if tachycardia/arrhythmias are noted.
♦ Ensure that patient who is ambulatory is protected from sun when spending time outdoors.

♦ Weigh patient 2–3 times a week, at same time of day, on same scale, if possible. Rapid weight gain or evidence of edema should be reported to physician immediately. Record I&O.
♦ Ensure that patient is protected from injury. Provide supervision and assistance when ambulating if dizziness and drowsiness are problems. Pad siderails and headboard for patient who experiences seizures.
♦ Give hard candy, gum, or frequent sips of water if dry mouth is a problem.
♦ Administer oral medication with food to minimize GI upset.
♦ Ensure that patient swallows tablet and does not "cheek" to avoid medication or to hoard for later use.
♦ Tablet may be crushed and mixed with food or fluid for patient who has difficulty swallowing.
♦ Store medication at controlled temperatures of 15°–30°C (59°–86°F).

Patient/Family Education

♦ Therapeutic effect may not be seen for as long as 4 weeks. If after this length of time no improvement is noted, physician may prescribe a different medication. Continue to take medication even though symptoms have not subsided.
♦ Use caution when driving or operating dangerous machinery. Drowsiness and dizziness can occur. If these side effects become persistent or interfere with daily activities, report to physician. Dosage adjustments may be necessary.
♦ Do not stop taking the drug abruptly. To do so might produce withdrawal symptoms, such as: • nausea • vertigo • insomnia • headache • malaise • nightmares.
♦ Use sunscreens and wear protective clothing when spending time outdoors. Skin may be sensitive to sunburn.
♦ Report occurrence of any of the following symptoms to physician imme-

diately: • sore throat • fever • malaise • unusual bleeding • easy bruising • persistent nausea/vomiting • severe headache • rapid heart rate • difficulty urinating.

♦ Rise slowly from a sitting or lying position to prevent a sudden drop in blood pressure.

♦ If dry mouth is a problem, take frequent sips of water, chew sugarless gum, or suck on hard candy. Good oral care (frequent brushing, flossing) is very important.

♦ Avoid smoking while on amoxapine therapy. Smoking increases metabolism of amoxapine, requiring adjustment in dosage to achieve therapeutic effect.

♦ Do not drink alcohol while on amoxapine therapy. These drugs potentiate each other's effects.

♦ Do not consume other medications (including over-the-counter meds) without physician's approval while taking amoxapine. Many medications contain substances that, in combination with tricyclics, could precipitate a life-threatening hypertensive crisis.

♦ Be aware of possible risks of taking amoxapine during pregnancy. Safe use during pregnancy and lactation has not been established. It is known that amoxapine readily crosses the placental barrier, so fetus could experience adverse effects of the drug. Inform physician immediately if pregnancy occurs, is suspected, or is planned.

♦ Be aware of side effects of amoxapine. Refer to written materials furnished by healthcare providers for safe self-administration.

♦ Carry card or other identification at all times describing medications being taken.

Evaluation

♦ Patient demonstrates a subsiding/resolution of the symptoms for which amoxapine was prescribed (depressed mood, suicidal ideation, anxiety).

♦ Patient verbalizes understanding of side effects and regimen required for prudent self-administration of amoxapine.

AMPHETAMINE SULFATE

(am-fet′ a-meen)
Racemic Amphetamine Sulfate

Classification(s):
CNS stimulant; Amphetamine; Anorexigenic
Schedule C II
Pregnancy Category C

INDICATIONS

♦ Narcolepsy ♦ Attention deficit disorder with hyperactivity in children ♦ Exogenous obesity.

ACTION

♦ Exact mechanism of action in CNS not known ♦ Amphetamines are sympathomimetic amines that stimulate the central nervous system, possibly by increasing synaptic release of norepinephrine, dopamine, and (at higher doses) serotonin in the brain; this is also accomplished by blocking reuptake at presynaptic membranes ♦ Central action occurs through cortical stimulation and may also be due to stimulation of the reticular activating system ♦ Action may also be due in part to the inhibition of amine oxidase ♦ Peripheral action is thought to be due to release of nonrepinephrine from adrenergic nerve stores and to direct effects on alpha- and beta-receptor sites.

PHARMACOKINETICS

Absorption: Rapid and complete absorption within 3 hours following oral administration.
Distribution: Widely distributed, with

high concentrations in the brain and CSF. Crosses placental barrier; enters breast milk.

Metabolism and Excretion: Metabolized by the liver and excreted in the urine. Elimination is enhanced by acidic urine, slowed by alkaline urine.

Half-Life: 7–33.6 hours (depending on pH of the urine).

CONTRAINDICATIONS AND PRECAUTIONS

Contraindicated in: ✦ Hypersensitivity to sympathomimetic amines ✦ Advanced arteriosclerosis ✦ Symptomatic cardiovascular disease ✦ Moderate to severe hypertension ✦ Hyperthyroidism ✦ Glaucoma ✦ Agitation or hyperexcitability ✦ History of drug abuse ✦ During or within 14 days of therapy with MAO inhibitors ✦ Children under 3 years of age ✦ Pregnancy.

Use Cautiously in: ✦ Lactation ✦ Psychotic children ✦ Tourette's disorder ✦ Patients with mild hypertension ✦ Anorexia ✦ Insomnia ✦ Elderly, debilitated, or asthenic patients ✦ Patients with a history of suicidal or homicidal tendencies.

ADVERSE REACTIONS AND SIDE EFFECTS*

CNS: overstimulation, restlessness, dizziness, insomnia, dyskinesia, euphoria, dysphoria, tremor, headache, symptoms of Tourette's disorder, psychoses (rare), disorientation, hallucinations, seizures, nervousness, increased motor activity, blurred vision, mydriasis.

CV: palpitations, tachycardia, elevation of blood pressure, pallor or flushing, arrhythmias.

Derm: urticaria.

Endo: changes in libido.

GI: dry mouth, metallic taste, diarrhea, constipation, anorexia, weight loss, nausea, vomiting, abdominal cramps.

Other: tolerance, physical and psychological dependence, cyanosis, chilliness, excessive sweating.

INTERACTIONS

Drug-Drug: ✦ **Furazolidone, MAO inhibitors (during treatment or within 14 days following administration):** hypertensive crisis, headache, hyperpyrexia, intracranial hemorrhage, bradycardia ✦ **Insulin:** alteration in requirements ✦ **Guanethidine:** decreased antihypertensive effects ✦ **Phenothiazines:** possible decreased effects of both drugs ✦ **Urinary alkalinizers (e.g., acetazolamide, sodium bicarbonate, potassium citrate, sodium acetate, sodium citrate, sodium lactate, tromethamine):** decreased amphetamine excretion, increased amphetamine effects, excess CNS stimulation, cardiovascular effects ✦ **Urinary acidifiers (e.g., ammonium chloride, potassium phosphate, sodium acid phosphate):** increased amphetamine excretion, decreased amphetamine effects.

Drug-Food: ✦ **Caffeinated foods and drinks:** increased effects of amphetamine.

ROUTE AND DOSAGE

Narcolepsy

✦ **PO (Adults and Children 12 Years and Older):** Initial dosage: 10 mg/day. May be increased in increments of 10 mg/day at weekly intervals until desired results are achieved, or adverse effects, such as anorexia or insomnia, appear. Usual dosage range: 5–60 mg/day.

✦ **PO (Children 6–12 Years):** 5 mg/day. May be increased in increments of 5 mg/day at weekly intervals until desired response is achieved. Maximum dose: 60 mg/day. With tablets or elixir, give first dose on awakening; additional doses (1 or 2) at intervals of 4–6 hours. Sustained-release forms may be used for once-a-day dosage.

*Underlines indicate most frequent; CAPITALS indicate life-threatening.

Attention Deficit Disorder in Children

- **PO (Children 3–5 Years):** 2.5 mg/day. May be increased in increments of 2.5 mg/day at weekly intervals until desired response is achieved.
- **PO (Children 6 Years and Older):** 5 mg daily or bid. May be increased in increments of 5 mg/day at weekly intervals until desired response is achieved. Dosage will rarely exceed 40 mg/day. Give first dose of tablets or elixir on awakening; additional doses (1 or 2) at intervals of 4–6 hours. Sustained-release forms may be used for once-a-day dosage.

Exogenous Obesity

- **PO (Adults and Children 12 Years or Older):** 5–30 mg/day in divided doses of 5–10 mg, 30–60 minutes before meals. Sustained-release forms: 10–15 mg in the morning (10–14 hours before bedtime).

PHARMACODYNAMICS

Route	Onset	Peak	Duration
PO	30–60 min	1–3 hr*	4–24 hr*

*Varies with individual, dosage form, number of doses, and pH of urine.

NURSING IMPLICATIONS

Assessment

- Assess and record baseline temperature, pulse, respiration, blood pressure, and weight for comparison during therapy.
- In diabetic patients, assess blood sugar bid or tid. Insulin adjustments may be required due to alteration in eating patterns and possibility of hyperactivity.
- For overweight patients, assess knowledge of sound nutritional, calorie-reduced diet, with program of regular exercise using amphetamine as an anorexigenic.
- Assess growth rate of children on amphetamine therapy carefully. A decrease in rate of development may be observed.
- Assess mental status for changes in mood, level of activity, degree of stimulation, aggressiveness.
- Assess sleeping patterns carefully. Insomnia may occur.
- Assess history of allergies, sensitivity to this drug or to other amphetamines.
- Assess history of glaucoma.
- Assess for presence of adverse reactions or side effects.
- Assess date of last menses (possible pregnancy), use of contraceptives.
- Assess if currently breast-feeding a child.
- Assess current and past alcohol and drug consumption.
- Assess usual amount of caffeine consumed.
- Assess for operation of automobile and/or other dangerous machinery.
- Assess patient/family knowledge about illness and need for medication.
- In collaboration with physician, assess CBC, urinalysis, and liver function tests periodically in patients on amphetamine therapy.
- **Lab Test Alterations:** Elevated serum thyroxine (T_4) levels; altered plasma and urinary steroid concentrations.
- **Withdrawal:** Assess for symptoms of withdrawal: • extreme fatigue • lethargy • increased dreaming • mental depression • suicidal ideations • changes on the sleep EEG.
- **Withdrawal Management:** Monitor vital signs.
  ◊ Place in quiet room with low stimuli.
  ◊ Allow patient to sleep as much as desired.
  ◊ Observe closely (every 15 minutes).
  ◊ Institute suicide precautions.
  ◊ Some physicians may elect to prescribe antidepressants to counteract feelings of depression and lethargy.
- **Toxicity and Overdose:** Therapeutic

blood levels of amphetamine range from 5–10 mcg/dL.

◇ Assess for symptoms of intoxication: • severe dermatoses • marked insomnia • irritability • hyperactivity • tachycardia • dilated pupils • elevated blood pressure • personality changes • hyperpyrexia • disorganization of thoughts • poor concentration • visual hallucinations • compulsive, stereotyped behavior • psychosis with manifestations similar to paranoid schizophrenia.

◇ Assess for symptoms of overdose: • restlessness • hyperirritability • insomnia • tremor • hyperreflexia • diaphoresis • mydriasis • flushing or pallor • profuse perspiration • hyperactivity • confusion • hypertension • extrasystoles • tachypnea • fever • hallucinations • panic state • paranoid ideations • delirium • marked hypertension • arrhythmias • heart block • seizures • coma • circulatory collapse • death.

♦ **Overdose Management:** Place in cool room.

◇ Monitor vital signs.

◇ Induce emesis or initiate gastric lavage (although gastric emptying is usually ineffective more than 4 hours after ingestion).

◇ Administer activated charcoal.

◇ Administer saline cathartic.

◇ Administer urinary acidifier, such as ammonium chloride.

◇ Administer diuretic.

◇ Give short-acting barbiturates for hyperactivity.

◇ Chlorpromazine has been effective in decreasing CNS stimulation.

◇ Administer IV phentolamine for severe hypertension.

◇ Administer fluid replacement and a vasopressor to prevent cardiovascular collapse.

◇ Give oxygen and artificial respiration, if necessary.

◇ Hemodialysis or peritoneal dialysis may be effective.

Potential Nursing Diagnoses

♦ High risk for injury due to overstimulation and hyperactivity; abrupt amphetamine withdrawal; overdose.

♦ High risk for self-directed violence related to suicidal ideations resulting from abrupt amphetamine withdrawal.

♦ High risk for violence directed at others related to aggressiveness as side effect of amphetamine.

♦ Alteration in nutrition, more than body requires, related to excessive intake in relation to metabolic needs.

♦ Alteration in nutrition, less than body requires, related to amphetamine side effects of anorexia and weight loss.

♦ Sleep pattern disturbance related to overstimulation by amphetamine.

♦ Alteration in thought processes related to adverse amphetamine effects of overstimulation and difficulty concentrating.

♦ Knowledge deficit related to medication regimen.

Plan/Implementation

♦ Monitor medication effects. Tolerance develops rapidly. If anorexic effects begin to diminish, notify physician immediately. Patient should be on reduced-calorie diet and program of regular exercise in addition to the medication.

♦ Monitor and record vital signs at regular intervals (bid) throughout therapy.

♦ Encourage use of gum, hard candy, or frequent sips of water for patient who experiences dry mouth. Ensure that patient practices good oral care (frequent brushing, flossing).

♦ Ensure that patient is protected from injury. Keep stimuli low and environment as quiet as possible to discourage overstimulation.

♦ Observe frequently for signs of impending violence to self or others. Institute suicide precautions if necessary. Assess level of anxiety often to prevent onset of physical aggression as agitation increases.

♦ In children with behavior disorders, a drug "holiday" should be attempted periodically under direction of physician to determine effectiveness of the medication and need for continuation.

♦ Ensure that tablet or capsule has been swallowed and not "cheeked" to avoid medication or to hoard for later use.

♦ Tablets may be crushed and mixed with food or fluid for patient who has difficulty swallowing.

♦ To prevent insomnia, give last dose at least 6 hours before retiring.

♦ As an anorexigenic, drug should be administered 30–60 minutes before meals.

♦ Store medication at controlled room temperature between 15° and 30°C (59°–86°F). Protect from heat and moisture.

Patient/Family Education

♦ Use caution in driving or operating dangerous machinery. Level of alertness may be diminished due to hyperactivity and stimulation. Dizziness may occur as a side effect.

♦ Do not stop taking the drug abruptly. Can produce serious withdrawal symptoms.

♦ Do not take other medications (including over-the-counter drugs) without physician's approval. Many medications contain substances that, in combination with amphetamine, can be harmful.

♦ Diabetic patient: Monitor blood sugar bid or tid or as instructed by physician. Be aware of need for possible alteration in insulin requirements due to changes in food intake, weight, and activity.

♦ Avoid consumption of large amounts of caffeinated products (coffee, tea, colas, chocolate), as they may enhance the stimulant effect of amphetamine.

♦ Follow reduced-calorie diet provided by dietitian and a program of regular exercise if using amphetamine as an appetite suppressant. **Do not exceed recommended dose if appetite suppressant effect diminishes. Contact physician.**

♦ Notify physician if restlessness, insomnia, anorexia, or dry mouth become severe, or if rapid, pounding heartbeat becomes evident.

♦ Be aware of possible risks of taking amphetamine during pregnancy. Safe use in pregnancy and lactation has not been established. It is known that amphetamine crosses placental barrier, so fetus could experience adverse effects of the drug. Inform physician immediately if pregnancy occurs, is suspected, or is planned.

♦ Be aware of potential side effects of amphetamine. Refer to written materials furnished by healthcare providers for safe self-administration.

♦ Carry card or other identification at all times describing medications being taken.

Evaluation

♦ Patient demonstrates a subsiding/resolution of the symptoms for which amphetamine sulfate was prescribed (inability to prevent falling asleep, obesity, behavior problems/hyperactivity in children).

♦ Patient verbalizes understanding of side effects and regimen required for prudent self-administration of amphetamine.

APROBARBITAL

(a-proe-bar'bi-tal)
Alurate

Classification(s)
Sedative-hypnotic; Barbiturate; CNS
depressant
Schedule C III
Pregnancy Category D

INDICATIONS

♦ Anxiety ♦ Insomnia.

ACTION

♦ Depresses the central nervous system ♦ Interferes with transmission through the reticular formation, which is concerned with arousal ♦ Causes imbalance in inhibitory and facilitatory mechanisms that influence the cerebral cortex and reticular formation ♦ Action on neurotransmitters is not well defined ♦ All levels of CNS depression can occur, from mild sedation to hypnosis to coma to death.

PHARMACOKINETICS

Absorption: Readily absorbed following oral administration.
Distribution: Rapidly and widely distributed. Crosses blood–brain and placental barriers; excreted in breast milk.
Metabolism and Excretion: Metabolized by the liver; excreted by the kidney as inactive metabolites and unchanged drug.
Half-Life: 14–40 hours.

CONTRAINDICATIONS AND PRECAUTIONS

Contraindicated in: ♦ Hypersensitivity to the drug ♦ Severe hepatic, renal, cardiac, or respiratory disease ♦ Individuals with a history of previous addiction ♦ Individuals with a history of porphyria ♦ Children (safety and effectiveness have not been established).

Use Cautiously in: ♦ Elderly and debilitated patients ♦ Patients with hepatic, renal, cardiac, or respiratory dysfunction ♦ Depressed/suicidal patients ♦ Patients with ammonia intoxication ♦ Pregnancy and lactation.

ADVERSE REACTIONS AND SIDE EFFECTS*

CNS: drowsiness, headache, lethargy, dizziness, mental depression, ataxia, residual sedation ("hangover"), confusion, paradoxical excitement and/or euphoria.
CV: hypotension, bradycardia.
Derm: skin rashes, urticaria, dermatitis (may precede potentially fatal reactions).
GI: nausea/vomiting, constipation.
Hemat: AGRANULOCYTOSIS, THROMBOCYTOPENIA.
Resp: hypoventilation, apnea, LARYNGOSPASM, BRONCHOSPASM.
Other: tolerance, physical and psychological dependence.

INTERACTIONS

Drug-Drug: ♦ **Other CNS depressants (including alcohol, benzodiazepines, antihistamines, opiates):** additive CNS depression ♦ **Chloramphenicol, MAO inhibitors, valproic acid, cimetidine, disulfiram:** increased effects of aprobarbital ♦ **Phenytoin:** increased or decreased effects of either drug (close monitoring of serum levels is required to control seizure activity) ♦ **Oral contraceptives:** decreased effectiveness of oral contraceptives ♦ **Oral anticoagulants:** decreased anticoagulant effects ♦ **Corticosteroids, digitoxin, doxycycline:** decreased effects of these drugs ♦ **Furosemide:** orthostatic hypotension ♦ **Griseofulvin:** decreased griseofulvin levels.
Drug-Food: ♦ **Vitamin D:** increased vitamin D metabolism, possible deficiency ♦ **Folic acid:** decreased absorption of folic acid, possible deficiency.

*Underlines indicate most frequent; CAPITALS indicate life-threatening.

ROUTE AND DOSAGE
Anxiety
- ✦ **PO (Adults):** 40 mg tid.
Insomnia
(Limit use to 2 weeks.)
- ✦ **PO (Adults):** 40–160 mg at bedtime.

PHARMACODYNAMICS

Route	Onset	Peak	Duration
PO	60 min	3 hr	6–8 hr

NURSING IMPLICATIONS
Assessment
- ✦ Assess level of anxiety. Symptoms include: • restlessness • pacing • insomnia • inability to concentrate • increased heart rate • increased respiration • elevated blood pressure • confusion • tremors • rapid speech.
- ✦ Assess sleep patterns. Keep records for adequate baseline data before initiation of therapy.
- ✦ Assess for suicidal ideation in depressed patients.
- ✦ Assess history of allergies, sensitivity to this drug or to other barbiturates.
- ✦ Assess date of last menses (possible pregnancy), use of contraceptives.
- ✦ Assess if currently breast-feeding a child.
- ✦ Assess current and past alcohol and drug consumption.
- ✦ Assess for operation of automobile and/or dangerous machinery.
- ✦ Assess for presence of adverse reactions or side effects.
- ✦ Assess patient/family knowledge about illness and need for medication.
- ✦ In collaboration with physician, assess renal and liver function tests and CBC in patients on prolonged therapy.
- ✦ **Lab Test Alterations:** Increased values of bromsulphalein (BSP) retention and protein-bound iodine (PBI).
- ◇ Elevated blood ammonia.
- ✦ **Withdrawal:** Assess for symptoms of withdrawal: • anxiety • tremors • in-

somnia • nausea/vomiting • weakness • diaphoresis • orthostatic hypotension • delirium • convulsions.
- ✦ **Withdrawal Management:** Monitor vital signs.
- ◇ Place in quiet room with low stimuli.
- ◇ Institute seizure precautions.
- ◇ A long-acting barbiturate, such as phenobarbital, may be ordered to suppress withdrawal symptoms.
- ◇ Phenytoin may be ordered to prevent seizures.
- ◇ Some physicians may order oxazepam, as needed, for objective withdrawal symptoms, gradually decreasing the dosage until the drug is discontinued.
- ✦ **Toxicity and Overdose:** Assess for symptoms of toxicity: • confusion • drowsiness • dyspnea • slurred speech • staggering.
- ◇ Assess for symptoms of overdose: • CNS and respiratory depression • hypoventilation • hypothermia • hypotension • oliguria • tachycardia • coma.
- ◇ May progress to respiratory arrest, circulatory collapse, and death.
- ✦ **Overdose Management:** Monitor vital signs.
- ◇ Ensure maintenance of airway.
- ◇ Induce vomiting in conscious patient or initiate gastric lavage in unconscious patient.
- ◇ Administer activated charcoal to minimize absorption of drug.
- ◇ Administer IV fluids.
- ◇ For severe intoxication, forced diuresis or hemodailysis may be used.

Potential Nursing Diagnosis
- ✦ Ineffective breathing pattern related to side effects of hypoventilation and apnea.
- ✦ High risk for injury related to abrupt withdrawal from long-term use; decreased mental alertness caused by side effect of residual sedation; side effects of dizziness, ataxia; effects of overdose.

- High risk for self-directed violence related to depressed mood.
- Anxiety (specify level) related to threats to physical integrity and/or self-concept.
- Sleep pattern disturbance related to situational crises; physical condition; severe level of anxiety.
- Activity intolerance, high risk for, related to side effects of residual sedation, drowsiness, dizziness.
- Knowledge deficit related to medication regimen.

Plan/Implementation

- Monitor vital signs before beginning therapy and at regular intervals (bid) throughout therapy.
- Ensure that patient is protected from injury. Supervise and assist with ambulation if dizziness and drowsiness are problems. Ensure that patient avoids participation in any activity that requires mental alertness (including smoking). Raise siderails, and instruct patient to remain in bed following administration.
- To minimize nausea, medication may be given with food or milk.
- Store medication at controlled room temperatures of 15°–30°C (59°–86°F). Protect from heat and moisture.

Patient/Family Education

- Use caution in driving or operating dangerous machinery. Drowsiness and dizziness can occur.
- Do not stop taking the drug abruptly. Can produce serious (even life-threatening) withdrawal symptoms. If a dose is missed, take it as close as possible to prescribed time. If it is already close to time for next dose, wait until then; do not double dose at next prescribed time.
- Do not consume other CNS depressants (including alcohol).
- Be aware of the risks of taking barbiturates during pregnancy (congenital malformations may be associated with use during the first trimester).

Also, evidence of withdrawal symptoms have been observed in neonates born to mothers who had ingested barbiturates regularly during the last trimester of pregnancy. Notify physician if pregnancy is suspected or planned.
- Because barbiturates decrease effectiveness of oral contraceptives, use alternative methods of birth control during aprobarbital therapy.
- Be aware of potential side effects. Refer to written materials furnished by healthcare providers regarding correct method of self-administration.
- Report symptoms of sore throat, fever, malaise, severe headache, conjunctivitis, rhinitis, urethritis, balanitis, easy bruising, petechiae, or epistaxis to physician immediately.
- Carry card or other identification at all times stating names of medications being taken.

Evaluation

- Patient demonstrates a subsiding/resolution of the symptoms for which aprobarbital was prescribed (anxiety, sleep disturbances).
- Patient verbalizes understanding of side effects and regimen required for prudent self-administration of aprobarbital.

ATROPINE SULFATE

(a′troe-peen)

Classification(s):
Anticholinergic; Antimuscarinic; Antispasmodic; Mydriatic
Pregnancy Category C

INDICATIONS

- Surgery and other procedures, including ECT (inhibits salivation and decreases respiratory tract secretions) ◆ Vagal stimulation during anesthesia (restores cardiac rate and arterial pressure) ◆ Peptic ulcer and other GI conditions ◆ Urinary frequency and urgency; nocturnal enuresis ♦ Bronchial asthma ♦ Poisoning by cholinergic drugs ♦ Treatment of parkinsonism rigidity and tremor.

ACTION

♦ Competitively inhibits the muscarinic actions of acetylcholine at postganglionic parasympathetic neuroeffector sites including smooth muscle, secretory glands, and sites within the central nervous system ♦ Specific anticholinergic responses are dose-related.

PHARMACOKINETICS

Absorption: Absorbed well from the GI tract, mucous membranes, skin, eyes, and following IM administration.
Distribution: Is widely distributed. Crosses blood–brain and placental barriers; thought to enter breast milk.
Metabolism and Excretion: Metabolized by the liver. Excreted mainly in urine; small amount excreted in expired air and feces.
Half-Life: 2–3 hours.

CONTRAINDICATIONS AND PRECAUTIONS

Contraindicated in: ♦ Hypersensitivity to anticholinergic drugs or tartrazine (contained in some preparations) ♦ Angle-closure glaucoma ♦ Adhesions between the iris and lens ♦ Tachycardia ♦ Acute hemorrhage with unstable cardiovascular status ♦ Myocardial ischemia ♦ Obstructive disease of the GI tract ♦ Paralytic ileus ♦ Intestinal atony of the elderly or debilitated patient ♦ Severe ulcerative colitis ♦ Toxic megacolon complicating ulcerative colitis ♦ Obstructive uropathy ♦ Myasthenia gravis ♦ Cardiospasm.
Use Cautiously in: ♦ Autonomic neuropathy ♦ Glaucoma ♦ Hepatic disease ♦ Mild to moderate ulcerative colitis ♦ Esophageal reflux ♦ Hiatal hernia associated with reflux esophagitis ♦ Renal disease ♦ Prostatic hypertrophy ♦ Hyperthy-

roidism ♦ Coronary artery disease ♦ Congestive heart failure ♦ Cardiac tachyarrhythmias ♦ Hypertension ♦ Chronic lung disease ♦ Infants and small children ♦ Down's syndrome ♦ Brain damage ♦ Patients exposed to elevated environmental temperatures ♦ Febrile patients ♦ Geriatric patients ♦ Gastric ulcer ♦ GI infections ♦ Patients with diarrhea ♦ Partial obstructive uropathy.

ADVERSE REACTIONS AND SIDE EFFECTS*

CNS: <u>headache</u>, flushing, nervousness, drowsiness, weakness, <u>dizziness</u>, insomnia, fever, mental confusion, excitement, restlessness, tremor.
CV: palpitations, bradycardia (with low doses), tachycardia (with high doses).
Derm: urticaria, other dermal manifestations.
GI: <u>xerostomia (dry mouth)</u>, altered taste perception, nausea, <u>vomiting</u>, dysphagia, heartburn, <u>constipation</u>, bloated feeling, PARALYTIC ILEUS, gastroesophageal reflux.
GU: urinary retention, <u>urinary hesitancy</u>, impotence.
Ocular: <u>blurred vision</u>, mydriasis, photophobia, cycloplegia, increased intraocular pressure.
Other: ANAPHYLAXIS, suppression of lactation, nasal congestion, decreased sweating.

INTERACTIONS

Drug-Drug: ♦ **Antihistamines, glutethimide, disopyramide, procainamide, quinidine, antipsychotics, antiparkinsonian agents, buclizine, meperidine, orphenadrine, amantadine, benzodiazepines, tricyclic antidepressants, MAO inhibitors:** enhanced anticholinergic effects ♦ **Nitrates, nitrites, alkalinizing agents, primidone, thioxanthenes, methylphenidate:** potentiation of adverse effects of atropine ♦ **Long-term cortico-**

---

*<u>Underlines</u> indicate most frequent; CAPITALS indicate life-threatening.

steroid or haloperidol therapy: increased intraocular pressure ✦ **Guanethidine, histamine, reserpine:** decreased effects of atropine ✦ **Phenothiazines, haloperidol:** possible decreased antipsychotic effects ✦ **Sympathomimetics, nitrofurantoin, thiazide diuretics:** increased effects of these drugs ✦ **Cholinesterase inhibitors, metoclopramide:** decreased effects of these drugs ✦ **Digitalis, slow-release digoxin tablets, anticholinergics, neostigmine:** increased potential for adverse effects ✦ **Antacids:** may interfere with absorption of anticholinergics ✦ **Cyclopropane anesthesia:** possible ventricular arrhythmias.

ROUTE AND DOSAGE
Preoperative or Preprocedural Medication
✦ **SC, IM, IV (Adults):** Usual dose: 0.4–0.6 mg 30–60 minutes before surgery or procedure (range 0.3–1.2 mg).
✦ **SC, IM (Children):** Dosage range: 0.1 mg (newborn) to 0.6 mg (12 years old) 30–60 minutes before surgery or procedure.

Vagally Mediated Bradycardia
✦ **IV (Adults):** Dosage range: 0.4–1.0 mg q 1–2 hours as needed. Larger doses, up to a total maximum dose of 2 mg, may be required.
✦ **IV (Children):** 0.02 mg/kg. Minimum dose 0.1 mg; maximum dose 1 mg. Maximum total dose: 1 mg children; 2 mg adolescents.

Cholinergic Drug Poisoning
✦ **IM, IV (Adults):** 1–2 mg; repeat with 2 mg IM or IV q 5–60 minutes until muscarinic signs and symptoms subside.
✦ **IM, IV (Children):** 0.05 mg/kg; repeat q 10–30 minutes until muscarinic signs and symptoms subside.

Bronchial Asthma
✦ **Inhaler (Adults):** 0.025 mg/kg diluted with 3–5 mL saline, administered through nebulizer tid or qid. Maximum dose 2.5 mg.
✦ **Inhaler (Children):** 0.05 mg/kg diluted in saline and administered through nebulizer tid or qid.

PHARMACODYNAMICS

Route	Onset	Peak	Duration
PO	30 min	30–60 min	4 hr
IM, SC	15 min	30 min	4 hr
IV	1 min	2–4 min	4 hr

NURSING IMPLICATIONS:
Assessment
✦ Assess mood daily in patient receiving ECT. Observe: • appearance • speech and thought patterns • behavior • interaction with others • somatic complaints • attendance in activities • evidence of excitement or agitation.
✦ Assess for symptoms of paralytic ileus: • constipation • abdominal pain and distention • absence of bowel sounds. Patients taking atropine concomitantly with other drugs that produce anticholinergic effects are particularly susceptible.
✦ Assess vital signs prior to administration. Record baseline values for comparison.
✦ Assess history of allergies, sensitivity to this drug or to other anticholinergic drugs.
✦ Assess date of last menses (possible pregnancy), use of contraceptives.
✦ Assess if currently breast-feeding a child.
✦ Assess current and past alcohol and drug consumption.
✦ Assess for operation of automobile and/or other dangerous machinery.
✦ Assess for presence of adverse reactions or side effects.
✦ Assess patient/family knowledge about illness and need for medication.
✦ **Toxicity and Overdose:** Assess for

symptoms of overdose: • dry mouth • thirst • dysphagia • vomiting • nausea • abdominal distention • muscular weakness • CNS stimulation followed by depression • delirium • drowsiness • restlessness • stupor • fever • dizziness • headache • seizures • tremor • hallucinations • anxiety • ataxia • psychotic behavior • rapid pulse and respiration • tachycardia with weak pulse • hypertension • palpitations • urinary retention • blurred vision • photophobia • dilated pupils • leukocytosis • flushed hot dry skin • rash over face, neck, and upper trunk • diminished or absent bowel sounds • hypotension • coma • skeletal muscle paralysis • respiratory failure • circulatory failure.

+ **Overdose Management:** Induce emesis or initiate gastric lavage.
◊ Administer activated charcoal slurry.
◊ Ensure adequate airway and ventilation.
◊ Monitor ECG continuously.
◊ Protect patient from injury due to seizures.
◊ Physostigmine by slow IV injection may reverse anticholinergic effects.
◊ Administer benzodiazepines or short-acting barbiturates to control excitement.
◊ Use fluid therapy and levarterenol to control hypotension and circulatory collapse.
◊ Use cold packs or other cooling measures to treat hyperpyrexia.
◊ Place patient in darkened room if photophobia occurs.

Potential Nursing Diagnoses

+ Decreased cardiac output related to vagal stimulation.
+ High risk for self-directed violence related to depressed mood.
+ High risk for injury related to atropine side effects of weakness, dizziness, blurred vision; overdose.
+ Hyperthermia related to anticholinergic effect of decreased sweating.

+ Altered thought processes related to atropine side effect of mental confusion.
+ Anxiety (moderate to severe) related to pending medical procedure (e.g., surgery, ECT).
+ Activity intolerance, high risk for, related to atropine's side effects of drowsiness, dizziness, weakness, mental confusion.
+ Knowledge deficit related to medication regimen.

Plan/Implementation:

+ **General Info:** Monitor vital signs daily. Report any changes to physician. Withhold dosage if pulse rate is markedly increased or decreased and contact physician immediately.
◊ Weigh patient 2–3 times a week, at same time of day, on same scale, if possible. A rapid weight gain or evidence of edema should be reported to physician immediately. Record I&O.
◊ Ensure that patient is protected from injury. Provide supervision and assistance when ambulating if dizziness and drowsiness are problems.
◊ Give hard candy, gum, or frequent sips of water if dry mouth is a problem, or treat with saliva substitute.
◊ Store medication at controlled room temperatures between 15° and 30°C (59°–86°F). Protect from heat, light, and moisture.
+ **PO:** Administer 30 minutes before meals.
◊ Do not give with antacids, as they may interfere with absorption of atropine.
+ **Parenteral:** May be administered subcutaneously (SC), IM, or IV.
◊ May be given undiluted.
◊ Administer IV at rate not exceeding 1 mg/min or less. Do not add to IV solutions. Administer through Y-tube or 3-way stopcock of infusion set.
◊ "Atropine flush" (intense flushing of the face and trunk) may occur 15–20 minutes following IM administration. This is not harmful.

Patient/Family Education

- Take atropine 30 minutes before meals.
- Use caution when driving or operating dangerous machinery. Drowsiness, dizziness, and blurred vision can occur.
- Report occurrence of any of the following symptoms to physician immediately: extreme dryness of mouth; difficulty urinating; constipation; fast, pounding heartbeat; eye pain; rash; visual disturbances; mental changes.
- Sensitivity to light can be relieved by wearing sunglasses and keeping room darkened.
- Stay indoors in air-conditioned room when weather is very hot. Perspiration is decreased with atropine and the body cannot cool itself as well. There is greater susceptibility to heat stroke. Inform physician if air-conditioned housing and/or work environment is not available.
- If dry mouth is a problem, take frequent sips of water, chew sugarless gum, or suck on hard candy. Saliva substitute may be used. Good oral care (frequent brushing, flossing) is very important.
- Do not consume other medications (including over-the-counter meds) without physician's approval. Many medications contain substances that interact with atropine in a way that may be harmful.
- Be aware of possible risks of taking atropine during pregnancy. Safe use during pregnancy and lactation has not been established. It is known that atropine readily crosses the placental barrier, and fetus could experience adverse effects of the drug. Inform physician immediately if pregnancy occurs, is suspected, or is planned.
- Be aware of side effects of atropine. Refer to written materials furnished by healthcare providers for safe self-administration.
- Carry card or other identification at all times describing medications being taken.

Evaluation

- Patient demonstrates a resolution/subsiding of the symptoms for which atropine was described (to decrease secretions prior to surgery or other procedures; bradyarrhythmias; cholinergic drug poisoning; bronchial asthma).
- Patient verbalizes understanding of side effects and regimen required for prudent self-administration of atropine.

BENZPHETAMINE

(benz-fet'a-meen)
Didrex

Classification(s):
Anorexigenic; CNS stimulant;
Sympathomimetic amine
Schedule C III
Pregnancy Category X

INDICATIONS

- Short-term management of exogenous obesity.

ACTION

- Exact mechanism of action is not known ◆ Sympathomimetic amines are thought to produce appetite suppression through direct stimulation of the satiety center in the hypothalamus and limbic system ◆ Pharmacologic effects are similar to those of amphetamines.

PHARMACOKINETICS

Absorption: Readily absorbed following oral administration.
Distribution: Is widely distributed. Crosses placental barrier. Not known if drug enters breast milk.
Metabolism and Excretion: Metabolized by the liver; excreted in urine. Elimination is enhanced by acidic urine; slowed by alkaline urine.

Half-Life: 7–33.6 hours (depending on pH of urine).

CONTRAINDICATIONS AND PRECAUTIONS

Contraindicated in: ♦ Hypersensitivity to sympathomimetic amines or tartrazine (contained in some preparations) ♦ Advanced arteriosclerosis ♦ Symptomatic cardiovascular disease ♦ Moderate to severe hypertension ♦ Hyperthyroidism ♦ Glaucoma ♦ Agitated states ♦ Patients with a history of drug abuse ♦ During or within 14 days of therapy with MAO inhibitors ♦ Concomitant use of other CNS stimulants ♦ Pregnancy and lactation ♦ Children under 12 years of age.

Use Cautiously in: ♦ Patients with mild hypertension ♦ Diabetes mellitus ♦ Elderly and debilitated patients.

ADVERSE REACTIONS AND SIDE EFFECTS*

CNS: <u>overstimulation</u>, <u>restlessness</u>, <u>dizziness</u>, <u>insomnia</u>, dyskinesia, <u>euphoria</u>, dysphoria, <u>tremor</u>, <u>headache</u>, drowsiness, mental depression, confusion, incoordination, fatigue, malaise, blurred vision, mydriasis, psychosis (rare).
CV: <u>palpitations</u>, <u>tachycardia</u>, hypertension.
Derm: urticaria, rash, allergic skin reactions.
Endo: impotence, changes in libido.
GI: <u>dry mouth</u>, unpleasant taste, nausea, vomiting.
Other: <u>tolerance</u>, physical and psychological dependence, alopecia, chills, fever, sweating.

INTERACTIONS

Drug-Drug: ♦ **Other CNS stimulants:** additive CNS stimulant effects ♦ **MAO inhibitors (during treatment or within 14 days following administration:** hypertensive crisis, headache, hyperpyrexia, intracranial hemorrhage, bradycardia ♦ **Insulin:** alteration in requirements ♦ **Guanethidine:** decreased antihypertensive effects ♦ **Barbiturates, phenothiazines:** decreased benzphetamine effects ♦ **General anesthetics:** cardiac arrhythmias.
Drug-Food: ♦ **Caffeinated foods and drinks:** increased effects of benzphetamine.

ROUTE AND DOSAGE
Exogenous Obesity
♦ **PO (Adults):** Initial dosage: 25–50 mg once daily. May be increased according to patient response. Usual dosages range from 25 to 50 mg daily to tid.

PHARMACODYNAMICS

Route	Onset	Peak	Duration
PO	30 min	1–3 hr	4 hr

NURSING IMPLICATIONS
Assessment
♦ Assess and record baseline data: • temperature • pulse • respiration • blood pressure • and weight for comparison during therapy.
♦ In diabetic patients, assess blood sugar bid or tid. Insulin adjustments may be required due to alteration in eating pattern; possibility of hyperactivity.
♦ Assess knowledge of sound nutritional, calorie-reduced diet and importance of regular exercise.
♦ Assess mental status for changes in mood, level of activity, degree of stimulation, aggressiveness.
♦ Assess sleeping patterns carefully. Insomnia may occur.
♦ Assess history of allergies, sensitivity to this drug, to other sympathomimetic amines, or to tartrazine.
♦ Assess history of glaucoma.
♦ Assess for presence of adverse reactions or side effects.
♦ Assess date of last menses (possible pregnancy), use of contraceptives.

*<u>Underlines</u> indicate most frequent; CAPITALS indicate life-threatening.

- Assess if currently breast-feeding a child.
- Assess current and past alcohol and drug consumption.
- Assess usual amount of caffeine consumed.
- Assess for operation of automobile and/or other dangerous machinery.
- Assess patient/family knowledge about condition and need for medication.
- In collaboration with physician, periodically assess CBC, urinalysis, and liver function tests.
- **Withdrawal:** Assess for symptoms of withdrawal: • nausea • vomiting • abdominal cramping • headache • fatigue • weakness • mental depression.
- **Withdrawal Management:** Monitor vital signs.
- ◇ Place patient in quiet room with low stimuli.
- ◇ Allow patient to sleep as much as desired.
- ◇ Maintain close observation (q15 min).
- ◇ Institute suicide precautions.
- ◇ Some physicians may prescribe antidepressants to counteract feelings of depression and lethargy.
- **Toxicity and Overdose:** Assess for symptoms of overdose: • restlessness • tremor • hyperreflexia • fever • rapid respiration • disorientation • belligerence • assaultiveness • hallucinations • panic states (stimulation is usually followed by fatigue and depression) • tachycardia • hypertension or hypotension • nausea • vomiting • diarrhea • abdominal cramping • seizures • coma • circulatory collapse • death.
- **Overdose Management:** Initiate gastric lavage.
- ◇ Maintain adequate airway.
- ◇ Initiate cardiac monitoring.
- ◇ Administer barbiturate for sedation.
- ◇ Administer phentolamine for severe acute hypertension.
- ◇ Administer IV fluids and a vasopressor for hypotension secondary to hypovolemia.

- ◇ Use urine acidifiers to promote urinary excretion of the drug.
- ◇ Hemodialysis and peritoneal dialysis are not effective.

Potential Nursing Diagnoses

- High risk for injury due to overstimulation and hyperactivity; abrupt benzphetamine withdrawal; overdose.
- High risk for self-directed violence related to suicidal ideations resulting from abrupt benzphetamine withdrawal.
- Alteration in nutrition, more than body requires, related to excessive intake in relation to metabolic needs.
- Sleep pattern disturbance related to overstimulation from benzphetamine use.
- Alteration in thought processes related to adverse benzphetamine effects of overstimulation and difficulty concentrating.
- Knowledge deficit related to medication regimen.

Plan/Implementation

- Monitor medication effects. Tolerance develops rapidly. If anorexic effects begin to diminish, notify physician immediately. Patient should be on reduced-calorie diet and program of regular exercise in addition to the medication.
- Monitor and record vital signs at regular intervals (bid) throughout therapy.
- Encourage use of sugarless gum, hard candy, or frequent sips of water for patient who experiences dry mouth. Ensure that patient practices good oral care (frequent brushing, flossing).
- Ensure that patient is protected from injury. Keep stimuli low and environment as quiet as possible to discourage overstimulation.
- Ensure that tablet has been swallowed and not "cheeked" to avoid medication or to hoard for later use.
- Store medication at controlled room

temperatures between 15° and 30°C (59°–86°F). Protect from heat, light, and moisture.

♦ Tablets may be crushed and mixed with food or fluid for patient who has difficulty swallowing.

♦ To prevent insomnia, give last dose at least 6 hours before retiring.

♦ Drug should be administered 30–60 minutes before meals.

Patient/Family Education

♦ Use caution in driving or operating dangerous machinery. Drowsiness, dizziness, and blurred vision can occur.

♦ Do not stop taking the drug abruptly. Can produce serious withdrawal symptoms.

♦ If insomnia is a problem, avoid taking medication late in the day. Take no later than 6 hours before bedtime.

♦ Do not take other medications (including over-the-counter drugs) without physician's approval. Many medications contain substances that, in combination with benzphetamine, can be harmful.

♦ Diabetic patient: Monitor blood sugar bid or tid or as instructed by physician. Be aware of need for possible alteration in insulin requirements due to changes in food intake, weight, and activity.

♦ Avoid consumption of large amounts of caffeinated products (coffee, tea, colas, chocolate), as they may enhance the stimulant effect of benzphetamine.

♦ Follow reduced-calorie diet provided by dietitian; maintain program of regular exercise. Do not exceed recommended dose if appetite suppressant effect diminishes. Contact physician.

♦ Notify physician if restlessness, insomnia, anorexia, or dry mouth become severe, or if rapid, pounding heartbeat becomes evident.

♦ Do not take benzphetamine during pregnancy. There is evidence of risk to fetus with this medication. Inform physician immediately if pregnancy is suspected or planned.

♦ Be aware of potential side effects of benzphetamine. Refer to written materials furnished by healthcare providers for safe self-administration.

♦ Carry card or other identification at all times describing medications being taken.

Evaluation

♦ Patient demonstrates a progressive weight loss with the use of benzphetamine as an adjunct to reduced caloric intake and a program of regular exercise.

♦ Patient verbalizes understanding of side effects and regimen required for prudent self-administration of benzphetamine.

BENZTROPINE

(benz'troe-peen)
Cogentin

Classification(s):
Antiparkinsonian; Anticholinergic
Pregnancy Category C

INDICATIONS

♦ Parkinsonism (used as adjunctive therapy in all forms) ♦ Extrapyramidal symptoms (except tardive dyskinesia) associated with antipsychotic drugs.

ACTION

♦ Acts to balance a dopamine deficiency and acetylcholine excess in the corpus striatum ♦ The acetylcholine receptor is blocked to diminish excess cholinergic effect.

PHARMACOKINETICS

Absorption: Well absorbed following oral and IM administration.
Distribution: Not completely understood. May cross placental barrier; may enter breast milk.

Metabolism and Excretion: Metabolized by the liver; excreted in urine.
Half-Life: Undetermined.

CONTRAINDICATIONS AND PRECAUTIONS

Contraindicated in: ✦ Hypersensitivity ✦ Angle-closure glaucoma ✦ Pyloric or duodenal obstruction ✦ Stenosing peptic ulcer ✦ Prostatic hypertrophy or bladder-neck obstruction ✦ Achalasia ✦ Myasthenia gravis ✦ Children under 3 years old ✦ Ulcerative colitis ✦ Toxic megacolon ✦ Tachycardia secondary to cardiac insufficiency or thyrotoxicosis.
Use Cautiously in: ✦ Narrow-angle glaucoma ✦ Elderly and debilitated patients ✦ Pregnancy and lactation (safety not established) ✦ Hepatic, renal, or cardiac insufficiency ✦ Tendency toward urinary retention ✦ Hyperthyroidism ✦ Hypertension ✦ Autonomic neuropathy ✦ Older children ✦ Patients exposed to high environmental temperature.

ADVERSE REACTIONS AND SIDE EFFECTS*

CNS: <u>drowsiness</u>, <u>dizziness</u>, <u>blurred vision</u>, disorientation, confusion, memory loss, agitation, nervousness, delirium, weakness, mydriasis, cycloplegia, headache, insomnia.
CV: orthostatic hypotension, hypotension, tachycardia, palpitations.
Derm: skin rashes, urticaria, other dermatoses.
GI: <u>dry mouth</u>, nausea, vomiting, epigastric distress, <u>constipation</u>, dilatation of the colon, PARALYTIC ILEUS.
GU: urinary retention, urinary hesitancy, dysuria, difficulty in achieving or maintaining an erection.
Psych: depression, delusions, hallucinations, paranoia.
Other: muscular weakness, muscular cramping, elevated temperature, flushing, decreased sweating, anaphylaxis, increased intraocular pressure.

INTERACTIONS

Drug-Drug: ✦ **Other drugs with anticholinergic properties (e.g., glutethimide, disopyramide, narcotic analgesics, phenothiazines, tricyclic antidepressants, antihistamines, quinidine salts, amantadine):** increased anticholinergic effects, potentially fatal paralytic ileus ✦ **Levodopa:** possible decreased levodopa absorption ✦ **Slow-dissolving digoxin:** decreased absorption of digoxin ✦ **CNS depressants (e.g., alcohol, barbiturates, narcotics, benzodiazepines):** increased CNS depressant effects ✦ **Ketoconazole:** decreased absorption of ketoconazole ✦ **Antacids:** decreased absorption of benztropine ✦ **Phenothiazines, haloperidol:** decreased antipsychotic effect.

ROUTE AND DOSAGE

Parkinsonism

✦ **PO, IM, IV (Adults):** Start with 0.5–1.0 mg at bedtime. Gradually increase in increments of 0.5 mg at 5- to 6-day intervals to the smallest amount necessary for optimal relief. Maximum dose: 6 mg/day.

✦ **Drug-Induced Extrapyramidal Symptoms**
✦ **PO (Adults):** 1–4 mg daily or bid. Withdraw drug after 1 or 2 weeks to determine need (symptoms may subside following initiation of therapy). Reinstitute therapy if symptoms recur.
✦ **IM, IV (Adults):** For acute dystonic reactions, give 1–2 mg for quick relief. If symptoms begin to return, dose may be repeated. Switch to oral form once acuity has subsided.

PHARMACODYNAMICS

Route	Onset	Peak	Duration
PO	1–2 hr	—	24 hr
IM, IV	15 min	—	6–10 hr

*Underlines indicate most frequent; CAPITALS indicate life-threatening.

NURSING IMPLICATIONS
Assessment

♦ Assess for symptoms of Parkinson's disease: • tremors • muscular weakness and rigidity • drooling • shuffling gait • disturbances of posture and equilibrium • flat affect • monotone speech.

♦ Assess for extrapyramidal symptoms: pseudoparkinsonism • tremors • shuffling gait • drooling • rigidity • akinesia (muscular weakness) • akathisia (continuous restlessness and fidgeting) • dystonia (involuntary muscular movements of face, arms, legs, and neck) • oculogyric crisis (uncontrolled rolling back of the eyes) • tardive dyskinesia (bizarre facial and tongue movements, stiff neck, difficulty swallowing). **Note:** Benztropine is not effective in alleviating symptoms of tardive dyskinesia.

♦ Assess for symptoms of paralytic ileus: • constipation • abdominal pain and distension • absence of bowel sounds. Patients taking benztropine concomitantly with other drugs that produce anticholinergic effects are particularly susceptible.

♦ Assess vital signs, weight. Record baseline values for comparison.

♦ Assess history of allergies, sensitivity to this drug.

♦ Assess date of last menses (possible pregnancy), use of contraceptives.

♦ Assess if currently breast-feeding a child.

♦ Assess current and past alcohol and drug consumption.

♦ Assess for operation of automobile and/or other dangerous machinery.

♦ Assess for presence of adverse reactions or side effects.

♦ Assess patient/family knowledge about illness and need for medication.

♦ In collaboration with physician, periodically assess CBC, liver function, and intraocular pressure in patients on long-term therapy.

♦ **Toxicity and Overdose:** Assess for symptoms of overdose: • CNS depression preceded or followed by stimulation • intensification of psychotic symptoms • anxiety • ataxia • seizures • incoherence • delusions • paranoia • anhydrosis • hyperpyrexia • hot, dry, flushed skin • dry mucous membranes • decreased bowel sounds • urinary retention • tachycardia • difficulty swallowing • cardiac arrhythmias • shock • coma • circulatory collapse • skeletal muscle paralysis • cardiac arrest • respiratory depression or arrest.

♦ **Overdose Management:** Monitor vital signs.

◊ Ensure adequate airway.

◊ Induce emesis in conscious patient (contraindicated in precomatose, convulsive, or psychotic states).

◊ Initiate gastric lavage.

◊ Administer activated charcoal to delay absorption.

◊ Administer pilocarpine, 5 mg PO, for peripheral effects.

◊ Administer physostigmine, 1–2 mg SC or slow IV to reverse anticholinergic effects (use only with availability of advanced life support).

◊ Use artificial respiration and oxygen for respiratory depression.

◊ Use tepid water sponges, cold packs, or other cooling applications for symptoms of hyperpyrexia.

◊ Darken room for symptoms of photophobia.

◊ Administer IV fluids and a vasopressor for prevention of circulatory collapse.

◊ Administer diazepam to control symptoms of acute psychosis.

Potential Nursing Diagnoses

♦ High risk for injury related to symptoms of Parkinson's disease or drug-induced extrapyramidal symptoms.

♦ Hyperthermia related to anticholinergic effect of decreased sweating.

♦ Sensory-perceptual alteration related to side effect of benztropine evidenced by hallucinations.

♦ Altered thought processes related to side effects of benztropine evidenced by delusional thinking, disorientation, confusion.

♦ Social isolation related to embarrassment from symptoms of Parkinson's disease.

♦ Activity intolerance, high risk for, related to benztropine side effects of drowsiness, dizziness, ataxia, weakness, confusion.

♦ Knowledge deficit related to medication regimen.

Plan/Implementation:

♦ **General Info:** Monitor vital signs daily. Be particularly alert for increase in pulse rate or temperature.

◊ Weigh patient 2–3 times a week, at same time of day, on same scale, if possible. A rapid weight gain or evidence of edema should be reported to physician immediately. Record I&O.

◊ Monitor for exacerbation of mental symptoms in patients who are receiving the drug to counteract extrapyramidal symptoms associated with antipsychotic medications.

◊ Ensure that patient is protected from injury. Provide supervision and assistance when ambulating if dizziness and drowsiness are problems.

◊ Give patient hard candy, gum, or frequent sips of water if dry mouth is a problem, or treat with saliva substitute.

◊ Store medication at controlled room temperatures between 15° and 30°C (59°–86°F). Protect from heat and moisture.

♦ **PO:** Ensure that patient swallows tablet and does not "cheek" to avoid medications or to hoard for later use.

◊ Administer with food to minimize gastric irritation.

◊ Tablet may be crushed and mixed with food or fluid for patient who has difficulty swallowing.

◊ Monitor vital signs before beginning therapy and at regular intervals (bid or tid) throughout therapy. Take BP lying and standing to monitor for possible hypotensive reaction; elderly are particularly susceptible. Dosage adjustment may be required.

♦ **Parenteral:** Benztropine injectable is useful for psychotic patients with acute dystonic reactions or other reactions that make oral administration difficult or impossible, or when a more rapid response is desired.

◊ Available as 1 mg/mL in 2-mL ampules. Prepared solution may be given undiluted.

◊ May be administered IM or IV.

◊ Because there is no significant difference in onset of action after IM or IV injection, IV route is seldom used except in acute drug reactions or psychotic patients.

◊ Administer IV at a rate not exceeding ≤1 mg/min.

◊ Switch to oral medication as soon as control of symptoms has been achieved.

Patient/Family Education

♦ May be taken with food if GI upset occurs.

♦ Use caution when driving or operating dangerous machinery. Drowsiness and dizziness can occur.

♦ Do not stop taking the drug abruptly. To do so might produce serious withdrawal symptoms.

♦ Report occurrence of any of the following symptoms to physician immediately: • pain or tenderness in area in front of ear • extreme dryness of mouth • difficulty urinating • abdominal pain • constipation • fast, pounding heartbeat • rash • visual disturbances • mental changes.

♦ Rise slowly from a sitting or lying position to prevent a sudden drop in blood pressure.

♦ Stay indoors in air-conditioned room when weather is very hot. Perspiration is decreased with benztropine and the body cannot cool itself as well. There is greater susceptibility to heat stroke. Inform physician if air-conditioned housing or work environment is not available.

♦ If dry mouth is a problem, take frequent sips of water, chew sugarless gum, or suck on hard candy. Good oral care (frequent brushing, flossing) is very important.

♦ Do not drink alcohol while on benztropine therapy.

♦ Do not consume other medications (including over-the-counter meds) without physician's approval. Many medications contain substances that interact with benztropine in a way that may be harmful.

♦ Be aware of possible risks of taking benztropine during pregnancy. Safe use during pregnancy and lactation has not been established. It is thought that benztropine readily crosses the placental barrier; if so, fetus could experience adverse effects of the drug. Inform physician immediately if pregnancy occurs, is suspected, or is planned.

♦ Be aware of side effects of benztropine. Refer to written materials furnished by healthcare providers for safe self-administration.

♦ Continue to take medication even if feeling well and as though it is not needed. Symptoms may return if medication is discontinued.

♦ Carry card or other identification at all times describing medications being taken.

Evaluation

♦ Patient demonstrates a subsiding of the symptoms for which benztropine was prescribed (parkinsonism; drug-induced extrapyramidal symptoms).

♦ Patient verbalizes understanding of side effects and regimen required for prudent self-administration of benztropine.

BETHANECHOL

(be-than'e-kole)
Duvoid, Myotonachol, Urecholine

Classification(s):
Cholinergic stimulant;
Parasympathomimetic
Pregnancy Category C

INDICATIONS

♦ Postoperative and postpartum nonobstructive (functional) urinary retention ♦ Neurogenic atony of the urinary bladder with retention ♦ **Investigational Uses:** ♦ Urinary retention associated with use of certain drugs, such as antidepressants and antipsychotics ♦ Reflux esophagitis.

ACTION

♦ Acts principally by stimulating the parasympathetic nervous system to contract the bladder, increase peristalsis in the ureters and GI tract, decrease bladder capacity, and increase pancreatic and GI secretion.

PHARMACOKINETICS

Absorption: Poorly absorbed from the GI tract. More rapid and complete absorption following subcutaneous administration.

Distribution: Distribution not fully understood. Does not cross blood–brain barrier in usual doses. Unknown if drug crosses placental barrier or enters breast milk.

Metabolism and Excretion: Not known.

Half-Life: Not well established.

CONTRAINDICATIONS AND PRECAUTIONS

Contraindicated in: ♦ Hypersensitivity to this drug or to tartrazine ♦ Hyperthyroidism ♦ Peptic ulcer ♦ Latent or active asthma ♦ Pronounced bradycardia ♦ Vasomotor instability ♦ Coronary artery disease ♦ Epilepsy ♦ Parkinsonism ♦ Coronary occlusion ✦ Hypotension ✦ Hypertension ✦ Mechanical GI or bladder obstruction ✦ Bladder-neck obstruction ✦ Spastic GI disturbances ✦ Acute inflammatory lesions of the GI tract ✦ Peritonitis ✦ Marked vagotonia ✦ Questionable strength or integrity of the GI or bladder wall ✦ Obstructive pulmonary disease ✦ Atrioventricular conduction defects ✦ Safe use in children and during pregnancy and lactation has not been established.

ADVERSE REACTIONS AND SIDE EFFECTS*

CNS: malaise, headache, blurred vision, dizziness, weakness, confusion, seizures.
CV: hypotension, orthostatic hypotension, reflex tachycardia, flushing of skin, transient complete HEART BLOCK, transient syncope with CARDIAC ARREST.
GI: abdominal cramps, nausea and vomiting, diarrhea, belching, salivation, borborygmi, fecal incontinence, urge to defecate, colicky pain.
GU: urinary urgency.
Resp: acute asthmatic attack, dyspnea, bronchial constriction.
Other: substernal pressure or pain (possibly due to bronchospasm or spasm of the esophagus), miosis (constricted pupils), sweating, lacrimation, hypothermia.

INTERACTIONS

Drug-Drug: ✦ **Quinidine, procainamide:** may antagonize cholinergic effects ✦ **Other cholinergic or anticholinesterase drugs (e.g., neostigmine, pyridostigmine, ambenonium):** additive cholinergic effects ✦ **Ganglionic blocking compounds (e.g., mecamylamine, trimethaphan):** critical fall in blood pressure, usually preceded by severe abdominal symptoms. ✦ **Atropine, epinephrine, other sympathomimetic amines:** antagonize bethanechol effects.

ROUTE AND DOSAGE

Urinary Retention

✦ **PO (Adults):** 10–50 mg bid to qid. Minimum effective dose is determined by giving 5–10 mg initially; same amount is repeated hourly to a maximum of 50 mg until satisfactory response occurs. An alternative dosage regimen is to give 10 mg initially, then 25 mg, then 50 mg at 6-hour intervals until the desired effect is achieved.
✦ **SC (Adults):** Usual dose is 2.5–5 mg. To determine minimum effective dose, inject 2.5 mg initially and repeat same amount at 15- to 30-minute intervals to a maximum of four doses, or until satisfactory response is achieved or adverse reactions appear. The minimum effective dose may be repeated tid or qid as required.

Phenothiazine-Related Bladder Dysfunction (Prevention)

✦ **PO (Adults):** 25 mg qid.

Phenothiazine-Related Bladder Dysfunction (Treatment)

✦ **PO (Adults):** 50–100 mg qid.

Tricyclic Antidepressant Related Bladder and Salivary Gland Inhibition

✦ **PO (Adults):** 25 mg tid.

PHARMACODYNAMICS

Route	Onset	Peak	Duration
PO	30–90 min	60–90 min	1–6 hr
SC	5–15 min	15–30 min	2 hr

NURSING IMPLICATIONS

Assessment

✦ Assess I&O and weight daily. Palpate for bladder distention. Monitor for urinary incontinence.
✦ Assess mood daily in patient receiving antidepressants and antipsychotics. Observe behavioral changes, level of participation in activities, withdrawal, restlessness, agitation.
✦ Assess vital signs prior to administra-

---

*Underlines indicate most frequent; CAPITALS indicate life-threatening.

tion. Record baseline values for comparison.

♦ Assess for signs of possible kidney infection: • chills • fever • flank pain • malaise. Infection can occur if the sphincter fails to relax as bethanechol contracts the bladder, thereby forcing urine (possibly with bacteria) up the ureter into the kidney pelvis.

♦ Assess history of allergies, sensitivity to this drug or to other cholinergic drugs.

♦ Assess date of last menses (possible pregnancy), use of contraceptives.

♦ Assess if currently breast-feeding a child.

♦ Assess current and past alcohol and drug consumption.

♦ Assess for operation of automobile and/or other dangerous machinery.

♦ Assess for presence of adverse reactions or side effects.

♦ Assess patient/family knowledge about illness and need for medication.

♦ **Lab Test Alterations:** Increased AST, serum lipase, amylase, and bilirubin.

♦ **Toxicity and Overdose:** Assess for symptoms of overdose: • abdominal discomfort and cramping • salivation • flushing of the skin ("hot feeling") • sweating • nausea and vomiting • substernal pressure or pain • involuntary defecation • urinary urgency • transient syncope • transient complete heart block • dyspnea • orthostatic hypotension • myocardial hypoxia • circulatory collapse • hypotension • diarrhea • shock • cardiac arrest.

♦ **Overdose Management:** Atropine is the specific antidote for bethanechol overdose. Recommended dosage for adults is 0.6–1.2 mg. For children under 12: 0.01 mg/kg q 2 hours until desired effect is achieved or adverse effects of atropine preclude further use. Maximum single dose should not exceed 0.4 mg.

◇ Subcutaneous injection of atropine is preferred except in emergencies, when the IV route may be used.

Potential Nursing Diagnosis

♦ Urinary retention related to use of medications that promote adverse effect of urinary retention.

♦ High risk for injury related to side effects of bethanechol, such as weakness, dizziness, blurred vision, confusion, seizures; overdose; inadvertent IM or IV injection.

♦ High risk for infection related to reflux of urine back into kidneys if sphincter fails to relax when bethanechol contracts the bladder.

♦ Activity intolerance, high risk for, related to bethanechol side effects of drowsiness, dizziness, weakness, mental confusion.

♦ Knowledge deficit related to medication regimen.

Plan/Implementation

♦ **General Info:** Monitor vital signs daily. Report any changes to physician. Monitor for orthostatic hypotension by measuring blood pressure both lying and standing.

◇ Weigh patient daily, and keep strict records of intake and output.

◇ Ensure that patient is protected from injury. Provide supervision and assistance when ambulating if dizziness and drowsiness are problems. Observe for seizure activity. May be necessary to pad headboard and siderails if patient experiences seizures during the night.

◇ Store medication at controlled room temperatures between 15° and 30°C (59°–86°F). Protect from heat, light, and moisture.

♦ **PO:** Administer when stomach is empty (1 hour before meals or 2 hours after meals). If taken soon after eating, nausea and vomiting may occur.

◇ Onset of action occurs within 30–90 minutes. Check vital signs every 1–2 hours for several hours following oral administration. Monitor for signs of overdose: abdominal discomfort, salivation, flushing of the skin ("hot feeling"), sweating, nausea, and vomiting. Contact physician immediately if any of these signs appear.

♦ **SC:** Parenteral form is for subcutaneous administration only. Do not administer IM or IV.

◊ If inadvertently given IM or IV, violent symptoms of cholinergic overstimulation may occur, such as circulatory collapse, drop in blood pressure, abdominal cramps, bloody diarrhea, shock, or sudden cardiac arrest.

◊ Rarely, these symptoms have occurred following SC administration. Always aspirate carefully before SC injection to ensure that medication will not be injected into a blood vessel.

◊ A syringe of atropine containing the appropriate adult or pediatric dosage (see "Overdose Management") should always be readily available when giving bethanechol SC, in the event that symptoms of cholinergic overstimulation appear.

◊ Onset of action occurs within 5–15 minutes. Check vital signs every 15–30 minutes following SC administration. Monitor for signs and symptoms of cholinergic overstimulation.

Patient/Family Education

♦ Take bethanechol 1 hour before or 2 hours after meals to prevent nausea and vomiting.

♦ Use caution when driving or operating dangerous machinery. Drowsiness, dizziness, and blurred vision can occur.

♦ Report occurrence of any of the following symptoms to physician immediately: • chills • fever • flank pain • malaise • abdominal discomfort • increased salivation, flushing of the skin, profuse sweating, persistent nausea and vomiting, diarrhea, dizziness.

♦ Rise slowly from a sitting or lying position in order to prevent sudden drop in blood pressure.

♦ Do not consume other medications (including over-the-counter meds) without physician's approval. Many medications contain substances that may interact with bethanechol in a way that could be harmful.

♦ Be aware of possible risks of taking bethanechol during pregnancy. Safe use during pregnancy and lactation has not been established. It is not known if bethanechol crosses the placental barrier. If it does, fetus could experience adverse effects of the drug. Inform physician immediately if pregnancy occurs, is suspected, or is planned.

♦ Be aware of side effects of bethanechol. Refer to written materials furnished by healthcare providers for safe self-administration.

♦ Carry card or other identification at all times describing medications being taken.

Evaluation

♦ Patient demonstrates a resolution/subsiding of the symptoms for which bethanechol was prescribed (urinary retention).

♦ Patient verbalizes understanding of side effects and regimen required for prudent self-administration of bethanechol.

BIPERIDEN

(bye-per′i-den)
Akineton

Classification(s):
Antiparkinsonian; Anticholinergic
Pregnancy Category C

INDICATION

♦ Parkinsonism (used as adjunctive therapy in all forms) ♦ Control of extrapyramidal symptoms (except tardive dyskinesia) associated with antipsychotic drugs ♦ **Investigational Uses:** ♦ Other disorders of extrapyramidal system ♦ Cerebral palsy ♦ Multiple sclerosis ♦ Spinal cord injuries.

ACTION

♦ Acts to balance a dopamine deficiency and acetylcholine excess in the corpus striatum ♦ The acetylcholine receptor is blocked to diminish excess cholinergic effect.

PHARMACOKINETICS

Absorption: Well absorbed following oral and IM administration.
Distribution: Not completely understood. May cross placental barrier; may enter breast milk.
Metabolism and Excretion: Metabolized by the liver. Excreted in urine.
Half-Life: Undetermined.

CONTRAINDICATIONS AND PRECAUTIONS

Contraindicated in: ♦ Hypersensitivity to this drug ♦ Angle-closure glaucoma ♦ Pyloric or duodenal obstruction ♦ stenosing peptic ulcer ♦ Prostatic hypertrophy or bladder-neck obstruction ♦ Achalasia ♦ Myasthenia gravis ♦ Ulcerative colitis ♦ Toxic megacolon ♦ Tachycardia secondary to cardiac insufficiency or thyrotoxicosis ♦ Safe use in children and in pregnant and lactating women not established.
Use Cautiously in: ♦ Narrow-angle glaucoma ♦ Elderly and debilitated patients ♦ Hepatic, renal, or cardiac insufficiency ♦ Tendency toward urinary retention ♦ Hyperthyroidism ♦ Hypertension ♦ Autonomic neuropathy ♦ Patients exposed to high environmental temperature.

ADVERSE REACTIONS AND SIDE EFFECTS*

CNS: drowsiness, dizziness, blurred vision, disorientation, confusion, memory loss, agitation, nervousness, delirium, weakness, mydriasis, cycloplegia, headache, insomnia; IV: postural hypotension, euphoria.
CV: orthostatic hypotension, hypotension, tachycardia, palpitations.
Derm: skin rashes, urticaria, other dermatoses.
GI: dry mouth, nausea, vomiting, epigastric distress, constipation, dilation of the colon, PARALYTIC ILEUS.
GU: urinary retention, urinary hesitancy, dysuria, difficulty in achieving or maintaining an erection, hematuria.
Psych: depression, delusions, hallucinations, paranoia.
Other: muscular weakness, muscular cramping, elevated temperature, flushing, decreased sweating, anaphylaxis, increased intraocular pressure.

INTERACTIONS

Drug-Drug: ♦ **Other drugs with anticholinergic properties (e.g., glutethimide, disopyramide, narcotic analgesics, phenothiazines, tricyclic antidepressants, antihistamines, quinidine salts, amantadine):** increased anticholinergic effects; potentially fatal paralytic ileus ♦ **Levodopa:** possible decreased levodopa absorption ♦ **Slow-dissolving digoxin:** decreased absorption of digoxin ♦ **CNS depressants (e.g., alcohol, barbiturates, narcotics, benzodiazepines):** increased CNS depressant effects ♦ **Ketoconazole:** decreased absorption of ketoconazole ♦ **Antacids:** decreased absorption of biperiden ♦ **Phenothiazines, haloperidol:** decreased antipsychotic effect.

ROUTE AND DOSAGE

Parkinsonism

♦ **PO (Adults):** 2 mg tid or qid. Maximum dosage: 16 mg/day.

---

*Underlines indicate most frequent; CAPITALS indicate life-threatening.

Drug-Induced Extrapyramidal Symptoms

♦ **PO (Adults):** 2 mg 1–3 times a day.
♦ **IM, IV (Adults):** 2 mg. Repeat every half hour until symptoms are resolved; maximum of four consecutive doses (8 mg) in 24 hours.

Substitution Therapy

To substitute for another antiparkinsonian drug, first drug is gradually withdrawn while biperiden is gradually increased.

PHARMACODYNAMICS

Route	Onset	Peak	Duration
PO	1 hr	2–4 hr	6–10 hr
IM, IV	15 min	—	6–10 hr

NURSING IMPLICATIONS

Assessment

♦ Assess for symptoms of Parkinson's disease: • tremors • muscular weakness and rigidity • drooling • shuffling gait • disturbances of posture and equilibrium • flat effect • monotone speech.
♦ Assess for extrapyramidal symptoms: • pseudoparkinsonian (tremors, shuffling gait, drooling, rigidity) • akinesia (muscular weakness) • akathisia (continuous restlessness and fidgeting) • dystonia (involuntary muscular movements of face, arms, legs, and neck) • oculogyric crisis (uncontrolled rolling back of the eyes) • tardive dyskinesia (bizarre facial and tongue movements, stiff neck, difficulty swallowing). **Note:** Biperiden is not effective in alleviating symptoms of tardive dyskinesia.
♦ Assess for symptoms of paralytic ileus: • constipation, abdominal pain and distention, absence of bowel sounds. Patients taking biperiden concomitantly with other drugs that produce anticholinergic effects are particularly susceptible.
♦ Assess vital signs, weight. Record baseline values for comparison.

♦ Assess history of allergies, sensitivity to this drug or to other anticholinergic drugs.
♦ Assess date of last menses (possible pregnancy), use of contraceptives.
♦ Assess if currently breast-feeding a child.
♦ Assess current and past alcohol and drug consumption.
♦ Assess for operation of automobile and/or other dangerous machinery.
♦ Assess for presence of adverse reactions or side effects.
♦ Assess patient/family knowledge about illness and need for medication.
♦ In collaboration with physician, periodically monitor CBC, liver function, and intraocular pressure in patients on long-term therapy.
♦ **Toxicity and Overdose:** Assess for symptoms of overdose: • CNS depression preceded or followed by stimulation • intensification of psychotic symptoms • anxiety • ataxia • seizures • incoherence • delusions • paranoia • anhydrosis • hyperpyrexia • hot, dry, flushed skin • dry mucous membranes • coma • skeletal muscle paralysis • urinary retention • tachycardia • difficulty swallowing • cardiac arrhythmias • circulatory collapse • cardiac arrest • respiratory depression or arrest.
♦ **Overdose Management:** Monitor vital signs.
◊ Ensure adequate airway.
◊ Induce emesis in conscious patient (contraindicated in precomatose, convulsive, or psychotic states).
◊ Initiate gastric lavage.
◊ Administer activated charcoal to delay absorption.
◊ Administer pilocarpine, 5 mg PO, for peripheral effects.
◊ Administer physostigmine, 1–2 mg SQ or slow IV to reverse anticholinergic effects (use only with availability of advanced life support).
◊ Use artificial respiration and oxygen for respiratory depression.

◊ Use tepid water sponges, cold packs, or other cooling applications for hyperpyrexia.

◊ Darken room for photophobia.

◊ Administer IV fluids and a vasopressor for circulatory collapse.

◊ Administer diazepam to control symptoms of acute psychosis.

Potential Nursing Diagnoses

♦ High risk for injury related to symptoms of Parkinson's disease or drug-induced extrapyramidal symptoms.

♦ Hyperthermia related to anticholinergic effect of decreased sweating.

♦ Sensory-perceptual alteration related to biperiden side effect of hallucinations.

♦ Altered thought processes related to biperiden side effects evidenced by delusional thinking, disorientation, confusion.

♦ Social isolation related to embarrassment from symptoms of Parkinson's disease.

♦ Activity intolerance, high risk for, related to biperiden side effects of drowsiness, dizziness, ataxia, weakness, confusion.

♦ Knowledge deficit related to medication regimen.

Plan/Implementation

♦ **General Info:** Monitor vital signs daily. Be particularly alert for increase in pulse rate or temperature.

◊ Weigh patient 2–3 times a week, at same time of day, on same scale, if possible. A rapid weight gain or evidence of edema should be reported to physician immediately. Record I&O.

◊ Monitor for exacerbation of mental symptoms in patients who are receiving the drug to counteract extrapyramidal symptoms associated with antipsychotic medications.

◊ Ensure that patient is protected from injury. Provide supervision and assistance when ambulating if dizziness and drowsiness are problems.

◊ Give hard candy, gum, or frequent sips of water if dry mouth is a problem, or treat with saliva substitute.

◊ Store medication in tight, light-resistant container at temperatures below 77°F.

♦ **PO:**

◊ Ensure that patient swallows tablet and does not "cheek" to avoid medication or to hoard for later use.

◊ May be administered with food to minimize gastric irritation.

◊ Tablet may be crushed and mixed with food or fluid for patient who has difficulty swallowing.

◊ Monitor vital signs before beginning therapy and at regular intervals (bid or tid) throughout therapy. Take BP lying and standing to monitor for possible hypotensive reactions. Elderly are particularly susceptible. Dosage adjustment may be required.

♦ **Parenteral:**

◊ Biperiden injectable is useful for psychotic patients with acute dystonic reactions or other reactions that make oral administration difficult or impossible, or when a more rapid response is desired.

◊ Available as 5 mg/mL in 1-mL ampules. Prepared solution may be given undiluted.

◊ May be administered IM or IV.

◊ Patient should be in recumbent position when parenteral biperiden is administered. Caution patient to move very slowly from recumbent to upright position following parenteral administration.

◊ Because there is no significant difference in onset of action after IM or IV injection, IV route is seldom used, except in acute drug reactions or psychotic patients.

◊ Administer IV at a rate not exceeding 2 mg/min.

◊ Switch to oral medication as soon as control of symptoms has been achieved.

Patient/Family Education

- ✦ May be taken with food if GI upset occurs.
- ✦ Use caution when driving or operating dangerous machinery. Drowsiness and dizziness can occur.
- ✦ Do not stop taking the drug abruptly. To do so might produce serious withdrawal symptoms.
- ✦ Report occurrence of any of the following symptoms to physician immediately: • pain or tenderness in area in front of ear • extreme dryness of mouth; difficulty urinating • abdominal pain; constipation • fast, pounding heartbeat • rash; visual disturbances • mental changes.
- ✦ Rise slowly from a sitting or lying position to prevent a sudden drop in blood pressure.
- ✦ Stay indoors in air-conditioned room when weather is very hot. Perspiration is decreased with biperiden and the body cannot cool itself as well. There is greater susceptibility to heat stroke. Inform physician if air-conditioned housing or work environment is not available.
- ✦ If dry mouth is a problem, take frequent sips of water, chew sugarless gum, or suck on hard candy. Good oral care (frequent brushing, flossing) is very important.
- ✦ Do not drink alcohol while on biperiden therapy.
- ✦ Do not consume other medications (including over-the-counter meds) without physician's approval. Many medications contain substances that interact with biperiden in a way that may be harmful.
- ✦ Be aware of possible risks of taking biperiden during pregnancy. Safe use during pregnancy and lactation has not been established. It is thought that biperiden readily crosses the placental barrier; if so, fetus could experience adverse effects of the drug. Inform physician immediately if pregnancy occurs, is suspected, or is planned.
- ✦ Be aware of side effects of biperiden. Refer to written materials furnished by healthcare providers for safe self-administration.
- ✦ Continue to take medication, even if feeling well and as though it is not needed. Symptoms may return if medication is discontinued.
- ✦ Carry card or other identification at all times describing medications being taken.

Evaluation

- ✦ Patient demonstrates a subsiding of the symptoms for which biperiden was prescribed (parkinsonism; drug-induced extrapyramidal symptoms).
- ✦ Patient verbalizes understanding of side effects and regimen required for prudent self-administration of biperiden.

BROMOCRIPTINE

(broe-moe-krip'teen)
Parlodel

Classification(s):
Antiparkinsonian; Dopamine receptor agonist; Prolactin inhibitor
Pregnancy Category C

INDICATIONS

✦ Idiopathic or postencephalitic Parkinson's disease ✦ Acromegaly. **Investigational Use:** ✦ Neuroleptic malignant syndrome ✦ Premenstrual breast symptoms ✦ Migraine.

ACTION

✦ Direct activation of postsynaptic dopamine receptors in the corpus striatum, resulting in correction of dopamine deficiency, a decrease in serum prolactin levels, and a reduction in elevated blood levels of growth hormone.

PHARMACOKINETICS

Absorption: Approximately 28% absorbed from GI tract.

Distribution: Not completely understood. 90–96% bound to serum albumin.

Metabolism and Excretion: Substantial first-pass metabolism. Only 6% reaches systemic circulation unchanged. Completely metabolized by the liver. Excreted via bile in the feces (85–98%); small amount excreted in urine (2.5–5.5%).

Half-Life: Initial phase: 4–4.5 hours. Terminal phase: 45–50 hours.

CONTRAINDICATIONS AND PRECAUTIONS

Contraindicated in: ♦ Hypersensitivity to this drug, other ergot alkaloids, or sulfites (contained in some preparations) ♦ Patients with severe ischemic heart disease or peripheral vascular disease ♦ Lactation ♦ Children under 15 (safety not established).

Use Cautiously in: ♦ Hepatic and renal insufficiency ♦ Patients with a history of myocardial infarction with residual atrial, nodal, or ventricular arrhythmia ♦ Patients with a history of mental disturbances ♦ Pregnancy ♦ Long-term therapy (more than 2 years) for Parkinson's disease (safety not established).

ADVERSE REACTIONS AND SIDE EFFECTS*

CNS: <u>headache</u>, <u>dizziness</u>, <u>fatigue</u>, <u>drowsiness</u>, <u>abnormal involuntary movements</u>, <u>confusion</u>, <u>fainting</u>, <u>visual disturbances</u>, <u>ataxia</u>, <u>insomnia</u>, <u>weakness</u>, seizures, sedation, nightmares, asthenia, anxiety, nervousness, numbness.

CV: <u>orthostatic hypotension</u>, digital vasospasm, hypotension, reduced tolerance to cold, syncope, exacerbation of angina, palpitations, arrhythmias, bradycardia, STROKE, VENTRICULAR TACHYCARDIA.

Derm: skin rash, skin mottling, urticaria, alopecia.

GI: <u>nausea</u>, <u>vomiting</u>, <u>abdominal cramps</u>, <u>constipation</u>, diarrhea, anorexia, <u>dry mouth</u>, indigestion, GI bleeding, dysphagia.

GU: urinary retention, urinary frequency, urinary incontinence.

Psych: <u>depression</u>, delusions, hallucinations, paranoia, mania.

Other: <u>nasal congestion</u>, leg cramps, blepharospasm, pulmonary infiltrates, pleural effusion, tingling fingers, cold feet.

INTERACTIONS

Drug-Drug: ♦ **Antihypertensives:** additive hypotensive effects ♦ **Phenothiazines, butyrophenones, reserpine, tricyclic antidepressants, methyldopa:** decreased efficacy of bromocriptine ♦ **Oral contraceptives:** interference with bromocriptine effects by increased stimulation of prolactin-secreting cells ♦ **Alcohol:** potentiation of the effects of alcohol; increased incidence of GI toxicity ♦ **Levodopa:** additive neurologic effects.

ROUTE AND DOSAGE

Parkinsonism

♦ **PO (Adults):** Initial dosage: 1.25 mg bid. Dosage may be increased q 2–4 weeks by 2.5 mg/day. Maximum dosage: 100 mg/day.

Acromegaly

♦ **PO (Adults):** Initial dosage: 1.25–2.5 mg for 3 days at HS. Add 1.25–2.5 mg q 3–7 days until optimal therapeutic benefit is achieved. Usual optimal therapeutic dosage range: 20–30 mg/day. Maximum dosage: 100 mg/day.

Neuroleptic Malignant Syndrome

♦ **PO (Adults):** 2.5–15 mg tid.

Migraine Headaches

♦ **PO (Adults):** 3 mg/day in divided doses.

---

*<u>Underlines</u> indicate most frequent; CAPITALS indicate life-threatening.

PHARMACODYNAMICS

Route	Onset	Peak	Duration
PO	0.5–1.5 hr	2 hr	4–8 hr

NURSING IMPLICATIONS
Assessment

- Assessment for symptoms of Parkinson's disease: • tremors • muscular weakness and rigidity • drooling • shuffling gait • disturbances of posture and equilibrium • flat affect • monotone speech.
- Assess for symptoms of neuroleptic malignant syndrome: • hyperpyrexia • muscle rigidity • altered mental status • irregular pulse or blood pressure.
- Assess vital signs. Record baseline values for comparison. Vital signs must be stable before beginning therapy.
- Assess for symptoms of mental disturbances: • depression (with or without suicidal ideations) • hallucinations • delusions • paranoia.
- Assess history of allergies, sensitivity to this drug or to other ergot alkaloids.
- Assess date of last menses (possible pregnancy), use of contraceptives.
- Assess whether currently breast-feeding a child.
- Assess current and past alcohol and drug consumption.
- Assess for operation of automobile and/or other dangerous machinery.
- Assess for presence of adverse reactions or side effects.
- Assess level of knowledge about illness and need for medication.
- In collaboration with physician, assess CBC and cardiac, renal, and liver function tests in patients on long-term therapy.
- **Lab Test Alterations:** Increased BUN, SGOT (AST), SGPT (ALT), GGPT, CPK, alkaline phosphatase, and uric acid.

Potential Nursing Diagnoses

- High risk for injury related to symptoms of Parkinson's disease (confusion, weakness, rigidity, disturbance in equilibrium) or side effects of bromocriptine (confusion, seizures, dizziness, fainting); neuroleptic malignant syndrome (see symptoms above).
- High risk for self-directed violence related to bromocriptine side effect of depressed mood.
- Pain related to migraine headaches.
- Sensory-perceptual alteration related to bromocriptine side effect of hallucinations.
- Altered thought processes related to bromocriptine side effects of delusional thinking, confusion.
- Social isolation related to embarrassment from symptoms of Parkinson's disease.
- Activity intolerance, high risk for, related to bromocriptine side effects of drowsiness, dizziness, weakness, confusion, fatigue.
- Knowledge deficit related to medication regimen.

Plan/Implementation

- Weigh patient 2–3 times a week, at same time of day, on same scale, if possible. A rapid weight gain or evidence of edema should be reported to physician immediately. Record I&O.
- Monitor for exacerbation of mental symptoms in patients who are receiving the drug for parkinsonism.
- Ensure that patient is protected from injury. Provide supervision and assistance when ambulating if dizziness and drowsiness are problems. Observe for seizure activity and ensure that precautions are instituted per hospital policy.
- Give hard candy, gum, or frequent sips of water if dry mouth is a problem, or treat with saliva substitute.
- Ensure that patient swallows tablet/capsule and does not "cheek" to avoid medication or to hoard for later use.
- Administer with food to minimize gastric irritation.
- Tablets may be crushed or contents of

capsules emptied and mixed with food or fluid for patient who has difficulty swallowing.

♦ First dose should be given with patient in recumbent position, as dizziness and fainting from hypotensive effects is more likely to occur at initiation of therapy.

♦ Monitor vital signs before beginning therapy and at regular intervals (bid or tid) throughout therapy. Take BP lying and standing to monitor for postural hypotensive reaction. Elderly are particularly susceptible. Dosage adjustment may be required.

♦ Dosage of levodopa or carbidopa/levodopa should be reduced when used concomitantly with bromocriptine.

♦ Evidence of pituitary tumor should be ruled out before initiating therapy for hyperprolactinemia.

♦ Store medication at controlled room temperature between 15° and 30°C (59°–86°F). Protect from heat and mositure.

Patient/Family Education

♦ Take medication with food to minimize GI upset.

♦ Use caution when driving or when operating dangerous machinery. Drowsiness and dizziness can occur.

♦ Report occurrence of any of the following symptoms to physician immediately: • a missed menstrual period • once menstruation has been reestablished • persistent nausea and vomiting • dizziness or fainting • severe headache • seizures • mental/behavioral changes • GI bleeding • difficulty urinating.

♦ Rise slowly from a sitting or lying position to prevent a sudden drop in BP.

♦ If dry mouth is a problem, take frequent sips of water, chew sugarless gum, or suck on hard candy. Good oral care (frequent brushing, flossing) is very important.

♦ Do not drink alcohol. Bromocriptine may potentiate the effects of alcohol.

♦ Do not consume other medications (including over-the-counter meds) without physician's approval.

♦ An increased sensitivity to cold may be noticeable. Avoid exposure and report tingling, paleness, or numbness of a body part to physician. Nose, fingers, and toes are most commonly affected.

♦ Be aware of possible risks of taking bromocriptine during pregnancy. Safe use during pregnancy has not been established. It is thought that bromocriptine crosses the placental barrier; if so, fetus could experience adverse effects of the drug. Discontinue therapy and inform physician immediately if pregnancy occurs, is suspected, or is planned.

♦ Contraceptive measures should be taken while on bromocriptine therapy. Barrier methods are recommended rather than oral contraceptives, as the latter interfere with the effects of bromocriptine by increasing stimulation of prolactin-secreting cells and may actually cause amenorrhea/galactorrhea.

♦ Be aware of side effects of bromocriptine. Refer to written materials furnished by healthcare providers for safe self-administration.

♦ Continue to take medication, even if feeling well and as though it is not needed. Symptoms may return if medication is discontinued.

♦ Carry card or other identification at all times describing medications being taken.

Evaluation

♦ Patient demonstrates a subsiding/resolution of the symptoms for which bromocriptine was prescribed (parkinsonism, migraine headache, neuroleptic malignant syndrome).

♦ Patient verbalizes understanding of side effects and regimen required for prudent self-administration of bromocriptine.

BUPROPION

(byoo-pro'pee-on)
Wellbutrin

Classification(s):
Unicyclic antidepressant
Pregnancy Category B

INDICATIONS

♦ Depression in patients who fail to respond adequately to or who cannot tolerate alternative antidepressant treatments. Not recommended as an antidepressant of first choice for most patients.

ACTION

♦ Exact mechanism of antidepressant effect is unknown ♦ Appears to be a weak blocker of the neuronal uptake of serotonin and norepinephrine ♦ Inhibits the neuronal reuptake of dopamine to some extent.

PHARMACOKINETICS

Absorption: Rapidly absorbed from the GI tract following oral administration.
Distribution: Is widely distributed. Crosses blood-brain and placental barriers. Unknown if excreted in breast milk.
Metabolism and Excretion: Metabolized by the liver. Excreted in urine (87%) and feces (10%).
Half-Life: 8–24 hours (average 14 hours).

CONTRAINDICATIONS AND PRECAUTIONS

Contraindicated in: ♦ Hypersensitivity to this drug ♦ Concomitant use of MAO inhibitors ♦ Patients with a history of seizure disorder or cranial trauma ♦ Children under 18 ♦ pregnancy and lactation (safety not established) ♦ Patients with current or prior diagnosis of bulimia or

anorexia nervosa (high incidence of seizures with bupropion in these individuals).
Use Cautiously in: ♦ Psychoses ♦ Suicidal patients ♦ Cardiovascular disorders ♦ Hepatic or renal insufficiency ♦ Elderly or debilitated patients.

ADVERSE REACTIONS AND SIDE EFFECTS*

CNS: agitation, insomnia, headache/migraine, tremors, seizures, psychotic behavior, mania, blurred vision, sedation, dizziness.
CV: palpitations, tachycardia.
Derm: skin rash, urticaria, pruritus.
GI: dry mouth, constipation, nausea, vomiting, weight loss, anorexia.
GU: dysmenorrhea, impotence, urinary frequency, urinary retention.
Hemat: LEUKOPENIA.
Other: flu-like symptoms, excessive sweating.

INTERACTIONS

Drug-Drug: ♦ **Drugs that alter hepatic enzyme activity (e.g., carbamazepine, phenytoin, cimetidine, phenobarbital):** decreased metabolism of bupropion ♦ **Levodopa:** increased incidence of adverse effects of bupropion ♦ **MAO inhibitors:** enhanced acute toxicity of bupropion ♦ **Drugs that lower seizure threshold (phenothiazines, lidocaine, tricyclic, antidepressants):** increased risk of seizures.

ROUTE AND DOSAGE

Depression

♦ **PO (Adults):** Initial dosage: 200 mg/day, given as 100 mg bid. Dosage may be increased to 300 mg/day, given as 100 mg tid no sooner than 3 days after beginning therapy. An increase in dosage, up to a maximum of 450 mg/day, given in divided doses (at least 4 hours apart) of not more than 150 mg each may be considered for patients

---

*Underlines indicate most frequent; CAPITALS indicate life-threatening.

in whom no clinical improvement is noted after several weeks of treatment at 300 mg/day.

PHARMACODYNAMICS

Route	Onset	Peak	Duration
PO	8 days*	1–3 hr	weeks†

*Up to 4 weeks may be required to achieve maximal clinical response.

†Allow up to 2 weeks following cessation of therapy for complete drug elimination.

NURSING IMPLICATIONS

Assessment

♦ Assess for suicidal ideation, plan, means. Assess for sudden lifts in mood, which could indicate patient's decision to commit suicide.

♦ Assess mental status daily: • mood • appearance • thought and communication patterns • symptoms of anxiety • restlessness • level of interest in the environment and in activities • suicidal ideation. Improvement in these behavior patterns and level of energy should be expected within 1–4 weeks following initiation of therapy.

♦ Assess for symptoms of blood dyscrasias: sore throat, fever, malaise.

♦ Assess vital signs, weight.

♦ Assess history of seizures.

♦ Assess history of allergies, sensitivity to this drug.

♦ Assess history of glaucoma.

♦ Assess date of last menses (possible pregnancy), use of contraceptives.

♦ Assess whether currently breast-feeding a child.

♦ Assess current and past alcohol and drug consumption.

♦ Assess for operation of automobile and/or other dangerous machinery.

♦ Assess for presence of adverse reactions or side effects.

♦ Assess patient/family knowledge about illness and need for medication.

♦ In collaboration with physician, assess CBC and liver function tests in patients on long-term therapy.

♦ **Toxicity and Overdose:** Range of therapeutic serum concentration is 50–100 ng/mL.

◊ Assess for symptoms of overdose: • dyspnea • ataxia • convulsions.

♦ **Overdose Management:** Monitor vital signs.

◊ Maintain adequate airway.

◊ Monitor ECG and EEG for 48 hours.

◊ Induce emesis in conscious patient.

◊ Initiate gastric lavage in unconscious patient.

◊ Administer activated charcoal to minimize absorption.

◊ Manage seizures with IV benzodiazepines.

Potential Nursing Diagnoses

♦ High risk for self-directed violence related to depressed mood.

♦ High risk for injury related to bupropion's side effects of sedation, dizziness, lowered seizure threshold; overdose.

♦ Social isolation related to depressed mood.

♦ High risk for activity intolerance related to bupropion's side effects of drowsiness, dizziness.

♦ Knowledge deficit related to medication regimen.

Plan/Implementation

♦ Monitor vital signs before beginning therapy and at regular intervals (bid or tid) throughout therapy. Take BP lying and standing in patients experiencing orthostatic hypotension. Elderly are particularly susceptible. Contact physician if tachycardia/arrhythmias are noted.

♦ Weigh patient 2–3 times a week, at same time of day, on same scale, if possible. A rapid weight gain or evidence of edema should be reported to physician immediately. Record I&O.

♦ Ensure that patient is protected from injury. Provide supervision and assistance when ambulating if dizziness and drowsiness are problems. Pad siderails and headboard for patient who experiences seizures. Institute seizure precautions according to hospital policy.

♦ Give hard candy, gum, or frequent sips of water if dry mouth is a problem.

♦ Administer oral medication with food to minimize GI upset.

♦ Ensure that patient swallows tablet and does not "cheek" to avoid medication or to hoard for later use.

♦ Tablet may be crushed and mixed with food or fluid for patient who has difficulty swallowing.

♦ Store medication at room temperature in tightly closed, light-resistant container. Protect from temperatures greater than 30°C (86°F).

Patient/Family Education

♦ Therapeutic effect may not be seen for as long as 4 weeks. If after this length of time no improvement is noted, physician may prescribe a different medication. Continue to take medication even though symptoms have not subsided.

♦ Do not "double up" on medication if a dose is missed unless advised to do so by physician. Taking bupropion in divided doses will decrease risk of seizures and other adverse effects.

♦ If insomnia becomes a problem, it may be beneficial to take last medication dose no later than 5 p.m. If insomnia persists, physician may prescribe an additional medication for a short period of time to aid sleep.

♦ Use caution when driving or when operating dangerous machinery. Drowsiness and dizziness can occur. If these side effects become persistent or interfere with daily activities, report to physician. Dosage adjustment may be necessary.

♦ Do not stop taking the drug abruptly.

To do so might cause a relapse of symptoms of depression.

♦ Report occurrence of any of the following symptoms to physician immediately: sore throat, fever, malaise, persistent nausea/vomiting, severe headache, rapid heart rate, difficulty urinating, seizure activity.

♦ If dry mouth is a problem, take frequent sips of water, chew sugarless gum, or suck hard candy. Good oral care (frequent brushing, flossing) is very important.

♦ Do not drink alcohol while on bupropion therapy. Alcohol may alter seizure threshold.

♦ Be aware of possible risks of taking bupropion during pregnancy. Safe use during pregnancy has not been established. Notify physician immediately if pregnancy occurs, is suspected, or is planned.

♦ It is unknown if bupropion is excreted in breast milk. Potential risk to infant should be considered and physician consulted before taking bupropion during lactation.

♦ Be aware of side effects of bupropion. Refer to written materials furnished by healthcare providers for safe self-administration.

♦ Carry card or other identification at all times describing medications being taken.

Evaluation

♦ Patient demonstrates a subsiding/resolution of the symptoms for which bupropion was prescribed (depression, suicidal ideation).

♦ Patient verbalizes understanding of side effects and regimen required for prudent self-administration of bupropion.

BUSPIRONE

(byoo-spy´rone)
BuSpar

Classification(s):
Antianxiety agent;
Azaspirodecanedione
Pregnancy Category B

INDICATIONS

♦ Generalized anxiety states. **Unlabeled Use:** Symptomatic management of PMS.

ACTION

♦ Unknown ♦ May produce desired effects through interactions with serotonin, dopamine, and other neurotransmitter receptors.

PHARMACOKINETICS

Absorption: Rapid absorption from the GI tract.
Distribution: Not yet established.
Metabolism and Excretion: Metabolized by the liver, producing active metabolites that are excreted in urine (60%) and feces (40%).
Half-Life: 2–3 hours.

CONTRAINDICATIONS AND PRECAUTIONS

Contraindicated in: ♦ Hypersensitivity to this drug.
Use Cautiously in: ♦ Patients using MAO inhibitors ♦ Elderly or debilitated patients ♦ Patients with hepatic or renal dysfunction ♦ Pregnancy and lactation ♦ Children under 18 years of age ♦ Buspirone will not block the withdrawal syndrome in patients with history of chronic benzodiazepine or other sedative/hypnotic use. Patients should be withdrawn gradually from these medications before beginning therapy with buspirone.

ADVERSE REACTIONS AND SIDE EFFECTS*

CNS: drowsiness, dizziness, headache, weakness, confusion, nervousness, fatigue, extrapyramidal symptoms, tardive dyskinesia, dysphoria, paradoxical excitement, blurred vision.
CV: tachycardia, hypotension, palpitations.
Derm: skin rash.
Endo: gynecomastia, galactorrhea.
GI: dry mouth, nausea, vomiting, diarrhea, anorexia, constipation.

INTERACTIONS

Drug-Drug: ♦ **MAO inhibitors:** elevated blood pressure.

ROUTE AND DOSAGE

Generalized Anxiety (Maintenance)
♦ **PO (Adults):** 5 mg tid. Dosage may be increased by 5 mg/day at intervals of 2–3 days, not to exceed 60 mg/day. Usually effective dose: 20–30 mg/day. Not recommended for p.r.n. administration due to delayed onset of therapeutic action. Long-term efficacy not established.

PHARMACODYNAMICS

Route	Onset	Peak	Duration
PO	7–10 days	40–90 min	UK

NURSING IMPLICATIONS
Assessment
♦ Assess extent of anxiety. Symptoms of generalized anxiety disorder include: ● motor tension (restlessness, fidgeting, trembling ● autonomic hyperactivity (sweating, dizziness, dry mouth, pounding heartbeat, cold and clammy skin, rapid pulse and respirations) ● apprehensive expectation (anxiety, worry, fear, anticipation of misfor-

*Underlines indicate most frequent; CAPITALS indicate life-threatening.

tune) • vigilance and scanning (hyperattentiveness to the environment). These symptoms have persisted for at least a month.

♦ Assess for suicidal ideation in depressed patients (depression and anxiety often are observed together).

♦ Assess history of allergies, sensitivity to this drug.

♦ Assess date of last menses (possible pregnancy), use of contraceptives.

♦ Assess whether currently breast-feeding a child.

♦ Assess current and past alcohol and drug consumption.

♦ Assess operation of automobile and/or other dangerous machinery.

♦ Assess for presence of adverse reactions or side effects. (**Note:** In comparison to benzodiazepines, there is less sedation and less interaction with alcohol, and clinical trials have demonstrated a lower addiction potential.)

♦ Assess patient/family knowledge about illness and need for medication.

♦ In collaboration with physician, assess renal and liver function tests in patients on long-term therapy.

♦ **Withdrawal:** Assess for symptoms of abrupt withdrawal from long-term use of benzodiazepines or other sedative/hypnotic drugs prior to beginning therapy with buspirone. • depression • insomnia • cramping • tremors • vomiting • sweating • convulsions • delirium

♦ **Withdrawal Management** (from symptoms of abrupt withdrawal from long-term use of benzodiazepines or other sedative-hypnotic drugs): Monitor vital signs.

◊ Place patient in quiet room with low stimuli.

◊ Institute seizure precautions.

◊ A long-acting barbiturate, such as phenobarbital, may be ordered to suppress withdrawal symptoms.

◊ Phenytoin may be ordered to prevent seizures.

◊ Some physicians may order oxazepam

as needed for objective withdrawal symptoms, gradually decreasing the dosage until the drug is discontinued.

♦ **Toxicity and Overdose:** Assess for symptoms of overdose: • nausea • vomiting • dizziness • drowsiness • miosis • gastric distress.

♦ **Overdose Management:** Monitor vital signs.

◊ Ensure adequate airway.

◊ Initiate symptomatic and supportive measures.

◊ Initiate gastric lavage.

◊ The effectiveness of hemodialysis in buspirone overdose has not been determined.

Potential Nursing Diagnoses

♦ High risk for injury related to panic anxiety; buspirone side effects of drowsiness, dizziness, and weakness.

♦ High risk for self-directed violence related to depressed mood.

♦ Anxiety (specify level) related to threats to physical integrity and/or self-concept.

♦ High risk for activity intolerance related to buspirone's side effects of: • fatigue • drowsiness • dizziness • muscular weakness.

♦ Knowledge deficit related to medication regimen.

Plan/Implementation

♦ Monitor vital signs before beginning therapy, and at regular intervals (bid) throughout therapy.

♦ To minimize nausea, give medication with food or milk.

♦ Ensure that patient practices good oral care. Offer hard, sugarless candy, gum, or frequent sips of water for dry mouth.

♦ Ensure that patient is protected from injury. Supervise and assist with ambulation if dizziness and muscular weakness are problems.

♦ Store medication at controlled room temperatures between 15° and 30°C (59°–86°F). Protect from heat and moisture.

Patient/Family Education

♦ Do not drive or operate dangerous machinery while taking buspirone. Drowsiness and dizziness can occur.

♦ Be aware of lag time between start of therapy and subsiding of symptoms. Relief is usually evident within 7–10 days. Be sure to take medication regularly as ordered so that it has sufficient time to take effect.

♦ Report any of the following symptoms to physician: motor restlessness, involuntary repetitive or spastic movements of face or neck.

♦ Do not take other medications, including over-the-counter medications, without physician's approval.

♦ Do not consume CNS depressants (including alcohol) with buspirone. Although there appears to be no interaction between buspirone and CNS depressants, individual responses cannot be predicted.

♦ Be aware of possible risks of taking buspirone during pregnancy. Use only if clearly required. Safety during pregnancy has not been fully established. Notify physician immediately if pregnancy is suspected or planned.

♦ Be aware of possible side effects of buspirone. Refer to written materials furnished by healthcare providers.

♦ Carry card or other identification at all times indicating medications being taken.

Evaluation

♦ Patient demonstrates a subsiding/resolution of the symptoms for which buspirone was prescribed (symptoms of generalized anxiety disorder).

♦ Patient verbalizes understanding of side effects and regimen required for prudent self-administration of buspirone.

BUTABARBITAL

(byoo-ta-bar'bi-tal)
Butisol, {Day-Barb, Neo-Barb}

Classification(s):
Sedative-hypnotic; Barbiturate; CNS depressant
Schedule C III
Pregnancy Category D

INDICATIONS

♦ Anxiety ♦ Insomnia ♦ Preoperative sedation.

ACTION

♦ Depresses the central nervous system ♦ Interferes with transmission through the reticular formation, which is concerned with arousal ♦ Causes imbalance in inhibitory and facilitatory mechanisms that influence the cerebral cortex and reticular formation ♦ Action on neurotransmitters is not well defined ♦ All levels of CNS depression can occur, from mild sedation to hypnosis to coma to death.

PHARMACOKINETICS

Absorption: Readily absorbed following oral administration.
Distribution: Rapidly and widely distributed. Crosses blood-brain and placental barriers; excreted in breast milk.
Metabolism and Excretion: Metabolized by the liver to inactive metabolites and excreted by the kidneys.
Half-Life: 32–44 hours.

CONTRAINDICATIONS AND PRECAUTIONS

Contraindicated in: ♦ Hypersensitivity to this drug or other barbiturates ♦ Severe hepatic, renal, cardiac, or respiratory disease ♦ Individuals with a history of previous addiction ♦ Patients with a history of porphyria.

{} = Only available in Canada.

Use Cautiously in: ♦ Elderly or debilitated patients ♦ Patients with hepatic, renal, cardiac, or respiratory dysfunction ♦ Depressed/suicidal patients ♦ Patients with ammonia intoxication ♦ Pregnancy and lactation.

ADVERSE REACTIONS AND SIDE EFFECTS*

CNS: <u>drowsiness</u>, headache, lethargy, <u>dizziness</u>, mental depression, ataxia, <u>residual sedation ("hangover")</u>, confusion, paradoxical excitement and/or euphoria.
CV: hypotension, bradycardia.
Derm: skin rashes, urticaria, dermatitis (may precede potentially fatal reactions).
GI: nausea/vomiting, constipation.
Hemat: AGRANULOCYTOSIS, THROMBOCYTOPENIA.
Resp: hypoventilation, apnea, LARYNGOSPASM, BRONCHOSPASM.
Other: tolerance, physical and psychological dependence.

INTERACTIONS

Drug-Drug: ♦ **Other CNS depressants (including alcohol, benzodiazepines, antihistamines, opiates):** additive CNS depression ♦ **Chloramphenicol, MAO inhibitors, valproic acid, cimetidine, disulfiram:** increased effects of butabarbital ♦ **Phenytoin:** increased or decreased effects of either drug (close monitoring of serum levels required to control seizure activity) ♦ **Oral contraceptives:** decreased effectiveness of oral contraceptives ♦ **Oral anticoagulants:** decreased anticoagulant effects ♦ **Corticosteroids, digitoxin, doxycycline:** decreased effects of these drugs ♦ **Furosemide:** orthostatic hypotension ♦ **Griseofulvin:** decreased griseofulvin levels.
Drug-Food: ♦ **Vitamin D:** increased vitamin D metabolism; possible deficiency ♦ **Folic acid:** decreased absorption of folic acid; possible deficiency.

ROUTE AND DOSAGE
Anxiety
♦ **PO (Adults):** 15–30 mg tid or qid.
♦ **PO (Children):** 6 mg/kg daily in 3 equally divided doses (range of 7.5–30 mg tid).

Insomnia
(Limit use to 2 weeks.)
♦ **PO (Adults):** 50–100 mg at bedtime.

Preoperative Sedation
♦ **PO (Adults):** 50–100 mg, administered 60–90 minutes before surgery.
♦ **PO (Children):** 2–6 mg/kg (maximum 100 mg).

PHARMACODYNAMICS

Route	Onset	Peak	Duration
PO	45–60 min	3–4 hr	6–8 hr

NURSING IMPLICATIONS
Assessment
♦ Assess level of anxiety. Symptoms include: • restlessness • pacing • insomnia • inability to concentrate • increased heart rate • increased respiration • elevated blood pressure • confusion • tremors • rapid speech.
♦ Assess sleep patterns. Keep records for adequate baseline data before the initiation of therapy.
♦ Assess for suicidal ideation in depressed patients.
♦ Assess history of allergies, sensitivity to this drug or to other barbiturates.
♦ Assess date of last menses (possible pregnancy), use of contraceptives.
♦ Assess whether currently breast-feeding a child.
♦ Assess current and past alcohol and drug consumption.
♦ Assess for operation of automobile and/or other dangerous machinery.
♦ Assess for presence of adverse reactions or side effects.

---

*Underlines indicate most frequent; CAPITALS indicate life-threatening.

♦ Assess patient/family knowledge about condition and need for medication.

♦ In collaboration with physician, assess CBC and renal and liver function tests in patients on prolonged therapy.

♦ **Lab Test Alterations:** Increased values of bromsulphalein (BSP) retention and protein-bound iodine (PBI).

◊ Elevation of blood ammonia.

♦ **Withdrawal:** Assess for symptoms of withdrawal: • anxiety • tremors • insomnia • nausea/vomiting • weakness • diaphoresis • orthostatic hypotension • delirium • convulsions.

♦ **Withdrawal Management:** Monitor vital signs.

◊ Place patient in quiet room with low stimuli.

◊ Institute seizure precautions.

◊ A long-acting barbiturate, such as phenobarbital, may be ordered to suppress withdrawal symptoms.

◊ Phenytoin may be ordered to prevent seizures.

◊ Some physicians may order oxazepam as needed for objective withdrawal symptoms, gradually decreasing the dosage until the drug is discontinued.

♦ **Toxicity and Overdose:** Assess for symptoms of toxicity: • confusion • drowsiness • dyspnea • slurred speech • staggering.

◊ Assess for symptoms of overdose: • CNS and respiratory depression • hypoventilation • hypothermia • hypotension • oliguria • tachycardia • coma. (May progress to respiratory arrest, circulatory collapse, and death.)

♦ **Overdose Management:** Monitor vital signs.

◊ Ensure maintenance of airway.

◊ Induce vomiting in conscious patient.

◊ Initiate gastric lavage in unconscious patient.

◊ Administer activated charcoal to minimize absorption of drug.

◊ Administer IV fluids.

◊ For severe intoxication, forced diuresis or hemodialysis may be used.

Potential Nursing Diagnoses

♦ Ineffective breathing pattern related to side effects of hypoventilation and apnea.

♦ High risk for injury related to abrupt withdrawal from long-term use; decreased mental alertness caused by side effect of residual sedation; side effects of dizziness, ataxia; effects of overdose.

♦ High risk for self-directed violence related to depressed mood.

♦ Anxiety (specify level) related to threats to physical integrity and/or self-concept.

♦ Sleep pattern disturbance related to situational crises; physical condition; severe level of anxiety.

♦ High risk for activity intolerance, related to side effects of residual sedation, drowsiness, dizziness.

♦ Knowledge deficit related to medication regimen.

Plan/Implementation

♦ Monitor vital signs before beginning therapy and at regular intervals (bid) throughout therapy.

♦ Ensure that patient is protected from injury. Supervise and assist with ambulation if dizziness and drowsiness are problems. Ensure that patient avoids participation in any activity that requires mental alertness (including smoking). Raise siderails and instruct patient to remain in bed following administration.

♦ To minimize nausea, medication may be given with food or milk.

♦ Ensure that tablet or capsule has been swallowed and not "cheeked" to avoid medication or to hoard for later use.

♦ Crush tablet or empty capsule and mix with food or fluid for patient who has difficulty swallowing or use elixir form.

Patient/Family Education

♦ Use caution in driving or when operating dangerous machinery. Drowsiness and dizziness can occur.

Do not stop taking the drug abruptly. To do so can produce serious (even life-threatening) withdrawal symptoms. If a dose is missed, take it as close as possible to the prescribed time. If it is close to time for next dose, wait until then; do not double up on dose at next prescribed time.

♦ Do not consume other CNS depressants (including alcohol).

♦ Be aware of the risks of taking barbiturates during pregnancy (congenital malformations may be associated with use during the first trimester). Also, evidence of withdrawal symptoms have been observed in neonates born to mothers who had ingested barbiturates regularly during the last trimester of pregnancy. Notify physician if pregnancy is suspected or planned.

♦ Because barbiturates decrease effectiveness of oral contraceptives, use alternative methods of birth control during butabarbital therapy.

♦ Be aware of potential side effects. Refer to written materials furnished by healthcare providers regarding correct method of self-administration.

♦ Report symptoms of sore throat, fever, malaise, severe headache, conjunctivitis, rhinitis, urethritis, balanitis, easy bruising, petechiae, or epistaxis to physician immediately.

♦ Carry card or other identification at all times stating names of medications being taken.

Evaluation

♦ Patient demonstrates a subsiding/resolution of the symptoms for which butabarbital was prescribed (anxiety, sleep disturbances).

♦ Patient verbalizes understanding of side effects and regimen required for prudent self-administration of butabarbital.

CARBAMAZEPINE

(kar-ba-maz′e-peen)
{Mazepine}, Tegretol

Classification(s):
Anticonvulsant; Iminostilbene derivative
Pregnancy Category C

INDICATIONS

♦ Tonic-clonic (grand mal) seizures ♦ Partial seizures with complex symptomatology (psychomotor) ♦ Mixed-type seizures refractory to other anticonvulsant medications ♦ Pain associated with trigeminal neuralgia. **Investigational Uses:** Neurogenic diabetes insipidus ♦ Bipolar affective disorder ♦ Schizoaffective disorder ♦ Resistant schizophrenia ♦ Rage reactions ♦ Alcohol withdrawal.

ACTION

♦ Unknown ♦ May reduce polysynaptic responses and block post-tetanic potentiation of synaptic transmission.

PHARMACOKINETICS

Absorption: Slowly absorbed from the GI tract.
Distribution: Is widely distributed. Crosses blood-brain and placental barriers; excreted in breast milk.
Metabolism and Excretion: Metabolized by the liver; metabolites excreted by the kidneys.
Half-Life: 25–65 hours (initial); 12–17 hours (repeated doses).

CONTRAINDICATIONS AND PRECAUTIONS

Contraindicated in: ♦ Hypersensitivity to this drug or to tricyclic antidepressants ♦ Previous bone marrow depression ♦ Concomitant use of MAO inhibitors ♦ Lactation.

{} = Only available in Canada.

Use Cautiously in: ♦ Elderly or debilitated patients ♦ Patients with hepatic, cardiac, or renal disease ♦ Increased intraocular pressure ♦ Pregnancy ♦ Children under 6 (safety not established). **Note:** Sole use of this medication in some patients with mixed-type epilepsy may increase incidence of tonic-clonic (grand mal) seizures.

ADVERSE REACTIONS AND SIDE EFFECTS*

CNS: drowsiness, dizziness, unsteadiness, confusion, headache, nystagmus, fatigue, blurred vision, speech disturbances, vertigo, ataxia.
CV: aggravation of hypertension, hypotension, syncope and collapse, aggravation of coronary artery disease, edema, thrombophlebitis, ARRHYTHMIAS, HEART BLOCK, CONGESTIVE HEART FAILURE.
Derm: skin rashes, alopecia, urticaria, photosensitivity, alterations in pigmentation, EXFOLIATIVE DERMATITIS, erythema multiforme.
GI: nausea/vomiting, diarrhea, constipation, anorexia, dry mouth, abdominal pain, glossitis, stomatitis.
GU: urinary retention, urinary frequency, impotence, elevated BUN, RENAL FAILURE, azotemia.
Hemat: BLOOD DYSCRASIAS (aplastic anemia, thrombocytopenia, agranulocytosis, leukopenia, leukocytosis, eosinophilia, purpura).
Resp: dyspnea.
Other: abnormal hepatic function, jaundice, hepatitis, conjunctivitis, painful joints and muscles, hypothyroidism, aggravation of systemic lupus erythematosus, diaphoresis, fever and chills, punctate lens opacities.

INTERACTIONS

Drug-Drug: ♦ **Erythromycin, verapamil, isoniazid, propoxyphene, troleandomycin, cimetidine:** increased effects of carbamazepine ♦ **Phensuximide, doxycycline, theophylline,** oral anticoagulants, oral contraceptives, phenytoin, ethosuximide, valproic acid, haloperidol: decreased effects of these drugs ♦ **Phenytoin, primidone, phenobarbital:** decreased effects of carbamazepine ♦ **Lithium:** increased risk of neurotoxicity.

ROUTE AND DOSAGE

Tonic-Clonic (Grand Mal), Psychomotor, and Mixed Seizures

♦ **PO (Adults and Children Over 12):** Initial dosage: 200 mg bid. At weekly intervals, increase dosage by 200 mg/day given tid or qid until control is achieved with minimal side effects. Maintenance dose: 800–1200 mg/day. Maximum dose: 1 g/day in children 13–15 years old; 1.2 g/day in patients older than 15 years.
♦ **PO (Children Ages 6–12):** Initial dosage: 100 mg bid. At weekly intervals, increase dosage by 100 mg/day given tid or qid until control is achieved with minimal side effects. Maintenance dose: 400–800 mg/day. Maximum dose: 1000 mg/day.

Trigeminal Neuralgia

♦ **PO (Adults):** Initial dosage: 100 mg bid. Increase dose by 200 mg/day, using increments of 100 mg every 12 hours until pain is relieved with minimal side effects. Maintenance dose: 200–1200 mg/day. Attempts to reduce dose or discontinue drug should be made at least once every 3 months. Maximum dose: 1.2 g/day.

Bipolar Affective Disorder

♦ **PO (Adults):** Initial dosage: 200 mg bid with food. Increase by 200 mg/day q 3–7 days. Watch patient response, tolerance, serum levels. Give in divided doses up to qid. Optimal serum level range is 8–12 mcg/mL.

Schizoaffective Disorder, Resistant Schizophrenia

♦ **PO (Adults):** 600–1200 mg/day in divided doses.

*Underlines indicate most frequent; CAPITALS indicate life-threatening.

Alcohol Withdrawal

* **PO (Adults):** 80 mg/day in divided doses, reduced until drug-free after 1 week.

Discontinuation of Therapy

* Withdraw slowly to prevent precipitation of seizures or status epilepticus.

PHARMACODYNAMICS

Route	Onset	Peak	Duration
PO	Variable	2–8 hr	6–12 hr

NURSING IMPLICATIONS

Assessment

* Assess occurrence, characteristics, and duration of seizure activity.
* Assess frequency, duration, and intensity of trigeminal neuralgia pain.
* Assess baseline vital signs.
* Assess history of allergies, sensitivity to this drug or to tricyclic antidepressants.
* Assess history of glaucoma.
* Assess date of last menses (possible pregnancy), use of contraceptives.
* Assess whether currently breast-feeding a child.
* Assess current and past alcohol and drug consumption.
* Assess operation of automobile and/or other dangerous machinery.
* Assess for presence of adverse reactions or side effects.
* Assess patient/family knowledge about illness and need for medication.
* In collaboration with physician, assess CBC, liver function tests, complete urinalysis and BUN; baseline and periodic eye examinations before starting as well as during therapy.
* **Lab Test Alterations:** Decreased thyroid function tests.
* **Toxicity and Overdose:** Range of therapeutic serum concentration is 3–14 mcg/mL.
* ◇ Assess for symptoms of toxicity/overdose: • restlessness • twitching • tremor • ataxia • drowsiness • dizziness • nystagmus • stupor • agitation • involuntary movements • mydriasis • flushing • cyanosis • urinary retention • tachycardia • hypotension or hypertension • nausea/vomiting • convulsions • oliguria • shock • respiratory depression • coma.
* **Overdose Management:** Monitor vital signs.
* ◇ Induce emesis in conscious patient.
* ◇ Initiate gastric lavage in unconscious patient.
* ◇ Administer activated charcoal to minimize absorption.
* ◇ Administer IV fluids and ensure maintenance of adequate airway.
* ◇ Parenteral barbiturates may be used to combat convulsions and hyperirritability, but could induce respiratory depression.
* ◇ Ensure availability of resuscitation equipment.
* ◇ Barbiturates should not be used if MAO inhibitors have been consumed within 1 week.
* ◇ Dialysis may be useful only in cases of severe poisoning associated with renal failure.

Potential Nursing Diagnoses

* High risk for injury related to seizures; abrupt withdrawal from long-term carbamazepine use; effects of toxicity or overdose.
* Pain related to spasms of trigeminal nerve.
* Impaired adjustment related to difficulty accepting diagnosis of epilepsy or trigeminal neuralgia.
* Social isolation related to fear of experiencing a seizure in the presence of others.
* High risk for activity intolerance, related to carbamazepine's side effects of drowsiness, dizziness, ataxia.
* Knowledge deficit related to medication regimen.

Plan/Implementation

* Monitor vital signs before beginning therapy and at regular intervals (bid) throughout therapy.

♦ Ensure patient practices good oral care. Offer hard, sugarless candy, gum, or frequent sips of water for dry mouth.

♦ Observe patient frequently (every hour) for occurrence of seizure activity.

♦ Ensure that patient is protected from injury. Supervise and assist with ambulation if dizziness and ataxia are problems. Avoid or monitor activities which require mental alertness (including smoking). Pad siderails and headboard for patient who experiences seizures during the night.

♦ Monitor and record lab assessments of serum carbamazepine levels. Report the presence of sore throat, fever, malaise, unusual bleeding, easy bruising, yellowish skin or eyes, edema, mouth ulcers, pale stools, petechial or purpuric hemorrhage, or oliguria to physician immediately.

♦ To minimize nausea, give medication with food or milk.

♦ If patient has difficulty swallowing tablet, crush and mix with food or fluid. Chewable tablet should be chewed, not swallowed whole.

♦ Ensure tablet has been swallowed and not "cheeked" to avoid medication or to hoard for later use.

♦ Store medication at controlled room temperatures between 15° and 30°C (59°–86°F). Protect from heat, light, and moisture.

Patient/Family Education

♦ Do not drive or operate dangerous machinery until individual response has been determined. Drowsiness and dizziness can occur.

♦ Do not stop taking the drug abruptly. To do so can result in status epilepticus.

♦ Avoid alcohol intake and nonprescription medication without approval from physician.

♦ Be aware of risks of taking carbamazepine during pregnancy. There is an association between use of anticonvulsant drugs by women with epilepsy and the incidence of birth defects in their children. A patient who requires the medication to prevent seizures may be maintained on it; however, she must be fully aware of potential risks to her unborn child. If pregnancy occurs, is suspected, or is planned, notify physician immediately.

♦ Due to decreased effectiveness of oral contraceptives during carbamazepine therapy, alternative methods of birth control should be used.

♦ Report any of the following symptoms to physician promptly: sore throat, fever, malaise, unusual bleeding, easy bruising, yellow skin or eyes, decrease in urine output, fluid retention, pale stools, impotence, mouth ulcers, abdominal pain.

♦ Protect a patient during seizures. In the case of tonic-clonic (grand mal) seizure, do not restrain. Padding may be used (towels, blankets, pillows) to prevent bumping against hard objects. When convulsion has subsided, turn patient on side to allow secretions to drain and prevent aspiration. Keep records of occurrence, characteristics, and duration of seizures. Accurate reports given to the physician provide assistance in stabilization and control of seizures. If patient has difficulty breathing or continues to experience subsequent seizures, family should immediately call for emergency assistance.

♦ Be aware of potential side effects. Refer to written materials furnished by healthcare providers regarding correct method of self-administration.

♦ Carry card or other identification at all times stating illness and names of medications being taken. Include names of physician and medical facility to which patient should be transported in the event of an emergency.

Evaluation

♦ Patient demonstrates stabilization of seizure activity with regular administration of carbamazepine.

♦ Patient verbalizes understanding of necessity for, side effects of, and regimen required for prudent self-administration of carbamazepine.

CARBIDOPA/LEVODOPA

(kar-bi-doe′pa/lee-voe-doe′pa)
Sinemet, Sinemet CR

Classification(s):
Antiparkinsonian
Pregnancy Category C

INDICATIONS

♦ Idiopathic, arteriosclerotic, and post-encephalitic parkinsonism ♦ Symptoms of parkinsonism associated with injury to the nervous system by carbon monoxide or manganese intoxication. **Investigational Use:** To reduce peripheral metabolism of oxitriptan (L-5-hydroxytryptophan) in treating postanoxic intention myoclonus.

ACTION

♦ Levodopa is decarboxylated into dopamine in the basal ganglia and in the periphery, thus correcting the decrease in striatal dopamine that produces the symptoms of parkinsonism ♦ Carbidopa prevents peripheral decarboxylation of levodopa, thereby making more levodopa available for transport to the brain and decreasing by 70–80% the dosage requirements for levodopa in reducing symptoms of parkinsonism. Carbidopa has no therapeutic effect when given alone. It is indicated only for concomitant use with levodopa.

PHARMACOKINETICS

Absorption: Levodopa is well absorbed following oral administration. 40–70% of carbidopa is absorbed following oral administration. Absorption may be delayed when administered with food.

Distribution: Widely distributed. Carbidopa does not cross blood-brain barrier. Both drugs are thought to cross placental barrier and to enter breast milk.

Metabolism and Excretion: Levodopa is metabolized by the liver. Carbidopa is not extensively metabolized. Excreted in urine.

Half-Life: Levodopa: 2 hours when given with carbidopa; carbidopa: 1–2 hours.

CONTRAINDICATIONS AND PRECAUTIONS

Contraindicated in: ♦ Hypersensitivity to either drug or tartrazine ♦ Narrow-angle glaucoma ♦ Concomitant use of MAO inhibitors ♦ Patients with a history of melanoma or with suspicious, undiagnosed skin lesions ♦ Lactation.

Use Cautiously in: ♦ Patients with severe cardiovascular or pulmonary disease ♦ Bronchial asthma ♦ Emphysema ♦ Occlusive cerebrovascular disease ♦ Renal, hepatic, or endocrine disease ♦ A history of myocardial infarction ♦ A history of active peptic ulcer disease ♦ A history of seizure disorders ♦ Depressed and suicidal patients ♦ Psychotic patients ♦ Pregnancy, children under 18 (safety not established).

ADVERSE REACTIONS AND SIDE EFFECTS*

CNS: <u>choreiform, dyskinetic or dystonic movements</u>, <u>ataxia</u>, <u>increased hand tremor</u>, <u>headache</u>, <u>dizziness</u>, <u>numbness</u>, <u>weakness and faintness</u>, <u>teeth grinding</u>, <u>confusion</u>, <u>insomnia</u>, <u>nightmares</u>, <u>hallucinations and paranoid delusions</u>, <u>hypomania</u>, <u>agitation and anxiety</u>, <u>malaise</u>, <u>fatigue</u>, <u>euphoria</u>, mental depression with or without suicidal ideations, nervousness, restlessness, toxic delirium, numbness, decreased attention span, memory

---

*<u>Underlines</u> indicate most frequent; CAPITALS indicate life-threatening.

loss, dementia, diplopia, blurred vision, dilated pupils, hot flashes, convulsions, oculogyric crisis, NEUROLEPTIC MALIGNANT SYNDROME.

CV: orthostatic hypotension, palpitations, arrhythmias, hypertension, phlebitis, flushing, sinus tachycardia.

Derm: skin rash, alopecia.

GI: nausea and vomiting, anorexia, abdominal pain, dry mouth, dysphagia, bitter taste, excessive salivation, diarrhea, constipation, flatulence, weight gain or loss, GI bleeding, duodenal ulcer, hiccups, trismus, dysphagia.

GU: urinary retention, urinary incontinence, priapism.

Hemat: HEMOLYTIC OR NONHEMOLYTIC ANEMIA, AGRANULOCYTOSIS, LEUKOPENIA, THROMBOCYTOPENIA, phlebitis.

Resp: bizarre breathing patterns, hyperventilation.

Other: bradykinesia, muscle twitching, increased sweating, dark sweat or urine, edema, hoarseness, ACTIVATION OF MALIGNANT MELANOMA, blepharospasm, muscle cramping.

INTERACTIONS

Drug-Drug: ♦ **Anticholinergics, clonidine, reserpine, phenothiazines and other antipsychotics, benzodiazepines, phenytoin, papaverine, diazepam, chlordiazepoxide:** decreased therapeutic effect of carbidopa/levodopa ♦ **Furazolidone:** increased therapeutic and toxic effect of carbidopa/levodopa ♦ **Antihypertensives (e.g., guanethidine, methyldopa):** increased hypotensive effects ♦ **Methyldopa:** increased CNS toxicity (e.g., psychosis) ♦ **MAO inhibitors:** hypertensive crisis, increased therapeutic and toxic effects of carbidopa/levodopa ♦ **Sympathomimetic drugs (e.g., ephedrine, amphetamines, epinephrine, and isoproterenol):** increased effects of these drugs ♦ **Tricyclic antidepressants:** sympathetic hyperactivity resulting in sinus tachycardia, postural hypotension, hypertension, and dyskinesia ♦ **Hypoglycemic agents:** increased or decreased hypoglycemic effects ♦ **Anticholinergic agents:** decreased tremor, occasional increase in abnormal involuntary movements ♦ **Cyclopropane or halogenated hydrocarbon general anesthetics:** increased possibility of cardiac arrhythmias.

ROUTE AND DOSAGE

(Tablets contain 10/100, 25/100, or 25/250 mg of carbidopa and levodopa, respectively.)

Parkinsonism

♦ **PO Sinemet (Adults):** 75/300–150/1500 mg/day in 3–4 divided doses. Can increase up to 200/2000 mg/day.
♦ **PO Sinemet CR (Adults):** Usual dose is 1 tablet bid at intervals of not less than 6 hours. Doses of 2–8 tablets/day in divided doses at intervals of 4–8 hours while awake have been used. Add 3 days between dosage adjustments.

PHARMACODYNAMICS

Route	Onset	Peak	Duration
PO (carbidopa)	15–30 min	—	5–24 hr
PO (levodopa)	30–45 min	1 hr	2–5 hr

NURSING IMPLICATIONS
Assessment

♦ Assess for symptoms of Parkinson's disease: • tremors • muscular weakness and rigidity • drooling • shuffling gait • disturbances of posture and equilibrium • flat affect • monotone speech.
♦ Assess for symptoms of depression and potential for suicide.
♦ Assess vital signs, weight. Record baseline values for comparison.
♦ Assess history of allergies, sensitivity to this drug.
♦ Assess date of last menses (possible pregnancy), use of contraceptives.

♦ Assess for symptoms of blood dyscrasias: sore throat, fever, malaise.

♦ Assess for symptoms of mental changes: • psychosis • hallucinations • delusions • paranoid ideations • dementia • depression with or without suicidal tendencies.

♦ Assess for history of malignant melanoma. Check skin for suspicious undiagnosed lesions.

♦ Assess whether currently breast-feeding a child.

♦ Assess current and past alcohol and drug consumption.

♦ Assess for operation of automobile and/or other dangerous machinery.

♦ Assess for presence of adverse reactions or side effects.

♦ Assess patient/family knowledge about illness and need for medication.

♦ In collaboration with physician, assess CBC and hepatic and renal function tests in patients on long-term therapy.

♦ **Lab Test Alterations:** Positive Coombs' test.

◊ False-positive urine glucose tests (copper reduction method).

◊ False-negative urine glucose tests (glucose oxidase method).

◊ Elevated AST, ALT, LDH, bilirubin, alkaline phosphatase, and protein-bound iodine.

◊ Decrease in WBC, hemoglobin, and hematocrit.

◊ Increase in serum prolactin levels.

♦ **Toxicity and Overdose:** Assess for symptoms of toxicity/overdose: • muscle twitching and spasmodic winking (blepharospasm) • facial grimacing • exaggerated protrusion of the tongue • behavioral changes • cardiac arrhythmias.

♦ **Overdose Management:** Monitor vital signs.

◊ Maintain adequate airway.

◊ Monitor ECG.

◊ Initiate gastric lavage.

◊ Judiciously administer IV fluids.

◊ Institute antiarrhythmic therapy if required.

◊ Provide general supportive measures.

Potential Nursing Diagnoses

♦ High risk for injury related to symptoms of Parkinson's disease or side effects of carbidopa/levodopa (dizziness, weakness, confusion).

♦ High risk for self-directed violence related to side effect of depressed mood with suicidal ideations.

♦ Sensory-perceptual alteration related to side effect of carbidopa/levodopa (hallucinations).

♦ Altered thought processes related to side effects of carbidopa/levodopa (delusional thinking, dementia, confusion).

♦ Social isolation related to embarrassment by symptoms of Parkinson's disease.

♦ High risk for activity intolerance, related to carbidopa/levodopa side effects of dizziness, ataxia, weakness, confusion, fatigue.

♦ Knowledge deficit related to medication regimen.

Plan/Implementation

♦ Monitor vital signs tid. Be alert for increase in pulse rate, temperature, blood pressure. Notify physician of significant elevations, arrhythmias, palpitations, or changes in respiratory rate or rhythm.

♦ Weigh patient 2–3 times a week, at same time of day, on same scale, if possible. A rapid weight gain or evidence of edema should be reported to physician immediately. Record I&O.

♦ Ensure that patient is protected from injury. Provide supervision and assistance when ambulating if dizziness and ataxia are problems. Patient should change positions slowly to minimize effects of orthostatic hypotension.

♦ Monitor for signs of difficulty with voluntary movements. Dyskinesias can occur sooner with combined therapy than with levodopa alone. Notify physician if dyskinetic or spastic movements occur.

♦ Give hard candy, gum, or frequent sips

of water if dry mouth is a problem, or treat with a saliva substitute.

♦ Monitor urine glucose and ketones carefully. Notify physician of significant changes. Adjustment in dosage of hypoglycemic agent may be necessary.

♦ Ensure that patient swallows tablet/capsule and does not "cheek" to avoid medication or to hoard for later use.

♦ Administer medication with food to minimize gastric irritation.

♦ Discuss with pharmacist whether to crush tablet or empty contents of capsule and mix with fruit-based fluid for patient who has difficulty swallowing.

♦ Monitor vital signs before beginning therapy, and at regular intervals (bid or tid) throughout therapy. Take BP lying and standing to monitor for possible hypotensive reaction. Elderly are particularly susceptible. Dosage adjustment may be required.

♦ Store medication at controlled room temperatures between 15° and 30°C (59°–86°F). Protect from heat, light, and moisture.

Patient/Family Education

♦ Take medication with food to minimize GI upset.

♦ Use caution when driving or when operating dangerous machinery. Dizziness and confusion can occur.

♦ Do not stop taking the drugs abruptly. To do so might produce withdrawal symptoms, such as muscle rigidity, weakness, tremors, elevated temperature, mental changes.

♦ Report occurrence of any of the following symptoms to physician immediately: uncontrollable movements of the face, eyelids, mouth, tongue, neck, arms, hands, or legs; mood or mental changes; irregular heartbeats or palpitations; difficult urination; severe or persistent nausea and vomiting; fever.

♦ Rise slowly from a sitting or lying position to prevent a sudden drop in blood pressure.

♦ If dry mouth is a problem, take frequent sips of water, chew sugarless gum, or suck on hard candy. Good oral care (frequent brushing, flossing) is very important.

♦ Diabetic patients should notify physician of any abnormal results in self-testing before adjusting dosage of hypoglycemic medications.

♦ Do not consume other medications (including over-the-counter meds) without physician's approval. Many medications contain substances that interact with carbidopa/levodopa in a way that may be harmful.

♦ Urine and perspiration may appear dark. This change is not significant nor is it harmful.

♦ Be aware of possible risks of taking carbidopa/levodopa during pregnancy. Safe use during pregnancy and lactation has not been established. It is thought that carbidopa/levodopa crosses the placental barrier; if so, fetus could experience adverse effects of the drug. Inform physician immediately if pregnancy occurs, is suspected, or is planned. Use is not recommended in nursing mothers.

♦ Be aware of side effects of carbidopa/levodopa. Refer to written materials furnished by healthcare providers for safe self-administration.

♦ Continue to take medication, even if feeling well and as though it is not needed. Symptoms may return if medication is discontinued.

♦ Carry card or other identification at all times describing medications being taken.

Evaluation

♦ Patient demonstrates a subsiding of the symptoms for which carbidopa/levodopa was prescribed (symptoms of parkinsonism).

♦ Patient verbalizes understanding of side effects and regimen required for prudent self-administration of carbidopa/levodopa.

CHLORAL HYDRATE

(klor′al-hye′drate)
Aquachloral, Noctec,
{Novochlorhydrate}

Classification(s):
Sedative-hypnotic; CNS depressant
Schedule C IV
Pregnancy Category C

INDICATIONS

♦ Insomnia (short-term management) ♦ Moderate anxiety ♦ Preoperative sedation ♦ Premedication for EEG evaluation ♦ Anxiety associated with drug withdrawal.

ACTION

♦ Not completely known. It is rapidly reduced to active metabolite, trichloroethanol, which at sedative-hypnotic doses is responsible for decreasing neural impulses and producing a mild CNS depression.

PHARMACOKINETICS

Absorption: Readily absorbed following oral or rectal administration.
Distribution: Rapidly distributed; extent not completely known. Crosses blood-brain and placental barriers and is excreted in breast milk.
Metabolism and Excretion: Rapidly converted to active metabolite trichloroethanol, which is metabolized by the liver and excreted as inactive compounds in urine and feces.
Half-Life: 8–11 hours (trichloroethanol).

CONTRAINDICATIONS AND PRECAUTIONS

Contraindicated in: ♦ Hypersensitivity to this drug ♦ Severe hepatic, renal, or cardiac disease ♦ Pregnancy ♦ Gastritis, esophagitis, or ulcer disease (oral form).
Use Cautiously in: ♦ Elderly or debilitated patients ♦ Depressed/suicidal patients ♦ Patients with a history of porphyria ♦ Patients with a history of drug abuse ♦ Lactation.

ADVERSE REACTIONS AND SIDE EFFECTS*

CNS: drowsiness, dizziness, ataxia, headache, paradoxical excitement.
Derm: skin rashes, urticaria, angioedema.
GI: nausea, vomiting, diarrhea, flatulence, offensive taste and breath.
Hemat: LEUKOPENIA.
Other: tolerance, physical and psychological dependence.

INTERACTIONS

Drug-Drug: ♦ **Other CNS depressants (including alcohol, benzodiazepines, opiates):** additive CNS depression ♦ **Oral anticoagulants:** transient increased effects of anticoagulants ♦ **IV furosemide:** blood pressure changes, flushing, diaphoresis.

ROUTE AND DOSAGE

Anxiety, Sedation
♦ **PO, Rect (Adults):** 250 mg tid after meals.
♦ **PO, Rect (Children):** 8.3 mg/kg tid; maximum dose 500 mg tid.

Insomnia
♦ **PO, Rect (Adults):** 500–1000 mg 15–30 minutes before retiring.
♦ **PO, Rect (Children):** 50 mg/kg (maximum 1000 mg per single dose).

Alcohol Withdrawal
♦ **PO, Rect (Adults):** 500–1000 mg. May be repeated q 6 h (maximum 2 g/24 hours).

{} = Only available in Canada.
*Underlines indicate most frequent; CAPITALS indicate life-threatening.

Premedication for EEG
+ **PO (Children):** 20–25 mg/kg.

PHARMACODYNAMICS

Route	Onset	Peak	Duration
PO, Rect	30–60 min	—	4–8 hr

NURSING IMPLICATIONS
Assessment
+ Assess level of anxiety and agitation. Report and document behaviors.
+ Assess sleep patterns. Keep records for adequate baseline data before the initiation of therapy.
+ Assess for suicidal ideation in depressed patients.
+ Assess history of allergies, sensitivity to this drug.
+ Assess date of last menses (possible pregnancy), use of contraceptives.
+ Assess whether currently breast-feeding a child.
+ Assess current and past alcohol and drug consumption.
+ Assess for operation of automobile and/or other dangerous machinery.
+ Assess for presence of adverse reactions or side effects.
+ Assess patient/family knowledge about illness and need for medication.
+ In collaboration with physician, assess CBC and renal and liver function tests in patients who have been on prolonged therapy.
+ **Lab Test Alterations:** May interfere with urinary 17-hydroxycorticosteroid and catecholamine determinations.
◇ False positive for glucose (copper sulfate urine testing).
+ **Withdrawal:** Assess for symptoms of withdrawal: • anxiety • tremors • insomnia • nausea/vomiting • weakness • diaphoresis • orthostatic hypotension • hallucinations • delirium • convulsions.
+ **Withdrawal Management:** Monitor vital signs.
◇ Place patient in quiet room with low stimuli.

◇ Institute seizure precautions.
◇ A long-acting barbiturate, such as phenobarbital, may be ordered to suppress withdrawal symptoms.
◇ Phenytoin may be ordered to prevent seizures.
◇ Some physicians may order oxazepam as needed for objective withdrawal symptoms, gradually decreasing the dosage until the drug is discontinued.
+ **Toxicity and Overdose:** Assess for symptoms of toxicity: • confusion • drowsiness • dyspnea • slurred speech • staggering.
◇ Assess for symptoms of overdose: • vomiting • miosis • areflexia • muscle flaccidity • CNS and respiratory depression • hypoventilation • hypothermia • hypotension • oliguria • tachycardia • coma. (May progress to respiratory arrest, circulatory, collapse, and death.)
+ **Overdose Management:** Monitor vital signs.
◇ Ensure maintenance of airway.
◇ Induce vomiting in conscious patient.
◇ Initiate gastric lavage in unconscious patient.
◇ Administer charcoal to minimize absorption of drug.
◇ Administer IV fluids.
◇ For severe intoxication, hemodialysis may be used. Peritoneal dialysis is *not* effective.

Potential Nursing Diagnoses
+ High risk for injury related to abrupt withdrawal from long-term use; decreased mental alertness caused by side effects of drowsiness and dizziness; effects of overdose.
+ High risk for self-directed violence related to depressed mood.
+ Anxiety (specify level) related to threats to physical integrity and/or self-concept.
+ Sleep pattern disturbance related to situational crisis; physical condition; severe level of anxiety.
+ High risk for activity intolerance, re-

lated to side effects of drowsiness, dizziness.

♦ Knowledge deficit related to medication regimen.

Plan/Implementation

♦ **General Info:** Monitor vital signs before beginning therapy and at regular intervals (bid) throughout therapy.

◊ Ensure that patient is protected from injury. Supervise and assist with ambulation if dizziness and drowsiness are problems. Ensure that patient avoids participation in any activity that requires mental alertness (including smoking). Raise siderails and instruct patient to remain in bed following administration.

◊ Store medication at controlled room temperatures between 15° and 30°C (59°–86°F). Protect from heat, light, and moisture.

♦ **PO:** To minimize irritation to gastric membranes, administer after meals or with food.

◊ Capsule should be taken whole with full glass of water, fruit juice, or other liquid. The solution may be mixed with a half glass of same liquids to increase palatability.

◊ Ensure capsule has been swallowed and not "cheeked" to avoid medication or to hoard for later use.

♦ **Rect:** Moisten suppository and gloved inserting finger with water. Ensure that area is free of irritation. If sedation has not been achieved within 30 minutes, recheck to ensure suppository has been retained.

Patient/Family Education

♦ Use caution in driving or when operating dangerous machinery. Drowsiness and dizziness can occur.

♦ Do not stop taking the drug abruptly. Doing so can produce serious (even life-threatening) withdrawal symptoms. If a dose is missed, take it as close as possible to prescribed time. If it is close to time for next dose, wait

until then; do not double up on dose at next prescribed time.

♦ Do not consume other CNS depressants (including alcohol).

♦ Be aware of possible risks of taking chloral hydrate during pregnancy (safety during pregnancy has not been established). Notify physician if pregnancy is suspected or planned.

♦ Be aware of potential side effects. Refer to written materials furnished by healthcare providers regarding correct method of self-administration.

♦ Report symptoms of sore throat, fever, malaise to physician immediately.

♦ Carry card or other identification at all times stating names of medications being taken.

Evaluation

♦ Patient demonstrates a subsiding/resolution of the symptoms for which chloral hydrate was prescribed (anxiety, sleep disturbances).

♦ Patient verbalizes understanding of side effects and regimen required for prudent self-administration of chloral hydrate.

CHLORDIAZEPOXIDE

(klor-dye-az-e-pox′ide)
Libritabs, Librium, {Medilium, Novopoxide, Relaxil}

Classification(s):
Antianxiety agent; Benzodiazepine
Schedule C IV
Pregnancy Category D

INDICATIONS

♦ Anxiety disorders ♦ Temporary relief of anxiety ♦ Acute alcohol withdrawal ♦ Preoperative sedation and reduction of anxiety.

ACTION

♦ Depresses subcortical levels of the central nervous system, particularly the limbic system and reticular formation ◆ Some studies have shown that this class of drugs potentiates the effects of the powerful inhibitory neurotransmitter gamma-aminobutyric acid (GABA) in the brain, thereby producing a calmative effect ◆ All levels of CNS depression can be effected, from mild sedation to hypnosis to coma.

PHARMACOKINETICS

Absorption: Rapidly absorbed from the GI tract; IM absorption slow and inconsistent.

Distribution: Is widely distributed. Crosses blood-brain and placental barriers; excreted in breast milk.

Metabolism and Excretion: Metabolized by the liver; produces active metabolites that are responsible for effects and that are excreted for the most part by the kidneys.

Half-Life: 5–30 hours.

CONTRAINDICATIONS AND PRECAUTIONS

Contraindicated in: Hypersensitivity to this drug or other benzodiazepines ◆ Concomitant use of other CNS depressants ◆ Pregnancy and lactation ◆ Narrow-angle glaucoma ◆ Shock ◆ Coma.

Use Cautiously in: Elderly or debilitated patients ◆ Patients with hepatic or renal dysfunction ◆ Individuals with history of drug abuse/addiction ◆ Depressed/suicidal patients ◆ Infants.

ADVERSE REACTIONS AND SIDE EFFECTS*

CNS: drowsiness, fatigue, ataxia, dizziness, confusion, headache, syncope, paradoxical excitement.

CV: bradycardia; with IV use: hypotension, SHOCK, CARDIOVASCULAR COLLAPSE.

Derm: rash, dermatitis, itching, pain at injection site.

Endo: gynecomastia, galactorrhea.

GI: dry mouth, nausea/vomiting, diarrhea, constipation, anorexia, weight gain

or loss, swollen tongue, metallic or bitter taste.

GU: urinary retention, incontinence, irregular menses, libidinal changes.

Hemat: neutropenia, GRANULOCYTOPENIA.

Resp: RESPIRATORY DEPRESSION (with IV use).

Other: tolerance, physical and psychological dependence.

INTERACTIONS

Drug-Drug: ◆ **Other CNS depressants (including alcohol, barbiturates, narcotics), antipsychotics, antidepressants, antihistamines:** additive CNS depression ◆ **Cimetidine and valproic acid:** increased effects of chlordiazepoxide ◆ **Oral contraceptives:** increased or decreased effects of chlordiazepoxide ◆ **Cigarette smoking and caffeine:** decreased effects of chlordiazepoxide ◆ **Phenytoin:** increased phenytoin serum levels (risk of toxicity) ◆ **Levodopa:** decreased effects of levodopa ◆ **Neuromuscular blocking agents:** increased respiratory depression ◆ **Digoxin:** reduced excretion of digoxin; increased potential for toxicity ◆ **Antitubercular drugs:** may increase or decrease levels ◆ **Disulfiram:** decreased clearance of chlordiazepoxide ◆ **All drugs in solution or syringe:** may cause precipitation of parenteral chlordiazepoxide.

ROUTE AND DOSAGE

Anxiety, Anxiety Disorders

- ◆ **PO (Adults):** 5–25 mg tid or qid.
- ◆ **IM, IV (Adults):** 50–100 mg initially, then 25–50 mg tid or qid as needed.
- ◆ **Geriatric, Debilitated, or Pediatric Patients:** Lower dosage usually required.

Acute Alcohol Withdrawal

- ◆ **PO (Adults):** 50–100 mg. Repeat dose as needed up to 300 mg/day.
- ◆ **IM, IV (Adults):** 50–100 mg initially; repeat in 2–4 hours if necessary.

*Underlines indicate most frequent; CAPITALS indicate life-threatening.

PHARMACODYNAMICS

Route	Onset	Peak	Duration
PO	15–30 min	2–4 hr	*
IM	15–30 min	15–30 min	*
IV	1–5 min	3–30 min	0.25–1 hr

*Varies with individual, age, disease state, and number of doses.

NURSING IMPLICATIONS

Assessment

♦ Assess level of anxiety. Symptoms include: • restlessness • pacing • insomnia • inability to concentrate • increased heart rate • increased respiration • elevated blood pressure • confusion • tremors • rapid speech.

♦ Assess for suicidal ideation (CNS depressants aggravate symptoms in depressed patients).

♦ Assess history of allergies, sensitivity to this drug.

♦ Assess history of glaucoma.

♦ Assess date of last menses (possible pregnancy), use of contraceptives.

♦ Assess whether currently breast-feeding a child.

♦ Assess current and past alcohol and drug consumption.

♦ Assess operation of automobile and/or other dangerous machinery.

♦ Assess for presence of adverse reactions or side effects.

♦ Assess patient/family knowledge about illness and need for medication.

♦ In collaboration with physician, assess CBC and liver function tests in patients on long-term therapy.

♦ **Lab Test Alterations:** May increase serum bilirubin, AST, and ALT.

◊ Abnormal renal function tests.

♦ **Withdrawal:** Assess for symptoms of withdrawal: • depression • insomnia • increased anxiety • abdominal and muscle cramps • tremors • vomiting • sweating • convulsions • delirium.

♦ **Withdrawal Management:** Monitor vital signs.

◊ Place patient in quiet room with low stimuli.

◊ Institute seizure precautions.

◊ A long-acting barbiturate, such as phenobarbital, may be ordered to suppress withdrawal symptoms.

◊ Phenytoin may be ordered to prevent seizures.

◊ Some physicians may order oxazepam as needed for objective withdrawal symptoms, gradually decreasing the dosage until the drug is discontinued.

♦ **Toxicity and Overdose:** Assess for symptoms of intoxication: • euphoria • relaxation • drowsiness • slurred speech • disorientation • mood lability • incoordination • unsteady gait • disinhibition of sexual and aggressive impulses • judgment and/or memory impairment.

◊ Assess for symptoms of overdose: • shallow respirations • cold and clammy skin • hypotension • dilated pupils • weak and rapid pulse • hypnosis • coma • possible death.

♦ **Overdose Management:** Monitor vital signs.

◊ Ensure maintenance of adequate airway.

◊ Induce vomiting in conscious patient.

◊ Initiate gastric lavage in unconscious patient.

◊ Administer activated charcoal to minimize absorption.

◊ Administer IV fluids.

◊ Administer norepinephrine or metaraminol to combat hypotension.

◊ Physician may also order flumazenil, a benzodiazepine antagonist.

◊ Forced diuresis with osmotic diuretics may help to accelerate elimination of the drug.

Potential Nursing Diagnoses

♦ High risk for injury related to seizures, panic anxiety, abrupt withdrawal from long-term chlordiazepoxide use, agitation from acute alcohol withdrawal, effects of chlordiazepoxide intoxication or overdose.

♦ High risk for self-directed violence related to depressed mood intensified by chlordiazepoxide.

* Anxiety (specify level) related to threats to physical integrity and/or self-concept.
* High risk for activity intolerance related to chlordiazepoxide side effects of lethargy, drowsiness, dizziness, muscular weakness.
* Knowledge deficit related to medication regimen.

Plan/Implementation

* **General Info:** Monitor vital signs before beginning therapy, at regular intervals (bid) throughout therapy, and q 10 minutes during IV administration.
◊ Ensure that patient practices good oral care. Offer hard, sugarless candy, gum, or frequent sips of water for dry mouth.
◊ Ensure that patient is protected from injury. Supervise and assist with ambulation if dizziness and muscular weakness are problems. Pad siderails and headboard for patient who experiences seizures.
* **PO:** If patient experiences nausea, medication may be given with food or milk.
◊ If patient has difficulty swallowing, tablet may be crushed (or capsule emptied) and mixed with food or fluid.
◊ Ensure that patient has actually swallowed tablet/capsule and not "cheeked" it to avoid medication or to hoard it for later use.
◊ Store tablets/capsules at controlled room temperatures between 15° and 30°C (59°–86°F).
* **IM:** Mix only with diluent provided by manufacturer. Prepare immediately before administration. Use only if solution appears clear. Discard any unused solution.
◊ IM diluent should be stored in refrigerator.
◊ Do not mix IM chlordiazepoxide with any other drug solution in vial or syringe.

◊ IM chlordiazepoxide is painful, and absorption by this route is unpredictable. Administer deep into large muscle mass to minimize pain and enhance absorption. Use Z-track method.
* **IV:** Solution reconstituted with special IM diluent should not be given IV. Use saline or sterile water to dilute (100 mg chlordiazepoxide to 5 mL diluent).
◊ Prepare immediately prior to administration. Discard any unused portion.
◊ Do not mix IV chlordiazepoxide with any other drug or solution in syringe or IV infusion bag.
◊ Avoid use of small veins to minimize risk of thrombophlebitis.
◊ Administer slowly (up to 100 mg over a minimum of 1 minute in adults) to reduce risk of respiratory depression, phlebitis, and/or cardiovascular collapse. Have patient remain in bed and observe closely for 2–3 hours.
◊ Ensure availability of emergency respiratory assistance.
◊ If direct injection into vein is not possible, inject into IV tubing as close as possible to site of vein insertion.
◊ Store medication at controlled room temperatures between 15° and 30°C (59°–86°F).

Patient/Family Education

* Do not drive or operate dangerous machinery. Drowsiness and dizziness can occur.
* Do not stop taking the drug abruptly. Doing so can produce serious withdrawal symptoms.
* Do not consume other CNS depressants (including alcohol).
* Do not take nonprescription medication without approval from physician.
* Carry card or other identification at all times stating names of medications being taken.
* Be aware of risks of taking chlordiazepoxide during pregnancy (congenital malformations have been associated with use during first trimester).

Notify physician of desirability to discontinue drug if pregnancy is suspected or planned.

♦ Be aware of possible side effects. Refer to written materials furnished by healthcare provider regarding correct method of self-administration.

Evalution

♦ Patient demonstrates a subsiding/resolution of the symptoms for which chlordiazepoxide was prescribed (anxiety; agitation, tremors, hallucinosis associated with acute alcohol withdrawal).

♦ Patient verbalizes understanding of side effects and regimen required for prudent self-administration of chlordiazepoxide.

CHLORMEZANONE

(klor-mez′a-none)
Trancopal

Classification(s):
Antianxiety agent; Metathiazanone
Pregnancy Category C

INDICATIONS

♦ Mild anxiety and tension states.

ACTION

♦ Depresses activity in the subcortical levels of the central nervous system ♦ Effectiveness in long-term use (more than 4 months) has not been established.

PHARMACOKINETICS

Absorption: Rapidly absorbed from the GI tract.
Distribution: Widely distributed. Transmission across placenta and excretion in breast milk not established.
Metabolism and Excretion: Partially metabolized by the liver; metabolites and unchanged drug are excreted by the kidneys.
Half-Life: 24 hours.

CONTRAINDICATIONS AND PRECAUTIONS

Contraindicated in: ♦ Hypersensitivity to this drug ♦ Children under 5 years of age.
Use Cautiously in: ♦ Elderly or debilitated patients ♦ Patients with hepatic or renal dysfunction ♦ Individuals with a history of drug abuse/addiciton ♦ Depressed/suicidal patients ♦ Preganancy and lactation.

ADVERSE REACTIONS AND SIDE EFFECTS*

CNS: <u>drowsiness</u>, <u>dizziness</u>, confusion, headache, paradoxical excitement, depression, weakness, slurred speech, tremor.
CV: tachycardia, hypotension, palpitations.
Derm: <u>rash</u>.
GI: <u>dry mouth</u>, nausea, anorexia.
GU: urinary retention, incontinence, irregular menses, libidinal changes.
Other: tolerance, physical and psychological dependence, cholestatic jaundice (rare and reversible).

INTERACTIONS

Drug-Drug: ♦ **Other CNS depressants (including alcohol, barbituartes, narcotics):** additive CNS depression.

ROUTE AND DOSAGE

Mild Anxiety and Tension States

♦ **PO (Adults):** 100–200 mg tid or qid.
♦ **PO (Children):** Ages 5–12: 50–100 mg tid or qid.

PHARMACODYNAMICS

Route	Onset	Peak	Duration
PO	15–30 min	UK	6 hr

NURSING IMPLICATIONS
Assessment

♦ Assess level of anxiety. Symptoms include: • restlessness • pacing • insomnia • inability to concentrate • increased heart rate • increased respirations • elevated blood pressure • confusion • tremors • rapid speech.

♦ Assess for suicidal ideation (CNS depressants aggravate symptoms in depressed patients).

♦ Assess history of allergies, sensitivity to this drug.

♦ Assess history of glaucoma.

♦ Assess date of last menses (possible pregnancy), use of contraceptives.

♦ Assess whether currently breast-feeding a child.

♦ Assess current and past alcohol and drug consumption.

♦ Assess operation of automobile and/or other dangerous machinery.

♦ Assess for presence of adverse reactions or side effects.

♦ Assess patient/family knowledge about illness and need for medication.

♦ In collaboration with physician, assess CBC and liver function tests in patients on long-term therapy.

♦ **Toxicity and Overdose:** Assess for symptoms of intoxication: • slurred speech • lethargy • heavy sedation.

◊ Assess for symptoms of overdose: • absence of reflexes • flaccidity • hypotension • coma.

♦ **Overdose Management:** Monitor vital signs.

◊ Ensure maintenance of adequate airway.

◊ Induce vomiting in conscious patient.

◊ Initiate gastric lavage in unconscious patient.

◊ Administer activated charcoal to minimize absorption.

◊ Administer IV fluids.

◊ Use of a vasopressor may be necessary to counteract severe hypotension.

Potential Nursing Diagnoses

♦ High risk for injury related to anxiety, abrupt withdrawal from long-term use, effects of intoxication or overdose.

♦ High risk for self-directed violence related to depressed mood.

♦ Anxiety (specify level) related to threats to physical integrity and/or self-concept.

♦ High risk for activity intolerance, related to chlormezanone's side effects of lethargy, drowsiness, dizziness, muscular weakness.

♦ Knowledge deficit related to medication regimen.

Plan/Implementation

♦ Monitor vital signs before beginning therapy and at regular intervals (bid) throughout therapy.

♦ Ensure that patient practices good oral care. Offer hard, sugarless candy, gum, or frequent sips of water for dry mouth.

♦ Ensure that patient is protected from injury. Supervise and assist with ambulation if dizziness and muscular weakness are problems.

♦ Following long-term use, ensure that patient does not discontinue drug abruptly. Dose should be tapered gradually to prevent possibility of withdrawal symptoms.

♦ To minimize nausea, chlormezanone may be given with food or milk.

♦ If patient has difficulty swallowing, tablet form may be crushed and mixed with food or fluid.

♦ Ensure that tablet has been swallowed and not "cheeked" to avoid medication or to hoard for later use.

♦ Store medication at controlled room temperatures between 15° and 30°C (59°–86°F). Protect from heat and moisture.

Patient/Family Education

♦ Do not drive or operate dangerous machinery. Drowsiness and dizziness can occur.

♦ Do not stop taking the drug abruptly. Doing so can result in serious withdrawal symptoms.

* Do not consume other CNS depressants (including alcohol).
* Do not take nonprescription medication without approval from physician.
* Be aware of risks of taking chlormezanone during pregnancy (safe use has not been established). Notify physician of desirability to discontinue drug if pregnancy is suspected or planned.
* Be aware of potential side effects. Refer to written materials furnished by healthcare providers regarding correct method of self-administration.
* Carry card or other identification at all times stating names of medications being taken.

Evaluation

* Patient demonstrates a subsiding/resolution of the symptoms for which chlormezanone was prescribed (mild anxiety and tension).
* Patient verbalizes understanding of side effects and regimen required for prudent self-administration of chlormezanone.

CHLORPROMAZINE

(klor-proe'ma-zeen)
Clorazine, {Chlor-Promanyl, Largactil}, Ormazine, Promapar, Promaz, Sonazine, Thorazine, Thor-Prom

Classification(s):
Antipsychotic; Antiemetic;
Neuroleptic; Phenothiazine
Pregnancy Category C

INDICATIONS

* Management of psychotic disorders such as schizophrenia, manic phase of bipolar disorder (until slower-acting lithium takes effect), brief reactive psychoses, and schizoaffective disorder ◆ Anxiety and agitation ◆ Intractable hiccups ◆ Acute intermittent porphyria ◆ Hyperactive children who exhibit excessive motor activity ◆ Severe behavioral problems in children, associated with explosive hyperexcitable behavior or combativeness ◆ Severe nausea and vomiting ◆ Pre- and postoperative sedation ◆ Tetanus (adjunctive treatment).

ACTION

* The exact mechanism of antipsychotic action is not fully understood, but is probably related to antidopaminergic effects ◆ Antipsychotics may block postsynaptic dopamine receptors in the basal ganglia, hypothalamus, limbic system, brain stem, and medulla ◆ Antipsychotic effects also appear to be related to inhibition of dopamine-mediated neurotransmission at the synapses ◆ Antipsychotic effects may also result from the drug's alpha-adrenergic blocking, muscarinic blocking, and adrenergic activity, as well as effects on other amines (such as GABA) or peptides.

PHARMACOKINETICS

Absorption: Rapid absorption of oral tablet and timed-release capsule dosage forms. Genetic differences in rate of first-pass metabolism result in a wide range of individual bioavailability. Oral liquid preparations and IM administration result in more consistent absorption.
Distribution: Widely distributed. Highly lipophilic; accumulates in brain, lungs, and other tissue with high blood supply. Crosses placental barrier; enters breast milk.
Metabolism and Excretion: Metabolized by the liver and in the kidneys. Excreted through kidneys and enterohepatic circulation. Active metabolites accumulate and are stored in fatty tissues over a prolonged period of time, and may be detected in urine up to 3–6 months following discontinuation of the drug.
Half-Life: 8–35 hours.

{} = Only available in Canada.

CONTRAINDICATIONS AND PRECAUTIONS

Contraindicated in: ◆ Hypersensitivity to this drug, other phenothiazines, or sulfites or tartrazine (contained in some preparations) ◆ Comatose or severely CNS-depressed patients ◆ Presence of large amounts of CNS depressants ◆ Bone marrow depression ◆ Blood dyscrasias ◆ Subcortical brain damage ◆ Parkinson's disease ◆ Liver, renal, and/or cardiac insufficiency ◆ Severe hypotension or hypertension ◆ Children under 6 months of age and women during pregnancy and lactation (safe use not established).

Use Cautiously in: ◆ Patients with a history of seizures ◆ Respiratory, renal, hepatic, thyroid, or cardiovascular disorders (e.g., respiratory infection, COPD, thyrotoxicosis, mitral insufficiency, angina pectoris) ◆ Prostatic hypertrophy ◆ Glaucoma ◆ Diabetes ◆ Elderly or debilitated patients ◆ Patients exposed to high or low environmental temperatures or to organophosphate insecticides ◆ Hypocalcemia ◆ Patients with a history of severe reactions to insulin or ECT ◆ Pediatric patients with acute illnesses or dehydration.

ADVERSE REACTIONS AND SIDE EFFECTS*

CNS: sedation, headache, seizures, insomnia, dizziness, exacerbation of psychotic symptoms, extrapyramidal symptoms (pseudoparkinsonism, akathisia, akinesia, dystonia, oculogyric crisis), tardive dyskinesia, fatigue, cerebral edema, ataxia, blurred vision. NEUROLEPTIC MALIGNANT SYNDROME, restlessness, anxiety, depression, hyperthermia or hypothermia.
CV: hypotension, orthostatic hypotension, hypertension, tachycardia, bradycardia, CARDIAC ARREST, ECG changes, ARRHYTHMIAS, PULMONARY EDEMA, CIRCULATORY COLLAPSE.

Derm: skin rashes, urticaria, petechiae, seborrhea, photosensitivity, eczema, erythema, hyperpigmentation, contact dermatitis, EXFOLIATIVE DERMATITIS (rare).
Endo: galactorrhea, gynecomastia (men), changes in libido, impotence, hyperglycemia or hypoglycemia, amenorrhea, retrograde ejaculation.
GI: dry mouth, nausea, vomiting, increased appetite and weight gain, anorexia, dyspepsia, constipation, diarrhea, jaundice, polydipsia, PARALYTIC ILEUS.
GU: urinary retention, frequency, or incontinence, bladder paralysis, polyuria, enuresis, priapism.
Hemat: AGRANULOCYTOSIS, LEUKOPENIA, ANEMIA, THROMBOCYTOPENIA, PANCYTOPENIA.
OPHTH: lens deposition.
Resp: LARYNGEAL EDEMA, LARYNGOSPASM, BRONCHOSPASM, SUPPRESSION OF COUGH REFLEX.
Other: decreased sweating.

INTERACTIONS

Drug-Drug: ◆ **CNS depressants (including alcohol, barbiturates, narcotics, anesthetics):** additive CNS depressant effects ◆ **Anticholinergic agents (e.g., atropine):** additive anticholinergic effects; decreased antipsychotic effects ◆ **Barbiturate anesthetics:** increased incidence of excitatory effects and hypotension ◆ **Barbiturates:** possible decreased effects of phenothiazines ◆ **Metyrosine:** potentiation of extrapyramidal side effects ◆ **Levodopa:** decreased efficacy of levodopa ◆ **Quinidine:** additive cardiac depressive effects ◆ **Magnesium- or aluminum-containing antidiarrheal mixtures, antacids:** reduced phenothiazine absorption/effectiveness ◆ **Guanethidine:** decreased antihypertensive action ◆ **Propranolol, metoprolol:** increased plasma levels and effects of both drugs ◆ **Lithium:** decreased plasma levels and effects of an-

*Underlines indicate most frequent; CAPITALS indicate life-threatening.

tipsychotic drug; severe neurotoxicity reported ◆ **Epinephrine:** reversal of usual pressor action of epinephrine, resulting in decreased blood pressure and tachycardia ◆ **Bromocriptine:** impairment of prolactin-suppressing action ◆ **Angiotensin converting enzyme (ACE) inhibitors:** increased effects of ACE inhibitors ◆ **Phenytoin:** decreased phenytoin metabolism, increased risk of toxicity ◆ **Polypeptide antibiotics:** possible neuromuscular respiratory depression ◆ **Metrizamide:** seizures ◆ **Cimetidine:** decreased effect of phenothiazines ◆ **Clonidine:** possibility of severe hypotension ◆ **Piperazine:** increased seizure potential.
Drug-Food: ◆ **Caffeine-containing beverages (e.g., coffee, tea, colas):** counteracted antipsychotic effects.

ROUTE AND DOSAGE

Psychoses, Acute Agitation
- **PO (Adults):** 10 mg tid or qid, or 25 mg bid or tid. Increase daily dosage by 20–50 mg semiweekly until symptoms are controlled.
- **PO (Adults, Maintenance):** Usual dose is 200 mg/day. Some patients may require as much as 800 mg/day.
- **PO (Children 6 Months and Older):** Outpatient dose is 0.5 mg/kg q 4–6 hours, as needed. Hospitalized patients may receive 50–100 mg/day. In older children, 200–500 mg may be required.
- **Rect (Children 6 Months and Older):** 1.0 mg/kg q 6–8 hours, as needed.
- **IM (Adults):** 25 mg. An additional 25–50 mg may be given in 1 hour, if necessary. Increase dosage gradually over several days (up to 400 mg q 4–6 hours in severe cases) until patient is controlled. Patient usually becomes quiet and cooperative within 24–48 hours. Oral dosage (500 mg/day is usually sufficient) may then be substituted. Gradual increases to 2 g/day may be necessary, but little therapeutic gain is achieved by exceeding 1 g/day for extended periods.
- **IM (Children):** 0.5 mg/kg q 6–8 hours, as needed. Maximum IM dosage: 40 mg/day for children up to 5 years old and weighing less than 22.7 kg; 75 mg/day for children 5–12 years old and weighing 22.7–45.5 kg. Generally not used in children less than 6 months of age.

Acute Intermittent Porphyria
- **PO (Adults):** 25–50 mg tid or qid.
- **IM (Adults):** 25 mg tid or qid.

Tetanus
- **IM (Adults):** 25–50 mg tid or qid, usually with barbiturates.
- **IV (Adults):** 25–50 mg diluted to a concentration not greater than 1 mg/mL and administered at rate of 1 mg/min.
- **IM, IV (Children):** 0.5 mg/kg q 6–8 hours. Maximum daily dosage: 40 mg for children up to 22.7 kg; 75 mg for children 22.7–45.5 kg. Maximum concentration for IV administration in children: 1 mg/mL; maximum rate: 0.5 mg/min.

Nausea and Vomiting
- **PO (Adults):** 10–25 mg q 4–6 hours.
- **PO (Children 6 Months and Older):** 0.5 mg/kg q 4–6 hours.
- **Rect (Adults):** 50–100 mg q 6–8 hours as needed.
- **Rect (Children 6 Months and Older):** 1.0 mg/kg q 6–8 hours as needed.
- **IM (Adults):** 25–50 mg q 3–4 hours as needed until symptoms subside.
- **IM (Children 6 Months and Older):** 0.5 mg/kg q 6–8 hours as needed. Maximum IM dosage: 40 mg/day for children up to 5 years old and weighing less than 22.7 kg. 75 mg/day for children 5–12 years old and weighing 22.7–45.5 kg.

Intractable Hiccups
- **PO (Adults):** 25–50 mg tid or qid.
- **IM (Adults):** If symptoms persist 2–3 days, 25–50 mg.

- **IV (Adults):** If PO and IM therapy are ineffective, 25–50 mg. Dilute in 500–1000 mL of normal saline and give as a slow infusion.

Preoperative Sedation

- **PO (Adults):** 25–50 mg 2–3 hours before surgery.
- **PO (Children 6 Months and Older):** 0.5 mg/kg 2–3 hours before surgery.
- **IM (Adults):** 12.5–25 mg 1–2 hours before surgery.
- **IM (Children 6 Months and Older):** 0.5 mg/kg 1–2 hours before surgery.

Postoperative Sedation

- **PO (Adults):** 10–25 mg q 4–6 hours, as needed.
- **PO (Children 6 Months and Older):** 0.5 mg/kg q 4–6 hours, as needed.
- **IM (Adults):** 12.5–25 mg. May be repeated in 1 hour if necessary and no hypotension has occurred.
- **IM (Children 6 Months and Older):** 0.5 mg/kg. May be repeated in 1 hour if necessary and no hypotension has occurred.

PHARMACODYNAMICS

Route	Onset*	Peak†	Duration‡
PO	30–60 min	2–4 hr	4–6 hr
PO (time release)	30–60 min	—	10–12 hr
Rect	45–75 min	—	3–4 hr
IM	15–30 min	15–20 min	4–8 hr
IV	5 min	5 min	—

*Full clinical effects may not be observed for 4–8 weeks.

†Steady-state plasma levels are achieved in approximately 4–7 days.

‡Drug may be detected in urine for 3–6 months after last dose.

NURSING IMPLICATIONS

Assessment

- Assess mental status daily. Assess: • mood • appearance • thought and communication patterns • level of interest in the environment and in activities • level of anxiety or agitation, • presence of hallucinations or delusions • suspiciousness • interactions with others • ability to carry out activities of daily living.
- Assess for symptoms of blood dyscrasias: • sore throat • fever • malaise • unusual bleeding • easy bruising.
- Assess for extrapyramidal symptoms: • pseudoparkinsonism (tremors, shuffling gait, drooling, rigidity) • akinesia (muscular weakness) • akathisia (continuous restlessness and fidgeting) • dystonia (involuntary muscular movements of face, arms, legs, and neck) • oculogyric crisis (uncontrolled rolling back of the eyes) • tardive dyskinesia (bizarre facial and tongue movements, stiff neck, difficulty swallowing).
- Assess for symptoms of neuroleptic malignant syndrome: • hyperpyrexia up to 107°F • elevated pulse • increased or decreased blood pressure • severe parkinsonian muscle rigidity • elevated creatinine phosphokinase blood levels • elevated white blood count • altered mental status (including catatonic signs or agitation) • acute renal failure • varying levels of consciousness (including stupor and coma) • pallor diaphoresis • tachycardia • arrhythmias • rhabdomyolysis.
- Assess vital signs, weight. Record baseline values for comparison.
- Assess history of allergies, sensitivity to this drug or to other phenothiazines.
- Assess for signs and symptoms of cholestatic jaundice: • abdominal pain • nausea • rash • fever • yellow skin • flu-like symptoms • abnormal lab test results (eosinophilia, bile in urine, increased serum transaminases, bilirubin, alkaline phosphatase).
- Assess date of last menses (possible pregnancy), use of contraceptives.
- Assess whether currently breast-feeding a child.

- Assess current and past alcohol and drug consumption.
- Assess operation of automobile and/or other dangerous machinery.
- Assess for presence of adverse reactions or side effects.
- Assess patient/family knowledge about illness and need for medication.
- In collaboration with physician, assess CBC and liver function tests and ophthalmological exams in patients on long-term therapy.
- **Lab Test Alterations:** Increased serum alkaline phosphatase, transaminases, bilirubin.
- ◊ Increase in protein-bound iodine.
- ◊ False-positive urine pregnancy test, possibly caused by drug metabolite that discolors the urine (less likely to occur when serum test is used).
- ◊ Increased urinary glucose.
- ◊ Decreased urinary estrogen, progestin, and gonadotropin.
- ◊ Increased plasma cholesterol level.
- ◊ Increased serum prolactin.
- **Withdrawal:** Assess for symptoms of abrupt withdrawal from long-term therapy: • gastritis • nausea • vomiting • dizziness • headache • tachycardia • insomnia • termulousness • sweating.
- **Toxicity and Overdose:** No correlation has been established between blood level and therapeutic effect.
- ◊ Assess for symptoms of overdose: • CNS depression, from heavy sedation to deep sleep to coma • hypotension • confusion • excitement • extrapyramidal symptoms • agitation • restlessness • convulsions • fever • autonomic reactions • ECG changes • cardiac arrhythmias • tachycardia • hypothermia • tremor • seizures • cyanosis.
- **Overdose Management:** Monitor vital signs.
- ◊ Ensure maintenance of open airway.
- ◊ Initiate gastric lavage.
- ◊ Do not induce emesis (nuchal rigidity may result in aspiration of vomitus).
- ◊ Antiparkinsonian drugs or diphenhydramine may be given to counteract extrapyramidal symptoms.
- ◊ Administer IV fluids or a vasoconstrictor to maintain adequate blood pressure. **Note:** Epinephrine is not recommended because of interaction with phenothiazines, causing further drop in blood pressure.
- ◊ Administer IV phenytoin for ventricular arrhythmias.
- ◊ Administer phenobarbital or diazepam to control convulsions or hyperactivity.
- ◊ Dialysis does not appear to be a useful intervention.

Potential Nursing Diagnoses

- High risk for violence directed at others, related to mistrust and panic anxiety.
- High risk for injury related to chlorpromazine side effects of sedation, dizziness, ataxia, weakness, lowered seizure threshold; abrupt withdrawal after prolonged use; overdose.
- Sensory-perceptual alteration related to panic anxiety evidenced by hallucinations.
- Altered thought processes related to panic anxiety evidenced by delusional thinking.
- Social isolation related to inability to trust others.
- High risk for activity intolerance, related to chlorpromazine's side effects of drowsiness, dizziness, ataxia, weakness.
- Noncompliance with medication regimen related to suspiciousness and mistrust of others.
- Knowledge deficit related to medication regimen.

Plan/Implementation:

- **General Info:** monitor vital signs before beginning therapy, and at regular intervals (bid or tid) throughout therapy. Take BP lying and standing to monitor for possible hypotensive reaction. Elderly are particularly susceptible. Dosage adjustment may be required.

◇ Ensure that patient who is ambulatory is protected from sun when spending time outdoors.

◇ Weigh patient 2–3 times a week, at same time of day, on same scale, if possible. A rapid weight gain or evidence of edema should be reported to physician immediately. Record I&O.

◇ Ensure that patient is protected from injury. Provide supervision and assistance when ambulating if dizziness and drowsiness are problems. Pad siderails and headboard for patient who experiences seizures.

◇ Give patient hard candy, gum, or frequent sips of water if dry mouth is a problem.

◇ Store all forms of chlorpromazine at controlled room temperatures between 15° and 30°C (59°–86°F). Protect from heat, moisture, and freezing.

♦ **PO:** Administer oral medication with food to minimize GI upset.

◇ Ensure that patient swallows tablet/capsule and does not "cheek" to avoid medication or to hoard for later use.

◇ Crush tablet and mix with food or fluid for patient who has difficulty swallowing, or use concentrate in fluid of choice.

◇ Do not open, crush, or chew capsules. Swallow whole.

◇ Mix concentrate just prior to administration with juice, milk, water, coffee, tea, carbonated beverage, or with semisolid food.

◇ If concentrate is accidentally spilled on skin or clothing during preparation or administration, wash area immediately, as contact dermatitis can occur.

♦ **Rect:** To ensure that suppository has been retained, check patient 20–30 minutes following rectal administration.

◇ To ensure accurate dosage, do not divide suppositories.

♦ **IM:** IM injection may be irritating to tissues; avoid SC injection.

◇ Avoid contact with injectable liquid. A contact dermatitis can occur.

◇ Inject slowly and deeply into upper, outer quadrant of buttock. Massage site thoroughly following injection.

◇ Because of possible hypotensive effects, patient should remain in recumbent position for at least one-half hour following IM injection.

◇ Rotate sites when multiple injections are administered.

◇ Do not mix with other agents in the syringe.

◇ Potency is not altered when solution is slightly yellow in color. Discard if marked discoloration is evident.

◇ Avoid injecting undiluted drug into vein. Aspirate carefully before injecting.

◇ If tissue irritation or pain is a problem, request order from physician for possible dilution. Injection may be diluted with saline or 2% procaine.

♦ **IV:** Because of possible hypotensive effects, drug should be administered with patient in recumbent position.

◇ Monitor blood pressure every 10 minutes during IV administration. Physician may order vasopressor (other than epinephrine) if hypotension occurs.

◇ IV solution should be diluted with normal saline to a concentration of at least 1 mg/mL.

◇ Potency is not altered when solution is slightly yellow in color. Discard if marked discoloration is evident.

◇ Administer direct IV, each 1 mg or fraction thereof over 1–2 minutes in adults; no faster than 0.5 mg per minute in children.

◇ Solution may be diluted in 500 mL of normal saline and given as an IV infusion. Recommended for intractable hiccups only.

Patient/Family Education

♦ Use caution when driving or when operating dangerous machinery. Drowsiness and dizziness can occur.

* Do not stop taking the drug abruptly. To do so might produce withdrawal symptoms, such as nausea, vomiting, gastritis, headache, tachycardia, insomnia, tremulousness.
* Use sunscreens and wear protective clothing when spending time outdoors. Skin is more susceptible to sunburn.
* Report occurrence of any of the following symptoms to physician immediately: sore throat, fever, malaise, unusual bleeding, easy bruising, persistent nausea/vomiting, severe headache, rapid heart rate, difficulty urinating, muscle twitching, tremors, darkly colored urine, pale stools, yellow skin or eyes, muscular incoordination, or skin rash.
* Drug may turn urine pink to reddish-brown in color. This is not significant nor is it harmful.
* Rise slowly from a sitting or lying position to prevent a sudden drop in blood pressure.
* If dry mouth is a problem, take frequent sips of water, chew sugarless gum, or suck on hard candy. Good oral care (frequent brushing, flossing) is very important.
* If you spill some liquid concentrate on your skin, wash it off immediately. If not, a rash may appear on the skin.
* Consult physician regarding smoking while on chlorpromazine therapy. Smoking increases metabolism of chlorpromazine, requiring adjustment in dosage to achieve therapeutic effect.
* Dress warmly in cold weather, and avoid extended exposure to very high or low temperatures. Body temperature is harder to maintain with this medication.

* Do not drink alcohol while on chlorpromazine therapy. These drugs potentiate each other's effects.
* Do not consume other medications (including over-the-counter meds) without physician's approval. Many medications contain substances that interact with chlorpromazine in a way that may be harmful.
* Be aware of possible risks of taking chlorpromazine during pregnancy. Safe use during pregnancy and lactation has not been established. Chlorpromazine readily crosses the placental barrier, so the fetus could experience adverse effects of the drug. Inform physician immediately if pregnancy occurs, is suspected, or is planned.
* Be aware of side effects of chlorpromazine. Refer to written materials furnished by healthcare providers for safe self-administration.
* Continue to take medication, even if feeling well and as though it is not needed. Symptoms may return if medication is discontinued.
* Carry card or other identification at all times describing medications being taken.

Evaluation

* Patient demonstrates a subsiding/resolution of the symptoms for which chlorpromazine was prescribed (panic anxiety, altered thought processes, altered perceptions, hiccups, nausea, and vomiting).
* Patient verbalizes understanding of side effects and regimen required for prudent self-administration of chlorpromazine.

CHLORPROTHIXENE

(klor-proe-thix′een)
Taractan, {Tarasan}

Classification(s):
Antipsychotic; Neuroleptic;
Thioxanthene
Pregnancy Category C

INDICATIONS

♦ Manifestations of psychotic disorders.

ACTION

♦ The exact mechanism of action is not fully understood ♦ Antipsychotics block postsynaptic dopamine receptors in the hypothalamus, limbic system, and reticular formation ♦ Antipsychotic effects appear to be related to inhibition of dopamine release, increased neuronal cell firing rate in the midbrain, and an increased turnover rate of dopamine in the forebrain ♦ Also has autonomic nervous system effects.

PHARMACOKINETICS

Absorption: Partial absorption of oral tablet dosage forms. Oral liquid preparations and IM administration result in more complete absorption.
Distribution: Widely distributed. Highly lipophilic; accumulates in brain, lungs, and other tissues with high blood supply. Crosses placental barriers; enters breast milk.
Metabolism and Excretion: Not completely known. At least partially metabolized by the liver. Excreted mainly in feces. Active metabolites accumulate and are stored in fatty tissue over a prolonged period of time and may be detected in urine up to several weeks following discontinuation of the drug.
Half-Life: Not well established.

CONTRAINDICATIONS AND PRECAUTIONS

Contraindicated in: ♦ Hypersensitivity to thioxanthenes, phenothiazines, or tartrazine (contained in some preparations) ♦ Comatose or severely CNS-depressed patients ♦ Presence of large amounts of CNS depressants ♦ Bone marrow depression ♦ Blood dyscrasias ♦ Subcortical brain damage ♦ Parkinson's disease ♦ Hepatic, renal, and/or cardiac insufficiency ♦ Severe hypotension or hypertension ♦ Patients with circulatory collapse ♦ Children under age 6 (oral use) ♦ Children under age 12 (parenteral use) ♦ Pregnancy and lactation (safe use not established).
Use Cautiously in: ♦ Patients with a history of seizures ♦ Respiratory, renal, hepatic, thyroid, or cardiovascular disorders (e.g., respiratory infection, thyrotoxicosis, mitral insufficiency, angina pectoris) ♦ Prostatic hypertrophy ♦ Glaucoma ♦ Diabetes ♦ Elderly or debilitated patients ♦ Patients in alcohol withdrawal ♦ Patients exposed to extreme environmental heat ♦ Patients taking atropine or atropine-like drugs.

ADVERSE REACTIONS AND SIDE EFFECTS*

CNS: sedation, headache, seizures, insomnia, dizziness, exacerbation of psychotic symptoms, extrapyramidal symptoms (pseudoparkinsonism, akathisia, akinesia, dystonia, oculogyric crisis) tardive dyskinesia, fatigue, cerebral edema, ataxia, blurred vision, restlessness, agitation, hyperpyrexia.
CV: orthostatic hypotension, hypertension, tachycardia, bradycardia, CARDIAC ARREST, ECG changes, ARRHYTHMIAS, PULMONARY EDEMA, CIRCULATORY COLLAPSE.
Derm: skin rashes, urticaria, petechiae, seborrhea, photosensitivity, eczema,

---

{} = Only available in Canada.
*Underlines indicate most frequent; CAPITALS indicate life-threatening.

pruritis, contact dermatitis, EXFOLIATIVE DERMATITIS (rare).

Endo: galactorrhea, gynecomastia (men), changes in libido, hyperglycemia or hypoglycemia, amenorrhea, retrograde ejaculation, enlarged parotid glands, glycosuria.

GI: dry mouth, nausea, vomiting, increased appetite and weight gain, anorexia, dyspepsia, constipation, diarrhea, jaundice, polydipsia, PARALYTIC ILEUS.

GU: urinary retention, frequency or incontinence, bladder paralysis, polyuria, enuresis, priapism.

Hemat: AGRANULOCYTOSIS, LEUKOPENIA, ANEMIA, THROMBOCYTOPENIA, PANCYTOPENIA, leukocytosis.

Resp: LARYNGOSPASM, BRONCHOSPASM, SUPPRESSION OF COUGH REFLEX.

Other: NEUROLEPTIC MALIGNANT SYNDROME.

INTERACTIONS

Drug-Drug: ◆ **CNS depressants (including alcohol, barbiturates, narcotics, anesthetics):** additive CNS depressant effects ◆ **Anticholinergic agents (e.g., atropine):** additive anticholinergic effects; decreased antipsychotic effects ◆ **Barbiturate anesthetics:** increased incidence of excitatory effects and hypotension ◆ **Barbiturates:** possible decreased antipsychotic effects ◆ **Metyrosine:** potentiation of extrapyramidal side effects ◆ **Levodopa:** possible decreased efficacy of levodopa/chlorprothixene ◆ **Quinidine:** additive cardiac depressive effects ◆ **Guanethidine:** decreased antihypertensive action ◆ **Lithium:** decreased plasma levels of chlorprothixene ◆ **Epinephrine:** reversal of usual pressor action of epinephrine, resulting in decreased blood pressure and tachycardia ◆ **Bromocriptine:** impairment of prolactin-suppressing action ◆ **Angiotensin converting enzyme (ACE) inhibitors:** increased effects of ACE inhibitors ◆ **Phenytoin:** decreased phenytoin metabolism; increased risk of toxicity ◆ **Polypeptide antibiotics:** neuromuscular respiratory depression ◆ **Metrizamide:** seizures ◆ **Cimetidine:** decreased antipsychotic effect ◆ **Clonidine:** possibility of severe hypotension and acute organic brain syndrome ◆ **Piperazine:** possible increased seizure potential.

Drug-Food: ◆ **Caffeine-containing beverages (e.g., coffee, tea, colas):** counteracted antipsychotic effect.

ROUTE AND DOSAGE

Psychotic Disorders

◆ **PO (Adults):** Initial dosage: 25–50 mg tid or qid. Increase gradually as needed. Dosages exceeding 600 mg/day are rarely required.

◆ **PO (Geriatric or Debilitated Patients):** 10–25 mg tid or qid.

◆ **PO (Children Over Age 6):** Initial dosage: 10–25 mg tid or qid. Increase gradually as needed and as tolerated.

◆ **IM (Adults):** 25–50 mg tid or qid.

◆ **IM (Children Over Age 12):** 25–50 mg tid or qid. Adjust to oral preparation gradually, alternating IM and PO doses initially.

PHARMACODYNAMICS

Route	Onset*	Peak†	Duration‡
PO	30–60 min	2–4 hr	4–6 hr
IM	10–30 min	1–2 hr	6–24 hr

*Full antipsychotic effects may not be observed for 4–8 weeks.

†Steady-state plasma levels are achieved in approximately 4–7 days.

‡Drug may be detected in urine for 3–6 months after last dose.

NURSING IMPLICATIONS

Assessment

◆ Assess mental status daily. Assess: ● mood ● appearance ● thought and communication patterns ● level of interest in the environment and in activities ● level of anxiety or agitation ● presence of hallucinations or delusions ● suspiciousness ● interactions with others ● ability to carry out activities of daily living.

◆ Assess for symptoms of blood dyscrasias: • sore throat • fever • malaise • unusual bleeding • easy bruising.

♦ Assess for extrapyramidal symptoms: • pseudoparkinsonism (tremors, shuffling gait, drooling, rigidity) • akinesia (muscular weakness) • akathisia (continuous restlessness and fidgeting) • dystonia (involuntary muscular movements of face, arms, legs, and neck) • oculogyric crisis (uncontrolled rolling back of the eyes) • tardive dyskinesia (bizarre facial and tongue movements, stiff neck, difficulty swallowing).

♦ Assess for symptoms of neuroleptic malignant syndrome: • hyperpyrexia up to 107°F • elevated pulse • increased or decreased blood pressure • severe parkinsonian muscle rigidity • elevated creatinine phosphokinase blood levels • elevated white blood count • altered mental status (including catatonic signs or agitation) • acute renal failure • varying levels of consciousness (including stupor and coma) • pallor diaphoresis • tachycardia • arrhythmias • rhabdomyolysis.

♦ Assess vital signs, weight. Record baseline values for comparison.

♦ Assess history of allergies, sensitivity to this drug or to other thioxanthenes or phenothiazines.

♦ Assess for signs and symptoms of cholestatic jaundice: • abdominal pain • nausea • rash • fever • yellow skin • flu-like symptoms • abnormal lab test results (eosinophilia, bile in urine, increased serum transaminases, bilirubin, alkaline phosphatase).

♦ Assess date of last menses (possible pregnancy), use of contraceptives.

♦ Assess whether currently breast-feeding a child.

♦ Assess current and past alcohol and drug consumption.

♦ Assess for operation of automobile and/or other dangerous machinery.

♦ Assess for presence of adverse reactions or side effects.

♦ Assess patient/family knowledge about illness and need for medication.

♦ In collaboration with physician, assess CBC and liver function tests and ophthalmological exams in patients on long-term therapy.

♦ **Lab Test Alterations:** Increased serum alkaline phosphatase, transaminases, bilirubin.

◊ Increased protein-bound iodine.

◊ False-positive urine pregnancy test, possibly caused by drug metabolite that discolors the urine (less likely to occur when serum test is used.)

◊ Increased urinary glucose.

◊ Decreased urinary estrogen, progestin, and gonadotropin.

◊ Increased plasma cholesterol level.

◊ Increased serum prolactin.

♦ **Withdrawal:** Assess for symptoms of abrupt withdrawal from long-term therapy: • gastritis • nausea • vomiting • dizziness • headache • tachycardia • insomnia • tremulousness • sweating.

♦ **Toxicity and Overdose:** No correlation has been established between blood level and therapeutic effect.

◊ Assess for symptoms of overdose: • CNS depression, from heavy sedation to deep sleep to coma • hypotension • confusion • excitement • extrapyramidal symptoms • agitation • restlessness • convulsions • fever • autonomic reactions • ECG changes • cardiac arrhythmias • tachycardia • hypothermia • tremor • seizures • cyanosis.

♦ **Overdose Management:** Monitor vital signs.

◊ Ensure maintenance of open airway.

◊ Initiate gastric lavage.

◊ Do not induce emesis (nuchal rigidity may result in aspiration of vomitus).

◊ Antiparkinsonian drugs or diphenhydramine may be given to counteract extrapyramidal symptoms.

◊ Administer IV fluids or a vasoconstrictor to maintain adequate blood pressure.

◇ **Note:** Epinephrine is not recommended because of its interaction with antipsychotics, which causes further drop in blood pressure.

◇ Administer IV phenytoin for ventricular arrhythmias.

◇ Administer phenobarbital or diazepam to control convulsions or hyperactivity.

◇ Dialysis does not appear to be a useful intervention.

Potential Nursing Diagnoses

♦ High risk for violence directed at others related to mistrust and panic anxiety.

♦ High risk for injury related to chlorprothixene's side effects of sedation, dizziness, ataxia, weakness, lowered seizure threshold; abrupt withdrawal after prolonged use; overdose.

♦ Sensory-perceptual alteration related to panic anxiety, evidenced by hallucinations.

♦ Altered thought processes related to panic anxiety, evidenced by delusional thinking.

♦ Social isolation related to inability to trust others.

♦ High risk for activity intolerance, related to chlorprothixene's side effects of drowsiness, dizziness, ataxia, weakness.

♦ Noncompliance with medication regimen related to suspiciousness and mistrust of others.

♦ Knowledge deficit related to medication regimen.

Plan/Implementation

♦ **General Info:** Monitor vital signs before beginning therapy and at regular intervals (bid or tid) throughout therapy. Take BP lying and standing to monitor for possible hypotensive reaction—elderly are particularly susceptible. Dosage adjustment may be required.

◇ Ensure that patient who is ambulatory is protected from sun when spending time outdoors.

◇ Weigh patient 2–3 times a week, at same time of day, on same scale, if possible. A rapid weight gain or evidence of edema should be reported to physician immediately. Record I&O.

◇ Ensure that patient is protected from injury. Provide supervision and assistance when ambulating if dizziness and drowsiness are problems. Pad siderails and headboard for patient who experiences seizures.

◇ Give patient hard candy, gum, or frequent sips of water if dry mouth is a problem.

◇ Store medication at controlled room temperatures between 15°C and 30°C (59°–86°F). Protect from heat, light, and moisture.

♦ **PO:** Administer oral medication with food to minimize GI upset.

◇ Ensure patient swallows tablet and does not "cheek" to avoid medication or to hoard for later use.

◇ Crush tablet and mix with food or fluid for patient who has difficulty swallowing, or give liquid concentrate.

◇ Administer concentrate undiluted or mix with milk, water, fruit juice, coffee, or carbonated beverage.

◇ If concentrate is accidentally spilled on skin or clothing during preparation or administration, wash area immediately, as contact dermatitis can occur.

♦ **IM:** Avoid contact with injectable liquid. A contact dermatitis can occur.

◇ Inject slowly and deeply into upper, outer quadrant of buttock or other large muscle mass, such as midlateral thigh.

◇ Because of possible hypotensive effects, patient should remain in recumbent position for at least 1 hour following IM injection. Monitor blood pressure every 10 minutes during this time.

◇ Rotate sites when multiple injections are administered.

◇ Aspirate carefully to avoid injection directly into blood vessel.

◇ Switch to oral medication as soon as feasible. Gradually give oral and parenteral doses alternately on the same day, then oral doses only.

Patient/Family Education

+ Use caution when driving or when operating dangerous machinery. Drowsiness and dizziness can occur.
+ Do not stop taking the drug abruptly. To do so might produce withdrawal symptoms, such as nausea, vomiting, gastritis, headache, tachycardia, insomnia, tremulousness.
+ Use sunscreens and wear protective clothing when spending time outdoors. Skin is more susceptible to sunburn.
+ Report occurrence of any of the following symptoms to physician immediately: • sore throat • fever • malaise • unusual bleeding • easy bruising • persistent nausea/vomiting • severe headache • rapid heart rate • difficulty urinating • muscle twitching • tremors • darkly colored urine • pale stools • yellow skin or eyes • muscular inco-ordination or skin rash.
+ Drug may turn urine pink to reddish-brown in color. This is not significant, nor is it harmful.
+ Rise slowly from a sitting or lying position to prevent a sudden drop in blood pressure.
+ If dry mouth is a problem, take frequent sips of water, chew sugarless gum, or suck on hard candy. Good oral care (frequent brushing, flossing) is very important.
+ Liquid concentrate spilled on the skin should be washed off immediately. If not, a rash may appear on the skin.
+ Consult physician regarding smoking while on chlorprothixene therapy. Smoking increases metabolism of chlorprothixene, requiring adjustment in dosage to achieve therapeutic effect.

+ Dress warmly in cold weather and avoid extended exposure to very high or low temperatures. Body temperature is harder to maintain while taking this medication.
+ Do not drink alcohol while on chlorprothixene therapy. These drugs potentiate each other's effects.
+ Do not consume other medications (including over-the-counter meds) without physician's approval. Many medications contain substances that interact with chlorprothixene in a way that may be harmful.
+ Be aware of possible risks of taking chlorprothixene during pregnancy. Safe use during pregnancy and lactation has not been established. It is known that chlorprothixene readily crosses the placental barrier, so the fetus could experience adverse effects of the drug. Inform physician immediately if pregnancy occurs, is suspected, or is planned.
+ Be aware of side effects of chlroprothixene. Refer to written materials furnished by healthcare providers for safe self-administration.
+ Continue to take medication, even if feeling well and as though it is not needed. Symptoms may return if medication is discontinued.
+ Carry card or other identification at all times describing medications being taken.

Evaluation

+ Patient demonstrates a subsiding/resolution of the symptoms for which chlorprothixene was prescribed (panic anxiety, altered thought processes, altered perceptions).
+ Patient verbalizes understanding of side effects and regimen required for prudent self-administration of chlorprothixene.

CLOMIPRAMINE

(kloe-mi′ pra-meen)
Anafranil

Classification(s):
Tricyclic antidepressant
Pregnancy Category C

INDICATIONS

♦ Severe obsessive-compulsive disorder ♦ Patients currently maintained on the drug, for whom therapeutic benefit has been established (obsessive-compulsive disorder not a criterion for treatment with these individuals) **Investigational uses:** ♦ Depressive symptoms, panic disorder, or phobic disorder, but only if obsessive-compulsive disorder is the primary diagnosis and strongly dominates the clinical picture. Has been used for some time in Europe to treat symptoms of depression, but has not been approved in the U.S. due to apparent risk of seizures identified in controlled trials to date.

ACTION

♦ Exact mechanism of action unclear ♦ Clomipramine appears to block primarily serotonin reuptake, while its active metabolite, desmethylclomipramine (DMCL), blocks norepinephrine reuptake, resulting in increased levels of these biogenic amines.

PHARMACOKINETICS

Absorption: Well absorbed from the GI tract following oral administration.
Distribution: Widely distributed. Thought to cross placental barrier and to enter breast milk.
Metabolism and Excretion: Metabolized by the liver. Excreted in urine.
Half-Life: 12–84 hours.

CONTRAINDICATIONS AND PRECAUTIONS

Contraindicated in: ♦ Hypersensitivity to this drug or to other tricyclic antidepressants ♦ Concomitant use of MAO inhibitors ♦ Acute recovery period following myocardial infarction ♦ Pregnancy and lactation (safety not established).
Use Cautiously in: ♦ Patients with a history of seizures ♦ Urinary retention ♦ Glaucoma ♦ Cardiovascular disorders ♦ Hepatic or renal insufficiency ♦ Psychotic patients ♦ Elderly or debilitated patients ♦ Acute intermittent porphyria.

ADVERSE REACTIONS AND SIDE EFFECTS*

CNS: drowsiness, dizziness, weakness, headache, fatigue, confusion, lethargy, memory deficits, disturbed concentration, tremors, ataxia, tinnitus, extrapyramidal symptoms, paresthesias of extremities, lowered seizure threshold, blurred vision, agitation, excitement, restlessness, insomnia, exacerbation of psychosis, shift to manic behavior.
CV: orthostatic hypotension, tachycardia and other arrhythmias, hypertension, MYOCARDIAL INFARCTION, HEART BLOCK, CONGESTIVE HEART FAILURE, ECG changes, syncope, CARDIOVASCULAR COLLAPSE.
Derm: skin rash, urticaria, photosensitivity, erythema, petechiae.
GI: dry mouth, constipation, nausea, vomiting, anorexia, diarrhea, abdominal cramps, adynamic ileus, esophageal reflux, stomatitis, black tongue.
GU: urinary retention, gynecomastia (men), testicular swelling, menstrual irregularity, breast engorgement and galactorrhea (women), changes in libido, impotence, delayed micturation, delayed or absent orgasm.
Hemat: AGRANULOCYTOSIS, THROMBOCYTOPENIA, LEUKOPENIA, eosinophilia, purpura.
Hepat: jaundice, hepatitis.

---

*Underlines indicate most frequent; CAPITALS indicate life-threatening.

Other: weight gain, nasal conjestion, alopecia, hypothermia, peripheral neuropathy.

INTERACTIONS

Drug-Drug: ♦ **MAO inhibitors:** hyperpyretic crisis, hypertensive crisis, severe seizures, tachycardia, death ♦ **Guanethidine, clonidine, (possibly) guanabenz:** decreased effects of these medications ♦ **Cimetidine:** increased clomipramine serum levels ♦ **Amphetamines, sympathomimetics:** increased hypertensive and cardiac effects of these drugs ♦ **CNS depressants (including alcohol, barbiturates, benzodiazepines):** potentiation of CNS effects ♦ **Thyroid medications:** tachycardia, arrhythmias ♦ **Methylphenidate, phenothiazines, haloperidol:** increased serum clomipramine levels ♦ **Ethchlorvynol:** transient delirium ♦ **Quinidine, procainamide, disopyramide:** potentiates adverse cardiovascular effects of clomipramine ♦ **Oral contraceptives:** decreased effects of clomipramine ♦ **Smoking:** increased clomipramine metabolism ♦ **Disulfiram:** decreased clomipramine metabolism ♦ **Levodopa, phenylbutazone:** delayed or decreased absorption of these drugs ♦ **Warfarin:** increased prothrombin time ♦ **Dicumarol:** increased plasma dicumarol concentrations.

ROUTE AND DOSAGE

Obsessive-Compulsive Disorder

- **PO (Adults):** Initial dosage: 25 mg/day. Gradually increase dosage to 100 mg/day during the first 2 weeks. May increase gradually over next several weeks to maximum daily dosage of 250 mg. May be given once daily at HS to minimize daytime sedation.
- **PO (Children):** Initial dosage: 25 mg/day. Gradually increase during first 2 weeks up to maximum of 3 mg/kg or 100 mg, whichever is smaller. May increase gradually over next several weeks to a maximum daily dosage

of 3 mg/kg or 200 mg, whichever is smaller. May give single dose at bedtime to minimize daytime sedation.

Depression

- **PO (Adults):** 75–150 mg/day in 1–3 divided doses. Lower doses of 30–50 mg/day may be sufficient for some patients. Dosage should be started low and gradually increased.

PHARMACODYNAMICS

Route	Onset	Peak	Duration
PO (obs-comp)	5–10 wk	—	weeks*
PO (depression)	2–4 wk	—	weeks*

*Allow up to 2 weeks following cessation of therapy for complete drug elimination.

NURSING IMPLICATIONS

Assessment

- Assess for suicidal ideation, plan, means. Assess for sudden lifts in mood, which could indicate patient's decision to commit suicide.
- Assess mental status daily. Assess: • mood • appearance • thought and communication patterns • level of interest in the environment and in activities • suicidal ideation. Improvement in these behavior patterns and level of energy should be expected in 2–4 weeks following initiation of therapy.
- Assess for evidence of obsessions or compulsions. Note degree to which these thoughts and behaviors interfere with daily functioning.
- Assess for symptoms of blood dyscrasias: • sore throat • fever • malaise • unusual bleeding • easy bruising.
- Assess vital signs, weight.
- Assess history of allergies, sensitivity to this drug or to other tricyclic antidepressants.
- Assess for history of glaucoma.
- Assess data of last menses (possible pregnancy), use of contraceptives.
- Assess whether currently breast-feeding a child.
- Assess current and past alcohol and drug consumption.

♦ Assess operation of automobile and/or other dangerous machinery.

♦ Assess for presence of adverse reactions or side effects.

♦ Assess level of knowledge about illness and need for medication.

♦ In collaboration with physician, assess CBC and liver function tests in patients on long-term therapy.

♦ **Lab Test Alterations:** Increased serum bilirubin, alkaline phosphatase, transaminase, and glucose.

◊ Decreased urinary 5-hydroxyindole-acetic acid (HIAA) and vanillylmandelic acid (VMA) excretion.

♦ **Withdrawal:** Assess for symptoms of abrupt withdrawal from long-term therapy: • nausea • headache • vertigo • malaise • insomnia • nightmares.

♦ **Toxicity and Overdose:** Range of therapeutic serum concentration has not been well substantiated.

◊ Assess for symptoms of overdose: • confusion • agitation • irritability • hallucinations • seizures • flushing • dry mouth • dilated pupils • delirium • hyperpyrexia • hypotension or hypertension • coma • tachycardia • arrhythmias • respiratory depression • cardiac arrest • renal failure • shock • congestive heart failure • acid-base disturbances.

♦ **Overdose Management:** Monitor vital signs.

◊ Ensure maintenance of open airway.

◊ Monitor ECG.

◊ Induce emesis in conscious patient.

◊ Initiate gastric lavage in unconscious patient.

◊ Administer activated charcoal to minimize absorption.

◊ Administer IV physostigmine cautiously to reverse anticholinergic effects.

◊ Use sodium bicarbonate, vasopressors, propranolol, or lidocaine for cardiovascular effects.

◊ Administer IV diazepam or phenytoin for seizures.

Potential Nursing Diagnoses

♦ High risk for self-directed violence related to depressed mood.

♦ Ineffective individual coping (obsessive-compulsive behaviors) related to repressed anxiety.

♦ High risk for injury related to clomipramine's side effects of sedation, dizziness, ataxia, weakness, confusion, lowered seizure threshold; abrupt withdrawal after prolonged use; overdose.

♦ Social isolation related to depressed mood and/or obsessive-compulsive behaviors.

♦ High risk for activity intolerance related to clomipramine side effects of drowsiness, dizziness, ataxia, weakness, confusion.

♦ Knowledge deficit related to medication regimen.

Plan/Implementation

♦ Monitor vital signs before beginning therapy and at regular intervals (bid or tid) throughout therapy. Take BP lying and standing in patients experiencing orthostatic hypotension; elderly are particularly susceptible. Contact physician if tachycardia/arrhythmias are noted.

♦ Ensure that patient who is ambulatory is protected from sun when spending time outdoors.

♦ Weigh patient 2–3 times a week, at same time of day, on same scale, if possible. A rapid weight gain or evidence of edema should be reported to physician immediately. Record I&O.

♦ Ensure that patient is protected from injury. Provide supervision and assistance when ambulating if dizziness and drowsiness are problems. Pad siderails and headboard for patient who experiences seizures.

♦ Give patient hard candy, gum, or frequent sips of water if dry mouth is a problem.

♦ Administer oral medication with food to minimize GI upset.

• Ensure that patient swallows capsule and does not "cheek" to avoid medication or to hoard for later use.

• Capsule may be emptied and mixed with food or fluid for patient who has difficulty swallowing.

• Store medication at controlled room temperatures between 15° and 30°C (59°–86°F). Protect from heat and moisture.

Patient/Family Education

• Therapeutic effect may not be seen for several weeks. If improvement is not experienced within a few weeks, physician may prescribe a different medication. Continue to take medication even though symptoms have not subsided.

• Use caution when driving or when operating dangerous machinery. Drowsiness and dizziness can occur. If these side effects become persistent or interfere with daily activities, report to physician. Dosage adjustment may be necessary.

• Do not stop taking the drug abruptly. To do so might produce withdrawal symptoms, such as nausea, vertigo, insomnia, headache, malaise, nightmares.

• Use sunscreens and wear protective clothing when spending time outdoors. Skin may be sensitive to sunburn.

• Report occurrence of any of the following symptoms to physician immediately: sore throat, fever, malaise, unusual bleeding, easy bruising, persistent nausea/vomiting, severe headache, rapid heart rate, difficulty urinating.

• Rise slowly from a sitting or lying position to prevent a sudden drop in blood pressure.

• If dry mouth is a problem, take frequent sips of water, chew sugarless gum, or suck on hard candy. Good oral care (frequent brushing, flossing) is very important.

• Do not smoke while on clomipramine therapy. Smoking increases metabolism of clomipramine, requiring adjustment in dosage to achieve therapeutic effect.

• Do not drink alcohol while on clomipramine therapy. These drugs potentiate each other's effects.

• Do not consume other medications (including over-the-counter meds) without physician's approval. Many medications contain substances that, in combination with tricyclics, could precipitate a life-threatening hypertensive crisis.

• Be aware of possible risks of taking clomipramine during pregnancy. Safe use during pregnancy and lactation has not been established. It is thought that clomipramine readily crosses the placental barrier; if so, a fetus could experience adverse effects of the drug. Inform physician immediately if pregnancy occurs, is suspected, or is planned.

• Be aware of side effects of clomipramine. Refer to written materials furnished by healthcare providers for safe self-administration.

• Carry card or other identification at all times describing medications being taken.

Evaluation

• Patient demonstrates a subsiding/resolution of the symptoms for which clomipramine was prescribed (depressed mood, suicidal ideation, obsessive-compulsive behaviors).

• Patient verbalizes understanding of side effects and regimen required for prudent self-administration of clomipramine.

CLONAZEPAM

(kloe-na'ze-pam)
Klonopin

Classification(s):
Anticonvulsant; Benzodiazepine
derivative
Schedule C IV
Pregnancy Category C

INDICATIONS

✦ Absence (petit mal), Lennox-Gastaut (petit mal variant), akinetic, and myoclonic seizures (prophylactic treatment) ✦ Absence seizures refractory to succinimides. **Investigational Use:** ✦ Panic attacks. **Unlabeled Uses:** ✦ Periodic leg movements during sleep ✦ Parkinsonian dysarthria ✦ Acute manic episodes ✦ Multifocal tic disorders ✦ Adjunct treatment of schizophrenia.

ACTION

✦ Not completely understood ✦ May potentiate effects of inhibitory neurotransmitter gamma-aminobutyric acid (GABA) in the brain ✦ Appears to suppress spike and wave discharge in absence (petit mal) seizures and decreases frequency, amplitude, duration, and spread of discharge in minor motor seizures.

PHARMACOKINETICS

Absorption: Rapidly absorbed from the GI tract.
Distribution: Thought to be widely distributed. Crosses the blood-brain and placental barriers; excreted in breast milk.
Metabolism and Excretion: Metabolized by the liver; metabolites excreted by the kidneys.
Half-Life: 18–39 hours.

CONTRAINDICATIONS AND PRECAUTIONS

Contraindicated in: ✦ Hypersensitivity to this drug or to other benzodiazepines ✦ Acute angle-closure glaucoma ✦ Severe liver disease ✦ Lactation.
Use Cautiously in: ✦ Elderly or debilitated patients ✦ Patients with hepatic or renal dysfunction ✦ Individuals with a history of drug abuse/addiction ✦ Depressed/suicidal patients ✦ Pregnancy ✦ Long-term use with children (safety not established). **Note:** Sole use of this medication in some patients with mixed type of epilepsy may increase incidence of tonic-clonic (grand mal) seizures.

ADVERSE REACTIONS AND SIDE EFFECTS*

CNS: drowsiness, ataxia, behavior problems, dizziness, confusion, headache, lethargy, insomnia, abnormal eye movements, diplopia, choreiform movements, nystagmus, vertigo, slurred speech, tremor, psychosis.
CV: palpitations.
Derm: skin rashes, alopecia, hirsuitism.
GI: dry mouth, nausea/vomiting, diarrhea, constipation, anorexia, hepatomegaly, gastritis, sore gums, increased salivation.
GU: urinary retention, dysuria, enuresis.
Hemat: BLOOD DYSCRASIAS, anemia, leukopenia, eosinophilia, thrombocytopenia.
Resp: chest congestion, dyspnea, RESPIRATORY DEPRESSION.
Other: tolerance, physical and psychological dependence.

INTERACTIONS

Drug-Drug: ✦ **Other CNS depressants (including alcohol, barbiturates, narcotics), antipsychotics, antidepressants, antihistamines, anticonvulsants:** additive CNS depression ✦ **valproic acid:** absence (petit mal) status ✦ **Phenobarbital, phenytoin, carbamazepine:** decreased therapeutic effect of clonazepam ✦ **Disulfiram:** increased clonazepam effect, toxicity.

*Underlines indicate most frequent; CAPITALS indicate life-threatening.

ROUTE AND DOSAGE
Petit Mal, Petit Mal Variant, Akinetic, or Myoclonic Seizures
* **PO (Adults:)** Initial dosage: 1.5 mg/day in 3 divided doses. May be increased by 0.5–1 mg every 3 days until control is achieved with minimal side effects. Maximum dose: 20 mg/day.
* **PO (Children under Age 10):** Initial dosage: 0.01–0.03 mg/kg/day in 2–3 divided doses. Maximum initial dose: 0.05 mg/kg/day. May be increased by 0.25–0.5 mg every 3 days to a maintenance dose of 0.1–0.2 mg/kg, divided into 3 doses, or until control is achieved with minimal side effects.
* **Discontinuation of Therapy:** Decrease dosage gradually to prevent precipitation of seizures, status epilepticus, or withdrawal symptoms.

Panic Attacks
* **PO (Adults):** 2–9 mg/day, divided into 2 doses.

Periodic Leg Movements During Sleep
* **PO (Adults):** 0.5–2 mg at HS.

Parkinsonian Dysarthria
* **PO (Adults):** 0.25–0.5 mg daily.

Acute Manic Episode
* **PO (Adults):** 0.75–16 mg daily.

Multifocal Tic Disorders
* **PO (Adults):** 1.5–12 mg daily.

Adjunct Treatment of Schizophrenia
* **PO (Adults):** 0.5–2 mg daily.

PHARMACODYNAMICS

Route	Onset	Peak	Duration
PO	20–60 min	1–2 hr	6–12 hr
			6–8 hr (infants)

NURSING IMPLICATIONS
Assessment
* Assess occurrence, characteristics, and duration of seizure activity.
* Assess for suicidal ideation (CNS depressants aggravate symptoms in depressed patients).
* Assess baseline vital signs.
* Assess history of allergies, sensitivity to this drug or to other benzodiazepines.
* Assess history of glaucoma.
* Assess date of last menses (possible pregnancy), use of contraceptives.
* Assess whether currently breast-feeding a child.
* Assess current and past alcohol and drug consumption.
* Assess operation of automobile and/or other dangerous machinery.
* Assess for presence of adverse reactions or side effects.
* Assess patient/family knowledge about illness and need for medication.
* In collaboration with physician, assess CBC and liver function tests in patients on long-term therapy.
* **Lab Test Alterations:** Increased serum transaminase and alkaline phosphatase.
* **Withdrawal:** Assess for symptoms of withdrawal: • depression • insomnia • increased anxiety • abdominal and muscle cramps • tremors • vomiting • sweating • convulsions • delirium.
* **Withdrawal Management:** Monitor vital signs.
◊ Place patient in quiet room with low stimuli.
◊ Institute seizure precautions.
◊ A long-acting barbiturate, such as phenobarbital, may be ordered to suppress withdrawal symptoms.
◊ Phenytoin may be ordered to prevent seizures.
◊ Some physicians may order oxazepam as needed for objective withdrawal symptoms, gradually decreasing the dosage until the drug is discontinued.
* **Toxicity and Overdose:** Range of therapeutic serum concentration is thought to be 20–80 ng/mL.
◊ Assess for symptoms of intoxication: • euphoria • relaxation • drowsiness • slurred speech • disorientation •

mood lability • incoordination • unsteady gait • disinhibition of sexual and aggressive impulses • judgment and/or memory impairment.

◊ Assess for symptoms of overdose: • somnolence • confusion • ataxia • diminished reflexes • shallow respirations • cold and clammy skin • hypotension • dilated pupils • weak and rapid pulse • hypnosis • coma.

✦ **Overdose Management:** Monitor vital signs.

◊ Ensure maintenance of adequate airway.

◊ Induce vomiting in conscious patient.

◊ Initiate gastric lavage in unconscious patient.

◊ Administer activated charcoal to minimize absorption.

◊ IV fluids and vasopressors may be used to combat hypotension.

◊ Forced diuresis may be used to facilitate elimination of the drug.

Potential Nursing Diagnoses

✦ High risk for injury related to seizures; abrupt withdrawal from long-term clonazepam use; effects of clonazepam intoxication or overdose.

✦ High risk for self-directed violence related to depressed mood.

✦ Social isolation related to fear of experiencing a seizure in the presence of others.

✦ High risk for activity intolerance, related to clonazepam's side effects of lethargy, drowsiness, dizziness, ataxia.

✦ Knowledge deficit related to medication regimen.

Plan/Implementation

✦ Monitor vital signs before beginning therapy and at regular intervals (bid) throughout therapy.

✦ Ensure that patient practices good mouth care. Offer patient hard, sugarless candy; gum; frequent sips of water for dry mouth.

✦ Ensure that patient is protected from injury. Supervise and assist with ambulation if dizziness and muscular weakness are problems. Pad siderails and headboard for patient who experiences seizures.

✦ Monitor and record lab assessments of serum clonazepam levels.

✦ Report the presence of sore throat, fever, malaise, unusual bleeding, easy bruising, dark urine, jaundice to physician immediately.

✦ To minimize nausea, give medication with food or milk.

✦ If patient has difficulty swallowing, crush tablet and mix with food or fluid.

✦ Ensure that tablet has been swallowed and not "cheeked" to avoid medication or to hoard for later use.

✦ Store medication at controlled room temperatures between 15° and 30°C (59°–86°F). Protect from heat, light, and moisture.

Patient/Family Education

✦ Do not drive or operate dangerous machinery until individual response has been determined. Drowsiness and dizziness can occur.

✦ Do not stop taking the drug abruptly. Doing so can result in serious withdrawal symptoms or status epilepticus.

✦ Do not consume other CNS depressants (including alcohol).

✦ Do not take nonprescription medication without approval from physician.

✦ Be aware of risks of taking clonazepam during pregnancy. There is an association between use of anticonvulsant drugs by women with epilepsy and the incidence of birth defects in their offspring. A patient who requires the medication to prevent seizures may be maintained on it; however, she must be fully aware of potential risks to unborn child. If pregnancy occurs, is suspected, or is planned, notify physician immediately.

✦ Report any of the following symptoms to physician promptly: sore throat, fever, malaise, unusual bleeding, easy bruising, dark urine, yellow skin or eyes.

- Protect patient during seizure. In the case of tonic-clonic (grand mal) seizure, do not restrain. Padding may be used (towels, blankets, pillows) to prevent bumping against hard objects. When convulsion has subsided, turn patient on side to allow secretions to drain and to prevent aspiration. Keep records of occurrence, characteristics, and duration of seizures, so that accurate reports may be given to physician for providing assistance in stabilization and control of seizures. If patient has difficulty breathing or continues to experience subsequent seizures, family should immediately call for emergency assistance.
- Be aware of potential side effects. Refer to written materials furnished by healthcare providers regarding correct method of self-administration.
- Carry card or other identification at all times describing illness and names of medications being taken.

Evaluation

- Patient demonstrates stabilization of symptoms for which clonazepam was prescribed (seizures, panic attacks, manic behavior).
- Patient verbalizes understanding of necessity for, side effects of, and regimen required for prudent self-administration of clonazepam.

CLORAZEPATE

(klor-az′e-pate)
Tranxene, Tranxene-SD

Classification(s):
Antianxiety agent; Benzodiazepine;
Skeletal muscle relaxant;
Anticonvulsant
Schedule C IV
Pregnancy Category D

INDICATIONS

- Anxiety disorders and anxiety symptoms
- Partial seizures (adjunctive management therapy)
- Acute alcohol withdrawal.

ACTION

- Depresses subcortical levels of the central nervous system, particularly the limbic system and reticular formation
- May potentiate effects of the powerful inhibitory neurotransmitter gamma-aminobutyric acid (GABA) in the brain, thereby producing a calmative effect
- All levels of CNS depression can be effected, from mild sedation to hypnosis to coma.

PHARMACOKINETICS

Absorption: Hydrolyzed to active metabolite desmethyldiazepam prior to absorption. Rapidly absorbed from the GI tract.

Distribution: Is widely distributed. Crosses the blood-brain and placental barriers; excreted in breast milk.

Metabolism and Excretion: Metabolized by the liver; excreted by the kidneys.

Half-Life: 30–100 hours (half-life of metabolite).

CONTRAINDICATIONS AND PRECAUTIONS

Contraindicated in:
- Hypersensitivity to this drug or other benzodiazepines
- Combination with other CNS depressants
- Pregnancy and lactation
- Narrow-angle glaucoma
- Children under age 9.

Use Cautiously in: ✦ Elderly or debilitated patients ✦ Patients with hepatic or renal dysfunction ✦ Individuals with a history of drug abuse/addiction ✦ Depressed/suicidal patients.

ADVERSE REACTIONS AND SIDE EFFECTS*

CNS: <u>drowsiness</u>, <u>fatigue</u>, <u>ataxia</u>, <u>dizziness</u>, confusion, headache, blurred vision, paradoxical excitement, mental depression.
CV: hypotension, bradycardia.
Derm: skin rashes.
Endo: gynecomastia, galactorrhea.
GI: dry mouth, nausea/vomiting, diarrhea, constipation.
Resp: respiratory depression.
Other: tolerance, physical and psychological dependence.

INTERACTIONS

Drug-Drug: ✦ **Other CNS depressants (including alcohol, barbiturates, narcotics), antipsychotics, antidepressants, antihistamines, anticonvulsants:** additive CNS depression ✦ **Cimetidine:** increased effects of clorazepate ✦ **Cigarette smoking and caffeine:** decreased effects of clorazepate ✦ **Neuromuscular blocking agents:** increased respiratory depression ✦ **Digoxin:** reduced excretion of digoxin; increased potential for toxicity ✦ **Disulfiram:** decreased clearance of clorazepate ✦ **Antacids:** decreased hydrolysis of clorazepate to metabolite, with reduced effect.

ROUTE AND DOSAGE

Anxiety, Anxiety Disorders

✦ **PO (Adults):** 15–60 mg/day in divided doses.
✦ **PO (Geriatric or Debilitated Patients):** Initially, 7.5–15 mg/day in divided doses or as single HS dose.

Adjunct Anticonvulsant Therapy

✦ **PO (Adults and Children over 12):** 7.5 mg tid; increases no greater than 7.5 mg/week; maximum dose 90 mg/day.
✦ **PO (Children Ages 9–12):** 7.5 mg bid; increases no greater than 7.5 mg/week; maximum dose 60 mg/day.

Acute Alcohol Withdrawal

✦ **PO (Adults):** Day 1: 30 mg initially, followed by 30–60 mg in divided doses; Day 2: 45–90 mg in divided doses; Day 3: 22.5–45 mg in divided doses; Day 4: 15–30 mg in divided doses; thereafter, gradually decrease daily dose to 7.5–15 mg; discontinue when condition stabilizes.

PHARMACODYNAMICS

Route	Onset	Peak	Duration
PO	30–60 min	1–2 hr	*

*Varies with individual, age, disease state, number of doses.

NURSING IMPLICATIONS

Assessment

✦ Assess level of anxiety. Symptoms include: ● restlessness ● pacing ● insomnia ● inability to concentrate ● increased heart rate ● increased respiration ● elevated blood pressure ● confusion ● tremors ● rapid speech.
✦ Assess for suicidal ideation (CNS depressants aggravate symptoms in depressed patients).
✦ Assess history of allergies, sensitivity to this drug or to other benzodiazepines.
✦ Assess history of glaucoma.
✦ Assess date of last menses (possible pregnancy), use of contraceptives.
✦ Assess whether currently breast-feeding a child.
✦ Assess current and past alcohol and drug consumption.
✦ Assess operation of automobile and/or other dangerous machinery.
✦ Assess for presence of adverse reactions or side effects.

*<u>Underlines</u> indicate most frequent; CAPITALS indicate life-threatening.

♦ Assess patient/family knowledge about illness and need for medication.

♦ In collaboration with physician, assess CBC and liver function tests in patients on long-term therapy.

♦ **Lab Test Alterations:** Increased serum bilirubin, AST, and ALT.

◊ Abnormal renal function tests.

♦ **Withdrawal:** Assess for symptoms of withdrawal: • depression • insomnia • increased anxiety • abdominal and muscle cramps • tremors • vomiting • sweating • convulsions • delirium.

♦ **Withdrawal Management:** Monitor vital signs.

◊ Place patient in quiet room with low stimuli.

◊ Institute seizure precautions.

◊ A long-acting barbiturate, such as phenobarbital, may be ordered to suppress withdrawal symptoms.

◊ Phenytoin may be ordered to prevent seizures.

◊ Some physicians may order oxazepam as needed for objective withdrawal symptoms, gradually decreasing the dosage until the drug is discontinued.

♦ **Toxicity and Overdose:** Assess for symptoms of intoxication: • euphoria • relaxation • drowsiness • slurred speech • disorientation • mood lability • incoordination • unsteady gait • disinhibition of sexual and aggressive impulses • judgment and/or memory impairment.

◊ Assess for symptoms of overdose: • shallow respiration • cold and clammy skin • hypotension • dilated pupils • weak and rapid pulse • hypnosis • coma • possible death.

♦ **Overdose Management:** Monitor vital signs.

◊ Ensure maintenance of adequate airway.

◊ Induce vomiting in conscious patient.

◊ Initiate gastric lavage in unconscious patient.

◊ Administer activated charcoal to minimize absorption.

◊ IV fluids and vasopressors may be used to combat hypotension.

◊ Forced diuresis may be used to facilitate elimination of the drug.

Potential Nursing Diagnoses

♦ High risk for injury related to seizures, panic anxiety, abrupt withdrawal from long-term clorazepate use, acute alcohol withdrawal, effects of clorazepate intoxication or overdose.

♦ High risk for self-directed violence related to depressed mood.

♦ Anxiety (specify level) related to threats to physical integrity and/or self-concept.

♦ High risk for activity intolerance, related to clorazepate's side effects of lethargy, drowsiness, dizziness, muscular weakness.

♦ Knowledge deficit related to medication regimen.

Plan/Implementation

♦ Monitor vital signs before beginning therapy and at regular intervals (bid) throughout therapy.

♦ Ensure that patient practices good oral care. Offer patient hard, sugarless candy; gum; frequent sips of water for dry mouth.

♦ Ensure that patient is protected from injury. Supervise and assist with ambulation if dizziness and muscular weakness are problems. Pad siderails and headboard for patient who experiences seizures.

♦ To minimize nausea, medication may be given with food or milk.

♦ If patient has difficulty swallowing, tablet may be crushed (or capsule emptied) and mixed with food or fluid.

♦ Ensure that tablet/capsule has been swallowed and not "cheeked" to avoid medication or to hoard for later use.

♦ Store medication in light-resistant container at controlled room temperature between 15° and 30°C (59°–86°F).

Patient/Family Education

- Do not drive or operate dangerous machinery. Drowsiness and dizziness can occur.
- Do not stop taking the drug abruptly. Doing so can result in serious withdrawal symptoms.
- Do not consume other CNS depressants (including alcohol).
- Do not take nonprescription medication without approval from physician.
- Be aware of risks of taking clorazepate during pregnancy (congenital malformations have been associated with use during first trimester). Notify physician of desirability to discontinue drug if pregnancy is suspected or planned.
- Be aware of potential side effects. Refer to written materials furnished by healthcare providers regarding correct method of self-administration.
- Carry card or other identification at all times stating names of medications being taken.

Evaluation

- Patient demonstrates a subsiding/resolution of the symptoms for which clorazepate was prescribed (anxiety symptoms, anxiety disorders, partial seizures, acute alcohol withdrawal).
- Patient verbalizes understanding of side effects and regimen required for prudent self-administration of clorazepate.

CLOZAPINE

(cloz'a-peen)
Clozaril

Classification(s):
Antipsychotic; Tricyclic dibenzodiazepine derivative; Neuroleptic
Pregnancy Category B

INDICATIONS

- Management of severely ill schizophrenic patients who do not respond to or are unable to tolerate other antipsychotic drug therapy.

ACTION

- Binds to D-1 and D-2 dopamine receptors in the central nervous system, thus limiting the effects of dopamine in the brain. Also exhibits antagonist activity at adrenergic, cholinergic, histaminergic, and serotonergic receptors. It is more active at limbic than at striatal dopamine receptors, thus achieving relative freedom from extrapyramidal side effects.

PHARMACOKINETICS

Absorption: Well absorbed by the GI tract following oral administration.
Distribution: Widely distributed. 95% bound to plasma proteins. Is excreted in breast milk.
Metabolism and Excretion: Metabolized by the liver. Excreted in urine (50%) and feces (30%) in the form of inactive metabolites. Only trace amounts of unchanged drug can be detected.
Half-Life: 4–66 hours.

CONTRAINDICATIONS AND PRECAUTIONS

Contraindicated in: ◆ Hypersensitivity to this drug ◆ Patients with myeloproliferative disorders ◆ Patients with history of clozapine-induced agranulocytosis ◆ Patients with granulocytopenia ◆ Concomitant use with other drugs that are known to suppress bone marrow function ◆ Severe CNS depression ◆ Comatose patients ◆ Lactation ◆ Children (safety and effectiveness below age 16 have not been established) ◆ Pregnancy (safety not established).

Use Cautiously in: ◆ Patients with history of seizures ◆ Compromised cardiovascular or pulmonary function ◆ Hepatic and renal insufficiency ◆ Prostatic hypertrophy ◆ Narrow-angle glaucoma.

ADVERSE REACTIONS AND SIDE EFFECTS*

CNS: drowsiness, sedation, SEIZURES, dizziness, syncope, headache, restlessness, agitation, confusion, fatigue, weakness.
CV: tachycardia, orthostatic hypotension, ECG changes, hypertension, chest pain.
Derm: rash.
GI: constipation, salivation, nausea, vomiting, abdominal discomfort, diarrhea, anorexia, weight gain.
GU: urinary retention, frequency or incontinence, abnormal ejaculation.
Hemat: AGRANULOCYTOSIS, LEUKOPENIA, NEUTROPENIA, eosinophilia.
Ocular: visual disturbances.
Resp: dyspnea, shortness of breath, throat discomfort, nasal congestion.
Other: sweating, fever, numb or sore tongue, NEUROLEPTIC MALIGNANT SYNDROME, tardive dyskinesia.

INTERACTIONS

Drug-Drug: ◆ **Drugs with anticholinergic properties (e.g., antihistamines, antidepressants, antiparkinsonian agents):** additive anticholinergic effects ◆ **Drugs that suppress bone marrow function (e.g., antineoplastic agents):** increased risk and/or severity of bone marrow suppression ◆ **CNS active drugs:** additive effects on the central nervous system ◆ **Antihypertensives:** additive hypotensive effects ◆ **Benzodiazepines; other psychotropic drugs:** possible severe orthostatic

hypotension (may even be accompanied by respiratory and/or cardiac arrest) ◆ **Warfarin; digitoxin; other drugs highly bound to plasma proteins:** increased effects of these drugs ◆ **Cimetidine:** increased plasma levels of clozapine ◆ **Phenytoin:** decreased plasma levels of clozapine.

ROUTE AND DOSAGE

Schizophrenia

◆ **PO (Adults):** To minimize risk of agranulocytosis, only a 1-week supply of clozapine is dispensed at a time. Weekly WBC testing is required prior to delivery of the next week's supply of medication. If the WBC count falls below 3000 mm³ or the granulocyte count falls below 1500 mm³, clozapine therapy is discontinued. **Initial Dosage:** 12.5 mg daily or bid. If well tolerated, continue with daily dosage increments of 25–50 mg/day over a period of 2 weeks up to a target dose of 300–450 mg/day in divided doses. Additional dosage increments of no more than 100 mg may be made once or twice weekly, not to exceed 900 mg/day.

PHARMACODYNAMICS

Route	Onset	Peak	Duration
PO	UK	1–6 hr	4–12 hr

NURSING IMPLICATIONS

Assessment

◆ Assess mental status daily. Assess mood • appearance • thought and communication patterns • level of interest in the environment and in activities • level of anxiety or agitation • presence of hallucinations or delusions • suspiciousness • interactions with others • ability to carry out activities of daily living.
◆ Assess for symptoms of blood dyscrasias: sore throat • fever • malaise •

unusual bleeding • easy bruising. Flu-like complaints may indicate presence of infection and should be reported to physician immediately.

◆ Assess for extrapyramidal symptoms: Pseudoparkinsonism (tremors, shuffling gait, drooling rigidity) • akinesia (muscular weakness) • akathisia (continuous restlessness and fidgeting) • dystonia (involuntary muscular movements of face, arms, legs, and neck) • oculogyric crisis (uncontrolled rolling back of the eyes) • tardive dyskinesia (bizarre facial and tongue movements, stiff neck, difficulty swallowing). **Note:** Although these symptoms may be a possibility with clozapine, they are relatively low risk compared with other antipsychotics.

◆ Assess for symptoms of neuroleptic malignant syndrome (NMS): • hyperpyrexia up to 107°F • elevated pulse • increased or decreased blood pressure • severe parkinsonian muscle rigidity • elevated creatinine phosphokinase blood levels • elevated white blood count • altered mental status (including catatonic signs or agitation) • acute renal failure • varying levels of consciousness (including stupor and coma) • pallor diaphoresis, tachycardia, arrhythmias, rhabdomyolysis.

◆ **Treatment of NMS:** • discontinue antipsychotic drugs and other drugs not necessary to concurrent therapy • intensive symptomatic treatment and monitoring of VS, degree of muscle rigidity, I&O, and level of consciousness • physician may order bromocriptine (Parlodel) or dantrolene (Dantrium) to counteract the effects of NMS.

◆ Assess vital signs, weight. Record baseline values for comparison.

◆ Assess history of allergies, sensitivity to this drug.

◆ Assess date of last menses (possible pregnancy); use of contraceptives.

◆ Assess if currently breast-feeding a child.

◆ Assess current and past alcohol and drug consumption.

◆ Assess operation of automobile and/or other dangerous machinery.

◆ Assess for presence of adverse reactions or side effects. Monitor daily or weekly WBC and granulocyte values as ordered by physician.

◆ Assess patient/family knowledge about illness and need for medication.

◆ **Withdrawal:** No specific syndrome of symptoms has been correlated with abrupt withdrawal of clozapine. However, in the event of planned termination of the medication, gradual reduction in dose is recommended over a 1- to 2-week period. Should a patient's condition require abrupt discontinuation (e.g., leukopenia), he or she should be carefully observed for the recurrence of psychotic symptoms.

◆ **Toxicity and Overdose:** No correlation has been established between blood level and therapeutic effect.

◆ Assess for symptoms of overdose: • altered states of consciousness, including drowsiness, delirium, and coma • tachycardia • hypotension • respiratory depression • hypersalivation • seizures.

◆ **Overdose Management:** • monitor vital signs and cardiac status • ensure maintenance of open airway • ensure adequate oxygenation and ventilation • administer activated charcoal with sorbitol (may be as effective as or more effective than emesis or lavage) • provide general symptomatic and supportive measures • continue monitoring for several days due to risk of delayed effects • avoid use of epinepherine and its derivatives for hypotension, and quinidine and procainamide for cardiac arrhythmias • forced diuresis, dialysis, hemoperfusion, and exchange transfusion are not likely to be beneficial.

Potential Nursing Diagnoses

♦ High risk for violence directed at others related to mistrust and panic anxiety.

♦ High risk for injury related to clozapine's side effects of agranulocytosis, orthostatic hypotension, sedation, dizziness, weakness, lowered seizure threshold; abrupt withdrawal after prolonged use; overdose.

♦ Sensory-perceptual alteration related to panic anxiety evidenced by hallucinations.

♦ Altered thought processes related to panic anxiety evidenced by delusional thinking.

♦ Social isolation related to inability to trust others.

♦ High risk for activity intolerance related to clozapine side effects of drowsiness, dizziness, weakness.

♦ Noncompliance with medication regimen related to suspiciousness and mistrust of others; strict necessity for weekly blood evaluations to continue therapy.

♦ Knowledge deficit related to medication regimen.

Plan/Implementation

♦ Monitor vital signs before beginning therapy, and at regular intervals (bid or tid) throughout therapy. Take BP lying and standing to monitor for possible orthostatic reaction. Elderly are particularly susceptible. Dose adjustment may be required. Report fever immediately. May be a sign of infection. Tachycardia is common. *Low* pulse rates may be an indication of noncompliance.

♦ Weigh patient 2–3 times a week, at same time of day, on same scale, if possible. A rapid weight gain, or evidence of edema should be reported to physician immediately. Record I&O. Weight gain may also be a result of increased appetite caused by the drug.

♦ Ensure that patient is protected from injury. Provide supervision and assistance when ambulating if dizziness and drowsiness are problems. Pad siderails and headboard for patient who experiences seizures.

♦ Monitor laboratory results of serum WBC count and granulocytes prior to administration of the medication.

♦ A significant number of patients on clozapine therapy experience extreme salivation. Offer support to patient, as this may be an embarrassing situation. May even be a safety issue (e.g., aspiration) if problem is very severe.

♦ Administer with food to minimize GI upset, if necessary.

♦ Ensure patient swallows tablet and does not "cheek" to avoid medication or hoard for later use.

♦ Crush tablet and mix with food or fluid for patient who has difficulty swallowing.

♦ Store at controlled room temperatures between 15° and 30°C (59°–86°F). Protect from heat, moisture, and freezing.

Patient/Family Education

♦ Avoid use of hazardous machinery while on clozapine therapy. Drowsiness, dizziness, and seizures can occur.

♦ Do not stop taking the drug abruptly. To do so may cause reappearance of symptoms for which medication was prescribed.

♦ Report weekly for blood monitoring due to risk of agranulocytosis with clozapine. Be aware that medication will be dispensed in 1-week supply only. Additional weekly supplies will be provided based upon results of weekly laboratory blood evaluations.

♦ Report occurrence of any of the following symptoms to physician immediately: sore throat • fever • malaise • lethargy • weakness • mucous membrane ulceration • flu-like symptoms, persistent nausea/vomiting • severe headache • seizures • rapid or irregular heart rate • difficulty urinating • dizziness • lightheadedness.

♦ Rise slowly from a sitting or lying position to prevent a sudden drop in blood pressure.

♦ Report presence of severe salivation to physician.

♦ Do not drink alcohol while on clozapine therapy. These drugs potentiate the effects of each other.

♦ Do not consume other medications (including over-the-counter meds) without physician's approval. Many medications contain substances that interact with clozapine in a way that may be harmful.

♦ Be aware of possible risks of taking clozapine during pregnancy. Safe use during pregnancy and lactation has not been established. Inform physician immediately if pregnancy occurs or is suspected or planned. It is known that clozapine is excreted in breast milk; therefore, it may have an effect on the nursing infant.

♦ Be aware of side effects of clozapine. Refer to written materials furnished by healthcare providers for safe self-administration.

♦ Continue to take medication, even if feeling well and as though it is not needed. Symptoms may return if medication is discontinued.

♦ Carry card or other identification at all times describing medications being taken.

Evaluation

♦ Patient demonstrates a subsiding/resolution of the symptoms for which clozapine was prescribed (panic anxiety, altered thought processes, altered perceptions, social isolation, apathy).

♦ Patient verbalizes understanding of side effects and regimen required for prudent self-administration of clozapine.

DESIPRAMINE

(dess-ip'ra-meen)
Norpramin, Pertofrane

Classification(s):
Tricyclic antidepressant
Pregnancy Category C

INDICATIONS

♦ Major depression with melancholia or psychotic symptoms ♦ Depression associated with organic disease, alcoholism, schizophrenia, or mental retardation ♦ Depressive phase of bipolar disorder. **Investigational Use:** ♦ Attention deficit disorder in children.

ACTION

♦ Exact mechanism of action unclear ♦ Blocks the reuptake of the neurotransmitters norepinephrine and serotonin, increasing their concentration at the synapse and correcting the deficit that is thought to contribute to the melancholy mood of the depressed person.

PHARMACOKINETICS

Absorption: Thought to be readily absorbed from the GI tract following oral administration.

Distribution: Is widely distributed. Crosses blood-brain and placental barriers; enters breast milk.

Metabolism and Excretion: Metabolized by the liver. Excreted by the kidneys.

Half-Life: 7–62 hours.

CONTRAINDICATIONS AND PRECAUTIONS

Contraindicated in: ♦ Hypersensitivity to this drug or to other tricyclic antidepressants ♦ Concomitant use of MAO inhibitors ♦ Acute recovery period following myocardial infarction ♦ Untreated angle-closure glaucoma ♦ Children, pregnancy, and lactation (safety not established).

Use Cautiously in: ♦ Patients with a history of seizures ♦ Urinary retention ♦ Benign prostatic hypertrophy ♦ Glaucoma ♦ Thyroid disease ♦ Cardiovascular disorders ♦ Respiratory difficulties ♦ Hepatic or renal insufficiency ♦ Psychotic patients ♦ Elderly or debilitated patients.

ADVERSE REACTIONS AND SIDE EFFECTS*

CNS: drowsiness, dizziness, weakness, headache, fatigue, confusion, lethargy, memory deficits, disturbed concentration, tremors, ataxia, tinnitus, extrapyramidal symptoms, paresthesias of extremities, lowered seizure threshold, blurred vision, agitation, excitement, restlessness, insomnia, exacerbation of psychosis, shift to manic behavior.

CV: orthostatic hypotension, tachycardia and other arrhythmias, hypertension, MYOCARDIAL INFARCTION, HEART BLOCK, CONGESTIVE HEART FAILURE, ECG changes, syncope, CARDIOVASCULAR COLLAPSE.

Derm: skin rash, urticaria, photosensitivity, erythema, petechiae.

GI: dry mouth, constipation, nausea, vomiting, anorexia, diarrhea, abdominal cramps, adynamic ileus, esophageal reflux, stomatitis, black tongue.

GU: urinary retention, gynecomastia (males), testicular swelling, menstrual irregularity, breast engorgement and galactorrhea (females), changes in libido, impotence, delayed micturation.

Hemat: AGRANULOCYTOSIS, THROMBOCYTOPENIA, LEUKOPENIA, eosinophilia, purpura.

Hepat: jaundice, hepatitis.

Other: weight gain, nasal congestion, alopecia, hypothermia, peripheral neuropathy.

INTERACTIONS

Drug-Drug: ♦ **MAO inhibitors:** hyperpyretic crisis, hypertensive crisis, severe seizures, tachycardia, death ♦ **Guaneth-**idine, clonidine, (possibly) guanabenz: decreased effects of these medications ♦ **Cimetidine:** increased desipramine serum levels ♦ **Amphetamines, sympathomimetics:** increased hypertensive and cardiac effects of these drugs ♦ **CNS depressants (including alcohol, barbiturates, benzodiazepines):** potentiation of CNS effects ♦ **Thyroid medications:** tachycardia, arrhythmias ♦ **Methylphenidate, phenothiazines, haloperidol:** increased serum desipramine levels ♦ **Ethchlorvynol:** transient delirium ♦ **Quinidine, procainamide, disopyramide:** potentiation of adverse cardiovascular effects of desipramine ♦ **Oral contraceptives:** decreased effects of desipramine ♦ **Smoking:** increased desipramine metabolism ♦ **Disulfiram:** decreased desipramine metabolism ♦ **Levodopa, phenylbutazone:** delayed or decreased absorption of these drugs ♦ **Warfarin:** increased prothrombin time ♦ **Dicumarol:** increased plasma dicumarol concentrations.

ROUTE AND DOSAGE

Depression

♦ **PO (Adults):** Initiate with 75–150 mg/day, then adjust to 100–200 mg/day; maximum dose 300 mg/day. Total daily dose may be divided or given in a single dose, preferably at bedtime.

♦ **PO (Adolescents, Geriatric Patients):** Initiate with 25–50 mg/day, then adjust to 25–100 mg/day; maximum dose 150 mg/day. Total daily dose may be divided or given in a single dose, preferably at bedtime.

♦ **PO (Maintenance):** After symptoms are controlled, reduce to lowest dose that will maintain relief of symptoms.

Attention Deficit Disorder

♦ **PO (Children):** 1–6 mg/kg/day (mean: 3.5 mg/kg/day)

*Underlines indicate most frequent; CAPITALS indicate life-threatening.

PHARMACODYNAMICS

Route	Onset	Peak	Duration
PO	2–4 wk	4–6 hr	Weeks*

*Allow up to 2 weeks following cessation of therapy for complete drug elimination.

NURSING IMPLICATIONS
Assessment

✦ Assess for suicidal ideation, plan, means. Assess for sudden lifts in mood, which could indicate patient's decision to commit suicide.

✦ Assess mental status daily. Assess: • mood • appearance • thought and communication patterns • level of interest in the environment and in activities • suicidal ideation. Improvement in these behavior patterns and level of energy should be expected within 2–4 weeks of initiation of therapy.

✦ Assess for symptoms of attention deficit disorder: • easy distractibility • short attention span • excessive motor activity • restlessness • fidgetiness • difficulty sitting still • disruptive behavior.

✦ Assess for symptoms of blood dyscrasias: • sore throat • fever • malaise • unusual bleeding • easy bruising.

✦ Assess vital signs, weight.

✦ Assess history of allergies, sensitivity to this drug or to other tricyclic antidepressants.

✦ Assess for history of glaucoma.

✦ Assess date of last menses (possible pregnancy), use of contraceptives.

✦ Assess whether currently breast-feeding a child.

✦ Assess current and past alcohol and drug consumption.

✦ Assess for operation of automobile and/or other dangerous machinery.

✦ Assess for presence of adverse reactions or side effects.

✦ Assess patient/family knowledge about illness and need for medication.

✦ In collaboration with physician, assess CBC and liver function tests in patients on long-term therapy.

✦ **Lab Test Alterations:** Increased serum bilirubin, alkaline phosphatase, transaminase, and glucose.

◊ Decreased urinary 5-hydroxyindole-acetic acid (HIAA) and vanillylmandelic acid (VMA) excretion.

✦ **Withdrawal:** Assess for symptoms of abrupt withdrawal from long-term therapy: • nausea • headache • vertigo • malaise • insomnia • nightmares.

✦ **Toxicity and Overdose:** Range of therapeutic serum concentration is 125–300 ng/mL.

◊ Assess for symptoms of overdose: • confusion • agitation • irritability • hallucinations • seizures • flushing • dry mouth • dilated pupils • delirium • hyperpyrexia • hypotension or hypertension • coma • tachycardia • arrhythmias • respiratory depression • cardiac arrest • renal failure • shock • congestive heart failure • acid-base disturbances.

✦ **Overdose Management:** Monitor vital signs.

◊ Ensure maintenance of adequate airway.

◊ Monitor ECG.

◊ Use ice packs, cold baths, or other cooling measures to control hyperpyrexia.

◊ Induce emesis in alert patient.

◊ Follow emesis with gastric lavage.

◊ Administer activated charcoal to minimize absorption.

◊ IV physostigmine may be used cautiously to reverse anticholinergic effects.

◊ Use IV fluids, sodium bicarbonate, vasopressors, phenytoin, propranolol, or lidocaine for cardiovascular effects.

◊ Administer IV diazepam for seizures.

◊ Monitor cardiac function for at least 5 days.

Potential Nursing Diagnoses

✦ High risk for self-directed violence related to depressed mood.

- High risk for injury related to desipramine's side effects of sedation: • dizziness • ataxia • weakness • confusion • lowered seizure threshold; abrupt withdrawal after prolonged use; overdose.
- Social isolation related to depressed mood.
- Impaired social interaction related to short attention span and easy distractibility.
- High risk for activity intolerance, related to desipramine's side effects of: • drowsiness • dizziness • ataxia • weakness • confusion.
- Knowledge deficit related to medication regimen.

Plan/Implementation

- Monitor vital signs before beginning therapy and at regular intervals (bid or tid) throughout therapy. Take BP lying and standing in patients experiencing orthostatic hypotension; elderly are particularly susceptible. Contact physician if tachycardia/arrhythmias are noted.
- Ensure that patient who is ambulatory is protected from sun when spending time outdoors.
- Weigh patient 2–3 times a week, at same time of day, on same scale, if possible. A rapid weight gain or evidence of edema should be reported to physician immediately. Record I&O.
- Ensure that patient is protected from injury. Provide supervision and assistance when ambulating if dizziness and drowsiness are problems. Pad siderails and headboard for patient who experiences seizures.
- Give patient hard candy, gum, or frequent sips of water if dry mouth is a problem.
- Administer oral medication with food to minimize GI upset.
- Ensure that patient swallows tablet/capsule and does not "cheek" to avoid medication or to hoard for later use.

- Tablet may be crushed or contents of capsule emptied and mixed with food or fluid for patient who has difficulty swallowing.
- Store tablets at room temperature, preferably below 30°C (86°F). Protect from excessive heat.

Patient/Family Education

- Therapeutic effect may not be seen for as long as 4 weeks. If after this time no improvement is noted, physician may prescribe a different medication. Continue to take medication even though symptoms have not subsided.
- Use caution when driving or when operating dangerous machinery. Drowsiness and dizziness can occur. If these side effects become persistent or interfere with daily activities, report to physician. Dosage adjustment may be necessary.
- Do not stop taking the drug abruptly. To do so might produce withdrawal symptoms, such as nausea, vertigo, insomnia, headache, malaise, nightmares.
- Use sunscreens and wear protective clothing when spending time outdoors. Skin may be sensitive to sunburn.
- Report occurrence of any of the following symptoms to physician immediately: sore throat • fever • malaise • unusual bleeding • easy bruising • persistent nausea/vomiting • severe headache • rapid heart rate • difficulty urinating.
- Rise slowly from a sitting or lying position to prevent a sudden drop in blood pressure.
- If dry mouth is a problem, take frequent sips of water, chew sugarless gum, or suck on hard candy. Good oral care (frequent brushing, flossing) is very important.
- Do not smoke while on desipramine therapy. Smoking increases metabolism of desipramine, requiring adjustment in dosage to achieve therapeutic effect.

♦ Do not drink alcohol while on desipramine therapy. These drugs potentiate each other's effects.

♦ Do not consume other medications (including over-the-counter meds) without physician's approval. Many medications contain substances that, in combination with tricyclics, could precipitate a life-threatening hypertensive crisis.

♦ Be aware of possible risks of taking desipramine during pregnancy. Safe use during pregnancy and lactation has not be established. Desipramine readily crosses the placental barrier, so a fetus could experience adverse effects of the drug. Inform physician immediately if pregnancy occurs, is suspected, or is planned.

♦ Be aware of side effects of desipramine. Refer to written materials furnished by healthcare providers for safe self-administration.

♦ Carry card or other identification at all times describing medications being taken.

Evaluation

♦ Patient demonstrates a subsiding/resolution of the symptoms for which desipramine was prescribed (depressed mood, suicidal ideation, symptoms of attention deficit disorder).

♦ Patient verbalizes understanding of side effects and regimen required for prudent self-administration of desipramine.

DEXTROAMPHETAMINE SULFATE

(dex-troe-am-fet′a-meen)
Dexampex, Dexedrine, Ferndex, Oxydess II, Spancap #1

Classification(s):
CNS stimulant; Amphetamine; Anorexigenic
Schedule C II
Pregnancy Category C

INDICATIONS

♦ Narcolepsy ♦ Attention deficit disorder with hyperactivity in children ♦ Exogenous obesity.

ACTION

♦ Exact mechanism of action in CNS not known ♦ Amphetamines are sympathomimetic amines that stimulate the central nervous system, possibly by increasing synaptic release of norepinephrine, dopamine, and, at higher doses, serotonin in the brain. This is also accomplished by blocking reuptake at presynaptic membranes ♦ Central action occurs through cortical stimulation and may also be due to stimulation of the reticular activating system ♦ Action may also be due in part to the inhibition of amine oxidase ♦ Peripheral action is thought to be due to release of norepinephrine from adrenergic nerve stores and to direct effects on alpha- and beta-receptor sites.

PHARMACOKINETICS

Absorption: Rapid and complete absorption within 3 hours following oral administration.

Distribution: Widely distributed, with high concentrations in the brain and CSF. Crosses placental barrier; enters breast milk.

Metabolism and Excretion: Metabolized by the liver and excreted in urine. Elimination is enhanced by acidic urine, slowed by alkaline urine.

Half-Life: 7–33.6 hours (depending on pH of urine).

CONTRAINDICATIONS AND PRECAUTIONS

Contraindicated in: ✦ Hypersensitivity to sympathomimetic amines or tartrazine (in some preparations) ✦ Advanced arteriosclerosis ✦ Symptomatic cardiovascular disease ✦ Moderate to severe hypertension ✦ Hyperthyroidism ✦ Glaucoma ✦ Agitated states ✦ Patients with a history of drug abuse ✦ During or within 14 days of receiving therapy with MAO inhibitors ✦ Children under 3 years of age ✦ Pregnancy.

Use Cautiously in: ✦ Lactation ✦ Psychotic children ✦ Tourette's disorder ✦ Mild hypertension ✦ Anorexia ✦ Insomnia ✦ Elderly or debilitated patients.

ADVERSE REACTIONS AND SIDE EFFECTS*

CNS: <u>overstimulation</u>, <u>restlessness</u>, <u>dizziness</u>, <u>insomnia</u>, dyskinesia, <u>euphoria</u>, dysphoria, tremor, headache, symptoms of Tourette's disorder, psychoses (<u>rare</u>), disorientation, hallucinations, seizures, nervousness, increased motor activity, blurred vision, <u>mydriasis</u>.
CV: <u>palpitations</u>, <u>tachycardia</u>, elevation of blood pressure, pallor or flushing, cardiac arrhythmias.
Derm: urticaria.
Endo: changes in libido.
GI: <u>dry mouth</u>, metallic taste, diarrhea, constipation, <u>anorexia</u>, <u>weight loss</u>, nausea, vomiting, abdominal cramps.
Other: <u>tolerance</u>, physical and psychological dependence, cyanosis, RESPIRATORY FAILURE, chilliness, excessive sweating.

INTERACTIONS

Drug-Drug: ✦ **Furazolidone, MAO inhibitors (during or within 14 days following administration of):** hypertensive crisis, headache, hyperpyrexia, intracranial hemorrhage, bradycardia ✦

Insulin: alteration in requirements ✦ **Guanethidine:** decreased antihypertensive effects ✦ **Phenothiazines:** possible decreased effects of both drugs ✦ **Urinary alkalinizers (e.g., acetazolamide, sodium bicarbonate, potassium citrate, sodium acetate, sodium citrate, sodium lactate, tromethamine):** decreased dextroamphetamine excretion, increased dextroamphetamine effects, excess CNS stimulation, cardiovascular effects ✦ **Urinary acidifiers (e.g., ammonium chloride, potassium phosphate, sodium acid phosphate):** increased dextroamphetamine excretion, decreased dextroamphetamine effects.

Drug-Food: ✦ **Caffeinated foods and drinks:** increased effects of dextroamphetamine.

ROUTE AND USAGE

Narcolepsy
✦ **PO (Adults, Children 12 Years and Older): Initial dosage:** 10 mg/day. May be increased in increments of 10 mg/day at weekly intervals until desired results are achieved or adverse effects, such as anorexia or insomnia appear.
✦ **PO (Children 6–12 Years): Initial dosage:** 5 mg/day. May be increased in increments of 5 mg/day at weekly intervals until desired response is achieved. With tablets or elixir, give first dose on awakening; additional doses (1 or 2) at intervals of 4–6 hours. Sustained-release forms may be used for once-a-day dosage, given in the morning.

Attention Deficit Disorder (Children)
✦ **PO (Children 3–5 Years): Initial Dosage:** 2.5 mg/day. May be increased in increments of 2.5 mg/day at weekly intervals until desired response is achieved.
✦ **PO (Children 6 Years and Older):**

*Underlines indicate most frequent; CAPITALS indicate life-threatening.

Initial Dosage: 5 mg daily or bid. May be increased in increments of 5 mg/day at weekly intervals until desired response is achieved. Dosage will rarely exceed 40 mg/day. Give first dose of tablets or elixir forms on awakening; additional doses (1 or 2) at intervals of 4–6 hours. Sustained-release forms may be used for once-a-day dosage, given in the morning.

Exogenous Obesity

♦ **PO (Adults, Children 12 Years and Older):** 5–30 mg/day in divided doses of 5 to 10 mg 30 to 60 minutes before meals. Sustained-release forms: 10–15 mg in the morning (10–14 hours before bedtime).

PHARMACODYNAMICS

Route	Onset	Peak	Duration
PO	30–60 min	1–3 hr*	4–24 hr*

*Varies with individual, dosage form, number of doses, and pH of urine.

NURSING IMPLICATIONS

Assessment

♦ Assess and record baseline temperature, pulse, respiration, blood pressure, and weight for comparison during therapy.

♦ In diabetic patient, assess blood sugar bid–tid. Insulin adjustments may be required due to alteration in eating pattern as well as possible hyperactivity.

♦ For overweight patient using amphetamines as an anorexigenic, assess knowledge of sound, nutritional, calorie-reduced diet with program of regular exercise.

♦ Carefully assess growth rate of children on dextroamphetamine therapy. A decrease in rate of development may be observed.

♦ Assess mental status for changes in mood, level of activity, degree of stimulation, aggressiveness.

♦ Assess sleeping patterns carefully. Insomnia may occur.

♦ Assess history of allergies, sensitivity to this drug or to other amphetamines.

♦ Assess history of glaucoma.

♦ Assess for presence of adverse reactions or side effects.

♦ Assess date of last menses (possible pregnancy), use of contraceptives.

♦ Assess whether currently breast-feeding a child.

♦ Assess current and past alcohol and drug consumption.

♦ Assess usual amount of caffeine consumed.

♦ Assess for operation of automobile and/or other dangerous machinery.

♦ Assess patient/family knowledge about illness and need for medication.

♦ In collaboration with physician, assess CBC, urinalysis, and liver function tests periodically in patients on amphetamine therapy.

♦ **Lab Test Alterations:** Elevated serum thyroxine (T_4) levels.

♦ **Withdrawal:** Assess for symptoms of withdrawal: • extreme fatigue • lethargy • increased dreaming • mental depression • suicidal ideations • changes on the sleep EEG.

♦ **Toxicity and Overdose:** Assess for symptoms of intoxication: • severe dermatoses • marked insomnia • irritability • hyperactivity • tachycardia • dilated pupils • elevated blood pressure • personality changes • hyperpyrexia • disorganization of thoughts • poor concentration • visual hallucinations • compulsive, stereotyped behavior • psychosis with manifestations similar to paranoid schizophrenia.

◊ Assess for symptoms of overdose: • restlessness • hyperirritability • insomnia • tremor • hyperreflexia • diaphoresis • mydriasis • flushing or pallor • profuse perspiration • hyperactivity • confusion • hypertension • extrasystoles • tachypnea • fever • hallucinations • panic state • paranoid ideations • delirium • marked hypertension • arrhythmias • heart block •

convulsions • circulatory collapse • death.

♦ **Overdose Management:** Monitor vital signs.

◊ Induce emesis.

◊ Initiate gastric lavage.

◊ Administer activated charcoal to minimize absorption.

◊ Administer saline cathartic.

◊ Administer urinary acidifier, such as ammonium chloride.

◊ Administer diuretic.

◊ Place patient in cool room.

◊ Administer short-acting barbiturates to treat hyperactivity.

◊ Administer IV phentolamine to treat severe hypertension.

◊ Use fluid replacement and a vasopressor to combat cardiovascular collapse.

◊ Use oxygen and artificial respiration, if necessary.

◊ Hemodialysis or peritoneal dialysis may be effective.

Potential Nursing Diagnoses

♦ High risk for injury due to overstimulation and hyperactivity, abrupt amphetamine withdrawal, overdose.

♦ High risk for self-directed violence related to suicidal ideations resulting from abrupt amphetamine withdrawal.

♦ High risk for violence directed at others related to aggressiveness as side effect of amphetamine.

♦ Alteration in nutrition, more than body requires, related to excessive intake in relation to metabolic needs.

♦ Alteration in nutrition, less than body requires, related to amphetamine's side effects of anorexia and weight loss.

♦ Sleep pattern disturbance related to overstimulation resulting from amphetamine use.

♦ Alteration in thought processes related to adverse amphetamine effects of overstimulation and difficulty concentrating.

♦ Knowledge of deficit related to medication.

Plan/Implementation

♦ Monitor medication effects. Tolerance develops rapidly. If anorexigenic effects begin to diminish, notify physician immediately. Patient should be on reduced-calorie diet and program of regular exercise in addition to the medication.

♦ Monitor and record vital signs at regular intervals (bid) throughout therapy.

♦ Encourage use of gum, hard candy, or frequent sips of water for patient who experiences dry mouth. Ensure that patient practices good oral care (frequent brushing, flossing).

♦ Ensure that patient is protected from injury. Keep stimuli low and environment as quiet as possible to discourage overstimulation.

♦ Observe frequently for signs of impending violence to self or others. Institute suicide precautions, if necessary. Assess level of anxiety often to prevent onset of physical aggression as agitation increases.

♦ In children with behavior disorders, a drug "holiday" should be attempted periodically under direction of physician to assess effectiveness of medication and need for continuation.

♦ Ensure that tablet/capsule has been swallowed and not "cheeked" to avoid medication or to hoard for later use.

♦ Tablets may be crushed and mixed with food or fluid for patient who has difficulty swallowing, or elixir form may be administered.

♦ Sustained-released capsules should not be opened nor contents mixed with food. They should be swallowed whole.

♦ To prevent insomnia, give last dose at least 6 hours before retiring.

♦ As an anorexigenic, drug should be administered 30–60 minutes before meals. Sustained-release form should be taken early in the morning (10–14 hours before bedtime).

♦ Store medication at controlled room

temperatures between 15° and 30°C (59°–86°F). Protect from heat and moisture.

Patient/Family Education

* Use caution in driving or when operating dangerous machinery. Level of alertness may be diminished due to hyperactivity and stimulation. Dizziness may occur as a side effect.
* Do not stop taking the drug abruptly. Doing so can produce serious withdrawal symptoms.
* Do not take other medications (including over-the-counter drugs) without physician's approval. Many medications contain substances that, in combination with amphetamine, can be harmful.
* Diabetic patient: Monitor blood sugar bid or tid or as instructed by physician. Be aware of need for possible alteration in insulin requirements due to changes in food intake, weight, and activity.
* Avoid consumption of large amounts of caffeinated products (coffee, tea, colas, chocolate), as they may enhance the stimulant effect of dextroamphetamine sulfate.
* Follow reduced-calorie diet provided by dietitian as well as a program of regular exercise if using amphetamine as an appetite suppressant. Do not exceed recommended dose if appetite suppressant effect diminishes. Contact physician.
* Notify physician if restlessness, insomnia, anorexia, or dry mouth become severe, or if rapid, pounding heartbeat becomes evident.
* Be aware of possible risks of taking dextroamphetamine during pregnancy. Safe use in pregnancy and lactation has not been established. Dextroamphetamine crosses placental barrier, so a fetus could experience adverse effects of the drug. Inform physician immediately if pregnancy occurs, is suspected, or is planned.
* Be aware of potential side effects of dextroamphetamine. Refer to written materials furnished by healthcare providers for safe self-administration.
* Carry card or other identification at all times describing medications being taken.

Evaluation

* Patient demonstrates a subsiding/resolution of the symptoms for which dextroamphetamine sulfate was prescribed (inability to prevent falling asleep, obesity, behavior problems/hyperactivity in children).
* Patient verbalizes understanding of side effects and regimen required for prudent self-administration of dextroamphetamine sulfate.

DIAZEPAM

(dye-az′e-pam)
{D-Tran, E-Pam, Meval, Novodipam, Stress-Pam}, Valium, Val-release, Vazepam, Zetran

Classification(s):
Antianxiety agent; Anticonvulsant; Skeletal muscle relaxant; Benzodiazepine
Schedule C IV
Pregnancy Category D

INDICATIONS

* Anxiety disorders * Anxiety symptoms (efficacy for periods greater than 4 months has not been evaluated) * Acute alcohol withdrawal * Skeletal muscle spasms * Convulsive disorders (adjunctive therapy) * Status epilepticus * Preoperative sedation and relief of anxiety * Anterograde amnesia. **Investigational Use:** * Prevention of night terrors.

{} = Only available in Canada.

ACTION

♦ Depresses subcortical levels of the central nervous system, particularly the limbic system and reticular formation ♦ May potentiate the effects of the powerful inhibitory neurotransmitter gamma-aminobutyric acid (GABA) in the brain, thereby producing a calmative effect ♦ All levels of CNS depression can be effected, from mild sedation to hypnosis to coma.

PHARMACOKINETICS

Absorption: Rapidly absorbed from the GI tract; IM absorption slow and inconsistent.

Distribution: Is widely distributed. Crosses blood-brain and placental barriers; excreted in breast milk.

Metabolism and Excretion: Metabolized by the liver; active metabolites, which are responsible for effects, are excreted for the most part by the kidneys.

Half-Life: 20–50 hours.

CONTRAINDICATIONS AND PRECAUTIONS

Contraindicated in: ♦ Hypersensitivity to this drug or to other benzodiazepines ♦ Combination with other CNS depressants ♦ Pregnancy and lactation ♦ Narrow-angle glaucoma ♦ Shock ♦ Coma.

Use Cautiously in: ♦ Elderly or debilitated patients ♦ Patients with hepatic or renal dysfunction ♦ Individuals with a history of drug abuse/addiction ♦ Depressed/suicidal patients ♦ Infants.

ADVERSE REACTIONS AND SIDE EFFECTS*

CNS: drowsiness, fatigue, ataxia, dizziness, confusion, headache, syncope, paradoxical excitement.

CV: bradycardia; with IV use: hypotension, SHOCK, CARDIOVASCULAR COLLAPSE.

Derm: rash, dermatitis, itching, pain at injection site.

Endo: gynecomastia, galactorrhea.

GI: dry mouth, nausea/vomiting, diarrhea, constipation, anorexia, weight gain or loss, swollen tongue, metallic or bitter taste.

GU: urinary retention, incontinence, irregular menses, libidinal changes.

Hemat: neutropenia, GRANULOCYTOPENIA.

Resp: RESPIRATORY DEPRESSION (with IV use).

Other: tolerance, physical and psychological dependence.

INTERACTIONS

Drug-Drug: ♦ **Other CNS depressants (including alcohol, barbiturates, narcotics), antipsychotics, antidepressants, antihistamines:** additive CNS depression ♦ **Cimetidine and valproic acid:** increased effects of diazepam ♦ **Oral contraceptives:** increased or decreased effects of diazepam ♦ **Cigarette smoking and caffeine:** decreased effects of diazepam ♦ **Phenytoin:** increased phenytoin serum levels (risk of toxicity) ♦ **Levodopa:** decreased effects of levodopa ♦ **Neuromuscular blocking agents:** increased respiratory depression ♦ **Digoxin:** reduced excretion of digoxin, increased potential for toxicity ♦ **Antitubercular drugs:** may increase or decrease levels ♦ **Disulfiram:** decreased clearance of diazepam ♦ **All drugs in solution or syringe:** precipitation of parenteral diazepam.

ROUTE AND DOSAGE

Anxiety, Convulsive Disorders

♦ **PO (Adults):** 2–10 mg bid or qid.
♦ **PO Extended Release (Adults):** 15–30 mg once a day.
♦ **PO (Children over 6 Months):** 1–2.5 mg tid or qid.
♦ **IM, IV (Adults):** 2–10 mg tid or qid as needed; may be repeated as soon as 1 hour, to a maximum of 30 mg in an 8-hour period.

---

*Underlines indicate most frequent; CAPITALS indicate life-threatening.

Skeletal Muscle Spasms (Tetanus)

+ **PO (Adults):** 2–10 mg tid or qid.
+ **IM, IV (Adults):** 5–10 mg initially, then 5–10 mg in 3–4 hours if needed.
+ **IM, IV (Children 5 and Over):** 5–10 mg tid or qid.
+ **IM, IV (Infants over 30 Days):** 1–2 mg tid or qid.

Acute Alcohol Withdrawal

+ **PO (Adults):** 10 mg tid or qid for the first 24 hours, then decrease to 5 mg tid or qid as needed.
+ **PO Extended Release (Adults):** one 30-mg dose for first 24 hours, followed by 15-mg once daily as needed.
+ **IM, IV (Adults):** 10 mg initially, then 5–10 mg in 3–4 hours if needed (sometimes necessary to give as often as every hour).

Status Epilepticus

+ **IV (Adults):** 5–10 mg initially; repeat every 10–15 minutes to a maximum dose of 30 mg (IV push 5 mg/minute).
+ **IV (Children 5 Years or Older):** 1 mg every 2–5 minutes to a maximum of 10 mg (IV push over period of 3 minutes).
+ **IV (Children 30 Days to Age 5):** 0.2–0.5 mg every 2–5 minutes to a maximum of 5 mg (IV push over period of 3 minutes).

Preoperative Sedation

+ **IM (Adults):** 10 mg before surgery.

Night Terrors (Investigational Use)

+ **PO (Adults and Children):** 5–10 mg HS.

PHARMACODYNAMICS

Route	Onset	Peak	Duration
PO	30–60 min	1–2 hr	*
IM	15–30 min	1–2 hr	*
IV	1–5 min	15–30 min	15–60 min

*Varies with individual, age, disease state, number of doses.

NURSING IMPLICATIONS

Assessment

+ Assess level of anxiety. Symptoms include: • restlessness • pacing • insomnia • inability to concentrate • increased heart rate • increased respiration • elevated blood pressure • confusion • tremors • rapid speech.
+ Assess for suicidal ideation (CNS depressants aggravate symptoms in depressed patients).
+ Assess history of allergies, sensitivity to this drug or to other benzodiazepines.
+ Assess history of glaucoma.
+ Assess for presence of adverse reactions or side effects.
+ Assess date of last menses (possible pregnancy), use of contraceptives.
+ Assess whether currently breast-feeding a child.
+ Assess current and past alcohol and drug consumption.
+ Assess operation of automobile and/or other dangerous machinery.
+ Assess patient/family knowledge about illness and need for medication.
+ In collaboration with physician, assess CBC and liver function tests in patients on long-term therapy.
+ **Lab Test Alterations:** Elevations in serum LDH, alkaline phosphatase, AST, ALT.
◊ Abnormal renal function tests.
+ **Withdrawal:** Assess for symptoms of withdrawal: • depression • insomnia • increased anxiety • abdominal and muscle cramps • tremors • vomiting • sweating • convulsions • delirium.
+ **Withdrawal Management:** Monitor vitals signs.
◊ Place patient in quiet room with low stimuli.
◊ Institute seizure precautions.
◊ A long-acting barbiturate, such as phenobarbital, may be ordered to suppress withdrawal symptoms.
◊ Phenytoin may be ordered to prevent seizures.

◇ Some physicians may order oxazepam as needed for objective withdrawal symptoms, gradually decreasing the dosage until the drug is discontinued.

✦ **Toxicity and Overdose:** Assess for symptoms of intoxication: • euphoria • relaxation • drowsiness • slurred speech • disorientation • mood lability • incoordination • unsteady gait • disinhibition of sexual and aggressive impulses • judgment and/or memory impairment.

◇ Assess for symptoms of overdose: • shallow respirations • cold and clammy skin • hypotension • dilated pupils • weak and rapid pulse • hypnosis • coma • possible death.

✦ **Overdose Management:** Monitor vital signs.

◇ Maintain adequate airway.

◇ Induce vomiting in conscious patient.

◇ Initiate gastric lavage in unconscious patient.

◇ Administer activated charcoal to minimize absorption.

◇ Administer norepinephrine or metaraminol to treat hypotension.

◇ Forced diuresis, IV fluids, and electrolytes may accelerate elimination.

◇ Dialysis is of limited value.

Potential Nursing Diagnosis

✦ High risk for injury related to seizures, panic anxiety, abrupt withdrawal from long-term diazepam use, agitation from acute alcohol withdrawal, effects of diazepam intoxication or overdose.

✦ High risk for self-directed violence related to depressed mood intensified by diazepam.

✦ Anxiety (specify level) related to threats to physical integrity and/or self-concept.

✦ High risk for activity intolerance, related to diazepam's side effects of lethargy, drowsiness, dizziness, muscular weakness.

✦ Knowledge deficit related to medication regimen.

Plan/Implementation

✦ **General Info:** Monitor vital signs before beginning therapy, at regular intervals (bid) throughout therapy, and q 10 min during IV administration.

◇ Ensure that patient practices good oral care. Offer patient hard, sugarless candy; gum; or frequent sips of water for dry mouth.

◇ Ensure that patient is protected from injury. Supervise and assist with ambulation and activities if dizziness and muscular weakness are problems. Pad siderails and headboard for patient who experiences seizures.

◇ Oral and parenteral forms of diazepam should be stored in light-resistant containers at controlled room temperatures between 15° and 30°C (59°–86°F).

✦ **PO:** To minimize nausea, medication may be given with food or milk.

◇ Short-acting tablets may be crushed and mixed with food or fluid for patient who has difficulty swallowing.

◇ Patient should not chew or empty contents of timed-release capsules. They should be taken whole.

◇ Ensure that tablet/capsule has been swallowed and not "cheeked" to avoid medication or to hoard for later use.

✦ **IM:** Do not mix with any other drug or solution in vial or syringe.

◇ IM diazepam is painful and absorption by this route is unpredictable. Inject slowly and deeply into large muscle mass to minimize pain and enhance absorption. Use Z-track method.

◇ Rotate injection sites if multiple injections are administered.

◇ Aspirate carefully before injection. Inadvertent arterial administration may result in arteriospasm or gangrene.

◇ Patient should remain in bed with siderails up and be observed closely for at least 3 hours following IM administration. Monitor vital signs every 15–30 minutes during this time.

* **IV:** Do not mix with any other drug or solution in syringe or IV infusion bag.
◇ Avoid use of small veins to minimize risk of thrombophlebitis.
◇ Administer slowly (5 mg/min in adults; total dose over 3 minutes in children) to reduce risk of respiratory depression, phlebitis, and/or cardio-vascular collapse.
◇ Patient should be in recumbent position during IV administration and should remain in bed with siderails up for at least 3 hours following IV ad-ministration. Observe closely and monitor vital signs every 5 minutes for first 30 minutes, then every 15–30 minutes for 3 hours.
◇ Ensure availability of emergency re-suscitation equipment.
◇ If direct injection into vein is not pos-sible, inject into IV tubing as close as possible to site of vein insertion.

Patient/Family Education

* Do not drive or operate dangerous machinery. Drowsiness and dizziness can occur.
* Do not stop taking the drug abruptly. Doing so can produce serious with-drawal symptoms, such as depression, insomnia, anxiety, abdominal and muscle cramps, tremors, vomiting, sweating, convulsions, delirium.
* Do not consume other CNS depres-sants (including alcohol).
* Do not take nonprescription medica-tion without approval from physician.
* Be aware of risks of taking diazepam during pregnancy (congenital malfor-mations have been associated with use during first trimester). Notify physi-cian of desirability to discontinue drug if pregnancy is suspected or planned.
* Be aware of possible side effects. Re-fer to written materials furnished by healthcare providers regarding cor-rect method of self-administration.
* Carry card or other identification at all

times stating names of medications be-ing taken.

Evaluation

* Patient demonstrates a subsiding/res-olution of the symptoms for which di-azepam was prescribed (anxiety, con-vulsions, muscle spasms, night terrors).
* Patient verbalizes understanding of side effects and regimen required for prudent self-administration of diaze-pam.

DIETHYLPROPION

(dye-eth-il-proe'pee-on)
Depletite-25, {Nobesine, Regibon} Tenuate, Tepanil

Classification(s):
Anorexigenic, CNS stimulant, Sympathomimetic amine
Schedule C IV
Pregnancy Category C

INDICATIONS

* Exogenous obesity—short-term (a few weeks) management.

ACTION

* Exact mechanism of action is not known * Sympathomimetic amines are thought to produce appetite suppression through direct stimulation of the satiety center in the hypothalamus and limbic system * Pharmacologic effects are sim-ilar to the amphetamines.

PHARMACOKINETICS

Absorption: Readily absorbed following oral administration.
Distribution: Is widely distributed. Crosses placental barrier; enters breast milk.
Metabolism and Excretion: Metab-olized by the liver, excreted in urine.
Half-Life: 1–3.5 hours.

{} = Only available in Canada.

CONTRAINDICATIONS AND PRECAUTIONS

Contraindicated in: ♦ Hypersensitivity to sympathomimetic amines ♦ Advanced arteriosclerosis ♦ Symptomatic cardiovascular disease ♦ Moderate to severe hypertension ♦ Hyperthyroidism ♦ Glaucoma ♦ Agitated states ♦ History of drug abuse ♦ During or within 14 days of receiving therapy with MAO inhibitors ♦ Concomitant use of other CNS stimulants ♦ Pregnancy and lactation, children under 12 years of age (safe use has not been established).

Use Cautiously in: ♦ Mild hypertension ♦ Diabetes mellitus ♦ Patients with a history of seizures ♦ Elderly or debilitated patients.

ADVERSE REACTIONS AND SIDE EFFECTS*

CNS: overstimulation, restlessness, dizziness, nervousness, anxiety, insomnia, dyskinesia, euphoria, dysphoria, tremor, headache, drowsiness, mental depression, confusion, incoordination, fatigue, malaise, blurred vision, mydriasis, psychoses (rare), increase in convulsions in some epileptic patients.
CV: palpitations, tachycardia, arrhythmias, hypertension or hypotension, fainting, precordial pain.
Derm: urticaria, rash, erythma, burning sensation, ecchymosis.
Endo: impotence, changes in libido, menstrual irregularity, gynecomastia.
GI: dry mouth, unpleasant taste, nausea, vomiting, diarrhea, constipation, abdominal discomfort.
Hemat: BONE MARROW DEPRESSION, AGRANULOCYTOSIS, LEUKOPENIA.
Other: tolerance, physical and psychological dependence, alopecia, chills, fever, dyspnea, muscle pain, dysuria, polyuria.

INTERACTIONS

Drug-Drug: ♦ **Other CNS stimulants:** additive CNS stimulant effects ♦ **MAO inhibitors (during therapy or within 14 days after administration):** hypertensive crisis, headache, hyperpyrexia, intracranial hemorrhage, bradycardia ♦ **Insulin:** alteration in requirements ♦ **Guanethidine:** decreased antihypertensive effects ♦ **Phenothiazines:** decreased diethylpropion effects ♦ **General anesthetics:** cardiac arrhythmias.
Drug-Food: ♦ **Caffeinated food and drinks:** increased effects of diethylpropion.

ROUTE AND DOSAGE

Exogenous Obesity

♦ **PO (Adults):** 25 mg tid (1 hour before meals) and an additional 25 mg in mid-evening if needed to overcome night hunger. Sustained-release tablets: 75 mg once daily, in mid-morning.

PHARMACODYNAMICS

Route	Onset	Peak	Duration
PO	30–60 min	1–3 hr	4 hr
PO (sustained release)	Variable	—	10–14 hr

NURSING IMPLICATIONS

Assessment

♦ Assess and record baseline temperature, pulse, respiration, blood pressure, and weight for comparison during therapy.
♦ In diabetic patient, assess blood sugar bid to tid. Insulin adjustments may be required due to alteration in eating pattern, as well as possibility of hyperactivity.
♦ Assess knowledge of sound nutri-

*Underlines indicate most frequent; CAPITALS indicate life-threatening.

tional, calorie-reduced diet, and importance of regular exercise.

♦ Assess mental status for changes in mood, level of activity, degree of stimulation.

♦ Assess sleeping patterns carefully. Insomnia may occur.

♦ Assess history of allergies, sensitivity to this drug or to other sympathomimetic amines.

♦ Assess history of glaucoma.

♦ Assess for presence of adverse reactions or side effects.

♦ Assess date of last menses (possible pregnancy), use of contraceptives.

♦ Assess whether currently breast-feeding a child.

♦ Assess current and past alcohol and drug consumption.

♦ Assess usual amount of caffeine consumed.

♦ Assess for operation of automobile and/or other dangerous machinery.

♦ Assess patient/family knowledge about condition and need for medication.

♦ In collaboration with physician, periodically assess CBC, urinalysis, and liver function tests.

♦ **Withdrawal:** Assess for symptoms of withdrawal: • nausea • vomiting • abdominal cramping • headache • fatigue • weakness • mental depression • suicidal ideation.

♦ **Withdrawal Management:** Monitor vital signs.

◇ Place patient in quiet room with low stimuli.

◇ Allow patient to sleep as much as desired.

◇ Maintain close observation (q 15 min).

◇ Institute suicide precautions.

◇ Some physicians may elect to prescribe antidepressants to counteract feelings of depression and lethargy.

♦ **Toxicity and Overdose:** Assess for symptoms of overdose: • restlessness • tremor • hyperreflexia • fever • rapid respiration • disorientation • belligerence • assaultiveness • hallu-

cinations • panic states (stimulation is usually followed by fatigue and depression) • tachycardia • hypertension or hypotension • nausea • vomiting • diarrhea • abdominal cramping • convulsions • coma • circulatory collapse • death.

♦ **Overdose Management:** Monitor vital signs.

◇ Maintain adequate airway.

◇ Initiate cardiac monitoring.

◇ Use cooling measures to control hyperpyrexia.

◇ Initiate gastric lavage.

◇ Administer barbiturate for sedation.

◇ Administer phentolamine to treat severe acute hypertension.

◇ Use IV fluids and a vasopressor to control hypotension secondary to hypovolemia.

◇ Use urine acidifiers to promote urinary excretion of the drug.

◇ Hemodialysis and peritoneal dialysis are not effective.

Potential Nursing Diagnoses

♦ High risk for injury due to overstimulation and hyperactivity, abrupt diethylpropion withdrawal, overdose.

♦ High risk for self-directed violence related to suicidal ideations resulting from abrupt diethylpropion withdrawal.

♦ Alteration in nutrition, more than body requires, related to excessive intake in relation to metabolic needs.

♦ Sleep pattern disturbance related to overstimulation resulting from diethylpropion use.

♦ Alteration in thought processes related to adverse diethylpropion effects of overstimulation and difficulty concentrating.

♦ Knowledge deficit related to medication regimen.

Plan/Implementation

♦ Monitor medication effects. Tolerance develops rapidly. If anorexigenic effects begin to diminish, notify physician immediately. Patient should be on reduced-calorie diet and program of regular exercise in addition to the medication.

♦ Monitor and record vital signs at regular intervals (bid) throughout therapy.

♦ Encourage use of sugarless gum, hard candy, or frequent sips of water for patient who experiences dry mouth. Ensure that patient practices good oral care (frequent brushing, flossing).

♦ Ensure that patient is protected from injury. Keep stimuli low and environment as quiet as possible to discourage overstimulation. Pad siderails and headboard with towels or blankets to protect patient who experiences seizures, particularly at night.

♦ Ensure that tablet has been swallowed and not "cheeked" to avoid medication or to hoard for later use.

♦ Short-acting tablets may be crushed and mixed with food or fluid for patient who has difficulty swallowing.

♦ Last dose may be given in mid-evening if needed to control night hunger. (Insomnia is not usually a serious side effect of this drug.)

♦ Drug should be administered 1 hour before meals.

♦ Store medication at controlled room temperatures between 15° and 30°C (59°–86°F). Protect from heat and moisture.

Patient/Family Education

♦ Use caution in driving or when operating dangerous machinery. Drowsiness, dizziness, and blurred vision can occur.

♦ Do not stop taking the drug abruptly. Doing so can produce serious withdrawal symptoms.

♦ If insomnia is a problem, avoid taking medication late in the day. Take no later than 6 hours before bedtime.

♦ Do not take other medications (including over-the-counter drugs) without physician's approval. Many medications contain substances that, in combination with diethylpropion, can be harmful.

♦ Diabetic patient: Monitor blood sugar bid or tid, or as instructed by physician. Be aware of need for possible alteration in insulin requirements due to changes in food intake, weight, and activity.

♦ Avoid consumption of large amounts of caffeinated products (coffee, tea, colas, chocolate), as they may enhance the stimulant effect of diethylpropion.

♦ Follow reduced-calorie diet provided by dietitian and program of regular exercise. Do not exceed recommended dose if appetite suppressant effect diminishes. Contact physician.

♦ Notify physician if restlessness, insomnia, anorexia, or dry mouth become severe, or if rapid, pounding heartbeat becomes evident.

♦ Be aware of possible risks of taking diethylpropion during pregnancy. Safe use during pregnancy and lactation has not been established. Inform physician immediately if pregnancy is suspected or planned.

♦ Be aware of potential side effects of diethylpropion. Refer to written materials furnished by healthcare providers for safe self-administration.

♦ Carry card or other identification at all times describing medications being taken.

Evaluation

♦ Patient demonstrates a progressive weight loss with the use of diethylpropion as an adjunct to reduced caloric intake and a program of regular exercise.

♦ Patient verbalizes understanding of side effects and regimen required for prudent self-administration of diethylpropion.

DIPHENHYDRAMINE

(dye-fen-hye′dra-meen)
Allerdryl, AllerMax, Belix, Benadryl, Benaphen, Dormarex 2, Fenylhist, Nordryl, Valdrene

Classification(s):
Antiparkinsonian agent, Antihistamine, Antiemetic, Antitussive
Pregnancy Category B

INDICATIONS

♦Parkinsonism ♦ Drug-induced extrapyramidal reactions ♦ Motion sickness ♦ Allergy reactions ♦ Also used as a nighttime sedative and as a cough suppressant.

ACTION

♦ Blocks histamine release by competing with histamine for H-1 receptor sites. Decreased allergic response is effected by diminished histamine activity ♦ May decrease cholinergic activity and prolong dopamine action in the central nervous system to produce antiparkinsonian effects.

PHARMACOKINETICS

Absorption: Readily absorbed following oral and IM administration.
Distribution: Not fully known. Undergoes first-pass metabolism, with only 40–60% reaching systemic circulation. Crosses placental barrier; excreted in breast milk.
Metabolism and Excretion: Metabolized by the liver. Excreted in urine.
Half-Life: 2.4–9.3 hours.

CONTRAINDICATIONS AND PRECAUTIONS

Contraindicated in: ♦ Hypersensitivity to this drug, other antihistamines, or sulfites (contained in some preparations) ♦ Newborn or premature infants ♦ Con-

comitant use of MAO inhibitors ♦ Lactation.
Use Cautiously in: ♦ Narrow-angle glaucoma ♦ Peptic ulcer ♦ Prostatic hypertrophy ♦ Asthmatic attack ♦ Bladder-neck obstruction ♦ Pyloroduodenal obstruction ♦ Elderly or debilitated patients ♦ Pregnancy ♦ Seizure disorders ♦ Hypertension.

ADVERSE REACTIONS AND SIDE EFFECTS*

CNS: drowsiness, sedation, dizziness, disturbed coordination, fatigue, confusion, restlessness, tremor, headache, insomnia, blurred vision, tinnitus, convulsions, paradoxical excitement, delirium, vertigo, nervousness, toxic psychosis, faintness.
CV: hypotension, palpitations, bradycardia, tachycardia, extrasystoles.
Derm: skin rashes, urticaria, photosensitivity, eczema, pruritus, erythema.
GI: epigastric distress, dry mouth, dry nose and throat, anorexia, increased appetite and weight gain, nausea, vomiting, diarrhea, constipation.
GU: urinary frequency, dysuria, urinary retention, early menses, decreased libido, impotence.
Hemat: HEMOLYTIC ANEMIA, THROMBOCYTOPENIA, LEUKOPENIA, AGRANULOCYTOSIS, PANCYTOPENIA.
Resp: thickening of bronchial secretions, chest tightness, wheezing, nasal stuffiness, sore throat, RESPIRATORY DEPRESSION.
Other: tingling and/or heaviness and weakness of the hands, anaphylactic shock, photosensitivity, excessive perspiration, chills.

INTERACTIONS

Drug-Drug: ♦ **CNS depressants (including alcohol, hypnotics, sedatives, tranquilizers, antianxiety agents, narcotic analgesics), procar-**

---

*Underlines indicate most frequent; CAPITALS indicate life-threatening.

bazine: additive CNS depression ✦ **Oral anticoagulants:** diminished anticoagulant effects ✦ **Epinephrine:** enhanced effects of epinephrine ✦ **MAO inhibitors:** prolonged and more intense anticholinergic effects ✦ **Heparin:** decreased anticoagulant effect.

ROUTE AND DOSAGE

- ✦ **PO (Adults):** 25–50 mg tid or qid. For nighttime sedation: 50 mg HS.
- ✦ **PO (Children over 9.1 kg):** 12.5–25 mg tid or qid or 5 mg/kg/day or 150 mg/m²/day. **Maximum daily dose:** 300 mg.
- ✦ **IM, IV (Adults):** 10–50 mg; up to 100 mg, if required. **Maximum daily dose:** 400 mg.
- ✦ **IM, IV (Children):** 5 mg/kg/day or 150 mg/m²/day in divided doses. **Maximum daily dose:** 300 mg divided into four doses.

PHARMACODYNAMICS

Route	Onset	Peak	Duration
PO	30–60 min	1–3 hr	4–6 hr
IM	15–30 min	1–3 hr	4–6 hr
IV	Rapid	—	4–6 hr

NURSING IMPLICATIONS
Assessment

- ✦ Assess for symptoms of anaphylaxis: • fever • redness of skin • itching • urticaria • increased irritability • dyspnea • chest constriction • cyanosis • convulsions • unconsciousness.
- ✦ Assess for symptoms of Parkinson's disease: • tremors • muscular weakness and rigidity • drooling • shuffling gait • disturbances of posture and equilibrium • flat affect • monotone speech.
- ✦ Assess for extrapyramidal symptoms: • pseudoparkinsonism (tremors, shuffling gait, drooling, rigidity) • akinesia (muscular weakness) • akathisia (continuous restlessness and fidgeting) • dystonia (involuntary muscular movements of face, arms, legs, and neck) • oculogyric crisis

(uncontrolled rolling back of the eyes) • tardive dyskinesia (bizarre facial and tongue movements, stiff neck, difficulty swallowing). **Note:** Diphenhydramine is not effective in alleviating symptoms of tardive dyskinesia.

- ✦ Assess characteristics and productivity of cough. Note amount and type of sputum produced.
- ✦ Assess for symptoms of blood dyscrasias: • fever • sore throat • malaise • unusual bruising • easy bleeding.
- ✦ Assess vital signs, weight. Record baseline values for comparison.
- ✦ Assess history of allergies, sensitivity to this drug or to other antihistamines.
- ✦ Assess date of last menses (possible pregnancy), use of contraceptives.
- ✦ Assess whether currently breast-feeding a child.
- ✦ Assess current and past alcohol and drug consumption.
- ✦ Assess for operation of automobile and/or other dangerous machinery.
- ✦ Assess for presence of adverse reactions or side effects.
- ✦ Assess patient/family knowledge about illness and need for medication.
- ✦ In collaboration with physician, assess CBC and liver function tests in patients on long-term therapy.
- ✦ **Toxicity and Overdose:** Assess for symptoms of overdose: • drowsiness • dizziness • fever • excitation • ataxia • dilated pupils • flushing • dry mouth • hyperpyrexia • oral and facial dystonic reactions • tonic-clonic seizures • postictal depression • hallucinations • toxic psychosis • delirium tremens • respiratory depression • cardiovascular collapse.
- ✦ **Overdose Management:** Monitor vital signs.
- ◇ Ensure maintenance of adequate airway.
- ◇ Induce emesis in conscious patient not in seizure.
- ◇ Initiate gastric lavage if emesis is not possible.
- ◇ Administer activated charcoal and a

saline cathartic to minimize absorption.

◇ Administer IV fluids or a vasopressor (norepinephrine, phenylephrine, dopamine) to prevent cardiovascular collapse.

◇ Do not use epinephrine, which may worsen hypotension.

◇ Use propranolol to treat ventricular arrhythmias.

◇ Administer IV phenytoin, diazepam, or a short-acting barbiturate to control seizures.

◇ The fever commonly seen in children who overdose on antihistamines may be treated with cold packs and cooling sponge baths.

Potential Nursing Diagnoses

♦ High risk for injury related to symptoms of Parkinson's disease, drug-induced extrapyramidal symptoms, anaphylactic shock, overdose.

♦ Ineffective airway clearance related to thick, tenacious secretions.

♦ High risk for fluid volume deficit related to vomiting associated with motion sickness.

♦ Social isolation related to embarrassment by symptoms of Parkinson's disease.

♦ High risk for activity intolerance, related to diphenhydramine's side effects of drowsiness, dizziness, ataxia, weakness, confusion.

♦ Knowledge deficit related to medication regimen.

Plan/Implementation

♦ **General Info:** Weigh patient 2–3 times a week, at same time of day, on same scale, if possible. A rapid weight gain or evidence of edema should be reported to physician immediately. Record I&O.

◇ Ensure that patient is protected from injury. Provide supervision and assistance when ambulating if dizziness and drowsiness are problems.

◇ Give patient hard candy, gum, or frequent sips of water if dry mouth is a problem, or treat with a saliva substitute.

◇ In the patient for whom it is not contraindicated, encourage intake of fluids to liquify bronchial secretions.

◇ Store medication at controlled room temperatures between 15° and 30°C (59°–86°F). Protect from heat, light, and moisture.

♦ **PO:** Ensure that patient swallows tablet/capsule and does not "cheek" to avoid medication or to hoard for later use.

◇ May be administered with food or milk to minimize gastric irritation.

◇ Tablet may be crushed or contents of capsule emptied and mixed with food or fluid for patient who has difficulty swallowing, or patient may be given elixir form.

◇ Only the "syrup" form of diphenhydramine is indicated as a nonnarcotic cough suppressant to control cough due to colds or allergy.

◇ As an antiemetic, use full dosage prophylactically for motion sickness. First dose is given 30 minutes before exposure to motion, and subsequent doses are given before meals and at bedtime for duration of exposure.

◇ Monitor vital signs before beginning therapy and at regular intervals (bid or tid) throughout therapy. Take BP lying and standing to monitor for possible hypotensive reaction. Elderly are particularly susceptible. Dosage adjustment may be required.

♦ **IM, IV:** Diphenhydramine injectable is useful for psychotic patients with acute dystonic reactions, allergic reactions to blood or plasma, in anaphylactic shock, or in other reactions that make oral administration difficult or impossible, or when a more rapid response is desired.

◇ Available solutions of 10 mg/mL and 50 mg/mL in 1-mL ampules and in multidose vials. Prepared solution may be given undiluted.

◇ May be administered IM or IV.

◇ Monitor vital signs carefully and frequently during parenteral administration.

◇ Solution is irritating to tissues. Avoid subcutaneous or perivascular injection.

◇ IM injection should be administered deep in large muscle mass. When multiple injections are given, alternate injection sites.

◇ Administer IV at rate not exceeding 25 mg/min.

◇ Switch to oral medication as soon as control of symptoms has been achieved.

Patient/Family Education

♦ May be taken with food or milk if GI upset occurs.

♦ Use caution when driving or when operating dangerous machinery. Drowsiness and dizziness can occur.

♦ Report occurrence of any of the following symptoms to physician immediately: extreme dryness of mouth • difficulty urinating • rapid and pounding heartbeat • rash • fever • sore throat • malaise • easy bruising • unusual bleeding.

♦ Rise slowly from a sitting or lying position to prevent a sudden drop in blood pressure.

♦ If dry mouth is a problem, take frequent sips of water, chew sugarless gum, or suck on hard candy. Good oral care (frequent brushing, flossing) is very important.

♦ Do not drink alcohol while on diphenhydramine therapy.

♦ Do not consume other medications (including over-the-counter meds) without physician's approval. Many medications contain substances that interact with diphenhydramine in a way that may be harmful.

♦ Be aware of possible risks of taking diphenhydramine during pregnancy. Safe use during pregnancy and lactation has not been established. It is thought that diphenhydramine readily crosses the placental barrier; if so, a fetus could experience adverse effects of the drug. Inform physician immediately if pregnancy occurs, is suspected, or is planned.

♦ Be aware of side effects of diphenhydramine. Refer to written materials furnished by healthcare providers for safe self-administration.

♦ Continue to take medication, even if feeling well and as though it is not needed. Symptoms may return if medication is discontinued.

♦ Carry card or other identification at all times describing medications being taken.

Evaluation

♦ Patient demonstrates a subsiding of the symptoms for which diphenhydramine was prescribed (parkinsonism, drug-induced extrapyramidal symptoms, allergy reactions, cough, motion sickness).

♦ Patient verbalizes understanding of side effects and regimen required for prudent self-administration of diphenhydramine.

DISULFIRAM

(dye-sul′fi-ram)
Antabuse

Classification(s):
Enzyme inhibitor
Pregnancy Category C

INDICATIONS

♦ Chronic alcoholism (aids in the maintenance of sobriety in individuals who have chosen this type of deterrent therapy).

ACTION

♦ Inhibits aldehyde dehydrogenase, thereby blocking oxidation of alcohol at the acetaldehyde to acetate stage. Serum acetaldehyde concentration may be 5–10 times higher than with normal alcohol metabolism. This acetaldehyde accumulation is thought to produce the disulfiram-alcohol reaction, which persists as long as alcohol is being metabolized. Rate of alcohol elimination does not appear to be affected.

PHARMACOKINETICS

Absorption: 80–95% rapidly absorbed following oral administration.
Distribution: Highly lipid-soluble; initially deposited in adipose tissue.
Metabolism and Excretion: Partially metabolized by the liver; excreted in urine, feces, and breath. Unknown if drug crosses placental barrier.
Half-Life: Not well substantiated.

CONTRAINDICATIONS AND PRECAUTIONS

Contraindicated in: ◆ Hypersensitivity to disulfiram or to other thiuram derivatives used in pesticides and rubber vulcanization ◆ Severe myocardial disease ◆ Coronary occlusion ◆ Psychoses ◆ Patients receiving or who have recently received metronidazole, paraldehyde, alcohol, or alcohol-containing preparations.
Use Cautiously in: ◆ Hepatic or renal insufficiency ◆ Diabetes mellitus ◆ Seizure disorders ◆ Cerebral damage ◆ Pregnancy ◆ History of rubber-contact dermatitis ◆ Chronic or acute nephritis ◆ Hepatic cirrhosis ◆ Abnormal EEG results ◆ Multiple drug dependence ◆ Hypothyroidism.

ADVERSE REACTIONS AND SIDE EFFECTS*

CNS: drowsiness, fatigue, restlessness, headache, psychosis, confusion, peripheral neuropathy, optic neuritis, vertigo, irritability, insomnia, personality changes, tonic-clonic seizures, polyneuritis, delirium.

Derm: skin rash, acneiform eruptions, allergic dermatitis.
GI: metallic or garlic-like aftertaste, HEPATOTOXICITY.
Hemat: BLOOD DYSCRASIAS.
Other: arthropathy, acetonemia, impotence, abnormal gait, DISULFIRAM-ALCOHOL REACTION.

INTERACTIONS

Drug-Drug: ◆ **Alcohol-containing beverages and other liquids (including topical preparations):** mild to severe life-threatening physical reaction (see Nursing Implications section for assessing toxicity) ◆ **Diazepam, chlordiazepoxide:** increased effects of these drugs ◆ **Phenytoin and its congeners:** phenytoin intoxication ◆ **Oral anticoagulants:** prolonged prothrombin time ◆ **Isoniazid:** unsteady gait or marked changes in behavior ◆ **Metronidazole:** acute toxic psychosis ◆ **Marijuana:** additive CNS stimulation ◆ **Barbiturates, paraldehyde:** increased serum concentration and possible toxicity ◆ **Tricyclic antidepressants:** possible enhancement of disulfiram-alcohol reaction, acute organic brain syndrome.
Drug-Food: ◆ **Caffeine:** decreased clearance of caffeine.

ROUTE AND DOSAGE

Alcohol Deterrent Therapy

(**Note:** Do not administer until the patient has abstained from alcohol for at least 12 hours, and never without the patient's knowledge.)
◆ **PO (Adults): Initial Dosage:** 250–500 mg daily in a single dose for 1–2 weeks. **Maintenance:** 125–500 mg daily. Do not exceed 500 mg/day.

PHARMACODYNAMICS

Route	Onset	Peak	Duration
PO	3–12 hr	—	Up to 14 days

*Underlines indicate most frequent; CAPITALS indicate life-threatening.

NURSING IMPLICATIONS
Assessment

* Assess baseline vital signs and weight.
* Assess mood, general appearance, orientation, motor behavior.
* Assess for symptoms of alcohol withdrawal: • tremors • nausea and vomiting • malaise • tachycardia • diaphoresis • elevated blood pressure • fever • seizures • anxiety • depression • irritability • diarrhea • anorexia • insomnia • orthostatic hypotension.
* Assess alcohol and drug history. Determine time and amount of last drink.
* Assess history of allergies (drug, food, others).
* Assess history of diabetes, cardiac disease, epilepsy, hypothyroidism, liver disease, or psychosis.
* Assess level of knowledge about condition and desire for therapy with disulfiram.
* Assess history of ability to abstain from alcohol.
* Assess date of last menses (possible pregnancy), use of contraceptives.
* Assess whether currently breast-feeding a child.
* Assess for presence of adverse reactions or side effects.
* In collaboration with physician, assess baseline and follow-up (every 10–14 days) transaminase tests to detect hepatic dysfunction resulting from disulfiram therapy. A complete blood count (CBC) and sequential multiple analysis (SMA-12) should be performed every 6 months throughout therapy.
* **Lab Test Alterations:** Decreased protein-bound iodine (PBI) test results.
◊ Reduced uptake of I_{131}.
◊ Decreased urinary vanillylmandelic acid (VMA).
◊ Possible increased urinary homovanillic acid.
* **Toxicity and Overdose:** Assess for symptoms of disulfiram-alcohol reaction. Symptoms can occur within 5–

10 minutes of ingestion of alcohol. Mild reactions can occur at blood alcohol levels as low as 5–10 mg%. Symptoms are fully developed at ∼50 mg%, and unconsciousness usually occurs at ∼125–150 mg%. The reaction may last from 30 minutes to several hours. Symptoms include: • flushing • throbbing in head and neck • respiratory difficulty • nausea • copious vomiting • sweating • thirst • chest pain • palpitations • dyspnea • hyperventilation • tachycardia • hypotension • syncope • weakness • vertigo • blurred vision • confusion. Severe reactions can progress to: • respiratory depression • cardiovascular collapse • arrhythmias • myocardial infarction • acute congestive heart failure • unconsciousness • convulsions • death.

* **Management of Disulfiram-Alcohol Reaction:** Monitor vital signs.
◊ Ensure maintenance of adequate airway.
◊ Initiate fluid therapy to restore blood pressure and treat shock.
◊ Administer oxygen.
◊ Administer IV vitamin C (1 g).
◊ Administer antihistamines.
◊ Administer ephedrine sulfate to treat hypotension.
◊ Monitor potassium levels (hypokalemia has been reported).

Potential Nursing Diagnoses

* High risk for injury related to disulfiram-alcohol reaction; alcohol withdrawal; disulfiram's side effects of drowsiness and fatigue.
* Ineffective breathing pattern related to disulfiram-alcohol reaction.
* Decreased cardiac output related to disulfiram-alcohol reaction.
* Ineffective denial related to underdeveloped ego evidenced by failure to view alcohol as a problem in patient's life.
* Ineffective individual coping related to chronic abuse of alcohol.

♦ Knowledge deficit related to medication regimen.

Plan/Implementation

♦ Ensure that patient is fully informed and gives written consent to participate in disulfiram therapy.

♦ Ensure that patient understands potential for life-threatening situation should even a small amount of alcohol be ingested or applied topically while taking disulfiram.

♦ Do not administer disulfiram until certain that patient has abstained from alcoholic beverages or other alcohol-containing substances (including preparations which may be absorbed through the skin) for at least 12 hours.

♦ Tablet may be crushed and mixed with food or fluid for patient who has difficulty swallowing.

♦ Ensure that tablet has been swallowed and not "cheeked" to avoid taking the medication.

♦ Single dose may be taken in the morning, or at bedtime if drowsiness occurs.

♦ Notify physician if behavioral changes become evident. Psychoses have occurred in patients on disulfiram therapy.

♦ Ensure that patient is protected from injury. Supervise and assist with ambulation if drowsiness and fatigue are problems.

♦ Store medication at controlled room temperature between 15° and 30°C (59°–86°F). Protect from heat, light, and moisture.

Patient/Family Education

♦ Use caution in driving or when operating dangerous machinery. Drowsiness and fatigue can occur.

♦ Drug may be taken at bedtime if drowsiness is a problem.

♦ Do not consume alcohol in any form while on disulfiram therapy. To do so can produce symptoms such as severe nausea and vomiting, flushing, throbbing headache, fast heart rate, chest pain, difficulty breathing, even death. These symptoms can begin within 5–10 minutes following ingestion of alcohol. They may last from 30 minutes to several hours. Family members should seek assistance from physician or emergency personnel immediately should these symptoms occur.

♦ Learn to read labels. Many products contain alcohol, from which you MUST abstain. These products include: • cough liquids • vanilla extract • aftershave lotions • colognes • mouthwash • isopropyl rubbing alcohol • nail polish removers. Do not rub any of these products on your body, as they can be absorbed through your skin and may produce symptoms just as those that occur when alcohol is ingested.

♦ Be sure to tell any doctor, dentist, or other healthcare professional from whom care is sought that you are taking disulfiram.

♦ You may experience an unpleasant metallic or garlic-like taste in your mouth. This is not dangerous and will usually disappear after 2 weeks of therapy.

♦ If disulfiram is discontinued, be aware that the sensitivity to alcohol may last for as long as 2 weeks. Consuming alcohol or using alcohol-containing substances during this 2-week period may result in the serious disulfiram-alcohol reaction previously described.

♦ Always carry a card explaining your participation in disulfiram therapy, possible consequences of the therapy, and symptoms that may indicate an emergency situation. Be sure to include name of physician and/or institution to contact should a reaction occur.

♦ Because of possible toxicity to the liver, ensure that blood tests are taken at least every 6 months while on long-term disulfiram therapy.

♦ Be aware of possible risks of taking

disulfiram during pregnancy. It is unknown if disulfiram crosses the placental barrier, so effects to unborn child are not known. Notify physician immediately if pregnancy is suspected or planned.

♦ Be aware of potential side effects. Usually, side effects associated with taking disulfiram alone subside after approximately 2 weeks. Refer to written materials furnished by healthcare providers regarding correct method of self-administration.

♦ It is advised that, along with deterrent therapy, the patient seek other assistance with alcoholism, such as Alcoholics Anonymous or other support group to aid in recovery process.

Evaluation

♦ Patient is able to abstain from alcohol while on disulfiram therapy.

♦ Patient experiences no symptoms associated with consumption of disulfiram-alcohol combination.

♦ Patient verbalizes understanding of side effects and regimen required for prudent self-administration of disulfiram.

DOXEPIN

(dox′e-pin)
Adapin, Sinequan

Classifiction(s):
Tricyclic Antidepressant
Pregnancy Category C

INDICATIONS

♦ Major depression with melancholia or psychotic symptoms ♦ Depression associated with organic disease and alcoholism ♦ Depressive phase of bipolar disorder ♦ Psychoneurotic anxiety ♦ Mixed symptoms of anxiety and depression. **Investigational Use:** ♦ Peptic ulcer disease.

ACTION

♦ Exact mechanism of action unclear ♦ Blocks the reuptake of the neurotransmitters norepinephrine and serotonin, increasing their concentration at the synapse and correcting the deficit that is thought to contribute to the melancholy mood of the depressed person.

PHARMACOKINETICS

Absorption: Readily absorbed from the GI tract following oral administration.
Distribution: Is widely distributed. Crosses blood-brain and placental barriers. Enters breast milk.
Metabolism and Excretion: Metabolized by the liver. Excreted by the kidneys.
Half-Life: 6–8 hours.

CONTRAINDICATIONS AND PRECAUTIONS

Contraindicated in: ♦ Hypersensitivity to this drug or to other tricyclic antidepressants ♦ Concomitant use of MAO inhibitors ♦ Acute recovery period following myocardial infarction ♦ Untreated angle-closure glaucoma ♦ Patients with tendency toward urinary retention ♦ Children under age 12; pregnancy and lactation (safety not established).
Use Cautiously in: ♦ Patients with a history of seizures ♦ Benign prostatic hypertrophy ♦ Respiratory difficulties ♦ Cardiovascular disorders ♦ Hepatic or renal insufficiency ♦ Psychotic patients ♦ Elderly or debilitated patients.

ADVERSE REACTIONS AND SIDE EFFECTS*

CNS: <u>drowsiness</u>, <u>dizziness</u>, weakness, headache, fatigue, confusion, lethargy, memory deficits, disturbed concentration, tremors, ataxia, tinnitus, extrapyramidal symptoms, paresthesias of extremities, lowered seizure threshold, blurred vision, agitation, excitement, restlessness,

---

*<u>Underlines</u> indicate most frequent; CAPITALS indicate life-threatening.

insomnia, exacerbation of psychosis, shift to manic behavior.

CV: orthostatic hypotension, tachycardia and other arrhythmias, hypertension, MYOCARDIAL INFARCTION, HEART BLOCK, CONGESTIVE HEART FAILURE, ECG changes, syncope, CARDIOVASCULAR COLLAPSE.

Derm: skin rash, urticaria, photosensitivity, erythema, petechiae.

GI: dry mouth, constipation, nausea, vomiting, anorexia, diarrhea, abdominal cramps, adynamic ileus, esophageal reflux, stomatitis, black tongue.

GU: urinary retention, gynecomastia (men), testicular swelling, menstrual irregularity, breast engorgement, galactorrhea (women), changes in libido, impotence, delayed micturition.

Hemat: AGRANULOCYTOSIS, THROMBOCYTOPENIA, LEUKOPENIA, eosinophilia, purpura.

Hepat: jaundice, hepatitis.

Other: weight gain, nasal conjestion, alopecia, hypothermia, peripheral neuropathy.

INTERACTIONS

Drug-Drug: ✦ **MAO inhibitors:** hyperpyretic crisis, hypertensive crisis, severe seizures, tachycardia, death ✦ **Guanethidine, clonidine, (possibly) guanabenz:** decreased effects of these medications ✦ **Cimetidine:** increased doxepin serum levels ✦ **Amphetamines, sympathomimetics:** increased hypertensive and cardiac effects of these drugs ✦ **CNS depressants (including alcohol, barbiturates, benzodiazepines):** potentiation of CNS effects ✦ **Thyroid medications:** tachycardia, arrhythmias ✦ **Methylphenidate, phenothiazines, haloperidol:** increased serum doxepin levels ✦ **Ethchlorvynol:** transient delirium ✦ **Quinidine, procainamide, disopyramide:** potentiates adverse cardiovascular effects of doxepin ✦ **Oral contraceptives:** decreased effects of doxepin ✦ **Smoking:** increases doxepin metabolism ✦ **Disulfiram:** decreases doxepin metabolism ✦ **Levodopa, phenylbutazone:** delayed or decreased absorption of these drugs ✦ **Dicumarol:** increased plasma dicumarol concentrations.

ROUTE AND DOSAGE

Mild to Moderate Anxiety or Depression

✦ **PO (Adults): Initial Dosage:** 10–25 mg tid. Adjust dose according to patient response. Usual optimal dosage is 75–150 mg/day. Total amount may be taken as single dose at bedtime.

Severe Anxiety or Depression

✦ **PO (Adults): Initial Dosage:** 50 mg tid. May be gradually increased to a maximum of 300 mg/day. Up to 150 mg may be given as single dose at bedtime.

PHARMACODYNAMICS

Route	Onset	Peak	Duration
PO	2–4 wk	<2 hr	Weeks*

*Allow up to 2 weeks following cessation of therapy for complete drug elimination

NURSING IMPLICATIONS

Assessment

✦ Assess level of anxiety. Symptoms include: ● restlessness ● pacing ● insomnia ● inability to concentrate ● increased heart rate ● increased respiration ● elevated blood pressure ● confusion ● tremors ● rapid speech.

✦ Assess for suicidal ideation, plan, means. Assess for sudden lift in mood, which could indicate patient's decision to commit suicide.

✦ Assess mental status daily: ● mood ● appearance ● thought and communication patterns ● level of interest in the environment and in activities ● suicidal ideation. Improvement in these behavior patterns and level of energy should be expected within 2–4 weeks following initiation of therapy.

✦ Assess for symptoms of blood dyscrasias: ● sore throat ● fever ● malaise ● unusual bleeding ● easy bruising.

✦ Assess vital signs, weight.

♦ Assess history of allergies, sensitivity to this drug or to other tricyclic antidepressants.

♦ Assess for history of glaucoma.

♦ Assess date of last menses (possible pregnancy), use of contraceptives.

♦ Assess whether currently breast-feeding a child.

♦ Assess current and past alcohol and drug consumption.

♦ Assess for operation of automobile and/or other dangerous machinery.

♦ Assess for presence of adverse reactions or side effects.

♦ Assess patient/family knowledge about illness and need for medication.

♦ In collaboration with physician, assess CBC and liver function tests in patients on long-term therapy.

♦ **Lab Test Alterations:** Increased serum bilirubin, alkaline phosphatase, transaminase, and glucose.

◇ Decreased urinary 5-hydroxyindole-acetic acid (HIAA) and vanillylmandelic acid (VMA) excretion.

♦ **Withdrawal:** Assess for symptoms of abrupt withdrawal from long-term therapy: ● nausea ● headache ● vertigo ● malaise ● insomnia ● nightmares.

♦ **Toxicity and Overdose:** Range of therapeutic serum concentration not well substantiated.

◇ Assess for symptoms of overdose: ● confusion ● agitation ● irritability ● hallucinations ● seizures ● flushing ● dry mouth ● dilated pupils ● delirium ● hyperpyrexia ● hypotension or hypertension ● coma ● tachycardia ● arrhythmias ● respiratory depression ● cardiac arrest ● renal failure ● shock ● congestive heart failure ● acid-base disturbances.

♦ **Overdose Management:** Monitor vital signs.

◇ Ensure maintenance of adequate airway.

◇ Monitor ECG.

◇ Induce emesis in the alert patient.

◇ Follow emesis with gastric lavage.

◇ Administer activated charcoal to minimize absorption.

◇ Cautiously administer IV physostigmine to reverse anticholinergic effects.

◇ Administer sodium bicarbonate, vasopressors, phenytoin, propranolol, or lidocaine to treat cardiovascular effects.

◇ Administer IV diazepam to combat seizures.

Potential Nursing Diagnoses

♦ High risk for self-directed violence related to depressed mood.

♦ High risk for injury related to doxepin side effects of sedation, dizziness, ataxia, weakness, confusion, lowered seizure threshold, abrupt withdrawal after prolonged use; overdose.

♦ Anxiety (moderate to severe) related to threat to physical integrity or self-concept.

♦ Social isolation related to depressed mood.

♦ High risk for activity intolerance, related to doxepin's side effects of drowsiness, dizziness, ataxia, weakness, confusion.

♦ Knowledge deficit related to medication regimen.

Plan/Implementation

♦ Monitor vital signs before beginning therapy and at regular intervals (bid or tid) throughout therapy. Take BP lying and standing in patients experiencing orthostatic hypotension; elderly are particularly susceptible. Contact physician if tachycardia/arrhythmias are noted.

♦ Ensure that patient who is ambulatory is protected from sun when spending time outdoors.

♦ Weigh patient 2–3 times a week, at same time of day, on same scale, if possible. A rapid weight gain or evidence of edema should be reported to physician immediately. Record I&O.

♦ Ensure that patient is protected from injury. Provide supervision and assistance when ambulating if dizziness and drowsiness are problems. Pad siderails and headboard for patient who experiences seizures.

♦ Give patient hard candy, gum, or frequent sips of water if dry mouth is a problem.

♦ Administer oral medication with food to minimize GI upset.

♦ Ensure that patient swallows capsule and does not "cheek" to avoid medication or to hoard for later use.

♦ Contents of capsule may be emptied and mixed with food or fluid for patient who has difficulty swallowing.

♦ Dilute oral concentrate with 120 mL water, fruit juice, or milk just prior to administration. Do not dilute with carbonated beverages, as mixture is incompatible. Do not prepare and store bulk dilutions.

♦ Store medication at controlled room temperatures between 15° and 30°C (59°–86°F). Protect from heat and moisture.

Patient/Family Education

♦ Therapeutic effect may not be seen for as long as 4 weeks. If after this length of time no improvement is noted, physician may prescribe a different medication. Continue to take medication even though symptoms have not subsided.

♦ Use caution when driving or when operating dangerous machinery. Drowsiness and dizziness can occur. If these side effects become persistent or interfere with daily activities, report them to physician. Dosage adjustment may be necessary.

♦ Do not stop taking the drug abruptly. To do so might produce withdrawal symptoms, such as nausea, vertigo, insomnia, headache, malaise, nightmares.

♦ Use sunscreens and wear protective clothing when spending time outdoors. Skin may be sensitive to sunburn.

♦ Report occurrence of any of the following symptoms to physician immediately: sore throat ● fever ● malaise ● unusual bleeding ● easy bruising ● persistent nausea/vomiting ● severe headache ● rapid heart rate ● difficulty urinating.

♦ Rise slowly from a sitting or lying position to prevent a sudden drop in blood pressure.

♦ If dry mouth is a problem, take frequent sips of water, chew sugarless gum, or suck on hard candy. Good oral care (frequent brushing, flossing) is very important.

♦ Do not smoke while on doxepin therapy. Smoking increases metabolism of doxepin, requiring adjustment in dosage to achieve therapeutic effect.

♦ Do not drink alcohol while on doxepin therapy. These drugs potentiate each other's effects.

♦ Do not consume other medications (including over-the-counter meds) with doxepin without physician's approval. Many medications contain substances that, in combination with tricyclics, could precipitate a life-threatening hypertensive crisis.

♦ Be aware of possible risks of taking doxepin during pregnancy. Safe use during pregnancy and lactation has not been established. Doxepin readily crosses the placental barrier, so a fetus could experience adverse effects from the drug. Inform physician immediately if pregnancy occurs, is suspected, or is planned.

♦ Be aware of side effects of doxepin. Refer to written materials furnished by healthcare providers for safe self-administration.

♦ Carry card or other identification at all times describing medications being taken.

Evaluation

♦ Patient demonstrates a subsiding/resolution of the symptoms for which doxepin was prescribed (depressed mood, suicidal ideation, anxiety).

♦ Patient verbalizes understanding of

side effects and regimen required for prudent self-administration of doxepin.

DROPERIDOL

(droe-per′i-dole)
Inapsine

Classification(s):
Antipsychotic, Neuroleptic,
Antiemetic, Butyrophenone
Pregnancy Category C

INDICATIONS

♦ Tranquilizing effect and to reduce nausea and vomiting in surgical and diagnostic procedures ♦ Premedication for induction of and as an adjunct to general and regional anesthesia.

ACTION

♦ The exact mechanism of antipsychotic action is not fully understood ♦ Appears to depress the CNS at subcortical level of the brain, midbrain, and brain stem reticular formation • Thought to inhibit ascending reticular activating system of brain stem; may also inhibit catecholamine receptors as well as reuptake of various neurotransmitters in midbrain ♦ Also is a strong central antagonist of dopamine receptors.

PHARMACOKINETICS

Absorption: Well absorbed following IM administration.
Distribution: Distribution is not completely known. Crosses blood-brain and placental barriers. Unknown if drug enters breast milk.
Metabolism and Excretion: Metabolized mainly by the liver. Excreted in urine and feces.
Half-Life: 2.2 hours.

CONTRAINDICATIONS AND PRECAUTIONS

Contraindicated in: ♦ Hypersensitivity to this drug or to other butyrophenones ♦ Children under 2 years of age; pregnancy and lactation (safe use has not been established).
Use Cautiously in: ♦ Elderly or debilitated patients ♦ Hypotensive patients ♦ Hepatic, renal, or cardiac disease ♦ Parkinson's disease.

ADVERSE REACTIONS AND SIDE EFFECTS*

CNS: <u>sedation</u>, <u>dizziness</u>, <u>extrapyramidal symptoms</u> (pseudoparkinsonism, akathisia, akinesia, dystonia, oculogyric crisis), <u>tardive dyskinesia</u>, postoperative hallucinations, muscular rigidity, restlessness, hyperactivity, anxiety.
CV: <u>hypotension</u>, hypertension (in combination with parenteral analgesics), <u>tachycardia</u>.
Resp: apnea, RESPIRATORY DEPRESSION, LARYNGOSPASM, BRONCHOSPASM, RESPIRATORY ARREST.
Other: <u>chills</u>, <u>shivering</u>, facial sweating.

INTERACTIONS

Drug-Drug: ♦ **CNS depressants (including alcohol, barbiturates, benzodiazepines, opiates, sedative/hypnotics):** additive CNS depression ♦ **Narcotic analgesics:** increased respiratory depression ♦ **Epinephrine:** usual pressor effect of epinephrine is reversed, resulting in additional decrease in blood pressure.

ROUTE AND DOSAGE

Preanesthesia Medication

♦ **IM (Adults):** 2.5–10 mg 30–60 min preoperatively.
♦ **IM (Children 2–12 Years):** 1–1.5 mg/9–11 kg.

---

*<u>Underlines</u> indicate most frequent; CAPITALS indicate life-threatening.

Adjunct to General Anesthesia

✦ **IV (Adults):** For induction: 0.22–0.275 mg/kg; for maintenance: 1.25–2.5 mg.
✦ **IV (Children 2–12 Years):** For induction: 0.088–0.165 mg/kg.

Diagnostic Procedures

✦ **IM (Adults):** 2.5–10 mg 30–60 min before the procedure. Additional 1.25–2.5 mg may be administered (usually IV), if necessary.

Adjunct to Regional Anesthesia

✦ **IM, IV (Adults):** 2.5–5 mg.

PHARMACODYNAMICS

Route	Onset	Peak	Duration
IM, IV	3–10 min	30 min	2–12 hr

NURSING IMPLICATIONS

Assessment

✦ Assess degree of nausea/vomiting.
✦ Assess hydration: Note: • weight • condition of mucous membranes • skin turgor • color • amount and density of urine • vital signs.
✦ Assess level of anxiety. Symptoms include: • restlessness • pacing • insomnia • inability to concentrate • increased heart rate • increased respiration • elevated blood pressure • confusion • tremors • rapid speech.
✦ Assess for exrapyramidal symptoms: • psuedoparkinsonism (tremors, shuffling gait, drooling, rigidity) • akinesia (muscular weakness) • akathisia (continuous restlessness and fidgeting) • dystonia (involuntary muscular movements of face, arms, legs, and neck) • oculogyric crisis (uncontrolled rolling back of the eyes) • tardive dyskinesia (bizarre facial and tongue movements, stiff neck, difficulty swallowing).
✦ Assess for signs of respiratory depression (apnea, restlessness, muscular rigidity) in patients receiving this drug in combination with narcotic analgesics.
✦ Assess vital signs, weight. Record baseline values for comparison.
✦ Assess history of allergies, sensitivity to this drug or to other butyrophenones.
✦ Assess date of last menses (possible pregnancy) use of contraceptives.
✦ Assess whether currently breast-feeding a child.
✦ Assess current and past alcohol and drug consumption.
✦ Assess for operation of automobile and/or other dangerous machinery.
✦ Assess for presence of adverse reactions or side effects.
✦ Assess patient/family knowledge about illness and need for medication.
✦ **Toxicity and Overdose:** No correlation has been established between blood level and therapeutic effect.
◇ Assess for overdose symptoms of intensification of pharmacologic effects and adverse reactions.
✦ **Overdose Management:** Monitor vital signs.
◇ Administer oxygen if patient presents with hypoventilation or apnea.
◇ Maintain a patent airway.
◇ Observe patient for 24 hours.
◇ Ensure that body warmth is maintained and fluid intake is adquate.
◇ If hypotension is severe or persists, consider hypovolemia as a cause and manage with parenteral fluid therapy.

Potential Nursing Diagnoses

✦ High risk for fluid volume deficit related to vomiting.
✦ High risk for injury related to droperidol's side effects of sedation, dizziness, hypotension, respiratory depression, overdose.
✦ Anxiety (moderate to severe) related to pending surgery or diagnostic procedure.
✦ Sensory-perceptual alteration related to adverse effect of post-op hallucinations.
✦ High risk for activity intolerance, related to droperidol's side effects of drowsiness, dizziness.

- Knowledge deficit related to medication regimen.

Plan/Implementation

- **General Info:** Monitor pulse and blood pressure closely. A pressor agent may be indicated if hypotension is severe. Do not use epinephrine, as interaction with droperidol produces additive hypotensive effects.
- ◇ Ensure that patient is protected from injury. Provide supervision and assistance when ambulating if dizziness and drowsiness are problems.
- ◇ Store medication at controlled room temperatures between 15°C and 30°C (59°–86°F). Protect from heat and light.
- **IM:** Nurses may be responsible for IM administration of droperidol as adjunctive medication to preanesthesia.
- ◇ Take vital signs immediately prior to administration. If respiratory rate is below 13, withhold medication and contact physician.
- ◇ Inject slowly and deeply into large muscle mass.
- ◇ Because of possible hypotensive effects, patient should remain in recumbent position following IM injection.
- ◇ Continue to monitor vital signs closely (q 5–10 min) following administration until patient is taken to surgery or for diagnostic procedure.
- ◇ Should evidence of respiratory depression occur, administer oxygen, ensure maintenance of patent airway, and notify physician immediately.
- ◇ Do not mix with parenteral barbiturates. Precipitation may occur.
- ◇ Postoperatively, continue to monitor vital signs closely. Physician should be notified if hypotension, bradycardia, tachycardia, or respiratory depression occurs.

- ◇ If narcotic analgesics are required postoperatively, they should be given at only 25–30% of usual dose. The effects of CNS depressants are potentiated by droperidol.
- **IV:** IV administration of droperidol is used primarily by or under the direct observation of the anesthesiologist.
- ◇ Rate of administration should not exceed 10 mg/min.
- ◇ Ensure that resuscitation equipment and medication to manage hypotension are readily available.

Patient/Family Education

- Rise slowly from a sitting or lying position to prevent a sudden drop in blood pressure.
- Be aware of possible risks of taking droperidol during pregnancy. Safe use during pregnancy and lactation has not been established. Droperidol readily crosses the placental barrier, so a fetus could experience adverse effects of the drug. Inform physician immediately if pregnant.
- Be aware of side effects of droperidol. Contact healthcare workers regarding any information about which you are unclear.
- For future reference, keep record of all medications that have been administered to you, and your body's response to each.

Evaluation

- Patient verbalizes understanding of potential side effects and need for administration of droperidol.
- Patient demonstrates a subsiding/resolution of the symptoms for which droperidol was prescribed (preanesthesia medication, adjunct to anesthesia, nausea and vomiting).

ETHCHLORVYNOL

(eth-klor-vi'nole)
Placidyl

Classification(s):
Sedative-hypnotic, CNS depressant
Schedule C IV
Pregnancy Category C

INDICATIONS

✦ Insomnia (short-term management) ✦
Moderate anxiety.

ACTION

✦ Exact mechanism of action is unknown
✦ Produces a calming effect through depression of the central nervous system.

PHARMACOKINETICS

Absorption: Rapidly absorbed following oral administration.
Distribution: Extensive localization in adipose tissue, liver, kidneys, spleen, brain, bile, and cerebrospinal fluid. Crosses placental barrier.
Metabolism and Excretion: Metabolized by the liver and excreted by the kidneys.
Half-Life: 10–20 hours.

CONTRAINDICATIONS AND PRECAUTIONS

Contraindicated in: ✦ Hypersensitivity to this drug or to tartrazine (contained in 750 mg capsules) ✦ Porphyria ✦ Pregnancy and lactation ✦ Children (safety and effectiveness not determined).
Use Cautiously in: ✦ Elderly or debilitated patients ✦ Patients with hepatic or renal dysfunction ✦ Depressed/suicidal patients ✦ Patients with a history of drug abuse/dependence ✦ Patients sensitive to aspirin (may react to tartrazine in 750-mg capsules).

ADVERSE REACTIONS AND SIDE EFFECTS*

CNS: drowsiness, dizziness, hangover, ataxia, facial numbness, paradoxical excitement, blurred vision, fatigue, nightmares, toxic amblyopia.
CV: hypotension.
Derm: skin rashes.
GI: nausea, vomiting, gastric upset, unpleasant aftertaste.
Hemat: THROMBOCYTOPENIA (rare).
Other: tolerance, physical and psychological dependence, cholestatic jaundice (rare).

INTERACTIONS

Drug-Drug: ✦ **Other CNS depressants (including alcohol, benzodiazepines, opiates), MAO inhibitors:** additive CNS depression ✦ **Oral anticoagulants:** decreased effects of anticoagulants ✦ **Tricyclic antidepressants:** transient delirium.

ROUTE AND DOSAGE

Anxiety

✦ **PO (Adults):** 200 mg bid or tid.

Insomnia

(Limit use to 1 week.)
✦ **PO (Adults):** 500–1000 mg 15–30 min before retiring.

PHARMACODYNAMICS

Route	Onset	Peak	Duration
PO	15–30 min	1–2 hr	5 hr

NURSING IMPLICATIONS

Assessment

✦ Assess level of anxiety and agitation. Report and document behaviors.
✦ Assess sleep patterns. Keep records for adequate baseline data before the initiation of therapy.
✦ Assess for suicidal ideation in depressed patients.

---

*Underlines indicate most frequent; CAPITALS indicate life-threatening.

♦ Assess history of allergies, sensitivity to this drug.

♦ Assess date of last menses (possible pregnancy), use of contraceptives.

♦ Assess whether currently breast-feeding a child.

♦ Assess current and past alcohol and drug consumption.

♦ Assess for operation of automobile and/or other dangerous machinery.

♦ Assess for presence of adverse reactions or side effects.

♦ Assess patient/family knowledge about condition and need for medication.

♦ In collaboration with physician, assess CBC and renal and liver function tests in patients who have been on prolonged use.

♦ **Withdrawal:** Assess for symptoms of withdrawal: • anxiety • tremors • insomnia • nausea/vomiting • weakness • diaphoresis • orthostatic hypotension • agitation • irritability • severe hallucinations • confusion • memory loss • delirium • convulsions.

♦ **Withdrawal Management:** Monitor vital signs.

◊ Place patient in quiet room with low stimuli.

◊ Institute seizure precautions.

◊ A long-acting barbiturate, such as phenobarbital, may be ordered to suppress withdrawal symptoms.

◊ Phenytoin may be ordered to prevent seizures.

◊ Some physicians may order oxazepam as needed for objective withdrawal symptoms, gradually decreasing the dosage until the drug is discontinued.

♦ **Toxicity and Overdose:** Assess for symptoms of toxicity: • confusion • drowsiness • dyspnea • slurred speech • staggering.

◊ Assess for symptoms of overdose: • CNS and respiratory depression • mydriasis • areflexia • hypoventilation • hypothermia • hypotension • oliguria • bradycardia • coma. (May progress to respiratory arrest, circulatory collapse, and death.)

♦ **Overdose Management:** Monitor vital signs.

◊ Ensure maintenance of airway.

◊ Induce vomiting in conscious patient.

◊ Initiate gastric lavage in unconscious patient.

◊ Administer activated charcoal to minimize absorption of drug.

◊ Administer IV fluids.

◊ For severe intoxication, forced diuresis or hemodialysis may be used.

Potential Nursing Diagnosis

♦ High risk for injury related to abrupt withdrawal from long-term use; decreased mental alertness caused by side effects of drowsiness and dizziness, effects of overdose.

♦ High risk for self-directed violence related to depressed mood.

♦ Anxiety (specify level) related to threats to physical integrity and/or self-concept.

♦ Sleep pattern disturbance related to situational crises, physical condition, severe level of anxiety.

♦ High risk for activity intolerance, related to side effects of drowsiness, dizziness.

♦ Knowledge deficit related to medication regimen.

Plan/Implementation

♦ Monitor vital signs before beginning therapy and at regular intervals (bid) throughout therapy.

♦ Ensure that patient is protected from injury. Supervise and assist with ambulation if dizziness and drowsiness are problems. Ensure that patient avoids participation in any activity requiring mental alerness (including smoking). Raise siderails and instruct patient to remain in bed following administration.

♦ To minimize nausea, medication may be given with food or milk.

♦ Ensure that capsule has been swallowed and not "cheeked" to avoid medication or to hoard for later use.

♦ Empty capsule and mix contents with

food or fluid for patient who has difficulty swallowing.

♦ Store medication at controlled room temperatures between 15° and 30°C (59°–86°F). Protect from heat, light, and moisture.

Patient/Family Education

♦ Use caution in driving or when operating dangerous machinery. Drowsiness and dizziness can occur.

♦ Do not stop taking the drug abruptly. Doing so can produce serious (even life-threatening) withdrawal symptoms. If a dose is missed, take it as close as possible to the prescribed time. If it is already close to time for next dose, wait until then; do not double up on dose at the next prescribed time.

♦ Do not consume other CNS depressants (including alcohol).

♦ Be aware of possible risks of taking ethchlorvynol during pregnancy (safety during pregnancy has not been established). Notify physician if pregnancy is suspected or planned.

♦ Be aware of potential side effects. Refer to written materials furnished by healthcare providers regarding correct method of self-administration.

♦ Report symptoms of sore throat, fever, malaise, unusual bleeding, or easy bruising to physician immediately.

♦ Carry card or other identification at all times stating names of medications being taken.

Evaluation

♦ Patient demonstrates a subsiding/resolution of the symptoms for which ethchlorvynol was prescribed (anxiety, sleep disturbances).

♦ Patient verbalizes understanding of side effects and regimen required for prudent self-administration of ethchlorvynol.

ETHINAMATE

(e-thin′a-mate)
Valmid

Classification(s):
Sedative-hypnotic, CNS depressant
Schedule C IV
Pregnancy Category C

INDICATIONS

♦ Insomnia (short-term management).

ACTION

♦ Exact mechanism of action is unknown
♦ Produces a calming effect through depression of the central nervous system.

PHARMACOKINETICS

Absorption: Rapidly absorbed following oral administration.
Distribution: Unknown. Transmission across placental barrier and excretion in breast milk have not been determined.
Metabolism and Excretion: Metabolized by the liver; excreted by the kidneys.
Half-Life: 2.5 hours.

CONTRAINDICATIONS AND PRECAUTIONS

Contraindicated in: ♦ Hypersensitivity to the drug ♦ Patients with uncontrolled pain ♦ Children under age 15; pregnancy and lactation (safety and effectiveness have not been established).
Use Cautiously in: ♦ Elderly or debilitated patients ♦ Patients with hepatic, renal, or respiratory dysfunction ♦ Depressed/suicidal patients ♦ Patients with a history of drug abuse/dependence.

ADVERSE REACTIONS AND SIDE EFFECTS*

CNS: <u>drowsiness</u>, <u>dizziness</u>, paradoxical excitement in children.
Derm: skin rashes.

---

*Underlines indicate most frequent; CAPITALS indicate life-threatening.

GI: nausea.
Hemat: THROMBOCYTOPENIA (rare).
Other: tolerance, physical and psychological dependence, hypersensitivity reactions with fever (rare).

INTERACTIONS

Drug-Drug: ◆ **Other CNS depressants (including alcohol, barbiturates, benzodiazepines, opiates):** additive CNS depression.

ROUTE AND DOSAGE
Insomnia
(Effectiveness for durations longer than 7 days not proven.)
◆ **PO (Adults):** 500–1000 mg 20 min before retiring.
◆ **PO (Geriatric):** 500 mg 20 min before retiring.

PHARMACODYNAMICS

Route	Onset	Peak	Duration
PO	20 min	1 hr	3–5 hr

NURSING IMPLICATIONS
Assessment
◆ Assess sleep patterns. Keep records for adequate baseline data before the initiation of therapy.
◆ Assess for suicidal ideation in depressed patients.
◆ Assess history of allergies, sensitivity to this drug.
◆ Assess date of last menses (possible pregnancy), use of contraceptives.
◆ Assess whether currently breast-feeding a child.
◆ Assess current and past alcohol and drug consumption.
◆ Assess for operation of automobile and/or other dangerous machinery.
◆ Assess for presence of adverse reactions or side effects.
◆ Assess patient/family knowledge about condition and need for medication.
◆ In collaboration with physician, assess CBC and renal and liver function tests

in patients who have been on prolonged use.
◆ **Lab Test Alterations:** May show false increase in urinary 17-ketosteroid and 17-hydroxycorticosteroid levels.
◆ **Withdrawal:** Assess for symptoms of withdrawal: ● anxiety ● tremors ● severe insomnia ● nausea/vomiting ● weakness ● hyperactive reflexes ● agitation ● confusion ● syncope ● diaphoresis ● orthostatic hypotension ● severe hallucinations ● delirium ● convulsions.
◆ **Withdrawal Management:** Monitor vital signs.
◊ Place patient in quiet room with low stimuli.
◊ Institute seizure precautions.
◊ A long-acting barbiturate, such as phenobarbital, may be ordered to suppress withdrawal symptoms.
◊ Phenytoin may be ordered to prevent seizures.
◊ Some physicians may order oxazepam as needed for objective withdrawal symptoms, gradually decreasing the dosage until the drug is discontinued.
◆ **Toxicity and Overdose:** Assess for symptoms of toxicity: ● confusion ● drowsiness ● dyspnea ● slurred speech ● staggering.
◊ Assess for symptoms of overdose: ● CNS and respiratory depression ● hypoventilation ● hypothermia ● hypotension ● transient jaundice ● oliguria ● tachycardia ● coma. (May progress to respiratory arrest, circulatory collapse, and death.)
◆ **Overdose Management:** Monitor vital signs.
◊ Ensure maintenance of airway.
◊ Induce vomiting in conscious patient.
◊ Initiate gastric lavage in unconscious patient.
◊ Administer activated charcoal to minimize absorption of drug.
◊ Administer IV fluids.
◊ For severe intoxication, forced diuresis or hemodialysis may be used.

Potential Nursing Diagnoses

♦ High risk for injury related to abrupt withdrawal from long-term use; decreased mental alertness caused by side effects of drowsiness and dizziness; and effects of overdose.
♦ High risk for self-directed violence related to depressed mood.
♦ Anxiety (specify level) related to threats to physical integrity and/or self-concept.
♦ Sleep pattern disturbance related to situational crises, physical condition, severe level of anxiety.
♦ High risk for activity intolerance, related to side effects of drowsiness, dizziness.
♦ Knowledge deficit related to medication regimen.

Plan/Implementation

♦ Monitor vital signs before beginning therapy and at regular intervals (bid) throughout therapy.
♦ Ensure that patient is protected from injury. Supervise and assist with ambulation if dizziness and drowsiness are problems. Ensure that patient avoids participation in any activity requiring mental alertness (including smoking). Raise siderails and instruct patient to remain in bed following administration.
♦ To minimize nausea, medication may be given with food or milk.
♦ Ensure that capsule has been swallowed and not "cheeked" to avoid medication or to hoard for later use.
♦ Empty contents of capsule and mix with food or fluid for patient who has difficulty swallowing.
♦ Store medication at controlled room temperatures between 15° and 30°C (59°–86°F). Protect from heat and moisture.

Patient/Family Education

♦ Use caution in driving or operating dangerous machinery. Drowsiness and dizziness can occur.
♦ Do not stop taking the drug abruptly.

Doing so can produce serious (even life-threatening) withdrawal symptoms. If a dose is missed, take it as close as possible to the prescribed time. If it is already close to time for next dose, wait until then; do not double up on dose at the next prescribed time.
♦ Do not consume other CNS depressants (including alcohol).
♦ Be aware of the risks of taking ethinamate during pregnancy (safety during pregnancy has not been established). Notify physician if pregnancy is suspected or planned.
♦ Be aware of potential side effects. Refer to written materials furnished by healthcare providers regarding correct method of self-administration.
♦ Report symptoms of sore throat, fever, malaise, unusual bleeding, or easy bruising to physician immediately.
♦ Carry card or other identification at all times stating names of medications being taken.

Evaluation

♦ Patient demonstrates a subsiding/resolution of the symptoms for which ethinamate was prescribed (sleep disturbances).
♦ Patient verbalizes understanding of side effects and regimen required for prudent self-administration of ethinamate.

ETHOPROPAZINE

(eth-oh-proe'pa-zeen)
Parsidol

Classification(s):
Antiparkinsonian agent,
Anticholinergic, Phenothiazine
derivative
Pregnancy Category C

INDICATIONS

♦ Parkinsonism (all forms) ♦ Extrapyramidal symptoms (except tardive dyskinesia) associated with antipsychotic drugs.

ACTION

♦ Unknown ♦ Thought to produce effects by blocking actions of acetylcholine within the central nervous system ♦ Has a strong atropine-like effect to block peripheral structures innervated by the parasympathetic system.

PHARMACOKINETICS

Absorption: Rapidly absorbed following oral administration.
Distribution: Not completely understood. May cross placental barrier; may enter breast milk.
Metabolism and Excretion: Unknown. Thought to be at least partially metabolized by the liver and excreted in urine.
Half-Life: Undetermined.

CONTRAINDICATIONS AND PRECAUTIONS

Contraindicated in: ♦ Hypersensitivity to this drug or to other phenothiazines ♦ Angle-closure glaucoma ♦ Pyloric or duodenal obstruction ♦ Stenosing peptic ulcers ♦ Prostatic hypertrophy or bladder-neck obstructions ♦ Achalasia ♦ Myasthenia gravis ♦ Ulcerative colitis ♦ Toxic megacolon ♦ Tachycardia secondary to cardiac insufficiency or thyrotoxicosis ♦ Children; pregnancy and lactation (safe use not established).
Use Cautiously in: ♦ Narrow-angle glaucoma ♦ Elderly or debilitated patients ♦ Hepatic, renal, or cardiac insufficiency ♦ Tendency toward urinary retention ♦ Hyperthyroidism ♦ Hypertension ♦ Autonomic neuropathy ♦ Patients exposed to high environmental temperature.

ADVERSE REACTIONS AND SIDE EFFECTS*

CNS: drowsiness, dizziness, blurred vision, disorientation, confusion, memory loss, agitation, nervousness, delirium, weakness, lowered seizure threshold, forgetfulness, lassitude, diplopia, headache, ataxia.
CV: orthostatic hypotension, hypotension, tachycardia, palpitations, ECG abnormalities.
Derm: skin rashes, urticaria, other dermatoses.
GI: dry mouth, nausea, vomiting, epigastric distress, constipation, dilatation of the colon, PARALYTIC ILEUS.
GU: urinary retention, urinary hesitancy, dysuria, difficulty in achieving or maintaining an erection.
Hemat: BLOOD DYSCRASIAS (agranulocytosis, pancytopenia, purpura).
Psych: depression, delusions, hallucinations, paranoia.
Other: muscular weakness, muscular cramping, elevated temperature, flushing, decreased sweating, jaundice, endocrine disturbances, visual changes, paresthesia, pigmentation.

INTERACTIONS

Drug-Drug: ♦ **Other drugs with anticholinergic properties (e.g., glutethimide, disopyramide, narcotic analgesics, other phenothiazines, tricyclic antidepressants, antihistamines, quinidine salts, amantadine):** increased anticholinergic effects, potentially fatal paralytic ileus ♦ **Levodopa:** possible decreased levodopa absorption ♦ **Slow-dissolving digoxin:** decreased absorption of digoxin ♦ **CNS depressants (e.g., alcohol, barbiturates, narcotics, benzodiazepines):** increased CNS depressant effects ♦ **Ketoconazole:** decreased absorption of ketoconazole ♦ **Antacids:** decreased absorption of ethopropazine ♦ **Angiotensin converting enzyme inhibitors (e.g., Captopril, Enalapril, Lisinopril):** increased effects of ACE inhibitors ♦ **Bromocriptine:** impairment of pro-

---

*Underlines indicate most frequent; CAPITALS indicate life-threatening.

lactin secretion ◆ **Metrizamide:** increased predisposition to seizures.

ROUTE AND DOSAGE

Parkinsonism, Drug-Induced Extrapyramidal Symptoms

◆ **PO (Adults): Initial Dosage:** 50 mg once or twice daily. Increase gradually, if needed. For mild to moderate symptoms, 100–400 mg daily. For severe cases, gradually increase to 500–600 mg or more daily.

Substitution Therapy

To substitute for another antiparkinsonian drug, first drug is gradually withdrawn while second drug is gradually increased.

PHARMACODYNAMICS

Route	Onset	Peak	Duration
PO	0.5–1 hr	2 hr	4 hr

NURSING IMPLICATIONS

Assessment

◆ Assess for symptoms of Parkinson's disease: • tremors • muscular weakness and rigidity • drooling • shuffling gait • disturbances of posture and equilibrium • flat affect • monotone speech.

◆ Assess for extrapyramidal symptoms: • pseudoparkinsonism (tremors, shuffling gait, drooling, rigidity) • akinesia (muscular weakness) • akathisia (continuous restlessness and fidgeting) • dystonia (involuntary muscular movements of face, arms, legs, and neck) • oculogyric crisis (uncontrolled rolling back of the eyes) • tardive dyskinesia (bizarre facial and tongue movements, stiff neck, difficulty swallowing). **Note:** Ethopropazine is not effective in alleviating symptoms of tardive dyskinesia.

◆ Assess for symptoms of paralytic ileus (constipation, abdominal pain and distention, absence of bowel sounds). Patients taking ethopropazine while also taking other drugs that produce anticholinergic effects are particularly susceptible.

◆ Assess vital signs, weight. Record baseline values for comparison.

◆ Assess history of allergies, sensitivity to this drug or to other phenothiazines.

◆ Assess date of last menses (possible pregnancy), use of contraceptives.

◆ Assess whether currently breast-feeding a child.

◆ Assess current and past alcohol and drug consumption.

◆ Assess for operation of automobile and/or other dangerous machinery.

◆ Assess for presence of adverse reactions or side effects.

◆ Assess patient/family knowledge about illness and need for medication.

◆ In collaboration with physician, assess CBC and liver function test in patients on long-term therapy.

◆ **Toxicity and Overdose:** Assess for symptoms of overdose: • CNS depression preceded or followed by stimulation • intensification of psychotic symptoms • anxiety • ataxia • seizures • incoherence • delusions • paranoia • anhidrosis • hyperpyrexia • hot, dry, flushed skin • dry mucous membranes • decreased bowel sounds • shock • coma • skeletal muscle paralysis • urinary retention • tachycardia • difficulty swallowing • cardiac arrhythmias • circulatory collapse • cardiac arrest • respiratory depression or arrest.

◆ **Overdose Management:** Monitor vital signs.

◇ Ensure maintenance of adequate airway.

◇ Induce emesis in conscious patient (contraindicated in precomatose, convulsive, or psychotic states).

◇ Initiate gastric lavage.

◇ Administer activated charcoal.

◇ Administer pilocarpine, 5 mg PO, to treat peripheral effects.

◇ Administer physostigmine, 1–2 mg SQ or slow IV, to reverse anticholinergic effects (use only with availability of advanced life support).

◇ Use artificial respiration and oxygen to counteract respiratory depression.

◇ Use tepid water sponges, cold packs, or other cooling applications to treat hyperpyrexia.

◇ Darken room to counter photophobia.

◇ Administer fluids and a vasopressor to prevent circulatory collapse.

◇ Administer diazepam to control CNS excitement or convulsions.

Potential Nursing Diagnoses

♦ High risk for injury related to symptoms of Parkinson's disease or drug-induced extrapyramidal symptoms.

♦ Hyperthermia related to anticholinergic effect of decreased sweating.

♦ Sensory-perceptual alteration related to adverse effects of ethopropazine (hallucinations).

♦ Altered thought processes related to side effects of ethopropazine (delusional thinking, disorientation, confusion).

♦ Social isolation related to embarrassment from symptoms of Parkinson's disease.

♦ High risk for activity intolerance, related to ethopropazine's side effects of drowsiness, dizziness, ataxia, weakness, confusion.

♦ Knowledge deficit related to medication regimen.

Plan/Implementation

♦ Monitor vital signs daily. Be particularly alert for increase in pulse rate or temperature.

♦ Weigh patient 2–3 times a week, at same time of day, on same scale, if possible. A rapid weight gain or evidence of edema should be reported to physician immediately. Record I&O.

♦ Monitor for exacerbation of mental symptoms in patients who are receiving the drug to counteract extrapyramidal symptoms associated with antipsychotic medications.

♦ Ensure that patient is protected from injury. Provide supervision and assistance when ambulating if dizziness and drowsiness are problems.

♦ Give patient hard candy, gum, or frequent sips of water if dry mouth is a problem, or treat with saliva substitute.

♦ Ensure that patient swallows tablet and does not "cheek" to avoid medication or to hoard for later use.

♦ Medication may be administered with food to minimize gastric irritation.

♦ Tablet may be crushed and mixed with food or fluid for patient who has difficulty swallowing.

♦ Monitor vital signs before beginning therapy and at regular intervals (bid or tid) throughout therapy. Take BP lying and standing to monitor for possible hypotensive reaction; elderly are particularly susceptible. Dosage adjustment may be required.

♦ Store medication at controlled room temperatures between 15° and 30°C (59°–86°F). Protect from heat, light, and moisture.

Patient/Family Education

♦ Medication may be taken with food if GI upset occurs.

♦ Use caution when driving or when operating dangerous machinery. Drowsiness and dizziness can occur.

♦ Do not stop taking the drug abruptly. To do so might produce serious withdrawal symptoms.

♦ Report occurrence of any of the following symptoms to physician immediately: pain or tenderness in area in front of ear, extreme dryness of mouth, difficulty urinating, abdominal pain, constipation, fast and pounding heartbeat, rash, visual disturbances, mental changes.

♦ Rise slowly from a sitting or lying position to prevent a sudden drop in blood pressure.

♦ Stay indoors in air-conditioned room when weather is very hot. Perspiration is decreased with ethopropazine, and the body cannot cool itself as well.

There is greater susceptibility to heat stroke. Inform physician if air-conditioned housing or work environment is not available.

♦ If dry mouth is a problem, take frequent sips of water, chew sugarless gum, or suck on hard candy. Good oral care (frequent brushing, flossing) is very important.

♦ Do not drink alcohol while on ethopropazine therapy.

♦ Do not consume other medications (including over-the-counter medicines) without physician's approval. Many medications contain substances that interact with ethopropazine in a way that may be harmful.

♦ Be aware of possible risks of taking ethopropazine during pregnancy. Safe use during pregnancy and lactation has not been established. It is thought that ethopropazine crosses the placental barrier; if so, a fetus could experience adverse effects of the drug. Inform physician immediately if pregnancy occurs, is suspected, or is planned.

♦ Be aware of side effects of ethopropazine. Refer to written materials furnished by healthcare providers for safe self-administration.

♦ Continue to take medication even if feeling well and as though it is not needed. Symptoms may return if medication is discontinued.

♦ Carry card or other identification at all times describing medications being taken.

Evaluation

♦ Patient demonstrates a subsiding of the symptoms for which ethopropazine was prescribed (parkinsonism, drug-induced extrapyramidal symptoms).

♦ Patient verbalizes understanding of side effects and regimen required for prudent self-administration of ethopropazine.

ETHOSUXIMIDE

(eth-oh-sux′i-mide)
Zarontin

Classification(s):
Anticonvulsant, Succinimide
Pregnancy Category C

INDICATIONS

♦ Absence (petit mal) seizures.

ACTION

♦ Depresses motor cortex and elevates central nervous system seizure threshold
♦ Suppresses paroxysmal spike and wave activity common in absence seizures.

PHARMACOKINETICS

Absorption: Rapidly absorbed from the GI tract.

Distribution: Widely distributed. Unknown if drug crosses placental barrier or is excreted in breast milk.

Metabolism and Excretion: Partially metabolized by the liver and excreted in urine, bile, and feces.

Half-Life: ∼60 hours in adults; ∼30 hours in children.

CONTRAINDICATIONS AND PRECAUTIONS

Contraindicated in: ♦ Hypersensitivity to this drug or to other succinimides.

Use Cautiously in: ♦ Patients with severe hepatic or renal disease ♦ Acute intermittent porphyria ♦ **Note:** Sole use of this medication in some patients with mixed type of epilepsy may increase incidence of tonic-clonic seizures ♦ Pregnancy and lactation (safety has not been established).

ADVERSE REACTIONS AND SIDE EFFECTS*

CNS: <u>drowsiness</u>, headache, <u>dizziness</u>, ataxia, <u>lethargy</u>, <u>fatigue</u>, irritability, hyperactivity.

*<u>Underlines</u> indicate most frequent; CAPITALS indicate life-threatening.

Derm: skin rashes, urticaria, pruritus, hirsutism.

GI: nausea/vomiting, anorexia, abdominal cramps, diarrhea, constipation, hiccups.

Hemat: LEUKOPENIA, AGRANULOCYTOSIS, THROMBOCYTOPENIA, APLASTIC ANEMIA.

Other: gingival hypertrophy, swollen tongue, alopecia, vaginal bleeding, RENAL AND HEPATIC DAMAGE, diplopia, sleep disturbances, night terrors, aggressiveness, paranoid psychosis, SLE, myopia.

INTERACTIONS

Drug-Drug: ♦**Hydantoin anticonvulsants:** decreased metabolism and increased risk of toxic effects of hydantoins ♦ **Oral contraceptives:** decreased effectiveness of oral contraceptives ♦ **CNS depressants (including alcohol, sedative-hypnotics, narcotics, antihistamines):** additive CNS depression ♦ **Carbamazepine:** decreased concentration of ethosuximide.

ROUTE AND DOSAGE

Absence (Petit Mal) Seizures

♦ **PO (Children 3–6 Years): Initial Dosage:** 250 mg/day single dose.
♦ **PO (Adults and Children over 6 Years):** 500 mg/day in divided doses.
♦ **PO (Maintenance):** Increase dose by 250 mg/day every 4–7 days until control is achieved with minimal side effects. Doses exceeding 1.5 g/day should be administered only under the strictest supervision of a physician.

PHARMACODYNAMICS

Route	Onset	Peak	Duration
PO	Rapid	1–4 hr	UK

NURSING IMPLICATIONS

Assessment

♦ Assess occurrence, characteristics, duration of seizure activity.
♦ Assess baseline vital signs.
♦ Assess history of allergies, sensitivity to this drug.
♦ Assess date of last menses (possible pregnancy), use of contraceptives.
♦ Assess whether currently breast-feeding a child.
♦ Assess current and past alcohol and drug consumption.
♦ Assess operation of automobile and/or other dangerous machinery.
♦ Assess for presence of adverse reactions or side effects.
♦ Assess patient/family knowledge about illness and need for medication.
♦ In collaboration with physician, assess CBC and renal and liver function tests in patients on ethosuximide therapy. Periodic urinalysis should be performed.
♦ **Lab Test Alterations:** Increased direct Coombs test.
♦ **Toxicity and Overdose:** Range of therapeutic serum concentration is 40–100 mcg/mL.
◊ Assess for symptoms of toxicity/overdose: • bone marrow depression • nausea/vomiting • ataxia • diplopia • cardiovascular collapse • Stevens-Johnson syndrome.
♦ **Overdose Management:** Monitor vital signs.
◊ Ensure maintenance of adequate airway.
◊ Induce emesis in conscious patient.
◊ Initiate gastric lavage in unconscious patient.
◊ Administer activated charcoal to minimize absorption.
◊ Monitor electrolytes.

Potential Nursing Diagnoses

♦ High risk for injury related to seizures; abrupt withdrawal from long-term ethosuximide use; side effects of dizziness, sedation, ataxia.
♦ Social isolation related to fear of experiencing a seizure in the presence of others.

♦ Impaired adjustment related to difficulty accepting diagnosis of epilepsy.

♦ High risk for activity intolerance, related to ethosuximide's side effects of sedation, drowsiness, dizziness, ataxia.

♦ Knowledge deficit related to medication regimen.

Plan/Implementation

♦ Monitor vital signs at regular intervals (bid) throughout therapy.

♦ Monitor and record lab assessments of serum ethosuximide levels.

♦ Report presence of skin rash, joint pain, fever, unusual bleeding, easy bruising, dark urine, or jaundice to physician immediately.

♦ Observe frequently (every hour) for occurrence of seizure activity.

♦ Ensure that patient is protected from injury. Supervise and assist with ambulation if dizziness and drowsiness are problems. Ensure that patient avoids participation in any activity requiring mental alertness (including smoking). Pad siderails and head of bed with towels or blanket for patient who experiences seizures during the night.

♦ Administer medication with food or milk to minimize GI irritation.

♦ Store medication at controlled room temperatures between 15° and 30°C (59°–86°F). Protect from heat, light, and moisture. Do not freeze.

Patient/Family Education

♦ Do not drive or operate dangerous machinery until individual response is determined. Drowsiness and dizziness can occur.

♦ Do not stop taking drug abruptly. To do so might precipitate absence (petit mal) status.

♦ Avoid alcoholic beverages.

♦ Carry or wear identification informing others of illness and medication usage.

♦ Do not take any other medication without approval from physician. To do so may be harmful.

♦ Promptly report any of the following symptoms to physician: sore throat, fever, malaise, skin rash, joint pain, unusual bleeding, easy bruising, dark urine, yellow skin or eyes.

♦ Be aware of possible risks of taking ethosuximide during pregnancy. Patient who requires the medication to prevent seizures may be maintained on it; however, she must be fully aware of potential risks to unborn child. There is a strong association between the use of anticonvulsant drugs by women with epilepsy and the incidence of birth defects in their offspring. If pregnancy occurs, is suspected, or is planned, report it to physician immediately.

♦ Due to decreased effectiveness of oral contraceptives with ethosuximide, use alternative methods of birth control during therapy.

♦ Protect patient during a seizure. In the case of tonic-clonic (grand mal) seizure, do not restrain. Padding may be used (towels, blankets, pillows) to prevent bumping against hard objects. When convulsion has subsided, turn patient on side to allow secretions to drain and to prevent aspiration. Keep records of occurrence, characteristics, and duration of seizures, so that accurate reports may be given to physician for providing assistance in stabilization and control of seizures. If patient has difficulty breathing or continues to experience subsequent seizures, family should immediately call for emergency assistance.

♦ Be aware of possible side effects. Refer to written materials furnished by healthcare providers for assistance in self-administration.

Evaluation

♦ Patient demonstrates stabilization of seizure activity with regular administration of ethosuximide.

◆ Patient verbalizes understanding of necessity for, side effects of, and regimen required for prudent self-administration of ethosuximide.

ETHOTOIN

(eth′oh-toyin)
Peganone

Classification(s):
Antonvulsant, Hydantoin
Pregnancy Category D

INDICATIONS

● Tonic-clonic (grand mal) and partial seizures with complex symptomatology (psychomotor).

ACTION

◆ Hydantoins act by increasing the seizure threshold in the cerebral cortex. By promoting sodium efflux from neurons in the motor cortex, they encourage stabilization of the threshold against hyperexcitability ◆ Maximal activity of the brain stem centers responsible for the tonic phase of grand mal seizures is also reduced.

PHARMACOKINETICS

Absorption: Rapidly absorbed following oral administration. Extent of absorption is unknown.
Distribution: Rapidly and widely distributed. Crosses placental barrier; excreted in breast milk.
Metabolism and Excretion: Metabolized by the liver into metabolites that are excreted by the kidneys.
Half-Life: 3–9 hours.

CONTRAINDICATIONS AND PRECAUTIONS

Contraindicated in: ◆ Hypersensitivity to this drug or to other hydantoins ◆ Lac-

tation ◆ Hepatic disease ◆ Hematologic disorders ◆ Concomitant use of phenacemide.
Use Cautiously in: ◆ Pregnancy ◆ Elderly or debilitated patients.

ADVERSE REACTIONS AND SIDE EFFECTS*

CNS: nystagmus, ataxia, drowsiness, dizziness, headache, diplopia, insomnia, fatigue, depression, numbness.
Derm: skin rashes, EXFOLIATIVE DERMATITIS.
GI: nausea, vomiting, diarrhea, TOXIC HEPATITIS.
Hemat: BLOOD DYSCRASIAS (thrombocytopenia, leukopenia, agranulocytosis, neutropenia).
Other: lymphadenopathy, osteomalacia, hyperglycemia, gingival hyperplasia, chest pain, fever.

INTERACTIONS

Drug-Drug: ◆ **Trimethoprim, amiodarone, benzodiazepines, disulfiram, isoniazid, phenylbutazone, chloramphenicol, cimetidine, sulfonamides, salicylates, acute alcohol intake, phenothiazines:** increased effects of ethotoin (increased risk of toxicity) ◆ **Barbiturates, diazoxide, rifampin, antineoplastic agents, chronic alcohol abuse, antacids, calcium gluconate, carbamazepine:** decreased effects of ethotoin ◆ **Phenobarbital, valproic acid, sodium valproate:** increased or decreased effects of either drug ◆ **Coumarin anticoagulants:** increased effects of ethotoin; increased or decreased anticoagulant effects ◆ **Quinidine:** decreased antiarrhythmic effects ◆ **Corticosteroids:** decreased efficacy of corticosteroids ◆ **Oral contraceptives:** decreased efficacy of oral contraceptives ◆ **Digi-**

toxin: decreased effects of digitoxin ✦ **Furosemide:** decreased effects of furosemide ✦ **Theophylline:** decreased efficacy of both drugs ✦ **Doxycycline:** decreased effects of doxycycline ✦ **Levodopa:** decreased effects of levodopa ✦ **Primidone:** increased primidone effects ✦ **Dopamine:** decreased effects of dopamine.

Drug-Food: ✦ **Vitamin K, vitamin D:** Patient may need supplemental intake of these nutrients while on ethotoin ✦ **Folic acid:** alteration in metabolism of either or both (may result in decreased effects of ethotoin or serum folate deficiency).

ROUTE AND DOSAGE
Tonic-Clonic and Psychomotor Seizures

✦ **PO (Adults): Initially:** 1000 mg/day or less in 4–6 divided doses. Gradually increase dosage over period of several days until maintenance dose is achieved. **Maintenance:** 2–3 g/day in 4–6 divided doses.

✦ **PO (Children): Initially:** up to 750 mg/day (depending on size and age) in 4–6 divided doses. Maintenance: 500–1000 mg/day in 4–6 equal doses (determined by age and nature of seizures). Occasionally, some children may require larger maintenance doses of 2 g/day or rarely 3 g/day.

✦ **Replacement Therapy:** Dose of ethotoin is gradually increased each week as dose of drug being replaced is gradually decreased.

✦ **Discontinuation of Treatment:** Withdraw slowly to avoid precipitating seizures or status epilepticus.

PHARMACODYNAMICS

Route	Onset	Peak	Duration
PO	30 min	2–4 hr	UK

NURSING IMPLICATIONS
Assessment

✦ Assess occurrence, characteristics, and duration of seizure activity.

✦ Assess baseline vital signs.

✦ Assess history of allergies, sensitivity to this and/or other hydantoins.

✦ Assess date of last menses (possible pregnancy), use of contraceptives.

✦ Assess whether currently breast-feeding a child.

✦ Assess current and past alcohol and drug consumption.

✦ Assess for symptoms of possible blood dyscrasias: • sore throat • fever • malaise • unusual bleeding • easy bruising.

✦ Assess for presence of adverse reactions or side effects.

✦ Assess patient's and family's response to diagnosis of epilepsy.

✦ Assess patient/family knowledge about illness and need for medication.

✦ In collaboration with physician, assess CBC, and renal and liver function tests in patients on prolonged ethotoin therapy.

✦ **Lab Test Alterations:** May increase serum glucose, bromsulphalein, and alkaline phosphatase.

◇ May decrease protein-bound iodine and urinary steroid levels.

✦ **Toxicity and Overdose:** Range of therapeutic serum concentration is thought to be 15–50 mcg/mL.

◇ Assess for toxic skin and mucous membrane manifestations, such as rashes, dermatitis, or pigmentation changes.

◇ Assess for symptoms of toxicity/overdose: • ataxia • confusion • nausea • vomiting • slurred speech • dizziness.

✦ **Overdose Management:** Monitor vital signs.

◇ Ensure maintenance of airway.

◇ Induce emesis in conscious patient.

◇ Initiate gastric lavage in unconscious patient.

◇ Hemodialysis may be considered.

Potential Nursing Diagnoses

✦ High risk for injury related to seizures; ethotoin's side effects of dizziness, drowsiness, decreased mental alertness; possible toxic serum levels of ethotoin; abrupt withdrawal from ethotoin use.

♦ Impaired adjustment related to difficulty accepting diagnosis of epilepsy.

♦ Social isolation related to fear of experiencing a seizure in the presence of others.

♦ High risk for activity intolerance, related to ethotoin's side effects of drowsiness, dizziness, decreased mental alertness.

♦ Knowledge deficit related to medication regimen.

Plan/Implementation

♦ Monitor vital signs at regular intervals (bid or tid) throughout therapy.

♦ Monitor serum ethotoin levels. Record and report to physician.

♦ Observe frequently (every hour) for occurrence of seizure activity.

♦ Ensure that patient is protected from injury. Supervise and assist with ambulation if dizziness and drowsiness are problems. Ensure that patient avoids participation in any activity requiring mental alertness (including smoking). Pad siderails and head of bed with towels or blanket to protect patient who experiences seizures during the night.

♦ Perform urine checks daily following initiation of therapy to determine if hyperglycemia has occurred.

♦ Administer medication with food to minimize GI irritation and enhance absorption.

♦ For patient who has difficulty swallowing, crush tablet and mix with food or fluid.

♦ Store medication at controlled room temperatures between 15° and 30°C (59°–86°F). Protect from heat and moisture.

Patient/Family Education

♦ Do not drive or operate dangerous machinery until individual response is determined. Drowsiness and decreased mental alertness can occur.

♦ Do not stop taking drug abruptly. To do so could precipitate status epilepticus.

♦ Avoid alcoholic beverages.

♦ Maintain good care of the mouth to minimize side effect of gingival hyperplasia.

♦ Carry or wear at all times identification informing others of illness and medication usage.

♦ Do not take any other medication without approval from physician. Combining drugs may be harmful.

♦ Promptly report any of the following symptoms to physician: sore throat • fever • malaise • ataxia • skin rash • severe nausea or vomiting • swollen glands • yellow skin or eyes • unusual bleeding • easy bruising • dark urine.

♦ Be aware of possible risks of taking ethotoin during pregnancy. Patient who requires the medication to prevent seizures may be maintained on it; however, she must be fully aware of potential risks to unborn child. There is a strong association between the use of anticonvulsant drugs by women with epilepsy and the incidence of birth defects in their offspring. A possible association also has been suggested between maternal use of anticonvulsants and a neonatal coagulation defect that poses a threat of serious bleeding during the first 24 hours of life. Notify physician immediately if pregnancy occurs, is suspected, or is planned.

♦ Because ethotoin decreases the effectiveness of oral contraceptives, use alternative method of birth control during ethotoin therapy.

♦ To protect patient during a seizure, padding may be used (towels, blankets, pillows) to prevent bumping against hard objects. When convulsion has subsided, turn patient on side to allow secretions to drain and to prevent aspiration. Keep records of occurrence, characteristics, and duration of seizures, so that accurate reports may be given to physician for providing assistance in stabilization and control of seizures. If patient has difficulty breathing or continues to experience subsequent seizures, family should call for emergency assistance immediately.

♦ Be aware of possible side effects of ethotoin. Refer to written materials furnished by healthcare providers to assist in self-administration.

Evaluation

♦ Patient demonstrates stabilization of seizure activity with regular administration of ethotoin.

♦ Patient verbalizes understanding of necessity for, side effects of, and regimen required for prudent self-administration of ethotoin.

FELBAMATE*

(fel′ ba-mate)
Felbatol

Classification(s):
Anticonvulsant
Pregnancy Category C

---

*NOTE: At the time of the publication of this text, the manufacturer of felbamate was recommending to physicians that use of this medication be suspended. Nine domestic cases and one foreign case of aplastic anemia had been correlated with the use of felbamate. In the event that suspension of the drug would render the patient too great a risk for life-threatening seizures, cautious use with close monitoring for aplastic anemia is being suggested. Dispensing of the medication has not been prohibited; however, use should be curtailed when prudent, until further testing can be completed and additional guidelines have been established.

INDICATIONS

♦ **Adults:** Partial seizures with and without generalization (both monotherapy and adjunctive therapy) ♦ **Children:** Partial and generalized seizures associated with Lennox-Gastaut syndrome (adjunctive therapy).

ACTION

♦ Unknown. Exhibits weak inhibitory effects on GABA receptor binding and benzodiazepine receptor binding. Demonstrates antagonist activity at the strychnine-insensitive glycine recognition site of the NMDA receptor-inophore complex.

PHARMACOKINETICS

Absorption: Well absorbed following oral administration.
Distribution: Distribution is unclear. Has been detected in breast milk.
Metabolism and Excretion: Metabolized by the liver; excreted in urine (about one-half as unchanged drug and one-half as metabolites).
Half-Life: 20–23 hours.

CONTRAINDICATIONS AND PRECAUTIONS

Contraindicated in: ♦ Hypersensitivity to the drug or its ingredients ♦ Demonstrated hypersensitivity to other carbamates.
Use Cautiously in: ♦ Elderly and debilitated patients ♦ Patients with hepatic, cardiac, or renal disease ♦ Pregnancy ♦ Children (safety has not been established other than in those with Lennox-Gastaut syndrome).

ADVERSE REACTIONS AND SIDE EFFECTS*

CNS: insomnia, headache, dizziness, somnolence, anxiety, nervousness, depression, tremor, agitation, ataxia.
CV: palpitations, tachycardia.

---

*Underlines indicate most frequent; CAPITALS indicate life-threatening.

Derm: acne, rash, pruritus.
GI: anorexia, nausea, vomiting, dyspepsia, diarrhea, constipation, abdominal pain, hiccups.
GU: intramenstrual bleeding, urinary tract infection.
Hemat: purpura, leukopenia, APLASTIC ANEMIA.
MS: myalgia.
Resp: upper respiratory tract infection, rhinitis, sinusitis, pharyngitis, coughing.
Special Senses: diplopia, otitis media, taste perversion, abnormal vision.
Misc: fatigue, weight decrease, face edema, fever, chest pain, weight increase, asthenia, malaise, influenza-like symptoms, dry mouth.

INTERACTIONS

Drug-Drug: ◆ **Phenytoin:** increase in phenytoin concentration; decrease in felbamate concentration ◆ **Valproic acid:** increase in valproic acid concentration ◆ **Carbamazepine:** decrease in carbamazepine concentration, but increase in carbamazepine epoxide (metabolite) concentration; decrease in felbamate concentration.

ROUTE AND DOSAGE

Adults (14 and Over): Partial Seizures, with or without Generalization

◆ **PO (Monotherapy): Initial Dosage:** 1200 mg/day in divided doses tid or qid. May increase the dosage, under close clinical observation, in 600-mg increments every 2 weeks to 2400 mg/day based on clinical response, and thereafter to 3600 mg/day if clinically indicated.
◆ **PO (Conversion to Monotherapy): Initial Dosage:** 1200 mg/day in divided doses tid or qid.
◆ At initiation of felbamate therapy: Reduce dosage of concomitant anticonvulsant by one-third. At Week 2: Increase felbamate dosage to 2400 mg/day; reduce dosage of concomitant

anticonvulsant by additional one-third of original dosage. At Week 3: Increase felbamate dosage up to 3600 mg/day; continue to reduce dosage of concomitant anticonvulsant as clinically indicated.
◆ **PO (Adjunctive Therapy):** Initiate felbamate at 1200 mg/day in divided doses tid or qid, while reducing dosage of concomitant anticonvulsant by 20%. Increase dosage of felbamate by 1200 mg/day increments at weekly intervals to 3600 mg/day. Further reductions in dosage of concomitant anticonvulsant may be necessary to control side effects due to drug interactions.

Children with Lennox-Gastaut Syndrome (Ages 2–14) Years)

◆ **PO (Adjunctive Therapy):** Initiate felbamate at 15 mg/kg/day in divided doses tid or qid, while reducing concomitant anticonvulsant by 20%. Increase dosage of felbamate by 15 mg/kg/day increments at weekly intervals to 45 mg/kg/day. Further reductions in dosage of concomitant anticonvulsant may be necessary to control side effects due to drug interactions.

Discontinuation of Therpay

Withdraw slowly to prevent precipitation of seizures or status epilepticus.

PHARMACODYNAMICS*

Route	Onset	Peak	Duration
PO	Variable	Variable	Variable

*Pharmacodynamics are dose proportional. Little difference has been noted between the tablet and suspension forms of the drug.

NURSING IMPLICATIONS

Assessment

◆ Assess occurrence, characteristics, and duration of seizure activity.
◆ Assess baseline vital signs.
◆ Assess history of allergies, sensitivity to this drug or to other carbamates.

+ Assess date of last menses (possible pregnancy); use of contraceptives.
+ Assess if currently breast-feeding a child.
+ Assess current and past alcohol and drug consumption.
+ Assess operation of automobile and/ or other dangerous machinery.
+ Assess for presence of adverse reactions or side effects.
+ Assess patient/family knowledge about condition and need for medication.
+ In collaboration with physician, assess CBC, liver function tests, complete urinalysis and BUN, at the initiation of, as well as during long-term therapy.
+ **Lab Test Alterations:** Increased SGPT (ALT).
+ **Toxicity and Overdose:** No correlation has been established between blood level and therapeutic effect.
+ Assess for symptoms of overdose: Gastric distress; increased heart rate. No serious adverse reactions have been reported.
+ **Overdose Management:** • Monitor vital signs • provide general supportive measures • unknown if felbamate is dialyzable.

Potential Nursing Diagnoses

+ High risk for injury related to seizures; abrupt withdrawal from long-term felbamate use.
+ Impaired adjustment related to difficulty accepting diagnosis of epilepsy.
+ Social isolation related to fear of experiencing a seizure in the presence of others.
+ High risk for activity intolerance related to felbamate's side effects of drowsiness, dizziness, fatigue.
+ Knowledge deficit related to medication regimen.

Plan/Implementation

+ Monitor vital signs before beginning therapy and at regular (bid) intervals throughout therapy.
+ Ensure patient practices good mouth care. Offer hard, sugarless candy; gum; frequent sips of water for dry mouth.
+ Observe patient frequently (every hour) for occurrence of seizure activity.
+ Ensure patient is protected from injury. Supervise and assist with ambulation if dizziness and ataxia are problems. Avoid or monitor activities that require mental alertness (including smoking). Pad siderails and headboard for patient who experiences seizures during the night.
+ Monitor and record adverse side effects of felbamate. Report to physician: significant changes in vital signs; persistent nausea, vomiting, or diarrhea; severe headache; significant weight changes.
+ To minimize nausea, give with food or milk.
+ If patient has difficulty swallowing tablet, crush and mix with food or fluid, or administer oral suspension.
+ Ensure tablet has been swallowed and not "cheeked" to avoid medication or hoard for later use.
+ Store at controlled room temperatures between 15° and 30°C (59°–86°F). Protect from heat, light, and moisture.

Patient/Family Education

+ Do not drive or operate dangerous machinery until individual response has been determined. Drowsiness and dizziness can occur.
+ Do not stop taking the drug abruptly. May result in onset of seizure activity.
+ Avoid alcohol intake or nonprescription medication without approval from physician.
+ Be aware of possible risks to the fetus of taking felbamate during pregnancy. The effects of this drug during pregnancy are not known. Animal studies have shown that felbamate crosses the placental barrier. If pregnancy occurs, or is suspected or planned, notify physician immediately.
+ Report any of the following symptoms

to physician promptly: sore throat • fever • malaise • easy bruising • decrease in urine output • fluid retention • persistent nausea and vomiting or diarrhea • severe headache • significant changes in weight.

- ♦ To protect patient during seizure: In the case of tonic-clonic (grand mal) seizure, do not restrain. Padding may be used (towels, blankets, pillows) to prevent bumping against hard objects. When convulsion has subsided, turn patient on side to allow secretions to drain and prevent aspiration. Keep records of occurrence, characteristics, and duration of seizures, so that accurate reports may be given to physician for providing assistance in stabilization and control of seizures. If patient has difficulty breathing or continues to experience subsequent seizures, family should immediately call for emergency assistance.
- ♦ Be aware of potential side effects. Refer to written materials furnished by healthcare providers regarding correct method of self-administration.
- ♦ Carry card or other identification at all times stating condition and names of medications being taken. Include name of physician and medical facility to which patient should be transported in event of an emergency.

Evaluation
- ♦ Patient demonstrates stabilization of seizure activity with regular administration of felbamate.
- ♦ Patient verbalizes understanding of necessity for, side effects of, and regimen required for prudent self-administration of felbamate.

FENFLURAMINE

(fen-flure'a-meen)
{Ponderal}, Pondimin

Classification(s):
Anorexigenic, Sympathomimetic amine
Schedule C IV
Pregnancy Category C

INDICATIONS
♦ Exogenous obesity (short-term management). **Investigational Use:** ♦ Autism in children with elevated serotonin levels.

ACTION
♦ Exact mechanism of action is not known ♦ Differs from other anorexigenics in that it produces EEG effects more closely related to CNS depressants than to CNS stimulants ♦ Action may be related to turnover rates of serotonin or increased glucose utilization.

PHARMACOKINETICS
Absorption: Readily absorbed following oral administration.
Distribution: Widely distributed. Unknown if drug crosses placental barrier or enters breast milk.
Metabolism and Excretion: Metabolized by the liver; excreted in urine. Elimination is enhanced by acidic urine, slowed by alkaline urine.
Half-Life: 11–20 hours (depending on pH of urine).

CONTRAINDICATIONS AND PRECAUTIONS
Contraindicated in: ♦ Hypersensitivity to sympathomimetic amines ♦ Advanced arteriosclerosis ♦ Symptomatic cardiovascular disease ♦ Severe hypertension ♦ Hyperthyroidism ♦ Glaucoma ♦ Agitated states ♦ Patients with a history of drug abuse ♦ Alcoholism ♦ During or within 14 days of receiving therapy with MAO

{} = Only available in Canada.

inhibitors ♦ Concomitant use of other CNS stimulants ♦ Pregnancy and lactation; children under 12 years of age (safe use not established).

Use Cautiously in: ♦ Patients with mild hypertension ♦ Diabetes mellitus ♦ Elderly or debilitated patients.

ADVERSE REACTIONS AND SIDE EFFECTS*

CNS: drowsiness, dizziness, mental depression, insomnia, dyskinesia, euphoria, dysphoria, tremor, headache, anxiety, restlessness, weakness, confusion, incoordination, fatigue, malaise, nightmares, blurred vision, mydriasis, psychoses, incoordination, nervousness, tension, agitation.

CV: palpitations, tachycardia, arrhythmias, hypertension or hypotension, fainting, precordial pain.

Derm: urticaria, rash, burning sensation.

Endo: impotence, changes in libido, menstrual upset, gynecomastia.

GI: dry mouth, unpleasant taste, nausea, vomiting, diarrhea, constipation, abdominal discomfort.

GU: dysuria, urinary frequency.

Hemat: HEMOLYTIC ANEMIA.

Other: tolerance, physical and psychological dependence, alopecia, chills, fever, sweating.

INTERACTIONS

Drug-Drug: ♦ **Alcohol, tricyclic antidepressants, other CNS depressants:** additive CNS depressant effects ♦ **CNS stimulants:** additive stimulant effects ♦ **MAO inhibitors (during therapy or within 14 days of administration):** hypertensive crises, headache, hyperpyrexia, intracranial hemorrhage, bradycardia ♦ **Insulin:** alteration in insulin requirements ♦ **Guanethidine, methyldopa, reserpine:** enhanced antihypertensive effects ♦ **Barbiturates,** **phenothiazines:** decreased fenfluramine effects ♦ **General anesthetics:** cardiac arrhythmias.

Drug-Food: ♦ **Caffeinated foods and drinks:** increased effects of fenfluramine.

ROUTE AND DOSAGE
Exogenous Obesity

♦ **PO (Adults):** Initial dosage: 20 mg tid, before meals. Dosage may be increased at weekly intervals by 20 mg daily. Maximum dosage: 40 mg tid.

Autism in Children with Elevated Serotonin Levels

♦ **PO (Children):** 1.5 mg/kg/day.

PHARMACODYNAMICS

Route	Onset	Peak	Duration
PO	1–2 hr	2–4 hr	4–6 hr

NURSING IMPLICATIONS
Assessment

♦ Assess and record baseline temperature, pulse, respiration, blood pressure, and weight for comparison during therapy.

♦ In diabetic patient, assess blood sugar bid–tid. Insulin adjustments may be required due to alteration in eating pattern and activity.

♦ Assess knowledge of sound nutritional, calorie-reduced diet and importance of regular exercise.

♦ Assess mental status for changes in mood, level of activity, degree of stimulation, depression.

♦ Assess sleeping patterns carefully. Insomnia may occur.

♦ Assess history of allergies, sensitivity to this drug or to other sympathomimetic amines.

♦ Assess history of glaucoma.

♦ Assess for presence of adverse reactions or side effects.

*Underlines indicate most frequent; CAPITALS indicate life-threatening.

* Assess date of last menses (possible pregnancy), use of contraceptives.
* Assess whether currently breast-feeding a child.
* Assess current and past alcohol and drug consumption.
* Assess usual amount of caffeine consumed.
* Assess for operation of automobile and/or other dangerous machinery.
* Assess patient/family knowledge about illness and need for medication.
* In collaboration with physician, periodically assess CBC, urinalysis, and liver function tests.
* **Withdrawal:** Assess for symptoms of withdrawal: • irritability • ataxia • tremor • disturbed concentration and memory • loss of sense of reality • visual hallucinations • inverted visual field • mental depression • suicidal feelings.
* **Withdrawal Management:** Monitor vital signs.
◇ Place patient in quiet room with low stimuli.
◇ Allow patient to sleep as much as desired.
◇ Observe closely (q 15 min).
◇ Institute suicide precautions.
◇ Some physicians may elect to prescribe antidepressants to counteract feelings of depression and lethargy.
* **Toxicity and Overdose:** Assess for symptoms of overdose: • agitation • drowsiness • confusion • flushing • tremor • fever • sweating • abdominal pain • hyperventilation • dilated, nonreactive pupils • exaggerated or depressed reflexes • nystagmus • continuous tremor of the lower jaw • tachycardia • hyperpyrexia • increased muscle tone • convulsions • coma • cardiac arrest.
* **Overdose Management:** Emesis is not safe due to rapid induction of unconsciousness and seizures following ingestion.
◇ Gastric lavage may be performed (ad-

ministration of muscle relaxants may be required first to counteract trismus).
◇ Administer activated charcoal to minimize absorption.
◇ Initiate mechanical respiration, defibrillation, or cardioversion, if necessary.
◇ Administer diazepam or phenobarbital to control convulsions or muscular hyperactivity.
◇ Administer propranolol to treat severe tachycardia.
◇ Administer lidocaine to treat ventricular extrasystoles.
◇ Administer chlorpromazine to treat hyperpyrexia.

Potential Nursing Diagnoses

* High risk for self-directed violence related to suicidal ideations from abrupt fenfluramine withdrawal.
* High risk for injury due to abrupt fenfluramine withdrawal; overdose; side effects of drowsiness; dizziness.
* Alteration in nutrition, more than body requires, related to excessive intake in relation to metabolic needs.
* Sleep pattern disturbance related to fenfluramine's side effects of restlessness and nervousness.
* Alteration in thought processes related to adverse fenfluramine effects of confusion and anxiety.
* Knowledge deficit related to medication regimen.

Plan/Implementation

* Monitor medication's effects. Tolerance develops rapidly. If anorexigenic effects begin to diminish, notify physician immediately. Patient should be on reduced-calorie diet and program of regular exercise in addition to the medication.
* Monitor and record vital signs at regular intervals (bid) throughout therapy.
* Encourage use of sugarless gum, hard candy, or frequent sips of water for

patient who experiences dry mouth. Ensure that patient practices good oral care (frequent brushing, flossing).

♦ Ensure that patient is protected from injury. Assist with ambulation if patient experiences drowsiness or dizziness.

♦ Ensure that tablet has been swallowed and not "cheeked" to avoid medication or to hoard for later use.

♦ Tablets may be crushed and mixed with food or fluid for patient who has difficulty swallowing.

♦ To prevent insomnia, give last dose at least 6 hours before retiring.

♦ Drug should be administered 30–60 minutes before meals.

♦ Store medication at controlled room temperatures between 15° and 30°C (59°–86°F). Protect from heat and moisture.

Patient/Family Education

♦ Use caution in driving or when operating dangerous machinery. Drowsiness, dizziness, and blurred vision can occur.

♦ Do not stop taking the drug abruptly. To do so can produce serious withdrawal symptoms.

♦ If insomnia is a problem, avoid taking medication late in the day. Take no later than 6 hours before bedtime.

♦ Do not take other medications (including over-the-counter drugs) without physician's approval. Many medications contain substances that, in combination with fenfluramine, can be harmful.

♦ Diabetic patient's blood sugar should be monitored bid or tid or as instructed by physician. Be aware of need for possible alteration in insulin requirements while taking fenfluramine.

♦ Avoid consumption of large amounts of caffeinated products (coffee, tea, colas, chocolate), as they may enhance the stimulant effect of fenfluramine.

♦ Follow reduced-calorie diet provided by dietitian and program of regular

exercise. Do not exceed recommended dose if appetite suppressant effect diminishes. Contact physician.

♦ Notify physician if restlessness, insomnia, anorexia, diarrhea, mental depression, or dry mouth become severe, or if rapid and pounding heartbeat becomes evident.

♦ Do not take fenfluramine during pregnancy. Safe use of this medication during pregnancy has not been established. Inform physician immediately if pregnancy is suspected or planned.

♦ Be aware of potential side effects of fenfluramine. Refer to written materials furnished by healthcare providers for safe self-administration.

♦ Carry card or other identification at all times describing medications being taken.

Evaluation

♦ Patient demonstrates a progressive weight loss with the use of fenfluramine as an adjunct to reduced caloric intake and a program of regular exercise.

♦ Patient verbalizes understanding of side effects and regimen required for prudent self-administration of fenfluramine.

FLUOXETINE

(floo-ox′e-teen)
Prozac

Classification(s):
Bicyclic antidepressant serotonin enhancer
Pregnancy Category B

INDICATIONS

♦ Major depressive disorder. **Investigational Use:** ♦ Exogenous obesity; obsessive compulsive disorder.

ACTION

♦ Blocks the presynaptic reuptake of serotonin, increasing its concentration at the synapse and correcting the deficit that is thought to contribute to the melancholy mood of the depressed person.

PHARMACOKINETICS

Absorption: Slowly absorbed from the GI tract following oral administration.
Distribution: Appears to be widely distributed. Unknown if drug crosses placental barrier or enters breast milk.
Metabolism and Excretion: Metabolized by the liver to several metabolites, including active metabolite norfluoxetine. Excreted by the kidneys.
Half-Life: 2–3 days (fluoxetine); 7–9 days (norfluoxetine).

CONTRAINDICATIONS AND PRECAUTIONS

Contraindicated in: ♦ Hypersensitivity to the drug ♦ Children; pregnancy and lactation (safety not established).
Use Cautiously in: ♦ Patients with a history of seizures ♦ Underweight or anorexic patients ♦ Hepatic or renal insufficiency ♦ Elderly or debilitated patients ♦ Patients with a history of drug abuse ♦ Suicidal patients ♦ Recent MI ♦ Effectiveness in long-term use (more than 5–6 weeks) has not been evaluated.

ADVERSE REACTIONS AND SIDE EFFECTS*

CNS: headache, nervousness, insomnia, drowsiness, anxiety, tremors, dizziness, fatigue, decreased concentration, vision disturbances, convulsions.
CV: hot flushes, palpitations, migraine, orthostatic hypotension, ARRHYTHMIAS.
Derm: rash, pruritus, urticaria.
GI: nausea, diarrhea, dry mouth, anorexia, weight loss, constipation, abdominal cramping.
GU: dysmenorrhea, sexual dysfunction, urinary frequency, urinary tract infection, urinary retention, decreased libido.

Hemat: ANEMIA, THROMBOCYTOPENIA, LEUKOPENIA, THROMBOCYTHEMIA.
Other: excessive sweating, weakness, fever/chills, joint and muscle pain.

INTERACTIONS

Drug-Drug: ♦ **CNS-active drugs:** interactions not established; use with caution ♦ **Diazepam:** prolonged half-life of diazepam ♦ **MAO inhibitors:** potential for hypertensive crisis. Allow at least 14 days between MAOI discontinuation and initiation of fluoxetine ♦ **Tryptophan:** central and peripheral toxicity, agitation, restlessness, GI distress ♦ **Warfarin:** increased activity of warfarin.

ROUTE AND DOSAGE
Depression
♦ **PO (Adults):** Initial dosage: 20 mg/day given in the morning. Dosage may be increased after several weeks if no clinical improvement is observed. Doses above 20 mg/day should be administered bid (morning and noon). Maximum dose: 80 mg/day.

Exogenous Obesity
♦ **PO (Adults):** 60 mg/day. Dosage may be increased to 80 mg/day in some patients.

PHARMACODYNAMICS

Route	Onset	Peak	Duration
PO	3–5 hr	6–8 hr	weeks*

*Allow up to 4 weeks following cessation of therapy for complete drug elimination.

NURSING IMPLICATIONS
Assessment
♦ Assess for suicidal ideation, plan, means. Assess for sudden lifts in mood, which could indicate patient's decision to commit suicide.
♦ Assess mental status daily: • mood • appearance • thought and communication patterns • level of interest in the

*Underlines indicate most frequent; CAPITALS indicate life-threatening.

environment and in activities • suicidal ideation. Improvement in these behavior patterns and level of energy should be expected in 2–4 weeks following initiation of therapy.

♦ Assess for symptoms of blood dyscrasias: • sore throat • fever • malaise • unusual bleeding • easy bruising.

♦ Assess vital signs, weight.

♦ Assess history of allergies, sensitivity to this drug.

♦ Assess for history of glaucoma.

♦ Assess date of last menses (possible pregnancy), use of contraceptives.

♦ Assess whether currently breast-feeding a child.

♦ Assess current and past alcohol and drug consumption.

♦ Assess for operation of automobile and/or other dangerous machinery.

♦ Assess for presence of adverse reactions or side effects.

♦ Assess patient/family knowledge about illness and need for medication.

♦ In collaboration with physician, assess CBC and liver function tests in patients on long-term therapy.

♦ **Toxicity and Overdose:** Level of therapeutic serum concentration is still being studied.

◊ Assess for symptoms of overdose: • nausea • vomiting • agitation • restlessness • hypomania • seizures • other signs of CNS excitation.

♦ **Overdose Management:** Monitor cardiac and vital signs.

◊ Ensure adequate oxygenation and ventilation.

◊ Induce emesis in conscious patient.

◊ Initiate gastric lavage in unconscious patient.

◊ Administer activated charcoal to minimize absorption.

◊ Seizures that fail to remit spontaneously may respond to diazepam.

Potential Nursing Diagnoses

♦ High risk for self-directed violence related to depressed mood.

♦ High risk for injury related to overdose; fluoxetine's side effects of sedation, dizziness, weakness, confusion.

♦ Social isolation related to depressed mood.

♦ High risk for activity intolerance, related to fluoxetine's side effects of drowsiness, dizziness, weakness, confusion.

♦ Knowledge deficit related to medication regimen.

Plan/Implementation

♦ Monitor vital signs before beginning therapy and at regular intervals (bid or tid) throughout therapy. Take BP lying and standing in patients experiencing orthostatic hypotension; elderly are particularly susceptible. Contact physician if tachycardia/arrhythmias are noted.

♦ Weigh patient 2–3 times a week, at same time of day, on same scale, if possible. A rapid weight gain or evidence of edema should be reported to physician immediately. Record I&O.

♦ Ensure that patient is protected from injury. Provide supervision and assistance when ambulating if dizziness and drowsiness are problems. Pad siderails and headboard for patient who experiences seizures.

♦ Give patient hard candy, gum, or frequent sips of water if dry mouth is a problem.

♦ Administer oral medication with food to minimize GI upset.

♦ Ensure that patient swallows capsule and does not "cheek" to avoid medication or to hoard for later use.

♦ Empty contents of capsule and mix with food or fluid for patient who has difficulty swallowing.

♦ Store medication at controlled room temperatures between 15° and 30°C (59°–86°F). Protect from heat and moisture.

Patient/Family Education

♦ Therapeutic effect may not be seen for as long as 4 weeks. If after this length of time no improvement is noted, physician may prescribe a different medication. Continue to take medication even though symptoms have not subsided.

♦ Use caution when driving or when operating dangerous machinery. Drowsiness and dizziness can occur. If these side effects become persistent or interfere with daily activities, report to physician. Dosage adjustment may be necessary.

♦ Report occurrence of any of the following symptoms to physician immediately: rash or hives, sore throat, fever, malaise, unusual bleeding, easy bruising, persistent nausea/vomiting, severe headache, rapid heart rate, difficulty urinating, anorexia/weight loss (particularly in underweight patients).

♦ Rise slowly from a sitting or lying position to prevent a sudden drop in blood pressure.

♦ If dry mouth is a problem, take frequent sips of water, chew sugarless gum, or suck on hard candy. Good oral care (frequent brushing, flossing) is very important.

♦ Do not drink alcohol while on fluoxetine therapy. These drugs potentiate each other's effects.

♦ Do not consume other medications (including over-the-counter meds) with fluoxetine without physician's approval. Many medications contain substances that, in combination with fluoxetine, could precipitate a potentially life-threatening situation.

♦ Be aware of possible risks of taking fluoxetine during pregnancy. Safe use during pregnancy and lactation has not been established. Inform physician immediately if pregnancy occurs, is suspected, or is planned.

♦ Be aware of side effects of fluoxetine. Refer to written materials furnished by healthcare providers for safe self-administration.

♦ Carry card or other identification at all

times describing medications being taken.

Evaluation

♦ Patient demonstrates a subsiding/resolution of the symptoms for which fluoxetine was prescribed (depressed mood, suicidal ideation, obesity).

♦ Patient verbalizes understanding of side effects and regimen required for prudent self-administration of fluoxetine.

FLUPHENAZINE

(floo-fen′a-zeen)
{Modecate Decanoate, Moditen Enanthate, Moditen HCl}, Permitil, Prolixin

Classification(s):
Antipsychotic, Neuroleptic, Phenothiazine
Pregnancy Category C

INDICATIONS

♦ Acute and chronic psychotic disorders.

ACTION

♦ The exact mechanism of antipsychotic action is not fully understood but is probably related to antidopaminergic effects ♦ Antipsychotics may block postsynaptic dopamine receptors in the basal ganglia, hypothalamus, limbic system, brain stem, and medulla ♦ Antipsychotic effects also appear to be related to inhibition of dopamine-mediated neurotransmission at the synapses ♦ Antipsychotic effects may also result from the drug's alpha-adrenergic blocking, muscarinic blocking, and adrenergic activity, as well as effects on other amines (such as GABA) or peptides.

PHARMACOKINETICS

Absorption: Rapid absorption of oral dosage forms.
Distribution: Not completely known.

{} = Only available in Canada.

Appears to be widely distributed. Crosses blood-brain and placental barriers. Enters breast milk.

Metabolism and Excretion: Partially metabolized by the liver. Excreted in urine and feces. May be detected in urine up to 3–6 months following discontinuation of the drug.

Half-Life: Fluphenazine hydrochloride: 14.7–15.3 hours; fluphenazine enanthate: 3.6–3.7 days; fluphenazine decanoate: 6.8–9.6 days.

CONTRAINDICATIONS AND PRECAUTIONS

Contraindicated in: ◆ Hypersensitivity to this drug, other phenothiazines, or sulfites or tartrazine (contained in some preparations) ◆ Comatose or severely CNS-depressed patients ◆ Presence of large amounts of CNS depressants ◆ Bone marrow depression ◆ Blood dyscrasias ◆ Subcortical brain damage ◆ Parkinson's disease ◆ Hepatic, renal, and/or cardiac insufficiency ◆ Severe hypotension or hypertension ◆ Children under 12 years of age; pregnancy and lactation (safe use not established).

Use Cautiously in: ◆ Patients with a history of seizures ◆ Respiratory (i.e., infection; COPD), renal; hepatic; thyroid, (i.e., thyrotoxicosis); or cardiovascular disorders (i.e., mitral insufficiency, angina pectoris) ◆ Prostatic hypertrophy ◆ Glaucoma ◆ Diabetes ◆ Elderly or debilitated patients ◆ Patients exposed to high or low environmental temperatures or to organophosphate insecticides ◆ Hypocalcemia ◆ Patients with a history of severe reactions to insulin or ECT ◆ Pediatric patients with acute illnesses or dehydration.

ADVERSE REACTIONS AND SIDE EFFECTS*

CNS: sedation, headache, seizures, insomnia, dizziness, exacerbation of psychotic symptoms, extrapyramidal symptoms (pseudoparkinsonism, akathisia, akinesia, dystonia, oculogyric crisis), tardive dyskinesia, fatigue, cerebral edema, ataxia, blurred vision, NEUROLEPTIC MALIGNANT SYNDROME, restlessness, anxiety, depression, hyperthermia or hypothermia.

CV: hypotension, orthostatic hypotension, hypertension, tachycardia, bradycardia, CARDIAC ARREST, ECG changes, ARRHYTHMIAS, PULMONARY EDEMA, CIRCULATORY COLLAPSE.

Derm: skin rashes, urticaria, petechiae, seborrhea, photosensitivity, eczema, erythema, hyperpigmentation, contact dermatitis, EXFOLIATIVE DERMATITIS (rare).

Endo: galactorrhea, gynecomastia (men), changes in libido, impotence, hyperglycemia or hypoglycemia, amenorrhea, retrograde ejaculation.

GI: dry mouth, nausea, vomiting, increased appetite and weight gain, anorexia, dyspepsia, constipation, diarrhea, fecal impaction, jaundice, polydipsia, PARALYTIC ILEUS.

GU: urinary retention, frequency or incontinence, bladder paralysis, polyuria, enuresis, priapism.

Hemat: AGRANULOCYTOSIS, LEUKOPENIA, ANEMIA, THROMBOCYTOPENIA, PANCYTOPENIA.

Ophth: lens deposition, glaucoma.

Resp: LARYNGEAL EDEMA, LARYNGOSPASM, BRONCHOSPASM, SUPPRESSION OF COUGH REFLEX.

Other: decreased sweating.

INTERACTIONS

Drug-Drug: ◆ **CNS depressants (including alcohol, barbiturates, narcotics, anesthetics):** additive CNS depressant effects ◆ **Anticholinergic agents (e.g., atropine):** additive anticholinergic effects, decreased antipsychotic effects ◆ **Barbiturate anesthetics:** increased incidence of excitatory effects and hypotension ◆ **Barbiturates:** possible decreased effects of phenothiazines ◆ **Clonidine:** acute brain syndrome ◆ **Metyrosine:** potentiation of extrapy-

*Underlines indicate most frequent; CAPITALS indicate life-threatening.

ramidal side effects ♦ **Levodopa:** decreased efficacy of levodopa ♦ **Quinidine:** additive cardiac depressive effects ♦ **Magnesium- or aluminum-containing antidiarrheal mixtures, antacids:** reduced phenothiazine absorption/effectiveness ♦ **Guanethidine:** decreased antihypertensive action ♦ **Lithium:** decreased plasma levels and effect of antipsychotic drug; severe neurotoxicity reported ♦ **Epinephrine:** reversal of usual pressor action of epinephrine, resulting in decrease in blood pressure and tachycardia ♦ **Bromocriptine:** impairment of prolactin suppressing action ♦ **Angiotensin converting enzyme (ACE) inhibitors:** increased effects of ACE inhibitors ♦ **Phenytoin:** decreased phenytoin metabolism, increased risk of toxicity ♦ **Polypeptide antibiotics:** possible neuromuscular respiratory depression ♦ **Metrizamide:** seizures ♦ **Cimetidine:** decreased effects of phenothiazines ♦ **Clonidine:** possibility of severe hypotension ♦ **Piperazine:** increased seizure potential.

Drug-Food: ♦ **Caffeine-containing beverages (e.g., coffee, tea, colas):** counteracted antipsychotic effect.

ROUTE AND DOSAGE

Fluphenazine Hydrochloride

♦ **PO (Adults):** Initial dose: 0.5–10 mg/day in divided doses q 6–8 hr. Doses under 20 mg/day usually reach optimal effect; occasionally 40 mg/day is required. Maintenance dose: 1–5 mg, often given as a single daily dose.
♦ **PO (Geriatric):** 1–2.5 mg/day, adjusted according to response.
♦ **IM (Adults):** Average starting dose: 1.25 mg. Initial total daily dosage may range from 2.5 to 10 mg, divided and given at 6–8 hr intervals. Dosages exceeding 10 mg/day should be given with caution.

Fluphenazine Enanthate, Fluphenazine Decanoate

♦ **IM, SC (Adults):** 12.5–25 mg (enanthate q 1–3 weeks; decanoate q 4–6 weeks). Dosage should not exceed 100 mg. If doses greater than 50 mg are necessary, increase succeeding doses cautiously in increments of 12.5 mg.

PHARMACODYNAMICS

Route	Onset	Peak	Duration‡
PO HCl	60 min*	1.5–2 hr†	6–8 hr
IM HCl	60 min*	0.5 hr†	6–8 hr
IM (enanthate)	1–3 days	2–3 days	1–3 wk
IM (decanoate)	1–3 days	1–2 days	4–6 wk

*Full clinical effects may not be observed for 4–8 weeks.
†Steady-state plasma levels are achieved in approximately 4–7 days.
‡Drug may be detected in urine for 3–6 months after last dose.

NURSING IMPLICATIONS

Assessment

♦ Assess mental status daily: • mood • appearance • thought and communication patterns • level of interest in the environment and in activities • level of anxiety or agitation • presence of hallucinations or delusions • suspiciousness • interactions with others • ability to carry out activities of daily living.
♦ Assess for symptoms of blood dyscrasias: • sore throat • fever • malaise • unusual bleeding • easy bruising.
♦ Assess for extrapyramidal symptoms: • pseudoparkinsonism (tremors, shuffling gait, drooling, rigidity) • akinesia (muscular weakness) • akathisia (continuous restlessness and fidgeting) • dystonia (involuntary muscular movements of face, arms, legs, and neck) • oculogyric crisis (uncontrolled rolling back of the eyes) • tardive dyskinesia (bizarre facial and tongue movements, stiff neck, difficulty swallowing).
♦ Assess for symptoms of neuroleptic malignant syndrome: • hyperpyrexia up to 107°F (41.6° C) • elevated pulse

- increased or decreased blood pressure • severe parkinsonian muscle rigidity • elevated creatinine phosphokinase blood levels • elevated white blood count • altered mental status (including catatonic signs or agitation) • acute renal failure • varying levels of consciousness (including stupor and coma) • pallor diaphoresis • tachycardia • arrhythmias • rhabdomyolysis.
- ✦ Assess vital signs, weight. Record baseline values for comparison.
- ✦ Assess history of allergies, sensitivity to this drug or to other phenothiazines.
- ✦ Assess for signs and symptoms of cholestatic jaundice: • abdominal pain • nausea • rash • fever • yellow skin • flu-like symptoms • abnormal lab test results (eosinophilia, bile in urine, increased serum transaminases, bilirubin, alkaline phosphatase).
- ✦ Assess date of last menses (possible pregnancy), use of contraceptives.
- ✦ Assess whether currently breast-feeding a child.
- ✦ Assess current and past alcohol and drug consumption.
- ✦ Assess for operation of automobile and/or other dangerous machinery.
- ✦ Assess for presence of adverse reactions or side effects.
- ✦ Assess patient/family knowledge about illness and need for medication.
- ✦ In collaboration with physician, assess CBC, liver function tests, and ophthalmologic exams in patients on long-term therapy.
- ✦ **Lab Test Alterations:** Increased serum alkaline phosphatase, transaminases, bilirubin.
- ◇ Increased protein-bound iodine.
- ◇ False-positive urine pregnancy test, possibly caused by drug metabolite that discolors urine (less likely to occur when serum test is used).
- ◇ Increased urinary glucose.
- ◇ Decreased urinary estrogen, progestin, and gonadotropin.
- ◇ Increased plasma cholesterol level.
- ◇ Increased serum prolactin.

- ✦ **Withdrawal:** Assess for symptoms of abrupt withdrawal from long-term therapy: • gastritis • nausea • vomiting • dizziness • headache • tachycardia • insomnia • tremulousness • sweating.
- ✦ **Toxicity and Overdose:** No correlation has been established between blood level and therapeutic effect.
- ◇ Assess for symptoms of overdose: • CNS depression, from heavy sedation to deep sleep to coma • hypotension • confusion • excitement • extrapyramidal symptoms • agitation • restlessness • convulsions • fever • autonomic reactions • ECG changes • cardiac arrhythmias • tachycardia • hypothermia • tremor • seizures • cyanosis.
- ✦ **Overdose Management:** Monitor vital signs.
- ◇ Ensure maintenance of open airway.
- ◇ Initiate gastric lavage.
- ◇ Do not induce emesis (nuchal rigidity may result in aspiration of vomitus).
- ◇ Give patient antiparkinsonian drugs or diphenhydramine to counteract extrapyramidal symptoms.
- ◇ Administer IV fluids or a vasoconstrictor to maintain adequate blood pressure. Epinephrine is not recommended due to interaction with phenothiazines that causes further drop in blood pressure.
- ◇ Administer IV phenytoin to treat ventricular arrhythmias.
- ◇ Administer phenobarbital or diazepam to control convulsions or hyperactivity.
- ◇ Dialysis does not appear to be a useful intervention.

Potential Nursing Diagnoses

- ✦ High risk for violence directed at others related to mistrust and panic anxiety.
- ✦ High risk for injury related to fluphenazine's side effects of sedation, dizziness, ataxia, weakness, lowered seizure threshold; abrupt withdrawal after prolonged use; overdose.

♦ Sensory-perceptual alteration related to panic anxiety evidenced by hallucinations.
♦ Altered thought processes related to panic anxiety evidenced by delusional thinking.
♦ Social isolation related to inability to trust others.
♦ High risk for activity intolerance, related to fluphenazine's side effects of drowsiness, dizziness, ataxia, weakness.
♦ Noncompliance with medication regimen related to suspiciousness and mistrust of others.
♦ Knowledge deficit related to medication regimen.

Plan/Implementation
♦ **General Info:** Monitor vital signs before beginning therapy and at regular intervals (bid or tid) throughout therapy. Take BP lying and standing to monitor for possible hypotensive reaction; elderly are particularly susceptible. Dosage adjustment may be required.
◊ Ensure that patient who is ambulatory is protected from sun when spending time outdoors.
◊ Weigh patient 2–3 times a week, at same time of day, on same scale, if possible. A rapid weight gain or evidence of edema should be reported to physician immediately. Record I&O.
◊ Ensure that patient is protected from injury. Provide supervision and assistance when ambulating if dizziness and drowsiness are problems. Pad siderails and headboard for patient who experiences seizures.
◊ Give patient hard candy, gum, or frequent sips of water if dry mouth is a problem.
◊ Store medication at controlled room temperatures between 15° and 30°C (59°–86°F). Protect from heat, light, and moisture.
♦ **PO:** Oral medication may be administered with food to minimize GI upset.

◊ Ensure that patient swallows tablet and does not "cheek" to avoid medication or to hoard for later use.
◊ Crush tablet and mix with food or fluid for patient who has difficulty swallowing, or use liquid concentrate.
◊ Just prior to administration, mix concentrate with water, saline, milk, carbonated orange or lemon/lime beverage, or pineapple, apricot, prune, orange, tomato, or grapefruit juice. Do not mix with coffee, cola, tea, or apple juice, as physical incompatibility may result. Do not prepare and store bulk dilutions.
◊ If concentrate is accidentally spilled on skin or clothing during preparation or administration, wash area immediately, as contact dermatitis can occur.
♦ **IM:** Inject slowly and deeply into upper, outer quadrant of buttock. Massage site thoroughly following injection.
◊ Because of possible hypotensive effects, patient should remain in recumbent position for at least one-half hour following IM injection.
◊ Rotate sites when multiple injections are administered.
◊ Do not mix with other agents in the syringe.
◊ Avoid contact with injectable liquid. A contact dermatitis can occur.
◊ Potency is not altered when solution is slightly yellow in color. Discard if marked discoloration is evident.
◊ Avoid injecting undiluted drug into vein. Aspirate carefully before injecting.

Patient/Family Education
♦ Use caution when driving or when operating dangerous machinery. Drowsiness and dizziness can occur.
♦ Do not stop taking the drug abruptly. To do so might produce withdrawal symptoms, such as nausea, vomiting, gastritis, headache, tachycardia, insomnia, tremulousness.

♦ Use sunscreens and wear protective clothing when spending time outdoors. Skin is more susceptible to sunburn.

♦ Report occurrence of any of the following symptoms to physician immediately: • sore throat • fever • malaise • unusual bleeding • easy bruising • persistent nausea/vomiting • severe headache • rapid heart rate • difficulty urinating • muscle twitching • tremors • darkly colored urine • pale stools • yellow skin or eyes • muscular incoordination • skin rash.

♦ Drug may turn urine a pink to reddish-brown in color. This is not significant nor is it harmful.

♦ Rise slowly from a sitting or lying position to prevent a sudden drop in blood pressure.

♦ If dry mouth is a problem, take frequent sips of water, chew sugarless gum, or suck on hard candy. Good oral care (frequent brushing, flossing) is very important.

♦ If some liquid concentrate is spilled on your skin, wash it off immediately. Otherwise, a rash may appear on the skin.

♦ Consult physician regarding smoking while on fluphenazine therapy. Smoking increases metabolism of fluphenazine, requiring adjustment in dosage to achieve therapeutic effect.

♦ Dress warmly in cold weather and avoid extended exposure to very high or low temperatures. Body temperature is harder to maintain with this medication.

♦ Do not drink alcohol while on flu-

phenazine therapy. These drugs potentiate each other's effects.

♦ Do not consume other medications (including over-the-counter meds) without physician's approval. Many medications contain substances that interact with fluphenazine in a way that may be harmful.

♦ Be aware of possible risks of taking fluphenazine during pregnancy. Safe use during pregnancy and lactation has not been established. Fluphenazine readily crosses the placental barrier, so a fetus could experience adverse effects of the drug. Inform physician immediately if pregnancy occurs, is suspected, or is planned.

♦ Be aware of side effects of fluphenazine. Refer to written materials furnished by healthcare providers for safe self-administration.

♦ Continue to take medication even if feeling well and as though it is not needed. Symptoms may return if medication is discontinued.

♦ Carry card or other identification at all times describing medications being taken.

Evaluation

♦ Patient demonstrates a subsiding/resolution of the symptoms for which fluphenazine was prescribed (panic anxiety, altered thought processes, altered perceptions).

♦ Patient verbalizes understanding of side effects and regimen required for prudent self-administration of fluphenazine.

FLURAZEPAM

(flure-az′e-pam)
Dalmane, Durapam, {Somnol}

Classification(s):
Sedative-hypnotic, Benzodiazepine,
CNS depressant
Schedule C IV
Pregnancy Category NR

INDICATIONS

♦ Insomnia characterized by difficulty in falling asleep, frequent nocturnal awakening, and/or early morning awakening. For short-term (no longer than 4 weeks) and intermittent use only.

ACTION

♦Depresses subcortical levels of the central nervous system, particularly the limbic system and reticular formation ♦ May potentiate the effects of the powerful inhibitory neurotransmitter gamma-aminobutyric acid (GABA) in the brain, thereby producing a calmative effect ♦ All levels of CNS depression can be effected, from mild sedation to hypnosis to coma.

PHARMACOKINETICS

Absorption: Rapidly absorbed from the GI tract.
Distribution: Is widely distributed. Crosses blood-brain and placental barriers; excreted in breast milk.
Metabolism and Excretion: Metabolized by the liver; produces active metabolites that are excreted primarily by the kidneys.
Half-Life: 47–100 hours (flurazepam); 2–100 hours (active metabolites).

CONTRAINDICATIONS AND PRECAUTIONS

Contraindicated in: ♦ Hypersensitivity to the drug ♦ Pregnancy and lactation ♦

Narrow-angle glaucoma ♦ Children under 15.
Use Cautiously in: ♦ Elderly or debilitated patients ♦ Patients with hepatic or renal dysfunction ♦ Individuals with a history of drug abuse/addiction ♦ Depressed/suicidal patients ♦ Combination with other CNS depressants ♦ Patients with low serum albumin.

ADVERSE REACTIONS AND SIDE EFFECTS*

CNS: residual sedation, dizziness, confusion, headache, lethargy, weakness, paradoxical excitement, blurred vision, encephalopathy, mental depression.
CV: hypotension, bradycardia.
Derm: rashes.
GI: nausea, vomiting, diarrhea, constipation.
Hemat: agranulocytosis.
Resp: respiratory depression.
Other: tolerance, physical and psychological dependence.

INTERACTIONS

Drug-Drug: ♦ **Other CNS depressants (including alcohol, barbiturates, narcotics), antipsychotics, antidepressants, antihistamines, anticonvulsants, cimetidine:** additive CNS depression ♦ **Neuromuscular blocking agents:** increased respiratory depression ♦ **Disulfiram:** increased duration of action of flurazepam.

ROUTE AND DOSAGE

Insomnia

♦ **PO (Adults):** 15–30 mg at bedtime.
♦ **PO (Geriatric or Debilitated Patients):** Initially, 15 mg at bedtime. Adjust dosage as response is determined.

PHARMACODYNAMICS

Route	Onset	Peak	Duration
PO	15–45 min	30–60 min	7–8 hr

{} = Only available in Canada.
*Underlines indicate most frequent; CAPITALS indicate life-threatening.

NURSING IMPLICATIONS
Assessment

◆ Assess sleep patterns. Keep records for adequate baseline data before the initiation of therapy.

◆ Assess for suicidal ideation (CNS depressants aggravate symptoms in depressed patients).

◆ Assess history of allergies, sensitivity to this drug or other benzodiazepines.

◆ Assess history of glaucoma.

◆ Assess date of last menses (possible pregnancy), use of contraceptives.

◆ Assess whether currently breast-feeding a child.

◆ Assess current and past alcohol and drug consumption.

◆ Assess operation of automobile and/ or other dangerous machinery.

◆ Assess for presence of adverse reactions or side effects.

◆ Assess patient/family knowledge about illness and need for medication.

◆ In collaboration with physician, assess CBC and liver function tests in patients on long-term therapy.

◆ **Lab Test Alterations:** May cause increases in total and direct serum bilirubin, AST, ALT, LDH, and alkaline phosphatase, as well as abnormal renal function tests.

◆ **Withdrawal:** Assess for symptoms of withdrawal: • depression • insomnia • increased anxiety • abdominal and muscle cramps • tremors • vomiting • sweating • convulsions • delirium.

◆ **Withdrawal Management:** Monitor vital signs.

◇ Place patient in quiet room with low stimuli.

◇ Institute seizure precautions.

◇ A long-acting barbiturate, such as phenobarbital, may be ordered to suppress withdrawal symptoms.

◇ Phenytoin may be ordered to prevent seizures.

◆ **Toxicity and Overdose:** Assess for symptoms of intoxication: • euphoria • excessive drowsiness • slurred speech • disorientation • mood lability

• incoordination • unsteady gait • disinhibition of sexual and aggressive impulses • judgment and/or memory impairment.

◇ Assess for symptoms of overdose: • shallow respiration • cold and clammy skin • hypotension • dilated pupils • weak and rapid pulse • hypnosis • coma • possible death.

◆ **Overdose Management:** Monitor vital signs.

◇ Ensure maintenance of adequate airway.

◇ Induce emesis in conscious patient.

◇ Initiate gastric lavage in unconscious patient.

◇ Administer IV fluids to encourage diuresis.

◇ Vasopressor may be required to combat hypotension.

Potential Nursing Diagnoses

◆ High risk for injury related to abrupt withdrawal from long-term use; effects of drug intoxication or overdose; decreased mental alertness caused by residual sedation.

◆ High risk for self-directed violence related to depressed mood.

◆ Sleep pattern disturbance related to situational crises, physical condition, severe level of anxiety.

◆ High risk for activity intolerance, related to side effects of lethargy, drowsiness, dizziness, weakness.

◆ Knowledge deficit related to medication regimen.

Plan/Implementation

◆ Monitor vital signs before beginning therapy and at regular intervals (bid) throughout therapy.

◆ Ensure that patient is protected from injury. Supervise and assist with ambulation if dizziness and muscular weakness are problems. Pad siderails and headboard for patient who experiences seizures (withdrawal).

◆ Ensure that capsule has been swallowed and not "cheeked" to avoid medication or to hoard for later use.

+ Raise siderails and ensure that patient remains in bed following administration.
+ Discourage smoking following administration.
+ Store medication at controlled room temperatures between 15° and 30°C (59°–86°F). Protect from heat, light, and moisture.

Patient/Family Education

+ Do not drive or operate dangerous machinery if residual drowsiness and dizziness occur.
+ Do not stop taking the drug abruptly. To do so can produce serious withdrawal symptoms.
+ Do not consume other CNS depressants unless prescribed by physician. Do not consume alcohol.
+ Do not take nonprescription medication without approval from physician.
+ Be aware of risks of taking flurazepam during pregnancy (congenital malformations have been associated with use of benzodiazepines during first trimester). Notify physician of desirability to discontinue drug if pregnancy is suspected or planned.
+ Be aware of potential side effects. Refer to written materials furnished by healthcare providers regarding correct method of self-administration.
+ Carry card or other identification at all times stating names of medications being taken.

Evaluation

+ Patient demonstrates a subsiding/resolution of the symptoms for which flurazepam was prescribed (insomnia, sleep disturbances).
+ Patient verbalizes understanding of side effects and regimen required for prudent self-administration of flurazepam.

GLUTETHIMIDE

(gloo-teth′i-mide)
Doriden, Doriglute

Classification(s):
Sedative-hypnotic, CNS depressant
Schedule C II
Pregnancy Category C

INDICATIONS

+ Insomnia (short-term management) + Preoperative sedation.

ACTION

+ Exact mechanism of action is unknown
+ Produces a calming effect through depression of the central nervous system.

PHARMACOKINETICS

Absorption: Erratic absorption following oral administration.
Distribution: Extensive distribution, with localization in adipose tissue. Also found in liver, kidneys, brain, and bile. Crosses placental barrier and is excreted in breast milk.
Metabolism and Excretion: Metabolized by the liver; excreted in urine and feces.
Half-Life: First phase, 4 hours; second phase, 10–12 hours.

CONTRAINDICATIONS AND PRECAUTIONS

Contraindicated in: + Hypersensitivity to the drug + Pregnancy and lactation + Porphyria + Children (safety and effectiveness has not been established) + Severe renal impairment + Uncontrolled pain.
Use Cautiously in: + Elderly or debilitated patients + Patients with hepatic, renal, or respiratory dysfunction + Depressed/suicidal patients + Patients with a history of drug abuse/dependence + Patients with prostatic hypertrophy, peptic ulcer, bladder-neck obstruction, py-

loroduodenal obstruction, angle-closure glaucoma, or cardiac arrhythmias.

ADVERSE REACTIONS AND SIDE EFFECTS*

CNS: <u>drowsiness</u>, <u>dizziness</u>, <u>hangover</u>, ataxia, headache, paradoxical excitement, blurred vision.

Derm: <u>skin rashes</u>.

GI: nausea, vomiting, dry mouth, gastric irritation, hiccups, diarrhea.

Hemat: BLOOD DYSCRASIAS (rare).

Other: tolerance, physical and psychological dependence.

INTERACTIONS

Drug-Drug: ◆ **Other CNS depressants (including alcohol, barbiturates, benzodiazepines, opiates):** additive CNS depression ◆ **Oral anticoagulants:** decreased anticoagulant response ◆ **Tricyclic antidepressants (and other drugs that produce anticholinergic effects):** additive anticholinergic effects.

ROUTE AND DOSAGE

Insomnia

(Limit use to 7 days, with at least 7 days before retreatment.)

◆ **PO (Adults):** 250–500 mg at bedtime. Maximum daily dose: 1 g.

Sedation

◆ **PO (Adults):** 125–250 mg tid after meals.

Preoperative Sedation

◆ **PO (Adults):** 500 mg at bedtime the night before surgery, then 500–1000 mg 1 hour before surgery.

PHARMACODYNAMICS

Route	Onset	Peak	Duration
PO	30 min	1–6 hr	4–8 hr

NURSING IMPLICATIONS

Assessment

◆ Assess level of anxiety and agitation. Report and document behaviors.

◆ Assess sleep patterns. Keep records for adequate baseline data before the initiation of therapy.

◆ Assess for suicidal ideation in depressed patients.

◆ Assess history of allergies, sensitivity to this drug.

◆ Assess date of last menses (possible pregnancy), use of contraceptives.

◆ Assess whether currently breast-feeding a child.

◆ Assess current and past alcohol and drug consumption.

◆ Assess for operation of automobile and/or other dangerous machinery.

◆ Assess for presence of adverse reactions or side effects.

◆ Assess patient/family knowledge about illness and need for medication.

◆ In collaboration with physician, assess CBC and renal and liver function tests in patients who have been on prolonged use.

◆ **Withdrawal:** Assess for symptoms of withdrawal: • anxiety • tremors • insomnia • nausea/vomiting • weakness • abdominal cramps • fever • chills • dysphasia • numbness of extremities • diaphoresis • orthostatic hypotension • tachycardia • hallucinations • delirium • convulsions.

◆ **Withdrawal Management:** Monitor vital signs.

◇ Place patient in quiet room with low stimuli.

◇ Institute seizure precautions.

◇ A long-acting barbiturate, such as phenobarbital, may be ordered to suppress withdrawal symptoms.

◇ Phenytoin may be ordered to prevent seizures.

◇ Some physicians may order oxazepam as needed for objective withdrawal symptoms, gradually decreasing dosage until the drug is discontinued.

◆ **Toxicity and Overdose:** Assess for symptoms of toxicity: • confusion •

---

*<u>Underlines</u> indicate most frequent; CAPITALS indicate life-threatening.

drowsiness • dyspnea • slurred speech • staggering.

◊ Assess for symptoms of overdose: • CNS and respiratory depression • hypoventilation • dryness of mouth • adynamic ileus • urinary bladder atony • dilated pupils • hypothermia • hypotension • shock • oliguria • coma. (May progress to respiratory arrest, circulatory collapse, and death.)

♦ **Overdose Management:** Monitor vital signs.

◊ Ensure maintenance of adequate airway.

◊ Induce vomiting in conscious patient.

◊ Initiate gastric lavage in unconscious patient.

◊ Administer activated charcoal to minimize absorption of drug.

◊ Administer IV fluids.

◊ For severe intoxication, hemodialysis may be used.

Potential Nursing Diagnoses

♦ High risk for injury related to abrupt withdrawal from long-term use; decreased mental alertness caused by side effects of drowsiness and dizziness; effects of overdose.

♦ High risk for self-directed violence related to depressed mood.

♦ Anxiety (specify level) related to threats to physical integrity and/or self-concept.

♦ Sleep pattern disturbance related to situational crises, physical condition, severe level of anxiety.

♦ High risk for activity intolerance, related to side effects of drowsiness, dizziness.

♦ Knowledge deficit related to medication regimen.

Plan/Implementation

♦ Monitor vital signs before beginning therapy, and at regular intervals (bid) throughout therapy.

♦ Ensure that patient is protected from injury. Supervise and assist with ambulation if dizziness and drowsiness are problems. Ensure that patient avoids participation in any activity requiring mental alertness (including smoking). Raise siderails and instruct patient to remain in bed following administration.

♦ To minimize nausea, medication may be given with food or milk.

♦ Ensure that tablet/capsule has been swallowed and not "cheeked" to avoid medication or to hoard for later use.

♦ Crush tablet or empty contents of capsule and mix with food or fluid for patient who has difficulty swallowing.

♦ Discontinue drug if skin rash appears.

♦ Store medication at controlled room temperatures between 15° and 30°C (59°–86°F). Protect from heat and moisture.

Patient/Family Education

♦ Use caution in driving or when operating dangerous machinery. Drowsiness and dizziness can occur.

♦ Do not stop taking the drug abruptly. Doing so can produce serious (even life-threatening) withdrawal symptoms. If a dose is missed, take it as close as possible to the prescribed time. If it is already close to time for next dose, wait until then; do not double up on dose at the next prescribed time.

♦ Do not consume other CNS depressants (including alcohol).

♦ Be aware of possible risks of taking glutethimide during pregnancy (safety during pregnancy has not been established). Notify physician if pregnancy is suspected or planned.

♦ Be aware of potential side effects. Refer to written materials furnished by healthcare providers regarding correct method of self-administration.

♦ Report symptoms of sore throat, fever, malaise, skin rash, unusual bleeding, or easy bruising to physician immediately.

♦ Carry card or other identification at all times stating names of medications being taken.

Evaluation

- Patient demonstrates a subsiding/resolution of the symptoms for which glutethimide was prescribed (sleep disturbances).
- Patient verbalizes understanding of side effects and regimen required for prudent self-administration of glutethimide.

GLYCOPYRROLATE

(glye-koe-pye'roe-late)
Robinul, Robinul Forte

Classification(s):
Anticholinergic, Antimuscarinic
**Pregnancy Category C
(parenteral: B)**

INDICATIONS

♦ Peptic ulcer and other GI conditions ♦ Preoperative or preprocedural (including ECT) medication to decrease secretions and block cardiac vagal inhibitory reflexes.

ACTION

♦ Competitively inhibits the muscarinic actions of acetylcholine at postganglionic parasympathetic neuroeffector sites, including smooth muscle, secretory glands, and sites within the central nervous system ♦ Specific anticholinergic responses are dose-related.

PHARMACOKINETICS

Absorption: Incompletely absorbed from the GI tract. Absorption following IM injection is more complete.
Distribution: Not completely understood. Does not cross blood-brain barrier. Crosses placental barrier. Unknown if drug enters breast milk.
Metabolism and Excretion: Small amounts metabolized by the liver. Excreted mainly in feces via biliary elimination and also in urine.
Half-Life: Not well established.

CONTRAINDICATIONS AND PRECAUTIONS

Contraindicated in: ♦ Hypersensitivity to this drug or other anticholinergic drugs ♦ Angle-closure glaucoma ♦ Adhesions between the iris and lens ♦ Tachycardia ♦ Unstable cardiovascular status in acute hemorrhage ♦ Myocardial ischemia ♦ Obstructive disease ♦ Paralytic ileus ♦ Intestinal atony of the elderly or debilitated patient ♦ Severe ulcerative colitis ♦ Toxic megacolon complicating ulcerative colitis ♦ Obstructive uropathy ♦ Myasthenia gravis ♦ Concomitant use of cyclopropane anesthesia ♦ Children under age 12 (except in parenteral use with anesthesia) ♦ Pregnancy and lactation (safe use not established).

Use Cautiously in: ♦ Autonomic neuropathy ♦ Glaucoma ♦ Hepatic disease ♦ Mild to moderate ulcerative colitis ♦ Hiatal hernia associated with reflux esophagitis ♦ Renal disease ♦ Prostatic hypertrophy ♦ Hyperthyroidism ♦ Coronary artery disease ♦ Congestive heart failure ♦ Cardiac tachyarrhythmias ♦ Hypertension ♦ Chronic lung disease ♦ Infants and small children ♦ Down's syndrome ♦ Brain damage ♦ Patients exposed to elevated environmental temperatures ♦ Febrile patients ♦ Geriatric patients ♦ Gastric ulcer ♦ GI infections ♦ Patients with diarrhea ♦ Partial obstructive uropathy.

ADVERSE REACTIONS AND SIDE EFFECTS*

CNS: headache, flushing, nervousness, drowsiness, weakness, dizziness, insomnia, fever, mental confusion, excitement, restlessness, tremor.
CV: palpitations, tachycardia.
Derm: urticaria and other dermal manifestations.
GI: xerostomia, altered taste perception, nausea, vomiting, dysphagia, heartburn, constipation, bloated feeling, PARALYTIC ILEUS, gastroesophageal reflux.
GU: urinary retention, urinary hesitancy, impotence.

*Underlines indicate most frequent; CAPITALS indicate life-threatening.

Ophth: blurred vision, mydriasis, photophobia, cycloplegia, increased intraocular pressure.

Other: ANAPHYLAXIS, suppression of lactation, nasal congestion, decreased sweating.

INTERACTIONS

Drug-Drug: ♦ **Antihistamines, glutethimide, disopyramide, procainamide, quinidine, antipsychotics, antiparkinson agents, buclizine, meperidine, orphenadrine, amantadine, benzodiazepines, tricyclic antidepressants, MAO inhibitors:** enhanced anticholinergic effects ♦ **Nitrates, nitrites, alkalinizing agents, primidone, thioxanthenes, methylphenidate:** potentiation of adverse effects of glycopyrrolate ♦ **Corticosteroids or haloperidol (long-term therapy):** increased intraocular pressure ♦ **Guanethidine, histamine, reserpine:** decreased effects of glycopyrrolate ♦ **Phenothiazines, haloperidol:** possible decreased antipsychotic effects ♦ **Sympathomimeties, nitrofurantoin, thiazide diuretics:** increased effects of these drugs ♦ **Cholinesterase inhibitors, metoclopramide:** decreased effects of these drugs ♦ **Digitalis, slow-release digoxin tablets, anticholinergics, neostigmine:** increased potential for adverse effects ♦ **Antacids:** may interfere with absorption of anticholinergics ♦ **Cyclopropane anesthesia:** possible ventricular arrhythmias.

ROUTE AND DOSAGE

Peptic Ulcer (Adjunctive Therapy)

♦ **PO (Adults):** 1 mg tid or 2 mg bid–tid. Maintenance: 1 mg bid. Maximum: 8 mg/day.
♦ **IM, IV (Adults):** 0.1–0.2 mg tid or qid.
♦ Safe use in peptic ulcer disease in children less than 12 years old not established.

Preoperative/Preprocedural Medication

♦ **IM (Adults):** 0.004 mg/kg 30–60 min prior to anesthesia.
♦ **IM (Children 2 Years and Older):** 0.004 mg/kg 30–60 min prior to anesthesia.
♦ **IM (Children Under 2 Years Old):** 0.004–0.008 mg/kg 30–60 min prior to anesthesia.

PHARMACODYNAMICS

Route	Onset	Peak	Duration
PO	—	1 hr	8–12 hr
IM, SQ	15–30 min	30–45 min	2–7 hr
IV	1 min	10–15 min	4 hr

NURSING IMPLICATIONS

Assessment

♦ Assess mood daily in patient receiving ECT: ● observe appearance ● speech and thought patterns ● behavior ● interaction with others ● somatic complaints ● attendance in activities ● evidence of excitement or agitation.
♦ Assess for symptoms of paralytic ileus: ● constipation ● abdominal pain and distention ● absence of bowel sounds. Patients taking glycopyrrolate concomitantly with other drugs that produce anticholinergic effects are particularly susceptible.
♦ Assess vital signs prior to administration. Record baseline values for comparison.
♦ Assess history of allergies, sensitivity to this or to other anticholinergic drugs.
♦ Assess date of last menses (possible pregnancy), use of contraceptives.
♦ Assess whether currently breast-feeding a child.
♦ Assess current and past alcohol and drug consumption.
♦ Assess for operation of automobile and/or other dangerous machinery.
♦ Assess for presence of adverse reactions or side effects.

♦ Assess patient/family knowledge about illness and need for medication.

♦ **Toxicity and Overdose:** Assess for symptoms of overdose: • dry mouth • thirst • dysphagia • vomiting • nausea • abdominal distention • muscular weakness • CNS stimulation followed by depression • delirium • drowsiness • restlessness • stupor • fever • dizziness • headache • seizures • tremor • hallucinations • anxiety • ataxia • psychotic behavior • rapid pulse and respiration • tachycardia with weak pulse • hypertension • palpitations • urinary retention • blurred vision • photophobia • dilated pupils • leukocytosis • flushed, hot, dry skin • rash over face, neck, and upper trunk • diminished or absent bowel sounds • hypotension • coma • skeletal muscle paralysis • respiratory failure • circulatory failure.

♦ **Overdose Management:** Induce emesis or initiate gastric lavage.

◊ Administer activated charcoal slurry.

◊ Ensure maintenance of adequate airway and ventilation.

◊ Continuously monitor ECG.

◊ Protect patient from injury due to seizures.

◊ Physostigmine administered by slow IV injection may reverse anticholinergic effects.

◊ Administer benzodiazepines or short-acting barbiturates to control excitement.

◊ Use fluid therapy and levarterenol to control hypotension and circulatory collapse.

◊ Apply cold packs or other cooling measures to treat hyperpyrexia.

◊ Darken room if photophobia occurs.

Potential Nursing Diagnoses

♦ Decreased cardiac output related to vagal stimulation.

♦ High risk for self-directed violence related to depressed mood.

♦ High risk for injury related to side effects of glycopyrrolate such as weakness, blurred vision, and dizziness, or to overdose.

♦ Hyperthermia related to anticholinergic effect of decreased sweating.

♦ Altered thought processes related to side effects of glycopyrrolate evidenced by mental confusion.

♦ Anxiety (moderate to severe) related to pending medical procedure (surgery, ECT).

♦ High risk for activity intolerance, related to glycopyrrolate's side effects of drowsiness, dizziness, weakness, mental confusion.

♦ Knowledge deficit related to medication regimen.

Plan/Implementation

♦ **General Info:** Monitor vital signs daily. Report any changes to physician. Withhold dosage if pulse rate is markedly increased or decreased and contact physician immediately.

◊ Weigh patient 2–3 times a week, at same time of day, on same scale, if possible. A rapid weight gain or evidence of edema should be reported to physician immediately. Record I&O.

◊ Ensure that patient is protected from injury. Provide supervision and assistance when ambulating if dizziness and drowsiness are problems.

◊ Give patient hard candy, gum, or frequent sips of water if dry mouth is a problem, or treat with saliva substitute.

◊ Store medication at controlled room temperatures between 15° and 30°C (59°–86°F). Protect from heat and freezing.

♦ **PO:** May administer medication prior to or with meals to minimize gastric irritation.

◊ Do not give glycopyrrolate with antacids, as they may interfere with absorption.

♦ **IM, IV:** Glycopyrrolate may be administered IM or IV.

◊ Administer IV at rate not exceeding 0.2 mg over 1–2 minutes. Administer through Y-tube or 3-way stopcock of infusion set.

♦ Glycopyrrolate is not stable above a pH of 6.0. Therefore, do not mix in syringe with any of the following drugs: methohexital, chloramphenicol, dimenhydrinate, pentobarbital, thiopental, pentazocine, secobarbital, sodium bicarbonate, diazepam, dexamethasone, buffered solution of lactated Ringer's solution, or with any drug capable of raising the pH above 6. A gas may evolve or a precipitate may form.

Patient/Family Education

♦ May take medication with meals to minimize GI upset.

♦ Use caution when driving or when operating dangerous machinery. Drowsiness, dizziness, and blurred vision can occur.

♦ Report occurrence of any of the following symptoms to physician immediately: extreme dryness of mouth • difficulty urinating • constipation • fast and pounding heartbeat • eye pain • rash • visual disturbances • mental changes.

♦ Sensitivity to light can be relieved by wearing sunglasses and keeping room darkened.

♦ Stay indoors in air-conditioned room when weather is very hot. Perspiration is decreased with glycopyrrolate, and the body cannot cool itself as well. There is greater susceptibility to heat stroke. Inform physician if air-conditioned housing and/or work environment is not available.

♦ If dry mouth is a problem, take frequent sips of water, chew sugarless gum, suck on hard candy, or use saliva substitute. Good oral care (frequent brushing, flossing) is very important.

♦ Do not consume other medications (including over-the-counter meds) without physician's approval. Some medications may contain substances

that interact with glycopyrrolate in a way that could be harmful.

♦ Be aware of possible risks of taking glycopyrrolate during pregnancy. Safe use during pregnancy and lactation has not been established. Glycopyrrolate readily crosses the placental barrier, so a fetus could experience adverse effects of the drug. Inform physician immediately if pregnancy occurs, is suspected, or is planned.

♦ Be aware of side effects of glycopyrrolate. Refer to written materials furnished by healthcare providers for safe self-administration.

♦ Carry card or other identification at all times describing medications being taken.

Evaluation

♦ Patient demonstrates a resolution/subsiding of the symptoms for which glycopyrrolate was prescribed (peptic ulcer, to decrease secretions prior to surgery or other procedures).

♦ Patient verbalizes understanding of side effects and regimen required for prudent self-administration of glycopyrrolate.

HALAZEPAM

(hal-az′e-pam)
Paxipam

Classification(s):
Antianxiety agent, Benzodiazepine, Skeletal muscle relaxant, Anticonvulsant, CNS depressant
Schedule C IV
Pregnancy Category D

INDICATIONS

♦ Anxiety disorders ♦ Anxiety symptoms (efficacy for periods greater than 4 months has not been evaluated).

ACTION

♦ Depresses subcortical levels of the central nervous system, particularly the limbic system and reticular formation ♦ May potentiate the effects of the powerful inhibitory neurotransmitter gamma-aminobutyric acid (GABA) in the brain, thereby producing a calmative effect ♦ All levels of CNS depression can be effected, from mild sedation to hypnosis to coma.

PHARMACOKINETICS

Absorption: Rapidly absorbed from the GI tract.
Distribution: Is widely distributed. Crosses the blood-brain and placental barriers; excreted in breast milk.
Metabolism and Excretion: Metabolized by the liver; produces active metabolites that are excreted by the kidneys.
Half-Life: 14 hours.

CONTRAINDICATIONS AND PRECAUTIONS

Contraindicated in: ♦ Hypersensitivity to this drug or to other benzodiazepines ♦ Concomitant use of other CNS depressants ♦ Pregnancy and lactation ♦ Narrow-angle glaucoma ♦ Children under 18.
Use Cautiously in: ♦ Elderly or debilitated patients ♦ Patients with hepatic or renal dysfunction ♦ Individuals with a history of drug abuse/addiction ♦ Depressed/suicidal patients.

ADVERSE REACTIONS AND SIDE EFFECTS*

CNS: <u>drowsiness</u>, <u>fatigue</u>, <u>ataxia</u>, <u>dizziness</u>, confusion, headache, syncope, paradoxical excitement, blurred vision, mental depression.
CV: tachycardia, hypotension, bradycardia.
Endo: gynecomastia, galactorrhea.
GI: dry mouth, nausea/vomiting, constipation, diarrhea.
GU: libidinal changes.
Resp: respiratory depression.
Other: tolerance, physical and psychological dependence.

INTERACTIONS

Drug-Drug: ♦ **Other CNS depressants (including alcohol, barbiturates, narcotics), antipsychotics, antidepressants, antihistamines, anticonvulsants:** additive CNS depression ♦ **Cimetidine:** increased effects of halazepam ♦ **Cigarette smoking and caffeine:** decreased effects of halazepam ♦ **Neuromuscular blocking agents:** increased respiratory depression ♦ **Digoxin:** reduced excretion of digoxin, increased potential for toxicity ♦ **Disulfiram:** decreased clearance of halazepam.

ROUTE AND DOSAGE

Anxiety, Anxiety Disorders

♦ **PO (Adults):** 20–40 mg tid or qid.
♦ **PO (Geriatric or Debilitated Patients):** 20 mg daily or bid.

PHARMACODYNAMICS

Route	Onset	Peak	Duration
PO	30–60 min	1–3 hr	*

*Varies with individual age, disease state, number of doses.

NURSING IMPLICATIONS

Assessment

♦ Assess level of anxiety. Symptoms include: ● restlessness ● pacing ● insomnia ● inability to concentrate ● increased heart rate ● increased respiration ● elevated blood pressure ● confusion ● tremors ● rapid speech.
♦ Assess for suicidal ideation (CNS depressants aggravate symptoms in depressed patients).
♦ Assess history of allergies, sensitivity to this drug.
♦ Assess history of glaucoma.
♦ Assess date of last menses (possible pregnancy), use of contraceptives.
♦ Assess whether currently breast-feeding a child.
♦ Assess current and past alcohol and drug consumption.

*<u>Underlines</u> indicate most frequent; CAPITALS indicate life-threatening.

♦ Assess operation of automobile and/or other dangerous machinery.

♦ Assess for presence of adverse reactions or side effects.

♦ Assess patient/family knowledge about illness and need for medication.

♦ In collaboration with physician, assess CBC and liver function tests in patients on long-term therapy.

♦ **Lab Test Alterations:** Abnormal renal function tests.

♦ **Withdrawal:** Assess for symptoms of withdrawal: • depression • insomnia • increased anxiety • abdominal and muscle cramps • tremors • vomiting • sweating • convulsions • delirium.

♦ **Withdrawal Management:** Monitor vital signs.

◊ Place patient in quiet room with low stimuli.

◊ Institute seizure precautions.

◊ A long-acting barbiturate, such as phenobarbital, may be ordered to suppress withdrawal symptoms.

◊ Phenytoin may be ordered to prevent seizures.

◊ Some physicians may order oxazepam as needed for objective withdrawal symptoms, gradually decreasing dosage until the drug is discontinued.

♦ **Toxicity and Overdose:** Assess for symptoms of intoxication: • euphoria • relaxation • drowsiness • slurred speech • disorientation • mood lability • incoordination • unsteady gait • disinhibition of sexual and aggressive impulses • judgment and/or memory impairment.

◊ Assess for symptoms of overdose: • shallow respiration • cold and clammy skin • hypotension • dilated pupils • weak and rapid pulse • hypnosis • coma • possible death.

♦ **Overdose Management:** Ensure maintenance of adequate airway.

◊ Monitor vital signs.

◊ Induce emesis in conscious patient.

◊ Initiate gastric lavage in unconscious patient.

◊ Administer activated charcoal to minimize absorption of the drug.

◊ IV fluids and diuretics may accelerate elimination of benzodiazepines.

Potential Nursing Diagnoses

♦ High risk for injury related to seizures, panic anxiety, abrupt withdrawal from long-term halazepam use, effects of halazepam intoxication or overdose.

♦ High risk for self-directed violence related to depressed mood.

♦ Anxiety (specify level) related to threats to physical integrity and/or self-concept.

♦ High risk for activity intolerance, related to halazepam's side effects of lethargy, drowsiness, dizziness, muscular weakness.

♦ Knowledge deficit related to medication regimen.

Plan/Implementation

♦ Monitor vital signs before beginning therapy, and at regular intervals (bid) throughout therapy.

♦ Ensure that patient practices good oral care. Offer patient hard, sugarless candy; gum; or frequent sips of water for dry mouth.

♦ Ensure that patient is protected from injury. Supervise and assist with ambulation if dizziness and muscular weakness are problems. Pad siderails and headboard for patient who experiences seizures.

♦ To minimize nausea, medication may be given with food or milk.

♦ If patient has difficulty swallowing, tablet may be crushed and mixed with food or fluid.

♦ Ensure that tablet has been swallowed and not "cheeked" to avoid medication or to hoard for later use.

♦ Store medication at temperatures between 2° and 30°C (36°–86°F).

Patient/Family Education

♦ Do not drive or operate dangerous machinery. Drowsiness and dizziness can occur.

♦ Do not stop taking the drug abruptly.

Doing so can result in serious withdrawal symptoms.
* Do not consume other CNS depressants (including alcohol).
* Do not take nonprescription medication without approval from physician.
* Be aware of risks of taking halazepam during pregnancy (congenital malformations have been associated with use during first trimester). Notify physician of desirability to discontinue drug if pregnancy is suspected or planned.
* Be aware of potential side effects. Refer to written materials furnished by healthcare providers regarding correct method of self-administration.
* Carry card or other identification at all times stating names of medications being taken.

Evaluation
* Patient demonstrates a subsiding/resolution of the symptoms for which halazepam was prescribed (anxiety symptoms, anxiety disorders).
* Patient verbalizes understanding of side effects and regimen required for prudent self-administration of halazepam.

HALOPERIDOL

(ha-loe-per′i-dole)
Haldol

Classification(s):
Antipsychotic, Neuroleptic,
Butyrophenone
Pregnancy Category C

INDICATIONS

* Management of acute and chronic psychoses * Control of tics and vocal utterances of Tourette's disorder * Treating symptoms of dementia in the elderly * Control of hyperactivity and severe behavior problems in children. **Investigational Uses:** * Antiemetic (doses smaller than those used to control psychotic be-

havior) * Control in acute psychiatric situations.

ACTION
* The exact mechanism of antipsychotic action is not fully understood * Appears to depress the CNS at subcortical level of the brain, midbrain, and brain stem reticular formation * Thought to inhibit ascending reticular activating system of brain stem; may also inhibit catecholamine receptors as well as reuptake of various neurotransmitters in midbrain * Also is a strong central antagonist of dopamine receptors.

PHARMACOKINETICS
Absorption: Oral dosage well absorbed from GI tract. Appears to undergo first-pass metabolism and enterohepatic circulation. Final oral bioavailability is about 60%. IM absorption varies from patient to patient. Decanoate release from fatty tissues is slow.

Distribution: Distribution is not fully known. Thought to be distributed mainly to the liver, with lower concentrations in the brain, heart, lungs, kidneys, and spleen. Crosses placental barrier. Enters breast milk.

Metabolism and Excretion: Metabolized mainly by the liver. Excreted through the kidneys and enterohepatic circulation into feces. After oral doses, the drug and metabolites may be detected in urine up to 28 days following discontinuation of the drug.

Half-Life: 13–35 hours (oral, IM lactate); 3 weeks (IM decanoate).

CONTRAINDICATIONS AND PRECAUTIONS

Contraindicated in: * Hypersensitivity to this drug or to tartrazine (contained in some preparations) * Comatose or severely CNS-depressed patients * Presence of large amounts of CNS depressants * Bone marrow depression * Blood dyscrasias * Subcortical brain damage * Parkinson's disease * Hepatic, renal, and/or cardiac insufficiency ♦ Severe hypotension or hypertension ♦ Children under 3 years of age; pregnancy and lactation (safe use not established).

Use Cautiously in: ♦ Patients with a history of seizures ♦ Respiratory (e.g., infection; COPD), renal, hepatic, thyroid (e.g., thyrotoxicosis), or cardiovascular disorders (e.g., mitral insufficiency, angina pectoris) ♦ Prostatic hypertrophy ♦ Glaucoma ♦ Diabetes ♦ Elderly and debilitated patients ♦ Patients exposed to high or low environmental temperatures or to organophosphate insecticides ♦ Hypocalcemia ♦ History of severe reactions to insulin or ECT ♦ Pediatric patients with acute illnesses or dehydration.

ADVERSE REACTIONS AND SIDE EFFECTS*

CNS: sedation, headache, seizures, insomnia, dizziness, exacerbation of psychotic symptoms, extrapyramidal symptoms (pseudoparkinsonism, akathisia, akinesia, dystonia, oculogyric crisis), tardive dyskinesia, fatigue, cerebral edema, ataxia, blurred vision, NEUROLEPTIC MALIGNANT SYNDROME, restlessness, anxiety, depression, hyperthermia or hypothermia, hyperpyrexia, heat stroke, confusion.

CV: hypotension, orthostatic hypotension, hypertension, tachycardia, bradycardia, CARDIAC ARREST, ECG changes, ARRHYTHMIAS, PULMONARY EDEMA, CIRCULATORY COLLAPSE.

Derm: skin rashes, urticaria, petechiae, seborrhea, photosensitivity, eczema, erythema, hyperpigmentation, contact dermatitis, maculopapular and acneiform reactions, alopecia, EXFOLIATIVE DERMATITIS (rare).

Endo: galactorrhea, gynecomastia (men), changes in libido, impotence, hyperglycemia or hypoglycemia, amenorrhea, retrograde ejaculation, hyponatremia, menstrual irregularities.

GI: dry mouth, nausea, vomiting, increased appetite and weight gain, anorexia, dyspepsia, constipation, diarrhea, jaundice, polydipsia, PARALYTIC ILEUS, IMPAIRED LIVER FUNCTION, hypersalivation, dyspepsia.

GU: urinary retention, frequency or incontinence, bladder paralysis, polyuria, enuresis, priapism.

Hemat: AGRANULOCYTOSIS, LEUKOPENIA, ANEMIA, leukocytosis.

Ophth: cataracts, retinopathy.

Resp: LARYNGEAL EDEMA, LARYNGOSPASM, BRONCHOSPASM, SUPPRESSION OF COUGH REFLEX.

Other: diaphoresis.

INTERACTIONS

Drug-Drug: ♦ **CNS depressants (including alcohol, barbiturates, narcotics, anesthetics):** additive CNS depressant effects ♦ **Anticholinergic agents (e.g., atropine):** additive anticholinergic effects, decreased antipsychotic effects ♦ **Barbiturate anesthetics:** increased incidence of excitatory effects and hypotension ♦ **Barbiturates:** possible decreased antipsychotic effects ♦ **Metyrosine:** potentiation of extrapyramidal side effects ♦ **Levodopa:** decreased efficacy of levodopa ♦ **Quinidine:** additive cardiac depressive effects ♦ **Guanethidine:** decreased antihypertensive action ♦ **Propranolol, metoprolol:** increased hypotensive action ♦ **Lithium:** neurologic toxicity, encephalopathy ♦ **Epinephrine:** reversal of usual pressor action of epinephrine, resulting in decreased blood pressure ♦ **Bromocriptine:** impairment of prolactin-suppressing action ♦ **Angiotensin converting enzyme (ACE) inhibitors:** increased effects of ACE inhibitors ♦ **Phenytoin:** decreased effects of haloperidol ♦ **Polypeptide antibiotics:** possible neuromuscular respiratory depression ♦

---

*Underlines indicate most frequent; CAPITALS indicate life-threatening.

Metrizamide: seizures ✦ **Carbamazepine:** decreased therapeutic effect of haloperidol ✦ **Methyldopa:** increased sedation, abnormal mental symptoms.

Drug-Food: ✦ **Caffeine-containing beverages (e.g., coffee, tea, colas):** counteracted antipsychotic effect.

ROUTE AND DOSAGE

Moderate Symptoms, Geriatric/Debilitated Patients, Tourette's Disorder

✦ **PO (Adults):** 0.5–2 mg bid or tid.
✦ **PO (Children 3–12 Years or 15–40 kg):** For nonpsychotic behavior disorders and Tourette's disorder: 0.05–0.075 mg/kg/day in 2–3 divided doses.

Severe Symptoms, Chronic or Resistant Patients

✦ **PO (Adults):** 3–5 mg bid or tid. Daily dosages up to 100 mg may be necessary for severely resistant patients who remain inadequately controlled.
✦ **PO (Children 3–12 Years or 15–40 kg):** 0.05–0.15 mg/kg/day in 2–3 divided doses. Occasionally higher doses are required in severely disturbed patients. There is little evidence of additional benefit with doses greater than 6 mg/day.
✦ **IM (Adults):** 2–5 mg q 4–8 hr. In the severely agitated patient, may be administered as often as q 60 min, depending on response.

Maintenance

✦ **PO (Adults and Children):** When desired therapeutic effect has been achieved, gradually reduce dosage to lowest effective maintenance level.

Chronic Psychoses (Prolonged Therapy)

✦ **IM Decanoate (Adults):** Initial dose: 10–15 times the daily oral dosage, to a maximum of 100 mg per dose every 4 weeks. Individual adjustment is then made in dosage and/or interval, according to patient response.

PHARMACODYNAMICS

Route	Onset	Peak	Duration
PO	Erratic*	2–6 hr†	24–72 hr‡
IM	30–60 min	10–20 min	4–8 hr
IM (decanoate)	—	6–7 day§	3–4 wk

*Full antipsychotic effects may not be observed for 4–8 weeks.
†Steady-state plasma levels are achieved in approximately 4–7 days.
‡Drug may be detected in urine for 3–6 months after last dose.
§Steady-state plasma levels usually reached in about 3 months.

NURSING IMPLICATIONS

Assessment

✦ Assess mental status daily: • mood • appearance • thought and communication patterns • level of interest in the environment and in activities • level of anxiety or agitation • presence of hallucinations or delusions • suspiciousness • interactions with others • ability to carry out activities of daily living.
✦ Assess for presence of spastic facial movements (tics) or unusual vocal utterances.
✦ Assess for symptoms of blood dyscrasias: • sore throat • fever • malaise • unusual bleeding • easy bruising.
✦ Assess for extrapyramidal symptoms: • pseudoparkinsonism (tremors, shuffling gait, drooling, rigidity) • akinesia (muscular weakness) • akathisia (continuous restlessness and fidgeting) • dystonia (involuntary muscular movements of face, arms, legs, and neck) • oculogyric crisis (uncontrolled rolling back of the eyes) • tardive dyskinesia (bizarre facial and tongue movements, stiff neck, difficulty swallowing).
✦ Assess for symptoms of neuroleptic malignant syndrome: • hyperpyrexia up to 107°F (41.6° C) • elevated pulse • increased or decreased blood pressure • severe parkinsonian muscle ri-

gidity • elevated creatinine phospho-kinase blood levels • elevated white blood count • altered mental status (including catatonic signs or agitation) • acute renal failure • varying levels of consciousness (including stupor and coma) • pallor • diaphoresis • tachycardia • arrhythmias • rhabdomyolysis.

♦ Assess vital signs, weight. Record baseline values for comparison.

♦ Assess history of allergies, sensitivity to this drug or to other butyrophenones.

♦ Assess for signs and symptoms of cholestatic jaundice: • abdominal pain • nausea • rash • fever • yellow skin • flu-like symptoms • abnormal lab (eosinophilia, bile in urine, increased serum transaminases, bilirubin, alkaline phosphatase).

♦ Assess date of last menses (possible pregnancy), use of contraceptives.

♦ Assess whether currently breast-feeding a child.

♦ Assess current and past alcohol and drug consumption.

♦ Assess for operation of automobile and/or other dangerous machinery.

♦ Assess for presence of adverse reactions or side effects.

♦ Assess patient/family knowledge about illness and need for medication.

♦ In collaboration with physician, assess CBC, liver function tests, and ophthalmologic exams in patients on long-term therapy.

♦ **Lab Test Alterations:** Increased serum alkaline phosphatase, transaminases, bilirubin.

◇ Increased protein-bound iodine.

◇ False-positive urine pregnancy test, possibly caused by drug metabolite that discolors urine (less likely to occur when serum test is used).

◇ Increased urinary glucose.

◇ Decreased urinary estrogen, progestin, and gonadotropin.

◇ Increased plasma cholesterol level.

◇ Increased serum prolactin.

♦ **Withdrawal:** Assess for symptoms of abrupt withdrawal from long-term

therapy: • gastritis • nausea • vomiting • dizziness • headache • tachycardia • insomnia • tremulousness • extrapyramidal symptoms.

♦ **Toxicity and Overdose:** No correlation has been established between blood level and therapeutic effect.

◇ Assess for symptoms of overdose: • CNS depression, from heavy sedation to deep sleep to coma • hypotension • confusion • excitement • severe extrapyramidal symptoms • agitation • restlessness • convulsions • fever • autonomic reactions • ECG changes • cardiac arrhythmias • tachycardia • hypothermia • tremor • seizures • cyanosis • respiratory depression • atypical ventricular tachycardia.

♦ **Overdose Management:** Ensure maintenance of open airway.

◇ Initiate gastric lavage.

◇ Administer activated charcoal.

◇ Do not induce emesis (nuchal rigidity may result in aspiration of vomitus).

◇ Administer antiparkinsonian drugs or diphenhydramine to counteract extrapyramidal symptoms.

◇ Administer IV fluids or a vasoconstrictor to maintain adequate blood pressure. **Note:** Epinephrine is not recommended due to drug interaction that may cause further drop in blood pressure.

◇ Administer IV phenytoin to control ventricular arrhythmias.

◇ Administer phenobarbital or diazepam to control convulsions or hyperactivity.

◇ Dialysis does not appear to be a useful intervention.

Potential Nursing Diagnoses

♦ High risk for violence directed at others related to mistrust and panic anxiety.

♦ High risk for injury related to haloperidol's side effects of sedation, dizziness, ataxia, weakness, lowered seizure threshold; abrupt withdrawal after prolonged use; overdose.

♦ Sensory-perceptual alteration related

to panic anxiety evidenced by hallucinations.

♦ Altered thought processes related to panic anxiety evidenced by delusional thinking.

♦ Social isolation related to inability to trust others.

♦ High risk for activity intolerance, related to haloperidol's side effects of drowsiness, dizziness, ataxia, weakness.

♦ Noncompliance with medication regimen related to suspiciousness and mistrust of others.

♦ Knowledge deficit related to medication regimen.

Plan/Implementation

♦ **General Info:** Monitor vital signs before beginning therapy, and at regular intervals (bid or tid) throughout therapy. Take BP lying and standing to monitor for possible hypotensive reaction; elderly are particularly susceptible. Dosage adjustment may be required.

◊ Ensure that patient who is ambulatory is protected from sun when spending time outdoors.

◊ Weigh patient 2–3 times a week, at same time of day, on same scale, if possible. A rapid weight gain or evidence of edema should be reported to physician immediately. Record I&O.

◊ Ensure that patient is protected from injury. Provide supervision and assistance when ambulating if dizziness and drowsiness are problems. Pad siderails and headboard for patient who experiences seizures.

◊ Give patient hard candy, gum, or frequent sips of water if dry mouth is a problem, or treat with saliva substitute.

◊ Store medication at controlled room temperatures between 15° and 30°C (59°–86°F). Protect from heat, light, and moisture.

♦ **PO:** Administer oral medication with food to minimize GI upset.

◊ Ensure that patient swallows tablet and does not "cheek" to avoid medication or to hoard for later use.

◊ Tablet may be crushed and mixed with food or fluid for patient who has difficulty swallowing, or a liquid concentrate may be used.

◊ Just prior to administration, mix concentrate with juice, water, noncola beverage, soup, or pudding. Do not mix with coffee or tea (may form precipitate).

◊ If concentrate is spilled on skin or clothing during preparation or administration, wash area immediately, as contact dermatitis may occur.

♦ **IM:** Avoid contact with lactate injection. A contact dermatitis may occur.

◊ Inject slowly and deeply into large muscle mass.

◊ Because of possible hypotensive effects, patient should remain in recumbent position for at least one-half hour following IM injection.

◊ Rotate injection sites when multiple injections are administered.

◊ Do not mix with other agents in the syringe.

◊ Potency is not altered when solution is slightly yellow in color. Discard if marked discoloration is evident.

◊ Avoid injecting undiluted drug into vein. Aspirate carefully before injecting.

◊ Maximum volume of haloperidol decanoate per IM site is 3 mL.

Patient/Family Education

♦ Use caution when driving or when operating dangerous machinery. Drowsiness and dizziness can occur.

♦ Do not stop taking the drug abruptly. To do so might produce withdrawal symptoms, such as nausea, vomiting, gastritis, headache, tachycardia, insomnia, tremulousness.

♦ Use sunscreens and wear protective clothing when spending time outdoors. Skin is more susceptible to sunburn.

♦ Report occurrence of any of the following symptoms to physician immediately: sore throat • fever • malaise • unusual bleeding • easy bruising • persistent nausea/vomiting • severe headache • rapid heart rate • difficulty urinating • muscle twitching • tremors • darkly colored urine • pale stools • yellow skin or eyes • muscular incoordination • or skin rash.

♦ Rise slowly from a sitting or lying position to prevent a sudden drop in blood pressure.

♦ If dry mouth is a problem, take frequent sips of water, chew sugarless gum, or suck on hard candy. Good oral care (frequent brushing, flossing) is very important.

♦ If some liquid concentrate is spilled on the skin, wash it off immediately. If not, a rash may appear.

♦ Do not drink alcohol while on haloperidol therapy. These drugs potentiate each other's effects.

♦ Do not consume other medications (including over-the-counter meds) without physician's approval. Many medications contain substances that interact with haloperidol in a way that may be harmful.

♦ Be aware of possible risks of taking haloperidol during pregnancy. Safe use during pregnancy and lactation has not been established. Haloperidol readily crosses the placental barrier, so a fetus could experience adverse effects of the drug. Inform physician immediately if pregnancy occurs, is suspected, or is planned.

♦ Be aware of side effects of haloperidol. Refer to written materials furnished by healthcare providers for safe self-administration.

♦ Continue to take medication even if feeling well and as though it is not needed. Symptoms may return if medication is discontinued.

♦ Carry card or other identification at all times describing medications being taken.

Evaluation

♦ Patient demonstrates a subsiding/resolution of the symptoms for which haloperidol was prescribed (panic anxiety, altered thought processes, altered perceptions, symptoms of Tourette's disorder).

♦ Patient verbalizes understanding of side effects and regimen required for prudent self-administration of haloperidol.

HYDROXYZINE

(hye-drox'i-zeen)
Anxanil, Atarax, Vistaril, Vistazine

Classification(s):
Antianxiety agent, Antihistamine, Piperazine derivative
Pregnancy Category C

INDICATIONS

♦ Anxiety disorders ♦ Temporary relief of anxiety symptoms ♦ Acute alcohol withdrawal ♦ Allergic reactions producing pruritic or asthmatic conditions ♦ Antiemetic ♦ Reduction of narcotic requirement, alleviation of anxiety, and control of emesis in pre- and postoperative and pre- and postpartum patients.

ACTION

♦ Suppresses activity in the limbic system and subcortical levels of the brain.

PHARMACOKINETICS

Absorption: Readily absorbed following oral and IM administration.
Distribution: Distribution unclear; unknown whether drug crosses placental barrier or is excreted in breast milk.
Metabolism and Excretion: Metabolized by the liver and excreted in urine and feces.
Half-Life: 3 hours.

CONTRAINDICATIONS AND PRECAUTIONS

Contraindicated in: ✦ Hypersensitivity to the drug ✦ Pregnancy and lactation. **Use Cautiously in:** ✦ Elderly or debilitated patients ✦ Patients with hepatic or renal dysfunction ✦ Individuals with history of drug abuse/addiction ✦ Depressed/suicidal patients ✦ Concomitant use of other CNS depressants.

ADVERSE REACTIONS AND SIDE EFFECTS*

CNS: drowsiness, dizziness, headache, tremors, convulsions (rare).
Derm: pain and redness at site of IM injection, skin rash.
GI: dry mouth.
Resp: wheezing, chest tightness (hypersensitivity to the drug).

INTERACTIONS

Drug-Drug: ✦ **Other CNS depressants (including alcohol, barbiturates, opiates):** increased CNS depressant effects ✦ **Antipsychotics, antidepressants, antihistamines:** increased CNS depressant and anticholinergic effects ✦ **Anticholinergic agents:** increased anticholinergic effects ✦ **Epinephrine:** reversal of vasopressor effect of epinephrine.

ROUTE AND DOSAGE

Anxiety Symptoms/Disorders
✦ **PO (Adults):** 50–100 mg qid.
✦ **PO (Children 6 Years or Older):** 50–100 mg/day in divided doses.
✦ **PO (Children under 6):** 50 mg/day in divided doses.

Pruritus Due to Allergic Conditions
✦ **PO (Adults):** 25 mg tid or qid.
✦ **PO (Children 6 Years or Older):** 50–100 mg/day in divided doses.
✦ **PO (Children under 6):** 50 mg/day in divided doses.

Pre- and Postoperative Sedation
✦ **PO (Adults):** 50–100 mg.
✦ **IM (Adults):** 25–100 mg.
✦ **PO (Children):** 0.6 mg/kg.
✦ **IM (Children):** 1.1 mg/kg.

Acute Alcohol Withdrawal
✦ **IM (Adults):** 50–100 mg initially, and every 4–6 hours as needed.

Nausea and Vomiting
✦ **IM (Adults):** 25–100 mg.
✦ **IM (Children):** 1.1 mg/kg.

Pre- and Postpartum Adjunctive Therapy
✦ **IM (Adults):** 25–100 mg.

PHARMACODYNAMICS

Route	Onset	Peak	Duration
PO, IM	15–30 min	2–4 hr	4–6 hr

NURSING IMPLICATIONS
Assessment
✦ Assess level of anxiety. Symptoms include: • restlessness • pacing • insomnia • inability to concentrate • increased heart rate • increased respiration • elevated blood pressure • confusion • tremors • rapid speech.
✦ Assess for suicidal ideation (CNS depressants may aggravate symptoms in depressed patients).
✦ Assess history of allergies, sensitivity to this drug.
✦ Assess date of last menses (possible pregnancy), use of contraceptives.
✦ Assess whether currently breast-feeding a child.
✦ Assess current and past alcohol and drug consumption.
✦ Assess for symptoms of alcohol withdrawal: • tremors • nausea/vomiting • malaise • tachycardia • diaphoresis • elevated blood pressure • fever • seizures • anxiety • depression • irritability • diarrhea • anorexia • insomnia • orthostatic hypotension.

---

*Underlines indicate most frequent; CAPITALS indicate life-threatening.

- Assess operation of automobile and/or other dangerous machinery.
- Assess for presence of adverse reactions or side effects.
- Assess patient/family knowledge about illness and need for medication.
- In collaboration with physician, assess renal and liver function tests in patients on long-term therapy.
- **Toxicity and Overdose:** Assess for symptoms of overdose: • hypersedation • hypotension.
- **Overdose Management:** Monitor vital signs.
- ◇ Ensure maintenance of adequate airway.
- ◇ Induce emesis in conscious patient.
- ◇ Initiate gastric lavage in unconscious patient.
- ◇ Control hypotension with IV fluids and norepinephrine or metaraminol. Do not use epinephrine, as hydroxyzine counteracts its pressor action.

Potential Nursing Diagnoses

- High risk for injury related to panic anxiety, agitation from acute alcohol withdrawal.
- High risk for self-directed violence related to depressed mood intensified by hydroxyzine.
- High risk for fluid volume deficit related to nausea and vomiting.
- Alteration in comfort related to itching resulting from allergic pruritus, pain at IM injection site.
- Anxiety (specify level) related to threats to physical integrity and/or self-concept.
- Activity intolerance related to hydroxyzine's side effects of drowsiness, dizziness.
- Knowledge deficit related to medication regimen.

Plan/Implementation

- **General Info:** Monitor vital signs before beginning therapy and at regular intervals (bid) throughout therapy.
- ◇ Ensure that patient practices good oral care. Offer patient hard, sugarless candy; gum; or frequent sips of water for dry mouth.
- ◇ Ensure that patient is protected from injury. Supervise and assist with ambulation if dizziness and sedation are problems. Pad siderails and headboard for patient who experiences seizures.
- ◇ Observe and record amount and frequency of emesis when administered for nausea and vomiting.
- ◇ Store medication in light-resistant container at controlled room temperatures between 15° and 30°C (59°–86°F).
- **PO:** Tablet may be crushed or capsule emptied and mixed with food or fluid for patient having difficulty swallowing.
- **IM:** Administer IM injection deeply into large muscle mass. Parenteral solution is for IM administration only. Use Z-track method to prevent back-tracking of medication into tissues. Injection into subcutaneous, intravenous, or intra-arterial tissues may result in pain, thrombophlebitis, and/or tissue necrosis.

Patient/Family Education

- Do not drive or operate dangerous machinery. Drowsiness and dizziness can occur.
- Do not consume other CNS depressants (including alcohol).
- Do not take over-the-counter medications without approval from physician. Many contain alcohol or antihistamines, which would compound the CNS depressant effects of hydroxyzine.
- Be aware of the risks of taking hydroxyzine during pregnancy (congenital malformations may be associated with use during the first trimester). Notify physician if pregnancy is suspected or planned.
- Be aware of potential side effects. Refer to written materials furnished by healthcare providers regarding correct method of self-administration.

• Carry card or other identification at all times stating names of medications being taken.

Evaluation

• Patient demonstrates a subsiding/resolution of the symptoms for which hydroxyzine was prescribed (anxiety, nausea/vomiting, pruritus, acute alcohol withdrawal).
• Patient verbalizes understanding of side effects and regimen required for prudent self-administration of hydroxyzine.

IMIPRAMINE

(im-ip′ra-meen)
{Impril}, Janimine, SK-Pramine, Tipramine, Tofranil

Classification(s):
Tricyclic antidepressant
Pregnancy Category C

INDICATIONS

• Major depression with melancholia or psychotic symptoms • Depression associated with organic disease, alcoholism, schizophrenia, or mental retardation • Depressive phase of bipolar disorder • Enuresis in children age 6 and older. **Investigational Uses:** • Attention deficit disorder in children • Chronic pain • Eating disorders • Panic disorder.

ACTION

• Exact mechanism of action unclear • Blocks the reuptake of the neurotransmitters norepinephrine and serotonin, increasing their concentration at the synapse and correcting the deficit that is thought to contribute to the melancholy mood of the depressed person.

PHARMACOKINETICS

Absorption: Readily absorbed from the GI tract following oral administration.
Distribution: Is widely distributed. Crosses blood-brain and placental barriers. Enters breast milk.
Metabolism and Excretion: Metabolized by the liver to active and inactive metabolites. Excreted in urine; small amounts excreted in feces.
Half-Life: 8–16 hours.

CONTRAINDICATIONS AND PRECAUTIONS

Contraindicated in: • Hypersensitivity to this drug or to other tricyclic antidepressants • Hypersensitivity to tartrazine dye (in Tofranil-PM 100- and 125-mg capsules and in Janimine 10- and 25-mg tablets) • Concomitant use of MAO inhibitors • Acute recovery period following myocardial infarction • Children under age 6 • Pregnancy and lactation (safety not established).

Use Cautiously in: • Patients with a history of seizures • Urinary retention • Glaucoma • Cardiovascular disorders • Hepatic or renal insufficiency • Psychotic patients • Elderly or debilitated patients • Acute intermittent porphyria.

ADVERSE REACTIONS AND SIDE EFFECTS*

CNS: drowsiness, dizziness, weakness, headache, fatigue, confusion, lethargy, memory deficit, disturbed concentration, tremors, ataxia, tinnitus, extrapyramidal symptoms, paresthesias of extremities, lowered seizure threshold, blurred vision, agitation, excitement, restlessness, insomnia, exacerbation of psychosis, shift to manic behavior.
CV: orthostatic hypotension, tachycardia and other arrhythmias, hypertension,

---

{} = Only available in Canada.
*Underlines indicate most frequent; CAPITALS indicate life-threatening.

MYOCARDIAL INFARCTION, HEART BLOCK, CONGESTIVE HEART FAILURE, ECG changes, syncope, CARDIOVASCULAR COLLAPSE.

Derm: skin rash, urticaria, photosensitivity, erythema, petechiae.

GI: dry mouth, constipation, nausea, vomiting, anorexia, diarrhea, abdominal cramps, adynamic ileus, esophageal reflux, stomatitis, black tongue.

GU: urinary retention, gynecomastia (men), testicular swelling, menstrual irregularity, breast engorgement and galactorrhea (women), changes in libido, impotence, delayed micturition.

Hemat: AGRANULOCYTOSIS, THROMBOCYTOPENIA, LEUKOPENIA, EOSINOPHILIA, PURPURA.

Hepat: jaundice, hepatitis.

Other: weight gain, nasal congestion, alopecia, hypothermia, peripheral neuropathy.

INTERACTIONS

Drug-Drug: ◆ **MAO inhibitors:** hyperpyretic crisis, hypertensive crisis, severe seizures, tachycardia, death ◆ **Guanethidine, clonidine, (possibly) guanabenz:** decreased effects of these medications ◆ **Cimetidine:** increased imipramine serum levels ◆ **Amphetamines, sympathomimetics:** increased hypertensive and cardiac effects of these drugs ◆ **CNS depressants (including alcohol, barbiturates, benzodiazepines):** potentiation of CNS effects ◆ **Thyroid medications:** tachycardia, arrhythmias ◆ **Methylphenidate, phenothiazines, haloperidol:** increased serum imipramine levels ◆ **Ethchlorvynol:** transient delirium ◆ **Quinidine, procainamide, disopyramide:** potentiates adverse cardiovascular effects of imipramine ◆ **Oral contraceptives:** decreased effects of imipramine ◆ **Smoking:** increased imipramine metabolism ◆ **Disulfiram:** decreased imipramine metabolism ◆ **Levodopa, phenylbutazone:** delayed or decreased absorption of these drugs ◆ **Warfarin:** increased prothrombin time ◆ **Dicumarol:** increased plasma dicumarol concentrations.

ROUTE AND DOSAGE

Depression

◆ **PO (Hospitalized Adults):** Initial dose: 100–150 mg/day in divided doses. Gradually increase to 200 mg/day. After 2 weeks, if symptomatic relief not achieved, increase dose to 250–300 mg/day. Total daily dose may be administered once a day, preferably at bedtime.

◆ **PO (Outpatient Adults):** Initial dose: 75 mg/day. Gradually increase to 150 mg/day. Maximum Daily Dose: 200 mg/day. Total daily dose may be administered once a day at bedtime.

◆ **PO (Adolescents, Geriatrics):** Initial dose: 30–40 mg/day. Rarely exceeds 100 mg/day.

◆ **IM (Adults):** Used only when initiating therapy with patients who are unable or unwilling to use the oral medication. 100 mg/day in divided doses. (Switch to oral form as soon as possible.)

◆ **PO (Children under 12, Investigational):** Initial dose: 1.5 mg/kg daily. Increase by approximately 1 mg/kg q 3–4 days. Maximum 5 mg/kg.

Enuresis

◆ **PO (Children 6–11):** Initial dose: 25 mg/day, given 1 hour before bedtime. If desired response is not achieved in 1 week, increase to 50 mg. Maximum: 2.5 mg/kg/day.

◆ **PO (Children 12 and Over):** Initial dose: 25 mg/day, given 1 hour before bedtime. If desired response is not achieved in 1 week, increase to 75 mg.

Attention Deficit Disorder in Children

◆ **PO (Children):** 2.5–5 mg/kg/day (investigational use only).

Chronic Pain

◆ **PO (Adults):** 50–200 mg/day (investigational use only).

PHARMACODYNAMICS

Route	Onset	Peak	Duration
PO	2–4 wk	1–2 hr	Weeks*
IM	2–4 wk	30 min	Weeks*

*Allow up to 2 weeks following cessation of therapy for complete drug elimination.

NURSING IMPLICATIONS

Assessment

♦ Assess for suicidal ideation, plan, means. Assess for sudden lifts in mood, which could indicate patient's decision to commit suicide.

♦ Assess mental status daily: • mood • appearance • thought and communication patterns • level of interest in the environment and in activities • suicidal ideation. Improvement in these behavior patterns and level of energy should be expected within 2–4 weeks following initiation of therapy.

♦ Assess for symptoms of blood dyscrasias: • sore throat • fever • malaise • unusual bleeding • easy bruising.

♦ Assess vital signs, weight.

♦ Assess history of allergies, sensitivity to this drug or to other tricyclic antidepressants.

♦ Assess for history of glaucoma.

♦ Assess date of last menses (possible pregnancy), use of contraceptives.

♦ Assess whether currently breast-feeding a child.

♦ Assess current and past alcohol and drug consumption.

♦ Assess operation of automobile and/ or other dangerous machinery.

♦ Assess for presence of adverse reactions or side effects.

♦ Assess patient/family knowledge about illness and need for medication.

♦ In collaboration with physician, assess CBC and liver function tests in patients on long-term therapy.

♦ **Lab Test Alterations:** Increased serum bilirubin, alkaline phosphatase, transaminase, and glucose.

◊ Decreased urinary 5-hydroxyindole-acetic acid (HIAA) and vanillylmandelic acid (VMA) excretion.

♦ **Withdrawal:** Range of therapeutic serum concentration is 150–300 ng/mL.

◊ Assess for symptoms of abrupt withdrawal from long-term therapy: • nausea • headache • vertigo • malaise • insomnia • nightmares.

♦ **Toxicity and Overdose:** Assess for symptoms of overdose: • confusion • agitation • irritability • hallucinations • seizures • flushing • dry mouth • dilated pupils • delirium • hyperpyrexia • hypotension or hypertension • coma • tachycardia • arrhythmias • respiratory depression • cardiac arrest • renal failure • shock • congestive heart failure • acid-base disturbances.

♦ **Overdose Management:** Monitor vital signs.

◊ Ensure maintenance of adequate airway.

◊ Monitor ECG.

◊ Induce emesis in conscious patient.

◊ Initiate gastric lavage in unconscious patient.

◊ Administer activated charcoal to minimize absorption.

◊ IV physostigmine may be used cautiously to reverse anticholinergic effects.

◊ Administer sodium bicarbonate, vasopressors, phenytoin, propranolol, or lidocaine to treat cardiovascular effects.

◊ Administer IV diazepam to control seizures.

Potential Nursing Diagnoses

♦ High risk for self-directed violence related to depressed mood.

♦ High risk for injury related to imipramine's side effects of sedation, dizziness, ataxia, weakness, confusion, lowered seizure threshold; abrupt withdrawal after prolonged use; overdose.

♦ Social isolation related to depressed mood.

- High risk for activity intolerance, related to imipramine's side effects of drowsiness, dizziness, ataxia, weakness, confusion.
- Knowledge deficit related to medication regimen.

Plan/Implementation

- **General Info:** Monitor vital signs before beginning therapy and at regular intervals (bid or tid) throughout therapy. Take BP lying and standing in patients experiencing orthostatic hypotension; elderly are particularly susceptible. Contact physician if tachycardia/arrhythmias are noted.
- For children, at investigational doses of 3.5 mg/kg/day or greater, monitor supine and standing blood pressure, ECG, and CBC before therapy is initiated and before any dosage increase.
- Ensure that patient who is ambulatory is protected from sun when spending time outdoors.
- Weigh patient 2–3 times a week, at same time of day, on same scale, if possible. A rapid weight gain or evidence of edema should be reported to physician immediately. Record I&O.
- Ensure that patient is protected from injury. Provide supervision and assistance when ambulating if dizziness and drowsiness are problems. Pad siderails and headboard for patient who experiences seizures.
- Give patient hard candy, gum, or frequent sips of water if dry mouth is a problem.
- Store medication at controlled room temperature of 15°–30°C (59°–86°F).
- **PO:** Administer oral medication with food to minimize GI upset.
- Ensure that patient swallows tablet/capsule and does not "cheek" to avoid medication or to hoard for later use.
- Crush tablet or empty capsule and mix with food or fluid for patient who has difficulty swallowing.
- **IM:** If crystals form in solution, immerse ampule in hot tap water for 1 minute. Does not affect therapeutic efficacy.
- Administer IM only if patient is unwilling or unable to use oral medication.
- Do not administer parenteral solution intravenously.
- Replace with oral maintenance therapy as soon as possible.

Patient/Family Education

- Therapeutic effect may not be seen for as long as 4 weeks. If after this length of time no improvement is noted, physician may prescribe a different medication. Continue to take medication even though symptoms have not subsided.
- Use caution when driving or operating dangerous machinery. Drowsiness and dizziness can occur. If these side effects become persistent or interfere with daily activities, report to physician. Dosage adjustment may be necessary.
- Do not stop taking the drug abruptly. To do so might produce withdrawal symptoms, such as nausea, vertigo, insomnia, headache, malaise, nightmares.
- Use sunscreens and wear protective clothing when spending time outdoors. Skin may be sensitive to sunburn.
- Report occurrence of any of the following symptoms to physician immediately: • sore throat • fever • malaise • unusual bleeding • easy bruising • persistent nausea/vomiting • severe headache • rapid heart rate • difficulty urinating.
- Rise slowly from a sitting or lying position to prevent a sudden drop in blood pressure.
- If dry mouth is a problem, take frequent sips of water, chew sugarless gum, or suck on hard candy. Good oral care (frequent brushing, flossing) is very important.

* Do not smoke while on imipramine therapy. Smoking increases metabolism of imipramine, requiring adjustment in dosage to achieve therapeutic effect.
* Do not drink alcohol while on imipramine therapy. These drugs potentiate each other's effects.
* Do not consume other medications (including over-the-counter meds) with imipramine without physician's approval. Many medications contain substances that, in combination with tricyclics, could precipitate a life-threatening hypertensive crisis.
* Be aware of possible risks of taking imipramine during pregnancy. Safe use during pregnancy and lactation has not been established. Imipramine readily crosses the placental barrier, so a fetus could experience adverse effects of the drug. Inform physician immediately if pregnancy occurs, is suspected, or is planned.
* Be aware of side effects of imipramine. Refer to written materials furnished by healthcare providers for safe self-administration.
* Carry card or other identification at all times describing medications being taken.

Evaluation
* Patient demonstrates a subsiding/resolution of the symptoms for which imipramine was prescribed (depressed mood, suicidal ideation, attention deficit disorder, chronic pain).
* Patient verbalizes understanding of side effects and regimen required for prudent self-administration of imipramine.

ISOCARBOXAZID

(eye-soe-kar-box′a-zid)
Marplan

Classification(s):
Antidepressant, Monoamine oxidase inhibitor, Hydrazine
Pregnancy Category C

INDICATIONS

* Depression in patients unresponsive to other antidepressive therapy (e.g., tricyclics, serotonin enhancers, ECT) or for whom tricyclic antidepressants are contraindicated. It is rarely a drug of first choice. **Investigational Use:** * Bulimia (with characteristics of atypical depression) * Panic disorder.

ACTION

* Exact mechanism of action on depression unknown * Inhibits the enzyme monoamine oxidase, which normally inhibits the activity of epinephrine, norepinephrine, dopamine, and serotonin. The concentration of these biogenic amines is then increased in storage sites throughout the nervous system. These increases in biogenic amines are thought to reduce symptoms of depression.

PHARMACOKINETICS

Absorption: Well absorbed from the GI tract following oral administration.
Distribution: Is widely distributed. Thought to cross placental barrier and to enter breast milk.
Metabolism and Excretion: Metabolized by the liver. Excreted in urine as metabolites and unchanged drug.
Half-Life: Not well established.

CONTRAINDICATIONS AND PRECAUTIONS

Contraindicated in: * Hypersensitivity to this drug or to other MAO inhibitors * Pheochromocytoma * Congestive heart failure * History of liver disease * Severe renal impairment ♦ Cerebrovascular defect ♦ Paranoid schizophrenic disorder ♦ Cardiovascular disease ♦ Hypertension ♦ History of severe or frequent headaches ♦ Patients over 60 ♦ Children less than 16 years of age. Pregnancy and lactation (safety not established).

Use Cautiously in: ♦ Patients with a history of seizures ♦ Diabetes mellitus ♦ Renal insufficiency ♦ Suicidal patients ♦ Schizophrenia ♦ Agitated or hypomanic patients ♦ History of angina pectoris or hyperthyroidism.

ADVERSE REACTIONS AND SIDE EFFECTS*

CNS: dizziness, vertigo, headache, overactivity, tremors, muscle twitching, mania, confusion, memory impairment, insomnia, drowsiness, blurred vision, restlessness, weakness, agitation.

CV: orthostatic hypotension, disturbances in cardiac rate and rhythm, tachycardia, palpitations, peripheral edema.

Derm: skin rashes.

GI: dry mouth, constipation, anorexia, body weight changes, nausea, vomiting, diarrhea, abdominal pain.

GU: dysuria, incontinence, urinary retention, changes in libido, transient impotence.

Hemat: spider telangiectases.

Other: excessive sweating, neuritis, arthralgia, weight gain, FATAL PROGRESSIVE NECROTIZING HEPATOCELLULAR DAMAGE (rare).

INTERACTIONS

Drug-Drug: ♦ **Sympathomimetic and catecholamine-releasing drugs (including amphetamines, methyldopa, levodopa, dopamine, tryptophan, epinephrine, norepinephrine):** increased hypertensive effects, headache, hyperpyrexia ♦ **CNS depressants (e.g., alcohol and certain narcotics such as meperidine):** possible hypo/hypertension, convulsions, coma, death ♦

Other MAO inhibitors, tricylic antidepressants, and other dibenzazepines (carbamazepine, cyclobenzaprine): hypertensive crisis, convulsions, coma, circulatory collapse ♦ **Antihypertensive drugs, thiazide diuretics:** hypotension ♦ **Guanethidine:** decreased antihypertensive effects ♦ **Doxapram:** potentiation of adverse cardiovascular effects ♦ **Insulin, oral hypoglycemics:** increased hypoglycemic effects ♦ **Methylphenidate:** increased effect of methylphenidate ♦ **Anesthetics:** increased hypotensive and CNS depressant effects ♦ **Disulfiram:** increased toxicity ♦ **Metrizamide:** increased risk of seizures.

Drug-Food: ♦ **Foods containing high concentrations of tryptophan, tryamine or other vasopressors** (aged cheeses or other aged, overripe, or fermented foods; broad beans; pickled herring; beef/chicken livers; preserved sausages; beer; wine, especially chianti; yeast products; chocolate; caffeinated drinks; canned figs; sour cream; yogurt; soy sauce; OTC cold medications; diet pills; avocados; raisins; bananas): hypertensive crisis. **Caution:** Can occur several weeks after MAOI therapy has been discontinued.

ROUTE AND DOSAGE

Depression

♦ **PO (Adults):** Usual starting dose is 30 mg/day in single or divided doses. Daily dose larger than 30 mg is not recommended. Many patients show favorable response within a week, but some may not achieve a beneficial effect for 3–4 weeks. Maintenance: As soon as clinical improvement is observed, reduce dosage to a maintenance level of 10–20 mg (or less) daily.

Bulimia

(With characteristics of atypical depression.)

---

*Underlines indicate most frequent; CAPITALS indicate life-threatening.

♦ **PO (Adults):** 10–50 mg/day (investigational use only). Adjust dosage with patient's response.

PHARMACODYNAMICS

Route	Onset	Peak	Duration
PO	7–10 days*	—	Weeks†

*3–4 weeks may be required to achieve maximal clinical response.
†Allow up to 2 weeks following cessation of therapy for complete drug elimination.

NURSING IMPLICATIONS

Assessment

♦ Assess for suicidal ideation, plan, means. Assess for sudden lifts in mood, which could indicate patient's decision to commit suicide.
♦ Assess mental status daily: • mood • appearance • thought and communication patterns • level of interest in the environment and in activities • suicidal ideation. Improvement in these behavior patterns and level of energy should be expected within 2–4 weeks following initiation of therapy.
♦ Assess vital signs, weight.
♦ Assess dieting pattern and consult dietitian.
♦ Assess history of allergies, sensitivity to this drug or to other MAO inhibitors.
♦ Assess for history of glaucoma.
♦ Assess date of last menses (possible pregnancy), use of contraceptives.
♦ Assess whether currently breast-feeding a child.
♦ Assess current and past alcohol and drug consumption.
♦ Assess for operation of automobile and/or other dangerous machinery.
♦ Assess for presence of adverse reactions or side effects.
♦ Assess patient/family knowledge about illness and need for medication.
♦ In collaboration with physician, assess CBC and liver and renal function tests in patients on long-term therapy.
♦ **Withdrawal:** Assess for symptoms of

abrupt withdrawal from long-term therapy: • headache • excitability • hallucinations • depression.

♦ **Hypertensive Crisis:** Assess for symptoms of hypertensive crisis: • severe occipital headache • palpitations • sharp rise in blood pressure • nuchal rigidity • chest pain • sweating • fever • nausea • vomiting • coma.
♦ **Management of Hypertensive Crisis:** Discontinue drug immediately.
◊ Monitor vital signs.
◊ Institute therapy to lower blood pressure.
◊ Do not use parenteral reserpine.
◊ Administer antihypertensives slowly to avoid producing an excessive hypotensive effect.
◊ Use external cooling measures to control hyperpyrexia.
♦ **Toxicity and Overdose:** Relationship between blood level and therapeutic response has not been established.
◊ Assess for symptoms of overdose: • excitement • irritability • anxiety • flushing • sweating • tachypnea • tachycardia • exaggerated tendon reflexes • hypotension • hypertension • convulsions • coma • cardiorespiratory arrest.
♦ **Overdose Management:** Monitor vital signs.
◊ Ensure maintenance of adequate airway.
◊ Initiate gastric lavage.
◊ Administer activated charcoal to minimize absorption.
◊ Monitor electrolytes.
◊ Protect against aspiration.
◊ Utilize supplemental oxygen and mechanical ventilatory assistance as needed.
◊ Administer IV diazepam to control convulsions.
◊ Use IV fluids to treat hypotension and cardiovascular collapse.
◊ Follow up with liver function evaluation.

Potential Nursing Diagnoses

- High risk for self-directed violence related to depressed mood.
- High risk for injury related to isocarboxazid's side effects of sedation, dizziness, fatigue, confusion, lowered seizure threshold; eating foods that contain tyramine or tryptophan; abrupt withdrawal after prolonged use; overdose.
- Social isolation related to depressed mood.
- High risk for activity intolerance, related to isocarboxazid's side effects of drowsiness, dizziness, fatigue, confusion.
- Knowledge deficit related to medication regimen.

Plan/Implementation

- Monitor vital signs before beginning therapy, and at regular intervals (bid or tid) throughout therapy. Take BP lying and standing in patients experiencing orthostatic hypotension; elderly are particularly susceptible. Contact physician if tachycardia/arrhythmias are noted.
- Weigh patient 2–3 times a week, at same time of day, on same scale, if possible. A rapid weight gain or evidence of edema should be reported to physician immediately. Record I&O.
- Ensure that patient is protected from injury. Provide supervision and assistance when ambulating if dizziness and drowsiness are problems. Pad siderails and headboard for patient who experiences seizures. Ensure that ambulatory patient is protected from the sun.
- Order low-tyramine diet for patient.
- Give patient hard candy, gum, or frequent sips of water if dry mouth is a problem.
- Administer oral medication with food to minimize GI upset.
- Ensure that patient swallows tablet and does not "cheek" to avoid medication or to hoard for later use.

- Tablet may be crushed and mixed with food or fluid for patient who has difficulty swallowing.
- Store medication at controlled room temperatures between 15° and 30°C (59°–86°F). Protect from heat, light, and moisture.

Patient/Family Education

- Therapeutic effect may be seen in 1–2 weeks. However, it may take as long as 6 weeks after upper dose is reached. If after this length of time no improvement is noted, physician may prescribe a different medication. Continue to take medication even though symptoms have not subsided.
- Do not consume the following foods/meds while on isocarboxazid: aged cheese • wine (especially chianti) • beer • chocolate • colas • coffee • tea • sour cream • beef/chicken livers • canned figs • soy sauce • overripe or fermented foods • pickled herring • preserved sausages • bananas • avocados • raisins • yogurt • yeast products • broad beans • cold remedies • diet pills.
- Use caution when driving or when operating dangerous machinery. Drowsiness and dizziness can occur. If these side effects become persistent or interfere with daily activities, report to physician. Dosage adjustment may be necessary.
- Do not stop taking the drug abruptly. To do so might produce withdrawal symptoms, such as headache, excitability, hallucinations, and depression.
- Report occurrence of any of the following symptoms to physician immediately: persistent nausea/vomiting • severe or frequent headaches • rapid heart rate • difficulty urinating • skin rash • stiff or sore neck • palpitations • chest pain.
- Rise slowly from a sitting or lying position to prevent a sudden drop in blood pressure.
- Avoid overexertion if you have a his-

tory of angina pectoris or coronary artery disease.

♦ Take medication with food to minimize GI upset.

♦ If dry mouth is a problem, take frequent sips of water, chew sugarless gum, or suck on hard candy. Good oral care (frequent brushing, flossing) is very important.

♦ Do not drink alcohol while on isocarboxazid therapy. Profound CNS depression can occur and be life-threatening.

♦ Do not consume other medications (including over-the-counter meds) with isocarboxazid without physician's approval. Many medications contain substances that, in combination with MAO inhibitors, could precipitate a life-threatening hypertensive crisis.

♦ Be aware of possible risks of taking isocarboxazid during pregnancy and lactation. Safe use during pregnancy and lactation has not been established. The drug is thought to enter breast milk, so possible effect on nursing child should be considered.

♦ Be aware of side effects of isocarboxazid. Refer to written materials furnished by healthcare providers for safe self-administration.

♦ Carry card or other identification at all times describing medications being taken.

Evaluation

♦ Patient demonstrates a subsiding/resolution of the symptoms for which isocarboxazid was prescribed (depressed mood, suicidal ideation, binge-and-purge syndrome).

♦ Patient verbalizes understanding of side effects and regimen required for prudent self-administration of isocarboxazid.

LEVODOPA

(lee-voe-doe′pa)
Dopar, Larodopa

Classification(s):
Antiparkinsonian agent
Pregnancy Category C

INDICATIONS

♦ Idiopathic, arteriosclerotic, and postencephalic parkinsonism ♦ Symptoms of parkinsonism associated with injury to the nervous system by carbon monoxide or manganese intoxication **Investigational Uses:** ♦ Pain resulting from herpes zoster (shingles) ♦ Bone pain resulting from metastatic carcinoma ♦ Postanoxic myoclonus ♦ Restless leg syndrome.

ACTION

♦ Levodopa is decarboxylated into dopamine in the basal ganglia and in the periphery, thus correcting the decrease in striatal dopamine that produces the symptoms of parkinsonism.

PHARMACOKINETICS

Absorption: Rapidly and well absorbed following oral administration. Slower and lower peak concentrations when taken with food.

Distribution: Is widely distributed. Thought to cross placental barrier and to enter breast milk.

Metabolism and Excretion: Extensively metabolized in the GI tract and by the liver. Excreted primarily in urine; small amounts in feces.

Half-Life: 1–3 hours.

CONTRAINDICATIONS AND PRECAUTIONS

Contraindicated in: ♦ Hypersensitivity to the drug or to tartrazine (contained in some preparations) ♦ Narrow-angle glaucoma ♦ Concomitant use of MAO inhibitors ♦ Patients with a history of melanoma or with suspicious, undiagnosed skin lesions ♦ lactation.

Use Cautiously in: ♦ Patients with severe cardiovascular or pulmonary disease ♦ Bronchial asthma ♦ Emphysema ♦ Occlusive cerebrovascular disease ♦ Renal, hepatic, or endocrine disease ♦ History of myocardial infarction ♦ History of active peptic ulcer disease ♦ History of seizure disorders ♦ Depressed and suicidal patients ♦ Psychotic patients ♦ Geriatric patients ♦ Pregnancy and children under 12 (safety not established).

ADVERSE REACTIONS AND SIDE EFFECTS*

CNS: choreiform, dyskinetic, or dystonic movements, ataxia, increased hand tremor, headache, dizziness, numbness, weakness and faintness, teeth grinding, confusion, insomnia, nightmares, hallucinations and paranoid delusions, hypomania, agitation and anxiety, malaise, fatigue, euphoria, mental depression with or without suicidal ideations, nervousness, restlessness, toxic delirium, numbness, decreased attention span, memory loss, dementia, diplopia, blurred vision, dilated pupils, hot flashes, convulsions, oculogyric crisis, NEUROLEPTIC MALIGNANT SYNDROME.

CV: orthostatic hypotension, palpitations, arrhythmias, hypertension, phlebitis, flushing, sinus tachycardia.

Derm: skin rash, alopecia.

GI: nausea and vomiting, anorexia, abdominal pain, dry mouth, dysphagia, bitter taste, excessive salivation, diarrhea, constipation, flatulence, weight gain or loss, GI bleeding, duodenal ulcer, hiccups, trismus, dysphagia.

GU: urinary retention, urinary incontinence, priapism.

Hemat: HEMOLYTIC OR NONHEMOLYTIC ANEMIA, AGRANULOCYTOSIS, LEUKOPENIA, THROMBOCYTOPENIA, phlebitis.

Resp: bizarre breathing patterns, hyperventilation.

Other: bradykinesia, muscle twitching, increased sweating, dark sweat or urine, edema, hoarseness, ACTIVATION OF MALIGNANT MELANOMA, blepharospasm, muscle cramping.

INTERACTIONS

Drug-Drug: ♦ **Anticholinergics, clonidine, reserpine, phenothiazines and other antipsychotics, benzodiazepines, phenytoin, papaverine, diazepam, chlordiazepoxide:** decreased therapeutic effect of levodopa ♦ **Furazolidone:** increased therapeutic and toxic effects of levodopa ♦ **Antihypertensives (e.g., guanethidine, methyldopa):** increased hypotensive effects ♦ Methyldopa: increased CNS toxicity (e.g., psychosis) ♦ **MAO inhibitors:** hypertensive crisis, increased therapeutic and toxic effects of levodopa ♦ **Sympathomimetic drugs (e.g., ephedrine, amphetamines, epinephrine, and isoproterenol):** increased effects of these drugs ♦ **Tricyclic antidepressants:** sympathetic hyperactivity resulting in sinus tachycardia, postural hypotension, hypertension, and dyskinesia ♦ **Hypoglycemic agents:** increased or decreased hypoglycemic effects ♦ **Anticholinergic agents:** decreased tremor, occasional increase in abnormal involuntary movements ♦ **Cyclopropane or halogenated hydrocarbon general anesthetics:** increased possibility of cardiac arrhythmias.

Drug-Food: ♦ **Pyridoxine HCl (vitamin B₆):** decreased therapeutic effects of levodopa.

ROUTE AND DOSAGE

Parkinsonism

♦ **PO (Adults):** Initial dosage; 0.5–1 g daily, divided into 2 or more equal doses. Dosage may be increased gradually in increments of 100–750 mg/day every 3–7 days. Maximum dosage: 8 g/day. Usual optimal dosage

*Underlines indicate most frequent; CAPITALS indicate life-threatening.

(reached after 6–8 weeks of therapy) is 3–6 g/day in 3 or more equally divided doses.

PHARMACODYNAMICS

Route	Onset	Peak	Duration
PO	30–45 min	1 hr	2–5 hr*

*A significant therapeutic response may not be obtained for 3–6 months.

NURSING IMPLICATIONS

Assessment

* Assess for symptoms of Parkinson's disease: • tremors • muscular weakness and rigidity • drooling • shuffling gait • disturbances of posture and equilibrium • flat affect • monotone speech.
* Assess for symptoms of depression and potential for suicide.
* Assess vital signs, weight. Record baseline values for comparison.
* Assess history of allergies, sensitivity to this drug.
* Assess date of last menses (possible pregnancy), use of contraceptives.
* Assess for symptoms of blood dyscrasias: • sore throat • fever • malaise • unusual bleeding • easy bruising.
* Assess for symptoms of mental changes: • psychosis • hallucinations • delusions • paranoid ideations • dementia • depression with or without suicidal tendencies.
* Assess for history of malignant melanoma. Check skin for suspicious, undiagnosed lesions.
* Assess whether currently breast-feeding a child.
* Assess current and past alcohol and drug consumption.
* Assess for operation of automobile and/or other dangerous machinery.
* Assess for presence of adverse reactions or side effects.
* Assess patient/family knowledge about illness and need for medication.
* In collaboration with physician, assess CBC and hepatic and renal function tests in patients on long-term therapy.

* **Lab Test Alterations:** Positive Coombs' test.
◊ False-positive urine glucose tests with copper reduction method.
◊ False-negative urine glucose tests with glucose oxidase method.
◊ Increased serum uric acid levels with colorimetric method.
◊ Elevated BUN, AST, ALT, LDH, bilirubin, alkaline phosphatase, and protein-bound iodine.
◊ Decreased WBC, hemoglobin, and hematocrit.
* **Toxicity and Overdose:** Assess for symptoms of toxicity/overdose: • muscle twitching and spasmodic winking (blepharospasm) • facial grimacing • exaggerated protrusion of the tongue • behavioral changes • cardiac arrhythmias.
* **Overdose Management:** Monitor vital signs.
◊ Monitor ECG.
◊ Maintain adequate airway.
◊ Initiate gastric lavage.
◊ Judiciously administer IV fluids.
◊ Initiate antiarrhythmic therapy if required.
◊ Employ general supportive measures.

Potential Nursing Diagnoses

* High risk for injury related to symptoms of Parkinson's disease or side effects of levodopa (dizziness, weakness, confusion).
* High risk for self-directed violence related to side effect of depressed mood with suicidal ideations.
* Sensory-perceptual alteration related to side effect of levodopa evidenced by hallucinations.
* Altered thought processes related to side effects of levodopa evidenced by delusional thinking, dementia, confusion.
* Social isolation related to embarrassment by symptoms of Parkinson's disease.
* High risk for activity intolerance, related to levodopa's side effects of diz-

ziness, ataxia, weakness, confusion, fatigue.

♦ Knowledge deficit related to medication regimen.

Plan/Implementation

♦ Monitor vital signs tid. Be alert for increase in pulse rate, temperature, blood pressure. Notify physician of significant elevations, arrhythmias, palpitations, or changes in respiratory rate or rhythm.

♦ Weigh patient 2–3 times a week, at same time of day, on same scale, if possible. A rapid weight gain or evidence of edema should be reported to physician immediately. Record I&O.

♦ Ensure that patient is protected from injury. Provide supervision and assistance when ambulating if dizziness and ataxia are problems. Patient should change positions slowly to minimize effects of orthostatic hypotension.

♦ Give patient hard candy, gum, or frequent sips of water if dry mouth is a problem, or treat with a saliva substitute.

♦ Monitor urine glucose and ketones carefully. Notify physician of significant changes. Adjustment in dosage of hypoglycemic agent may be necessary.

♦ Ensure that patient swallows tablet/ capsule and does not "cheek" to avoid medication or to hoard for later use.

♦ Administer with food to minimize gastric irritation.

♦ Discuss with pharmacist the advisability of crushing tablet or emptying contents of capsule and mixing with fruit-based fluid for patient who has difficulty swallowing.

♦ Monitor vital signs before beginning therapy and at regular intervals (bid or tid) throughout therapy. Take BP lying and standing to monitor for possible hypotensive reaction; elderly are particularly susceptible. Dosage adjustment may be required.

♦ Store medication at controlled room temperatures between 15° and 30°C (59°–86°F). Protect from heat, light, and moisture.

Patient/Family Education

♦ Take medication with food to minimize GI upset.

♦ Use caution when driving or when operating dangerous machinery. Dizziness and confusion can occur.

♦ Do not stop taking the drug abruptly. To do so might produce withdrawal symptoms, such as muscle rigidity, weakness, tremors, elevated temperature.

♦ Report occurrence of any of the following symptoms to physician immediately: uncontrollable movements of the face, eyelids, mouth, tongue, neck, arms, hands, or legs ● mood or mental changes ● irregular heartbeats or palpitations ● difficult urination ● severe or persistent nausea and vomiting ● fever.

♦ Rise slowly from a sitting or lying position to prevent a sudden drop in blood pressure.

♦ If dry mouth is a problem, take frequent sips of water, chew sugarless gum, or suck on hard candy. Good oral care (frequent brushing, flossing) is very important.

♦ Diabetic patients should notify physician of any abnormal results in self-testing before adjusting dosage of hypoglycemic medications.

♦ Do not consume other medications (including over-the-counter meds) without physician's approval. Many medications contain substances that interact with levodopa in a way that may be harmful.

♦ Do not take vitamin preparations without first discussing with physician. Some preparations contain vitamin B_6, which can reduce the effectiveness of levodopa.

♦ Urine and perspiration may appear dark. This change is not significant nor is it harmful.

* Be aware of possible risks of taking levodopa during pregnancy. Safe use during pregnancy and lactation has not been established. It is thought that levodopa crosses the placental barrier; if so, a fetus could experience adverse effects of the drug. Inform physician immediately if pregnancy occurs, is suspected, or is planned. Use is not recommended in nursing mothers.
* Be aware of side effects of levodopa. Refer to written materials furnished by healthcare providers for safe self-administration.
* Continue to take medication even if feeling well and as though it is not needed. Symptoms may return if medication is discontinued.
* Carry card or other identification at all times describing medications being taken.

Evaluation

* Patient demonstrates a subsiding of the symptoms for which levodopa was prescribed (symptoms of parkinsonism, pain, myoclonus).
* Patient verbalizes understanding of side effects and regimen required for prudent self-administration of levodopa.

LITHIUM CARBONATE

(li'thee-um)
{Carbolith, Duralith}, Eskalith, Lithane, {Lithizine}, Lithobid, Lithonate, Lithotabs

LITHIUM CITRATE

Cibalith-S

Classification(s):
Antimanic
Pregnancy Category D

INDICATIONS

* Manic episodes associated with bipolar disorder * Maintenance therapy to prevent or diminish intensity of subsequent manic episodes * Depression associated with bipolar disorder. **Investigational Uses:** * Major depression * Neutropenia * Cluster or migraine headaches (prophylaxis) * Schizoaffective or schizophrenic disorder * Alcohol dependence * Children with apparent mixed bipolar disorder, aggressive behavior, hyperactivity with psychotic or neurotic components.

ACTION

* Specific mechanism of action is unknown * Theories relate effectiveness to an alteration in sodium metabolism within nerve and muscle cells, as well as an enhancement of the reuptake of biogenic amines in the brain, lowering levels in the body, resulting in decreased hyperactivity * May block development of sensitive dopamine receptors in the CNS of manic patients.

PHARMACOKINETICS

Absorption: Oral administration results in rapid and complete absorption

---

{} = Only available in Canada.

through the GI tract; extended-release forms are 60–90% absorbed.

Distribution: Is widely distributed. Crosses blood-brain barrier, resulting in cerebrospinal fluid concentrations approximately 30–50% of plasma levels. Crosses placental barrier (at approximately equal levels and is excreted in breast milk (30–50% of plasma levels).

Metabolism and Excretion: Not metabolized. Remains in the body in its ionic form. Approximately 95–99% excreted by the kidneys.

Half-Life: 21–30 hours.

CONTRAINDICATIONS AND PRECAUTIONS

Contraindicated in: ◆ Severe cardiovascular disease ◆ Severe renal disease ◆ Severe dehydration ◆ Sodium depletion ◆ Brain damage ◆ Pregnancy and lactation.

Use Cautiously in: ◆ Elderly patients ◆ Thyroid disorders ◆ Diabetes mellitus ◆ Urinary retention ◆ History of seizure disorder ◆ Children (safety and efficacy not established).

ADVERSE REACTIONS AND SIDE EFFECTS*

CNS: <u>fine hand tremors</u>, twitching, <u>fatigue</u>, confusion, <u>dizziness</u>, muscular weakness, restlessness, <u>headache</u>, <u>lethargy</u>, <u>drowsiness</u>, epileptiform seizures.

CV: arrhythmias, hypotension, <u>ECG changes</u>.

Derm: <u>acne</u>, drying and thinning of hair, anesthesia of skin, rash.

Endo: <u>hypothyroidism</u>, transient hyperglycemia, excessive weight gain.

GI: <u>anorexia</u>, <u>nausea</u>, <u>vomiting</u>, <u>diarrhea</u>, abdominal pain, <u>dry mouth</u>, thirst.

GU: <u>polyuria</u>, glycosuria, nephrogenic diabetes insipidus, oliguria, albuminuria.

Hemat: <u>reversible leukocytosis</u> (WBC 10,000–15,000).

INTERACTIONS

Drug-Drug: ◆ **Aminophylline, mannitol, acetazolamide, sodium bicar-**

bonate, drugs high in sodium content: increased renal elimination and decreased effectiveness of lithium ◆ **Haloperidol:** encephalopathic syndrome and resulting brain damage ◆ **Neuromuscular blocking agents:** prolonged effects of skeletal muscle relaxation ◆ **Paroxicam, indomethacin, and other nonsteroidal anti-inflammatory drugs:** significant (30–60%) increases in steady-state plasma lithium levels, increased risk of toxicity ◆ **Thiazide diuretics:** decreased renal clearance of lithium, increased risk of toxicity ◆ **Phenothiazines:** decreased antipsychotic effect and/or increased lithium excretion ◆ **Phenytoin, carbamazepine:** possible adverse neurologic effects ◆ **Iodides:** synergistic or additive hypothyroid effects.

Drug-Food: ◆ **Increased dietary sodium intake:** increased renal elimination of lithium ◆ **Decreased dietary sodium intake:** decreased renal excretion of lithium, increased risk of toxicity.

ROUTE AND DOSAGE

Acute Mania
◆ **PO (Adults):** 600 mg tid or qid. Extended-release forms: 900 mg bid. Normalization of symptoms is usually achieved within 1–3 weeks.

Maintenance Therapy
◆ **PO (Adults):** 300–1200 mg/day in divided doses.

Investigational Uses
(Major depression, schizoaffective or schizophrenic disorder, alcohol dependence.)
◆ **PO (Adults):** 300 mg tid–qid.

Prophylaxis for Cluster Headaches
◆ **PO (Adults):** 600–1500 mg/day in divided doses.

Children with Apparent Mixed Bipolar Disorder
◆ **PO (Children):** Initial dosage: 15–

*<u>Underlines</u> indicate most frequent; CAPITALS indicate life-threatening.

60 mg/kg/day in 3 divided doses, not to exceed usual adult dosage. Adjust to serum lithium levels. Range is usually 150–300 mg/day in divided doses.

PHARMACODYNAMICS

Route	Onset	Peak	Duration
PO	Rapid	0.5–3 hr	*

*Varies with individual age, disease state, number of doses.

NURSING IMPLICATIONS

Assessment

- Assess for suicidal ideation.
- Assess for presence of adverse reactions or side effects.
- Assess mood and behavior frequently. Typical symptoms of mania include: • pressure of speech • motor hyperactivity • reduced need for sleep • flight of ideas • grandiosity • elation • poor judgment • aggressiveness • possible hostility.
- Assess patient/family knowledge about illness and need for medication.
- In collaboration with physician, assess renal and thyroid function, obtain baseline ECG.
- Assess for symptoms of infection or other conditions that result in fever, diaphoresis, diarrhea, and/or diuresis. Lithium and sodium are similar in chemical structure, behaving similarly and competing for various sites in the body. The conditions described deplete the body of its normal sodium, and lithium that would normally be excreted is reabsorbed by the kidneys, increasing its blood level and possibility of toxicity.
- **Lab Test Alterations:** Decreased serum potassium, T_3, T_4, PBI, VMA.
- ◇ Increased glucose (blood and urine), BUN, WBC, urine protein, and uric acid.
- **Toxicity and Overdose:** Lithium levels should be drawn weekly until therapeutic level is reached, then monthly during maintenance therapy. Therapeutic serum levels for acute mania: 1.0–1.5 mEq/L; for maintenance therapy: 0.6–1.2 mEq/L.
- ◇ Assess for signs and symptoms of lithium toxicity (symptoms intensify as level of toxicity increases). At serum levels of 1.5–2.0 mEq/L, symptoms include: • persistent nausea and vomiting • severe diarrhea • ataxia • blurred vision • tinnitus. At serum levels of 2.0–3.5 mEq/L: • excessive output of dilute urine • increasing tremors • muscular irritability • psychomotor retardation • mental confusion • giddiness. Serum levels above 3.5 mEq/L are potentially life-threatening and may result in: • impaired consciousness • nystagmus • seizures • coma • oliguria/anuria • arrhythmias • myocardial infarction • cardiovascular collapse. Withhold dosage and notify physician immediately should any of these symptoms occur.
- ◇ Assess for symptoms of overdose: • vomiting • agitation • tremors • hyperreflexia • muscle twitching • convulsions (may be followed by coma) • euphoria • confusion • hallucinations • delirium • sweating • headache • hyperpyrexia • tachycardia • palpitations • cardiac arrhythmias • hypertension • mydriasis • dry mucous membranes.
- **Overdose Management:** Monitor vital signs.
- ◇ Ensure adequate airway.
- ◇ Keep environmental stimuli to a minimum.
- ◇ Induce emesis or initiate gastric lavage if patient is conscious.
- ◇ If intoxication is severe, a short-acting barbiturate may be given prior to lavage.
- ◇ Maintain adequate circulation.
- ◇ Treat hypertension as required.
- ◇ External cooling measures may be required for hyperpyrexia.
- ◇ Dialysis may be initiated for severe intoxication.

Potential Nursing Diagnoses

♦ High risk for injury related to extreme hyperactivity; toxic levels of lithium.

♦ High risk for violence, self-directed or directed at others, related to biochemical alterations, excessive hyperactivity.

♦ High risk for fluid volume deficit, related to polyuria associated with lithium toxicity.

♦ High risk for alteration in nutrition, more than body requires, related to lithium-induced changes in glucose metabolism; excessive intake of high-calorie beverages in response to lithium's side effect of polydipsia.

♦ High risk for activity intolerance, related to lithium's side effects of lethargy, drowsiness, dizziness, muscular weakness.

♦ Knowledge deficit related to medication regimen.

Plan/Implementation

♦ Verify that lithium levels are drawn weekly until therapeutic level is reached, then monthly. Blood samples should be drawn 12 hours after the last dose.

♦ Monitor laboratory reports of serum lithium levels before giving medication. Withhold dosage and consult physician if level is above 1.5 mEq/L.

♦ Give with meals to minimize GI upset.

♦ Monitor for pulse irregularities and changes in blood pressure with routine assessment of vital signs.

♦ Monitor daily intake/output and weight. Report changes (e.g., altered ratio of I&O, sudden weight gain, or edema) to physician immediately.

♦ Ensure that tablet/capsule has been swallowed and not "cheeked" to avoid medication or to hoard for later use.

♦ Provide diet adequate in sodium.

♦ Encourage fluid intake of 2500 to 3000 mL/day.

♦ Monitor for signs and symptoms of lithium toxicity. Therapeutic level is highly individual; some patients may become toxic at levels ordinarily tolerated by others.

♦ Store medication at controlled room temperature between 15° and 30°C (59°–86°F). Protect tablets/capsules from moisture.

Patient/Family Education

♦ Take medication on a regular basis, even when feeling well. Discontinuation can result in return of symptoms.

♦ Do not drive or operate dangerous machinery until lithium levels are stabilized. Drowsiness and dizziness can occur.

♦ Do not skimp on dietary sodium intake. Choose foods from the four food groups. Avoid "junk" foods. Drink 6–8 large glasses of water each day. Avoid excessive use of beverages containing caffeine (coffee, tea, colas), which promote increased urine output.

♦ Notify physician if vomiting or diarrhea occurs. These symptoms can result in sodium loss and an increased risk of toxicity.

♦ Carry card or other identification noting patient is taking lithium.

♦ Be aware of appropriate diet should weight gain become a problem. Include adequate sodium and other nutrients while decreasing number of calories.

♦ Be aware of risks of becoming pregnant while on lithium therapy. Use information furnished by healthcare providers regarding methods of contraception. Notify physician as soon as possible if pregnancy is suspected or planned.

♦ Be aware of side effects and symptoms associated with toxicity. Notify physician if any of the following symptoms occur: persistent nausea and vomiting • severe diarrhea • ataxia • blurred vision • tinnitus.

♦ Refer to written materials furnished by healthcare providers regarding self-administered maintenance therapy.

Keep appointments for outpatient follow-up; have serum lithium level checked every 1–2 months, or as advised by physician.

Evaluation

* Patient demonstrates a subsiding/resolution of the symptoms associated with mania (hyperactivity, forceful and rapid speech, disrupted patterns of eating and sleeping, impaired thought processes).
* Patient verbalizes understanding of side effects, symptoms of toxicity, and required regimen for compliance with lithium therapy.

LORAZEPAM

(lor-a'ze-pam)
Ativan

Classification(s):
Antianxiety agent, Benzodiazepine, Skeletal muscle relaxant, Anticonvulsant, CNS depressant
Schedule C IV
Pregnancy Category D

INDICATIONS

* Treatment of anxiety disorders ♦ Temporary relief of anxiety symptoms ♦ Anxiety associated with depression ♦ Preoperative sedation ♦ Nausea/vomiting associated with chemotherapy in cancer patients.

ACTION

* Depresses subcortical levels of the central nervous system, particularly the limbic system and reticular formation ♦ May potentiate the effects of the powerful inhibitory neurotransmitter gamma-aminobutyric acid (GABA) in the brain, thereby producing a calmative effect ♦ All levels of CNS depression can be effected, from mild sedation to hypnosis to coma.

PHARMACOKINETICS

Absorption: Readily absorbed following oral and IM administration.
Distribution: Is widely distributed. Crosses blood-brain and placental barriers; excreted in breast milk.
Metabolism and Excretion: Metabolized by the liver, producing inactive metabolites that are excreted by the kidneys.
Half-Life: 10–20 hours.

CONTRAINDICATIONS AND PRECAUTIONS

Contraindicated in: ♦ Hypersensitivity to this drug or to other benzodiazepines ♦ Combination with other CNS depressants ♦ Pregnancy and lactation ♦ Narrow-angle glaucoma ♦ Shock ♦ Coma ♦ Children under 12 (oral preparations) ♦ Children under 18 (parenteral preparation).
Use Cautiously in: ♦ Elderly or debilitated patients ♦ Patients with hepatic or renal dysfunction ♦ Individuals with a history of drug abuse/addiction ♦ Depressed/suicidal patients.

ADVERSE REACTIONS AND SIDE EFFECTS*

CNS: <u>drowsiness</u>, <u>fatigue</u>, <u>ataxia</u>, <u>dizziness</u>, confusion, headache, syncope, paradoxical excitement.
CV: hypotension, hypertension.
Derm: skin rashes, pain and redness at site of IM injection.
Endo: gynecomastia, galactorrhea.
GI: dry mouth, nausea/vomiting, anorexia.
Resp: RESPIRATORY DEPRESSION (with IV use).
Other: tolerance, physical and psychological dependence.

INTERACTIONS

Drug-Drug: ♦ **Other CNS depressants (including alcohol, barbiturates,**

---

*Underlines indicate most frequent; CAPITALS indicate life-threatening.

narcotics), **antipsychotics, antidepressants, antihistamines, anticonvulsants:** additive CNS depression ◆
Cigarette smoking and caffeine: decreased effects of lorazepam ◆ **Neuromuscular blocking agents:** increased
respiratory depression ◆ **Digoxin:** reduced excretion of digoxin, increased
potential for toxicity.

ROUTE AND DOSAGE

Anxiety, Anxiety Disorders, Anxiety Associated with Depression

◆ **PO (Adults):** 2–3 mg bid or tid.
◆ **PO (Geriatric/Debilitated Patients):** 1–2 mg daily in 2–3 divided
doses.

Sedation, Anxiety Symptoms

◆ **IV (Adults):** 2 mg total, or 0.044 mg/
kg, whichever dosage is smaller.

Preoperative Sedation

◆ **PO (Adults):** 0.05 mg/kg, up to a
maximum of 4 mg.

PHARMACODYNAMICS

Route	Onset	Peak	Duration
PO	15–45 min	2 hr	*
IM	15–30 min	60–90 min	*
IV	5–15 min	60–90 min	16 hr

*Varies with individual age, disease state, number
of doses.

NURSING IMPLICATIONS

Assessment

◆ Assess level of anxiety. Symptoms include restlessness, pacing, insomnia,
inability to concentrate, increased
heart rate, increased respiration, elevated blood pressure, confusion,
tremors, rapid speech.
◆ Assess for suicidal ideation (CNS depressants aggravate symptoms in depressed patients).
◆ Assess history of allergies, sensitivity to
this drug or to other benzodiazepines.
◆ Assess history of glaucoma.
◆ Assess for presence of adverse reactions or side effects.

◆ Assess date of last menses (possible
pregnancy), use of contraceptives.
◆ Assess whether currently breast-feeding a child.
◆ Assess current and past alcohol and
drug consumption.
◆ Assess operation of automobile and/
or other dangerous machinery.
◆ Assess patient/family knowledge about
illness and need for medication.
◆ In collaboration with physician, assess
CBC and liver function tests in patients
on long-term therapy.
◆ **Withdrawal:** Assess for symptoms of
withdrawal: ● depression ● insomnia
● increased anxiety ● abdominal and
muscle cramps ● tremors ● vomiting
● sweating ● convulsions ● delirium.
◆ **Withdrawal Management:** Monitor
vital signs.
◇ Place patient in quiet room with low
stimuli.
◇ Institute seizure precautions.
◇ A long-acting barbiturate, such as phenobarbital, may be ordered to prevent
seizures.
◇ Some physicians may order oxazepam
as needed for objective withdrawal
symptoms, gradually decreasing dosage until the drug is discontinued.
◆ **Toxicity and Overdose:** Assess for
symptoms of intoxication: ● euphoria
● relaxation ● drowsiness ● slurred
speech ● disorientation ● mood lability
● incoordination ● unsteady gait ● disinhibition of sexual and aggressive impulses ● judgment and/or memory impairment.
◇ Assess for symptoms of overdose: ●
shallow respiration ● cold and clammy
skin ● hypotension ● dilated pupils ●
weak and rapid pulse ● hypnosis ●
coma ● possible death.
◆ **Overdose Management:** Monitor vital signs.
◇ Ensure maintenance of adequate airway.
◇ Induce vomiting in conscious patient.
◇ Initiate gastric lavage in unconscious
patient.

◊ Administer activated charcoal to minimize absorption.

◊ IV fluids and vasopressors may be used to combat hypotension.

◊ Forced diuresis may be used to facilitate elimination of the drug.

Potential Nursing Diagnoses

♦ High risk for injury related to seizures, panic anxiety, abrupt withdrawal from long-term lorazepam use, effects of lorazepam use, effects of lorazepam intoxication or overdose.

♦ High risk for self-directed violence related to depressed mood intensified by lorazepam.

♦ Anxiety (specify level) related to threats to physical integrity and/or self-concept.

♦ High risk for activity intolerance, related to lorazepam's side effects of lethargy, drowsiness, dizziness, muscular weakness.

♦ Knowledge deficit related to medication regimen.

Plan/Implementation

♦ **General Info:** Monitor vital signs before beginning therapy, at regular intervals (bid) throughout therapy, and q 10 minutes during IV administration.

◊ Ensure that patient practices good oral care. Offer hard, sugarless candy; gum; or frequent sips of water if dry mouth is a problem.

◊ Ensure that patient is protected from injury. Supervise and assist with ambulation if dizziness and muscular weakness are problems. Pad siderails and headboard for patient who experiences seizures.

♦ **PO:** To minimize nausea, medication may be given with food or milk.

◊ If patient has difficulty swallowing, tablet may be crushed and mixed with food or fluid.

◊ Ensure that tablet has been swallowed and not "cheeked" to avoid medication or to hoard for later use.

◊ Store medication at controlled room temperatures between 15° and 30°C (59°–86°F) in tightly closed container.

♦ **IM:** IM lorazepam is administered in its undiluted form.

◊ IM lorazepam should be administered deeply into large muscle mass to minimize pain and to enhance absorption. Use Z-track method.

◊ Store medication in refrigerator. Protect from light.

♦ **IV:** IV solution should be prepared immediately before use. Dilute drug with equal volume of D5W, sterile water, or saline for injection. Inject directly into vein or into IV infusion tubing.

◊ Avoid use of small veins to minimize risk of thrombophlebitis.

◊ Administer slowly (up to 2 mg/min) to reduce risk of respiratory depression, phlebitis, and/or cardiovascular collapse.

◊ Ensure availability of emergency respiratory assistance.

◊ Refrigerate unused diluted solution. Do not use if discolored or if precipitate is visible.

◊ Bed rest is required for 3 hours after IV administration; assistance may be required for up to 8 hours.

◊ Store medication in refrigerator. Protect from light.

Patient/Family Education

♦ Do not drive or operate dangerous machinery. Drowsiness and dizziness can occur.

♦ Do not stop taking the drug abruptly. Can produce serious withdrawal symptoms.

♦ Do not consume other CNS depressants (including alcohol).

♦ Do not take nonprescription medication without approval from physician.

♦ Carry card or other identification at all times stating names of medications being taken.

♦ Be aware of risks of taking lorazepam during pregnancy (congenital malformations have been associated with use during first trimester). Notify physician of desirability to discontinue drug if pregnancy is suspected or planned.

♦ Be aware of possible side effects. Refer to written materials furnished by healthcare providers regarding correct method of self-administration.

Evaluation

♦ Patient demonstrates a subsiding/resolution of the symptoms for which lorazepam was prescribed (anxiety symptoms, anxiety disorders, anxiety associated with depression, nausea and vomiting associated with cancer chemotherapy).

♦ Patient verbalizes understanding of side effects and regimen required for prudent self-administration of lorazepam.

LOXAPINE

(lox′a-peen)
{Loxapac}, Loxitane, Loxitane-C

Classification(s):
Antipsychotic, Neuroleptic,
Dibenzoxazepine
Pregnancy Category C

INDICATIONS

♦ Manifestations of psychotic disorders.

ACTION

♦ The exact mechanism of antipsychotic action is not fully understood ♦ Loxapine is thought to act primarily in the reticular formation ♦ It reduces firing threshold of CNS neurons.

PHARMACOKINETICS

Absorption: Absorption following oral and parenteral routes is rapid and virtually complete.
Distribution: Widely distributed, with highest concentrations in brain, heart, liver, and pancreas. Thought to cross placental barrier and to enter breast milk.
Metabolism and Excretion: Almost completely metabolized by the liver. Excreted in urine and feces.
Half-Life: Initial: 5 hours; terminal: 19 hours.

CONTRAINDICATIONS AND PRECAUTIONS

Contraindicated in: ♦ Hypersensitivity to this drug or to other antipsychotics ♦ Comatose or severely CNS-depressed patients ♦ Presence of large amounts of CNS depressants ♦ Bone marrow depression ♦ Blood dyscrasias ♦ Subcortical brain damage ♦ Parkinson's disease ♦ Hepatic, renal, and/or cardiac insufficiency ♦ Severe hypotension or hypertension ♦ Children under 16; pregnancy and lactation (safe use has not been established).
Use Cautiously in: ♦ Patients with a history of seizures ♦ Respiratory, renal, hepatic, thyroid, or cardiovascular disorders (e.g., respiratory infection, COPD, thyrotoxicosis, mitral insufficiency, angina pectoris) ♦ Prostatic hypertropy ♦ Glaucoma ♦ Diabetes ♦ Elderly or debilitated patients.

ADVERSE REACTIONS AND SIDE EFFECTS*

CNS: sedation, headache, seizures, insomnia, dizziness, extrapyramidal symptoms (pseudoparkinsonism, akathisia, akinesia, dystonia, oculogyric crisis), tardive dyskinesia, fatigue, cerebral edema, ataxia, blurred vision, NEUROLEPTIC MALIGNANT SYNDROME, confusion, tinnitus, hyperpyrexia.
CV: orthostatic hypotension, hypertension, tachycardia, bradycardia, ECG changes, ARRHYTHMIAS.
Derm: skin rashes, urticaria, petechiae, seborrhea, photosensitivity, eczema, fa-

---

{} = Only available in Canada.
*Underlines indicate most frequent; CAPITALS indicate life-threatening.

cial edema, dermatitis, EXFOLIATIVE DERMATITIS (rare).

Endo: galactorrhea, gynecomastia (men), changes in libido, hyperglycemia or hypoglycemia, amenorrhea, retrograde ejaculation.

GI: dry mouth, nausea, vomiting, increased appetite and weight gain, anorexia, dyspepsia, constipation, diarrhea, jaundice, polydipsia, PARALYTIC ILEUS.

GU: urinary retention, frequency or incontinence, bladder paralysis, polyuria, enuresis.

Hemat: AGRANULOCYTOSIS, LEUKOPENIA, ANEMIA, THROMBOCYTOPENIA.

Resp: LARYNGOSPASM, BRONCHOSPASM, SUPPRESSION OF COUGH REFLEX.

Other: nasal congestion.

INTERACTIONS

Drug-Drug: ◆ **CNS depressants (including alcohol, barbiturates, narcotics, anesthetics);** additive CNS depressant effects ◆ **Anticholinergic agents (e.g., atropine):** additive anticholinergic effects, decreased antipsychotic effects ◆ **Metyrosine:** potentiation of extrapyramidal side effects ◆ **Levodopa:** decreased efficacy of levodopa ◆ **Quinidine:** additive cardiac depressive effects ◆ **Guanethidine:** decreased antihypertensive action ◆ **Lithium:** decreased plasma levels of antipsychotic drug ◆ **Epineprine:** reversal of usual pressor action of epinephrine, resulting in decreased blood pressure ◆ **Phenytoin:** decreased phenytoin levels, possibly decreasing effects ◆ **Polypeptide antibiotics:** neuromuscular respiratory depression ◆ **Metrizamide:** seizures.

Drug-Food: ◆ **Caffeine-containing beverages (e.g., coffee, tea, colas):** counteracted antipsychotic effect.

ROUTE AND DOSAGE

Psychotic Disorders

◆ **PO (Adults):** Initial dosage: 10 mg bid. In severely disturbed patients, initial dosage of up to 50 mg/day may be required. Increase dosage fairly rapidly over the first 7–10 days until psychotic symptoms are controlled. Usual range: 60–100 mg/day in 2–4 divided doses. Maximum dosage: 250 mg/day.

◆ **IM (Adults):** 12.5–50 mg q 4–6 hr or longer. Some patients achieve control with bid administration. Switch to oral medication as soon as control has been achieved, usually within 5 days.

◆ **PO (Adults, Maintenance):** Dosage should be maintained at lowest level compatible with control of symptoms. Usual range: 20–60 mg/day in 2–4 divided doses.

PHARMACODYNAMICS

Route	Onset*	Peak	Duration
PO	20–30 min	1.5–3 hr	12 hr
IM	15–30 min	15–20 min	12 hr

*Full antipsychotic effects may not be observed for 4–8 weeks.

NURSING IMPLICATIONS

Assessment

◆ Assess mental status daily: mood ● appearance ● thought and communication patterns ● level of interest in the environment and in activities ● level of anxiety or agitation ● presence of hallucinations or delusions ● suspiciousness ● interactions with others ● ability to carry out ADL.

◆ Assess for symptoms of blood dyscrasias: sore throat ● fever, malaise ● unusual bleeding ● easy bruising.

◆ Assess for extrapyramidal symptoms: pseudoparkinsonism (tremors, shuffling gait, drooling, rigidity) ● akinesia (muscular weakness) ● akathisia (continuous restlessness and fidgeting) ● dystonia (involuntary muscular movements of face, arms, legs, and neck) ● oculogyric crisis (uncontrolled rolling back of the eyes) ● tardive dyskinesia (bizarre facial and tongue movements, stiff neck, difficulty swallowing).

♦ Assess for symptoms of neuroleptic malignant syndrome: hyperpyrexia up to 107°F (41.6°C) • elevated pulse • increased or decreased blood pressure • severe parkinsonian muscle rigidity • elevated creatinine phosphokinase blood levels • elevated white blood count • altered mental status (including catatonic signs or agitation) • acute renal failure • varying levels of consciousness (including stupor and coma) • pallor • diaphoresis • tachycardia • arrhythmias • rhabdomyolysis.

♦ Assess vital signs, weight. Record baseline values for comparison.

♦ Assess history of allergies, sensitivity to this drug.

♦ Assess date of last menses (possible pregnancy), use of contraceptives.

♦ Assess whether currently breast-feeding a child.

♦ Assess current and past alcohol and drug consumption.

♦ Assess for operation of automobile and/or other dangerous machinery.

♦ Assess for presence of adverse reactions or side effects.

♦ Assess patient/family knowledge about illness and need for medication.

♦ In collaboration with physician, assess CBC, liver function tests, and ophthalmologic exams in patients on long-term therapy.

♦ **Lab Test Alterations:** Increased serum alkaline phosphatase, transaminases, bilirubin.

◊ Increased protein-bound iodine.

◊ False-positive pregnancy test, possibly caused by drug metabolite that discolors urine (less likely to occur when serum test is used).

◊ Increased urinary glucose.

◊ Decreased urinary estrogen, progestin, and gonadotropin.

◊ Increased plasma cholesterol level.

◊ Increased serum prolactin.

♦ **Withdrawal:** Assess for symptoms of abrupt withdrawal from long-term therapy: • gastritis • nausea • vomiting

• dizziness • headache • tachycardia • insomnia • tremulousness.

♦ **Toxicity and Overdose:** No correlation has been established between blood level and therapeutic effect.

◊ Assess for symptoms of overdose: • seizures • CNS depression, from heavy sedation to deep sleep to coma • hypotension • severe extrapyramidal symptoms • agitation • restlessness • fever • autonomic reactions • ECG changes • cardiac arrhythmias.

♦ **Overdose Management:** Monitor vital signs.

◊ Ensure maintenance of open airway.

◊ Initiate gastric lavage.

◊ Do not induce emesis (nuchal rigidity may result in aspiration of vomitus).

◊ Antiparkinsonian drugs or diphenhydramine may be administered to counteract extrapyramidal symptoms.

◊ Administer IV fluids or a vasoconstrictor to maintain adequate blood pressure. **Note:** Epinephrine is not recommended due to interaction with antipsychotics that causes further drop in blood pressure.

◊ Administer IV phenytoin to control ventricular arrhythmias.

◊ Administer diazepam or pentobarbital to control convulsions or hyperactivity.

◊ Dialysis does not appear to be a useful intervention.

Potential Nursing Diagnoses

♦ High risk for violence directed at others related to mistrust and panic anxiety.

♦ High risk for injury related to abrupt withdrawal after prolonged use; overdose; loxapine's side effects of sedation, dizziness, ataxia, weakness, lowered seizure threshold.

♦ Sensory-perceptual alteration related to panic anxiety evidenced by hallucinations.

♦ Altered thought processes related to panic anxiety evidenced by delusional thinking.

♦ Social isolation related to inability to trust others.

♦ High risk for activity intolerance, related to loxapine's side effects of drowsiness, dizziness, ataxia, weakness.

♦ Noncompliance with medication regimen related to suspiciousness and mistrust of others.

♦ Knowledge deficit related to medication regimen.

Plan/Implementation

♦ **General Info:** Monitor vital signs before beginning therapy and at regular intervals (bid or tid) throughout therapy. Take BP lying and standing to monitor for possible hypotensive reaction; elderly are particularly susceptible. Dosage adjustment may be required.

◊ Ensure that patient who is ambulatory is protected from sun when spending time outdoors.

◊ Weigh patient 2–3 times a week, at same time of day, on same scale, if possible. A rapid weight gain or evidence of edema should be reported to physician immediately. Record I&O.

◊ Ensure that patient is protected from injury. Provide supervision and assistance when ambulating if dizziness and drowsiness are problems. Pad siderails and headboard for patient who experiences seizures.

◊ Give patient hard candy, gum, or frequent sips of water if dry mouth is a problem.

◊ Store medication at controlled room temperatures between 15° and 30°C (59°–86°F) in light-resistant containers. Protect from freezing.

♦ **PO:** Ensure that patient swallows capsule and does not "cheek" to avoid medication or to hoard for later use.

◊ Capsule may be opened and contents mixed with food or fluid for patient who has difficulty swallowing, or a liquid concentrate may be used.

◊ Administer concentrate in 60–90 mL

of orange or grapefruit juice just prior to administration.

◊ Do not store diluted concentrate.

♦ **IM:** IM injection is used for prompt symptomatic control in the acutely agitated patient and in patients whose symptoms render oral medication temporarily impractical.

◊ Inject slowly and deeply into upper, outer quadrant of buttock or other large muscle mass, such as midlateral thigh.

◊ Because of possible hypotensive effects, patient should remain in recumbent position for at least one-half hour following IM injection.

◊ Rotate sites when multiple injections are administered.

◊ Aspirate carefully to avoid injection directly into blood vessel.

◊ Switch to oral medication as soon as control of symptoms has been achieved.

◊ Do not administer injection IV.

Patient/Family Education

♦ Use caution when driving or when operating dangerous machinery. Drowsiness and dizziness can occur.

♦ Do not stop taking the drug abruptly. To do so might produce withdrawal symptoms, such as nausea, vomiting, gastritis, headache, tachycardia, insomnia, tremulousness.

♦ Use sunscreens and wear protective clothing when spending time outdoors. Skin is more susceptible to sunburn.

♦ Report occurrence of any of the following symptoms to physician immediately: sore throat • fever • malaise • unusual bleeding • easy bruising • persistent nausea/vomiting • severe headache • rapid heart rate • difficulty urinating • muscle twitching • tremors • darkly colored urine • pale stools • yellow skin or eyes • muscular incoordination • or skin rash.

♦ Rise slowly from a sitting or lying position to prevent a drop in blood pressure.

- If dry mouth is a problem, take frequent sips of water, chew sugarless gum, or suck on hard candy. Good oral care (frequent brushing, flossing) is very important.
- Do not drink alcohol while on loxapine therapy. These drugs potentiate each other's effects.
- Do not consume other medications (including over-the-counter meds) without physician's approval. Many medications contain substances that interact with loxapine in a way that may be harmful.
- Be aware of possible risks of taking loxapine during pregnancy. Safe use during pregnancy and lactation has not been established. It is thought that loxapine crosses the placental barrier, so it is possible a fetus could experience adverse effects of the drug. Inform physician immediately if pregnancy occurs, is suspected, or is planned.
- Be aware of side effects of loxapine. Refer to written materials furnished by healthcare providers for safe self-administration.
- Continue to take medication even if feeling well and as though it is not needed. Symptoms may return if medication is discontinued.
- Carry card or other identification at all times describing medications being taken.

Evaluation

- Patient demonstrates a subsiding/resolution of the symptoms for which loxapine was prescribed (panic anxiety, altered thought processes, altered perceptions).
- Patient verbalizes understanding of side effects and regimen required for prudent self-administration of loxapine.

MAPROTILINE

(ma-proe'ti-leen)
Ludiomil

Classification(s):
Tetracyclic antidepressant
Pregnancy Category B

INDICATIONS

- Major depression with melancholia or psychotic symptoms - Dysthymic disorder - Depressive phase of bipolar disorder - Mixed symptoms of anxiety and depression.

ACTION

- Exact mechanism of action unclear - Blocks the reuptake of the neurotransmitter norepinephrine, increasing its concentration at the synapse and correcting the deficit thought to contribute to the melancholy mood of the depressed person.

PHARMACOKINETICS

Absorption: Slowly but completely absorbed from the GI tract following oral administration.

Distribution: Widely distributed. May cross placental barrier. Is excreted in breast milk.

Metabolism and Excretion: Slowly metabolized by the liver. Excreted in urine and feces.

Half-Life: 27–58 hours.

CONTRAINDICATIONS AND PRECAUTIONS

Contraindicated in: - Hypersensitivity to this drug or to tricyclic antidepressants - Concomitant use of MAO inhibitors - Acute recovery period following myocardial infarction - Known or suspected seizure disorders - Prostatic hypertrophy - Children under age 18; pregnancy (safety not established).

Use Cautiously in: - Urinary retention

♦ Glaucoma ♦ Thyroid disease ♦ Cardiovascular disorders ♦ Hepatic or renal insufficiency ♦ Suicidal patients ♦ Lactation ♦ Elderly or debilitated patients.

ADVERSE REACTIONS AND SIDE EFFECTS*

CNS: drowsiness, dizziness, weakness, headache, fatigue, confusion, lethargy, memory deficits, disturbed concentration, tremors, ataxia, tinnitus, extrapyramidal symptoms, paresthesias of extremities, lowered seizure threshold, blurred vision, agitation, excitement, restlessness, insomnia, exacerbation of psychosis, shift to manic behavior.

CV: orthostatic hypotension, tachycardia and other arrhythmias, hypertension, MYOCARDIAL INFARCTION, HEART BLOCK, CONGESTIVE HEART FAILURE, ECG changes, syncope, CARDIOVASCULAR COLLAPSE.

Derm: skin rash, urticaria, photosensitivity, erythema, petechiae.

GI: dry mouth, constipation, nausea, vomiting, anorexia, diarrhea, abdominal cramps, adynamic ileus, esophageal reflux, stomatitis, black tongue.

GU: urinary retention, gynecomastia (men), testicular swelling, menstrual irregularity, breast engorgement and galactorrhea (women), changes in libido, impotence, delayed micturition.

Hemat: AGRANULOCYTOSIS, THROMBOCYTOPENIA, LEUKOPENIA, eosinophilia, purpura.

Hepat: jaundice, hepatitis.

Other: weight gain, nasal congestion, alopecia, hypothermia, peripheral neuropathy.

INTERACTIONS

Drug-Drug: ♦ **MAO inhibitors:** hyperpyretic crisis, hypertensive crisis ♦ **Guanethidine, clonidine:** decreased effects of these medications ♦ **Cimetidine:** increased maprotiline serum levels ♦ **Amphetamines:** increased hypertensive effects of these drugs ♦ **CNS depressants (including alcohol, barbiturates, benzodiazepines):** potentiation of CNS effects ♦ **Thyroid medications:** tachycardia, arrhythmias ♦ **Phenothiazines (or rapid withdrawal from benzodiazepines by persons taking maprotiline):** increased risk of seizures ♦ **Methylphenidate, phenothiazines:** increased serum maprotiline levels ♦ **Ethchlorvynol:** transient delirium ♦ **Quinidine, procainamide:** potentiation of adverse cardiovascular effects of maprotiline ♦ **Oral contraceptives:** decreased effects of maprotiline ♦ **Smoking:** increased maprotiline metabolism ♦ **Beta-adrenergic blockers:** increased effects of maprotiline ♦ **Sympathomimetics:** decreased alpha-adrenergic effects ♦ **Anticholinergic drugs (e.g., antihistamines, atropine):** additive anticholinergic effects.

ROUTE AND DOSAGE

Mild to Moderate Depression
♦ **PO (Adults):** Initial dosage: 75 mg/day. After 2 weeks, increase gradually in 25-mg increments as required and tolerated. 150 mg/day is usually adequate, but some patients may require as much as 225 mg/day. Total may be given in single daily dose or in divided doses.
♦ **PO (Geriatric):** Doses of 50–75 mg/day are usually adequate.

Severe Depression
♦ **PO (Adults):** Initial dosage: 100–150 mg/day. May be gradually increased as required and tolerated. Maximum dosage: 225 mg/day.

Maintenance Therapy
♦ **PO (Adults):** Lowest effective level: 75–150 mg/day, with adjustment depending upon therapeutic response.
♦ **PO (Geriatric):** 50–75 mg/day.

---

*Underlines indicate most frequent; CAPITALS indicate life-threatening.

PHARMACODYNAMICS

Route	Onset	Peak	Duration
PO	2–4 wk	8–12 hr	Weeks*

*Allow up to 2 weeks following cessation of therapy for complete drug elimination.

NURSING IMPLICATIONS

Assessment

- Assess for suicidal ideation, plan, means. Assess for sudden lifts in mood, which could indicate patient's decision to commit suicide.

- Assess mental status daily: • mood • appearance • thought and communication patterns • level of interest in the environment and in activities • suicidal ideation. Improvement in these behavior patterns and level of energy should be expected within 2–4 weeks following initiation of therapy.

- Assess for symptoms of blood dyscrasias: • sore throat • fever • malaise • unusual bleeding • easy bruising.

- Assess vital signs, weight.

- Assess history of allergies, sensitivity to this drug or to tricyclic antidepressants.

- Assess for history of glaucoma.

- Assess date of last menses (possible pregnancy), use of contraceptives.

- Assess whether currently breast-feeding a child.

- Assess current and past alcohol and drug consumption.

- Assess for operation of automobile and/or other dangerous machinery.

- Assess for presence of adverse reactions or side effects.

- Assess patient/family knowledge about illness and need for medication.

- In collaboration with physician, assess CBC and liver function tests in patients on long-term therapy.

- **Lab Test Alterations:** Increased serum bilirubin, alkaline phosphatase, and glucose.

- ◇ Decreased urinary 5-hydroxyindole-acetic acid (HIAA) and vanillylmandelic acid (VMA) excretion.

- **Withdrawal:** Assess for symptoms of abrupt withdrawal from long-term therapy: • nausea • headache • vertigo • malaise • insomnia • nightmares.

- **Toxicity and Overdose:** Range of therapeutic serum concentration not well substantiated.

- ◇ Assess for symptoms of overdose: • confusion • agitation • hallucinations • seizures • flushing • dry mouth • dilated pupils • hyperpyrexia • hypotension • coma • tachycardia • arrhythmias • cardiac arrest • renal failure.

- **Overdose Management:** Monitor vital signs.

- ◇ Ensure maintenance of adequate airway.

- ◇ Monitor ECG.

- ◇ Induce emesis in conscious patient.

- ◇ Initiate gastric lavage in unconscious patient.

- ◇ Administer activated charcoal to minimize absorption.

- ◇ IV physostigmine may be administered cautiously to reverse anticholinergic effects.

- ◇ Administer sodium bicarbonate, vasopressors, phenytoin, propranolol, or lidocaine to control cardiovascular effects.

- ◇ Administer IV diazepam to control seizures.

Potential Nursing Diagnoses

- High risk for self-directed violence related to depressed mood.

- High risk for injury related to abrupt withdrawal after prolonged use; overdose; maprotiline's side effects of sedation, dizziness, ataxia, weakness, confusion, lowered seizure threshold.

- Social isolation related to depressed mood.

- High risk for activity intolerance, related to maprotiline's side effects of drowsiness, dizziness, ataxia, weakness, confusion.

- Knowledge deficit related to medication regimen.

Plan/Implementation

* Monitor vital signs before beginning therapy and at regular intervals (bid or tid) throughout therapy. Take BP lying and standing in patients experiencing orthostatic hypotension; elderly are particularly susceptible. Contact physician if tachycardia/arrhythmias are noted.

* Ensure that patient who is ambulatory is protected from sun when spending time outdoors.

* Weigh patient 2–3 times a week, at same time of day, on same scale, if possible. A rapid weight gain or evidence of edema should be reported to physician immediately. Record I&O.

* Ensure that patient is protected from injury. Provide supervision and assistance when ambulating if dizziness and drowsiness are problems. Pad siderails and headboard for patient who experiences seizures.

* Give patient hard candy, gum, or frequent sips of water if dry mouth is a problem.

* Medication may be administered with food to minimize GI upset.

* Ensure that patient swallows tablet and does not "cheek" to avoid medication or to hoard for later use.

* Tablet may be crushed and mixed with food or fluid for patient who has difficulty swallowing.

* Store at controlled room temperatures between 15° and 30°C (59°–86°F). Protect from heat and moisture.

Patient/Family Education

* Therapeutic effect may not be seen for as long as 4 weeks. If after this length of time no improvement is noted, physician may prescribe a different medication. Continue to take medication even though symptoms have not subsided.

* Use caution when driving or when operating dangerous machinery. Drowsiness and dizziness can occur. If these side effects become persistent or interfere with activities of daily living, report to physician. Dosage adjustment may be necessary.

* Do not stop taking the drug abruptly. To do so might produce withdrawal symptoms, such as nausea, vertigo, insomnia, headache, malaise, nightmares.

* Use sunscreens and wear protective clothing when spending time outdoors. Skin may be sensitive to sunburn.

* Report occurrence of any of the following symptoms to physician immediately: sore throat • fever • malaise • unusual bleeding • easy bruising • persistent nausea/vomiting • severe headache • rapid heart rate • difficulty urinating • seizures.

* Rise slowly from a sitting or lying position to prevent a sudden drop in blood pressure.

* If dry mouth is a problem, take frequent sips of water, chew sugarless gum, or suck on hard candy. Good oral care (frequent brushing, flossing) is very important.

* Do not smoke while on maprotiline therapy. Smoking increases metabolism of maprotiline, requiring adjustment in dosage to achieve therapeutic effect.

* Do not drink alcohol while on maprotiline therapy. These drugs potentiate each other's effects.

* Do not consume other medications (including over-the-counter meds) without physician's approval. Many medications contain substances that, in combination with maprotiline, could precipitate a life-threatening hypertensive crisis.

* Be aware of possible risks of taking maprotiline during pregnancy. Safe use during pregnancy has not been established. Inform physician immediately if pregnancy occurs, is suspected, or is planned.

* Maprotiline is excreted in breast milk, so potential risk to infant should be

considered and discussed with physician before taking maprotiline during lactation.

♦ Be aware of side effects of maprotiline. Refer to written materials furnished by healthcare providers for safe self-administration.

♦ Carry card or other identification at all times describing medications being taken.

Evaluation

♦ Patient demonstrates a subsiding/resolution of the symptoms for which maprotiline was prescribed (depressed mood, suicidal ideation).

♦ Patient verbalizes understanding of side effects and regimen required for prudent self-administration of maprotiline.

MAZINDOL

(may′zin-dole)
Mazanor, Sanorex

Classification(s):
Anorexigenic, CNS stimulant,
Sympathomimetic amine
Schedule C IV
Pregnancy Category C

INDICATIONS

♦ Exogenous obesity (short-term management).

ACTION

♦ Exact mechanism of action is not known ♦ Sympathomimetic amines are thought to produce appetite suppression through direct stimulation of the satiety center in the hypothalamus and limbic system ♦ Pharmacologic effects are similar to the amphetamines.

PHARMACOKINETICS

Absorption: Readily absorbed following oral administration.

Distribution: Is widely distributed. Crosses placental barrier; enters breast milk.

Metabolism and Excretion: Partially metabolized by the liver; excreted in urine.

Half-Life: Not well substantiated.

CONTRAINDICATIONS AND PRECAUTIONS

Contraindicated in: ♦ Hypersensitivity to sympathomimetic amines ♦ Advanced arteriosclerosis ♦ Symptomatic cardiovascular disease ♦ Severe hypertension ♦ Hyperthyroidism ♦ Glaucoma ♦ Agitated states ♦ History of drug abuse ♦ Therapy with or within 14 days of receiving MAO inhibitors ♦ Concomitant use of other CNS stimulants ♦ Pregnancy and lactation ♦ Children under 12 years of age.

Use Cautiously in: ♦ Mild hypertension ♦ Diabetes mellitus ♦ Elderly or debilitated patients.

ADVERSE REACTIONS AND SIDE EFFECTS*

CNS: <u>overstimulation</u>, <u>restlessness</u>, <u>dizziness</u>, <u>insomnia</u>, dyskinesia, <u>euphoria</u>, <u>dysphoria</u>, tremor, headache, drowsiness, mental depression, confusion, incoordination, fatigue, malaise, blurred vision, mydriasis, psychoses (rare), nervousness, drowsiness, weakness, shivering.

CV: <u>palpitations</u>, <u>tachycardia</u>, arrhythmias, hypertension or hypotension, fainting.

Derm: urticaria, rash, erythema, burning sensation.

Endo: impotence, changes in libido, menstrual upset, gynecomastia.

GI: <u>dry mouth</u>, unpleasant taste, <u>nausea</u>, vomiting, diarrhea, constipation, <u>abdominal discomfort</u>.

Other: <u>tolerance</u>, physical and psychological dependence, fever, excessive sweating, pallor.

---

*<u>Underlines</u> indicate most frequent; CAPITALS indicate life-threatening.

INTERACTIONS

Drug-Drug: ✦ **Other CNS stimulants:** additive CNS stimulant effects ✦ **MAO inhibitors (during or within 14 days of administration):** hypertensive crisis, headache, hyperpyrexia, intracranial hemorrhage, bradycardia ✦ **Insulin:** alteration in insulin requirements ✦ **Guanethidine:** decreased antihypertensive effects ✦ **Barbiturates, phenothiazines:** decreased mazindol effects ✦ **General anesthetics:** cardiac arrhythmias ✦ **Exogenous catecholamines:** increased pressor effects of these drugs. ✦ **Lithium:** one case of lithium toxicity has been documented.

Drug-Food: ✦ **Caffeinated foods and drinks:** increased effects of mazindol.

ROUTE AND DOSAGE

Exogenous Obesity

✦ **PO (Adults):** Initial dosage: 1 mg daily. Adjust dose to patient response. Usual dose is 1 mg tid (1 hour before meals) or 2 mg once daily (1 hour before lunch).

PHARMACODYNAMICS

Route	Onset	Peak	Duration
PO	30–60 min	—	8–15 hr

NURSING IMPLICATIONS

Assessment

✦ Assess and record baseline temperature, pulse, respiration, blood pressure, and weight for comparison during therapy.
✦ In diabetic patient, assess blood sugar bid–tid. Insulin adjustments may be required due to alteration in eating pattern and possibility of hyperactivity.
✦ Assess patient knowledge of sound, nutritional, calorie-reduced diet and importance of regular exercise.
✦ Assess mental status for changes in mood, level of activity, degree of stimulation, aggressiveness.
✦ Assess sleeping patterns carefully. Insomnia may occur.
✦ Assess history of allergies, sensitivity to this drug or to other sympathomimetic amines.
✦ Assess history of glaucoma.
✦ Assess for presence of adverse reactions or side effects.
✦ Assess date of last menses (possible pregnancy), use of contraceptives.
✦ Assess whether currently breast-feeding a child.
✦ Assess current and past alcohol and drug consumption.
✦ Assess usual amount of caffeine consumed.
✦ Assess for operation of automobile and/or other dangerous machinery.
✦ Assess patient/family knowledge about condition and need for medication.
✦ In collaboration with physician, periodically assess CBC, urinalysis, and liver function tests.
✦ **Withdrawal:** Assess for symptoms of withdrawal: • nausea • vomiting • abdominal cramping • headache • fatigue • weakness • mental depression • suicidal ideations.
✦ **Withdrawal Management:** Monitor vital signs.
◊ Place patient in quiet room with low stimuli.
◊ Allow patient to sleep as much as desired.
◊ Observe patient closely (q 15 min).
◊ Institute suicide precautions.
◊ Some physicians may elect to prescribe antidepressants to counteract feelings of depression and lethargy.
✦ **Toxicity and Overdose:** Assess for symptoms of overdose: • restlessness • tremor • hyperreflexia • fever • rapid respiration • disorientation • belligerence • assaultiveness • hallucinations • panic states (stimulation is usually followed by fatigue and depression) • tachycardia • hypertension or hypotension • nausea • vomiting • diarrhea • abdominal cramping • convulsions • coma • circulatory collapse • death.

+ **Overdose Management:** Monitor vital signs.
◊ Maintain adequate airway.
◊ Initiate gastric lavage.
◊ Institute cardiac monitoring.
◊ Administer barbiturate for sedation.
◊ Administer phentolamine to combat severe acute hypertension.
◊ Administer IV fluids and a vasopressor to treat hypotension secondary to hypovolemia.
◊ Administer urine acidifiers to promote urinary excretion of the drug.
◊ Hemodialysis and peritoneal dialysis are not effective.

Potential Nursing Diagnoses

+ High risk for injury related to overstimulation and hyperactivity; abrupt mazindol withdrawal; overdose.
+ High risk for self-directed violence related to suicidal ideations resulting from abrupt mazindol withdrawal.
+ Alteration in nutrition, more than body requires, related to excessive intake in relation to metabolic needs.
+ Sleep pattern disturbance related to overstimulation from mazindol use.
+ Alteration in thought processes related to adverse mazindol effects of overstimulation and difficulty concentrating.
+ Knowledge deficit related to medication regimen.

Plan/Implementation

+ Monitor medication effects. Tolerance develops rapidly. If anorexigenic effects begin to diminish, notify physician immediately. Patient should be on reduced-calorie diet and program of regular exercise in addition to the medication.
+ Monitor and record vital signs at regular intervals (bid) throughout therapy.
+ Encourage use of sugarless gum, hard candy, or frequent sips of water for patient who experiences dry mouth. Ensure that patient practices good oral care (frequent brushing, flossing).

+ Ensure that patient is protected from injury. Keep stimuli low and environment as quiet as possible to discourage overstimulation.
+ Ensure that tablet has been swallowed and not "cheeked" to avoid medication or to hoard for later use.
+ Tablets may be crushed and mixed with food or fluid for patient who has difficulty swallowing.
+ To prevent insomnia, ensure that last dose is administered at least 6 hours before retiring.
+ Drug should be administered 60 minutes before meals. May be given with meals if GI discomfort occurs.
+ Store medication at controlled room temperatures between 15° and 30°C (59°–86°F). Protect from heat and moisture.

Patient/Family Education

+ Use caution in driving or when operating dangerous machinery. Drowsiness, dizziness, and blurred vision can occur.
+ Do not stop taking the drug abruptly. To do so can produce serious withdrawal symptoms.
+ Medication may be taken with meals if GI upset occurs.
+ If insomnia is a problem, avoid taking medication late in the day. Take no later than 6 hours before bedtime.
+ Do not take other medications (including over-the-counter drugs) without physician's approval. Many medications contain substances that, in combination with mazindol, can be harmful.
+ Monitor blood sugar of diabetic patient bid or tid, or as instructed by physician. Be aware of need for possible alteration in insulin requirements due to changes in food intake, weight, and activity.
+ Avoid consumption of large amounts of caffeinated products (coffee, tea, colas, chocolate), as they may enhance the stimulant effect of mazindol.
+ Follow reduced-calorie diet provided

by dietitian and a program of regular exercise. Do not exceed recommended dose if appetite suppressant effect diminishes. Contact physician.

♦ Notify physician if restlessness, insomnia, anorexia, or dry mouth become severe or if rapid and pounding heartbeat becomes evident.

♦ Do not take mazindol during pregnancy. There may be a risk to a fetus with this medication. Inform physician immediately if pregnancy is suspected or planned.

♦ Be aware of potential side effects of mazindol. Refer to written materials furnished by healthcare providers for safe self-administration.

♦ Carry card or other identification at all times describing medications being taken.

Evaluation

♦ Patient demonstrates a progressive weight loss with the use of mazindol as an adjunct to reduced caloric intake and a program of regular exercise.

♦ Patient verbalizes understanding of side effects and regimen required for prudent self-administration of mazindol.

MEPHENYTOIN

(me-fen′i-toyn)
Mesantoin

Classification(s):
Anticonvulsant, Hydantoin
Pregnancy Category C

INDICATIONS

♦ Tonic-clonic (grand mal) seizures ♦ Partial seizures with complex symptomatology (psychomotor) ♦ Partial seizures (focal) ♦ Partial seizures with motor symptoms (Jacksonian).

ACTION

♦ Hydantoins act by increasing the seizure threshold in the cerebral cortex. By promoting sodium efflux from neurons in the motor cortex, they encourage stabilization of the threshold against hyperexcitability. Maximal activity of the brainstem centers responsible for the tonic phase of grand mal seizures is also reduced.

PHARMACOKINETICS

Absorption: Rapidly absorbed following oral administration.
Distribution: Rapidly and widely distributed. Crosses placental barrier and is excreted in breast milk.
Metabolism and Excretion: Metabolized by the liver into active metabolites that are excreted by the kidneys.
Half-Life: 144 hours.

CONTRAINDICATIONS AND PRECAUTIONS

Contraindicated: ♦ Hypersensitivity to this drug or to other hydantoins ♦ Lactation ♦ Concomitant use of oxazolidinediones (paramethadione, trimethadione).
Use Cautiously in: ♦ Hepatic or renal dysfunction ♦ Pregnancy ♦ Elderly or debilitated patients.

ADVERSE REACTIONS AND SIDE EFFECTS*

CNS: nystagmus, ataxia, <u>drowsiness</u>, dizziness, headache, diplopia, insomnia, fatigue, depression, choreiform movements.
Derm: skin rashes, exfoliative dermatitis, erythema multiforme.
GI: <u>nausea</u>, vomiting, constipation, toxic hepatitis, jaundice.
Hemat: blood dyscrasias (thrombocytopenia, leukopenia, agranulocytosis, pancytopenia, neutropenia, aplastic anemia, hemolytic anemia).

---

*<u>Underlines</u> indicate most frequent; CAPITALS indicate life-threatening.

Other: lymphadenopathy, osteomalacia, hyperglycemia, conjunctivitis, weight gain, edema, photophobia, alopecia.

INTERACTIONS

Drug-Drug: ✦ **Trimethoprim, amiodarone, benzodiazepines, disulfiram, isoniazid, phenylbutazone, chloramphenicol, cimetidine, sulfonamides, salicylates, acute alcohol intake, phenothiazines:** increased effect of mephenytoin (increased risk of toxicity). ✦ **Barbiturates, diazoxide, rifampin, antineoplastic agents, chronic alcohol abuse, antacids, calcium gluconate, carbamazepine:** decreased effects of mephenytoin ✦ **Phenobarbital, valproic acid, sodium valproate:** increased or decreased effects of either drug ✦ **Coumarin anticoagulants:** increased effects of mephenytoin, increased or decreased anticoagulant effects ✦ **Quinidine:** decreased antiarrhythmic effects ✦ **Corticosteroids:** decreased efficacy of corticosteroids ✦ **Oral contraceptives:** decreased efficacy of oral contraceptives ✦ **Digitoxin:** decreased effects of digitoxin ✦ **Furosemide:** decreased effects of furosemide ✦ **Theophylline:** decreased efficacy of both drugs ✦ **Doxycycline:** decreased effects of doxycycline ✦ **Levodopa:** decreased effects of levodopa ✦ **Primidone:** increased primidone effects ✦ **Dopamine:** decreased effects of dopamine.

Drug-Food: ✦ **Vitamin K, vitamin D:** patient may need supplemental intake of these nutrients while on mephenytoin ✦ **Folic acid:** alteration in metabolism of either or both could result in decreased effects of mephenytoin or a serum folate deficiency.

ROUTE AND DOSAGE

(Usually administered with phenytoin, phenobarbital, or primidone.)

Tonic-Clonic, Psychomotor, Focal, and Jacksonian Seizures

✦ **PO (Adults):** Initially, 50–100 mg/day in single daily dose for first week;

increase dose by 50–100 mg/week until maintenance dose achieved. Maintenance: 200–600 mg/day in 3 equally divided doses (up to 800 mg/day may be required by some patients).

✦ **PO (Children):** Initially, 50–100 mg/day for first week; increase dose by 50–100 mg/week until maintenance dose achieved. Maintenance: 100–400 mg/day in 3 equally divided doses.

✦ **PO (Replacement Therapy):** 50–100 mg/day during first week. Dosage of mephenytoin is gradually increased each week as dosage of drug being replaced is gradually decreased, except when replacing phenobarbital, which should be continued at regular dosage until full dosage of mephenytoin is attained.

PHARMACODYNAMICS

Route	Onset	Peak	Duration
PO	30 min	2–4 hr	24–48 hr

NURSING IMPLICATIONS

Assessment

✦ Assess occurrence, characteristics, and duration of seizure activity.
✦ Assess baseline vital signs.
✦ Assess history of allergies, sensitivity to this drug and/or other drugs.
✦ Assess date of last menses (possible pregnancy), use of contraceptives.
✦ Assess whether currently breast-feeding a child.
✦ Assess current and past alcohol and drug consumption.
✦ Assess for symptoms of possible blood dyscrasias: ● sore throat ● fever ● malaise ● unusual bleeding ● easy bruising ● glandular swelling ● cutaneous reactions.
✦ Assess CBC. Blood dyscrasias have occurred as early as 2 weeks and as late as 30 months after initiation of therapy. Blood examinations are recommended on the following schedule: Before starting therapy; every 2 weeks until maintenance dose established and 2 weeks after establishment of

maintenance dose; monthly for 1 year after maintenance dose established; then every 3 months. If neutrophil level drops to between 1600 and 2500/mm³, counts should be taken every 2 weeks. Discontinue medication if count drops below 1600/mm³.

♦ Assess for presence of adverse reactions or side effects.

♦ Assess patient's and family's response to diagnosis of epilepsy.

♦ Assess patient/family knowledge about illness and need for medication.

♦ In collaboration with physician, assess CBC and renal and liver function tests in patients on prolonged mephenytoin therapy.

♦ **Lab Test Alterations:** May increase serum glucose, bromsulphalein, and alkaline phosphatase.

◊ May decrease protein-bound iodine and urinary steroid levels.

♦ **Toxicity Overdose:** Range of therapeutic serum concentration of mephenytoin and its major metabolite is 25–40 mcg/mL.

◊ Assess for toxic skin and mucous membrane manifestations, such as rashes, dermatitis, pigmentation changes.

◊ Assess for symptoms of toxicity/overdose: • ataxia • confusion • nausea • vomiting • slurred speech • dizziness • bone marrow depression.

♦ **Overdose Management:** Monitor vital signs.

◊ Maintain adequate airway.

◊ Induce vomiting in conscious patient.

◊ Initiate gastric lavage if patient is unconscious.

◊ Administer IV fluids and vasopressors to control hypotension.

◊ Use mechanical ventilation if required.

◊ Hemodialysis may be considered.

Potential Nursing Diagnoses

♦ High risk for injury related to seizures; mephenytoin's side effects such as dizziness, drowsiness, decreased mental alertness; possible toxic serum levels

of mephenytoin; abrupt withdrawal from mephenytoin use.

♦ Impaired adjustment related to difficulty accepting diagnosis of epilepsy.

♦ Social isolation related to fear of experiencing a seizure in the presence of others.

♦ High risk for activity intolerance related to mephenytoin's side effects of drowsiness, dizziness, decreased mental alertness.

♦ Knowledge deficit related to medication regimen.

Plan/Implementation

♦ Monitor vital signs at regular intervals (bid or tid) throughout therapy.

♦ Monitor serum mephenytoin levels. Record and report to physician.

♦ Observe frequently (every hour) for occurrence of seizure activity.

♦ Ensure that patient is protected from injury. Supervise and assist with ambulation if dizziness and drowsiness are problems. Ensure that patient avoids participation in any activity requiring mental alertness (including smoking). Pad siderails and head of bed with towels or blanket to protect patient who experiences seizures during the night.

♦ Perform urine checks daily following initiation of therapy to determine if hyperglycemia has occurred.

♦ Administer medication with food to minimize GI irritation and to enhance absorption.

♦ For patient who has difficulty swallowing, tablet may be crushed and mixed with food or fluid.

♦ Store medication at controlled room temperatures between 15° and 30°C (59°–86°F). Protect from heat and moisture.

Patient/Family Education

♦ Do not drive or operate dangerous machinery until individual response is determined. Drowsiness and decreased mental alertness can occur.

♦ Do not stop taking drug abruptly. To

do so could precipitate status epilepticus.

♦ Avoid alcoholic beverages.

♦ Maintain good oral care to minimize side effect of gingival hyperplasia.

♦ Carry or wear at all times identification informing others of illness and medication usage.

♦ Do not take any other medication without approval from physician. Combining drugs may be harmful.

♦ Promptly report any of the following symptoms to physician: sore throat • fever • malaise • ataxia • skin rash • severe nausea or vomiting • swollen glands, yellow skin or eyes • unusual bleeding • easy bruising • or dark urine.

♦ Be aware of possible risks of taking mephenytoin during pregnancy. Patient who requires the medication to prevent seizures may be maintained on it; however, she must be fully aware of potential risks to unborn child. There is a strong association between the use of anticonvulsant drugs by women with epilepsy and the incidence of birth defects in their children. A possible association has also been suggested between maternal use of anticonvulsants and a neonatal coagulation defect that poses a threat of serious bleeding during the first 24 hours of life. Notify physician immediately if pregnancy occurs, is suspected, or is planned.

♦ Because mephenytoin decreases the effectiveness of oral contraceptives, use alternative method of birth control during therapy.

♦ To protect patient during a seizure, padding (towels, blankets, pillows) may be used to prevent bumping against hard objects. When convulsion has subsided, turn patient on side to allow secretions to drain and to prevent aspiration. Keep records of occurrence, characteristics, and duration of seizures, so that accurate reports may be given to physician for providing assistance in stabilization and control of seizures. If patient has difficulty breathing or continues to experience subsequent seizures, family should immediately call for emergency assistance.

♦ Be aware of possible side effects of mephenytoin. Refer to written materials which have been furnished by healthcare providers to assist in self-administration.

Evaluation

♦ Patient demonstrates stabilization of seizure activity with regular administration of mephenytoin.

♦ Patient verbalizes understanding of necessity for, side effects of, and regimen required for prudent self-administration of mephenytoin.

MEPHOBARBITAL

(me-foe-bar'bi-tal)
Mebaral

Classification(s):
Anticonvulsant, Barbiturate, CNS depressant, Sedative/hypnotic agent
Schedule C IV
Pregnancy Category D

INDICATIONS

♦ Tonic-clonic (grand mal) and absence (petit mal) seizures (prophylactic management) ♦ Moderate anxiety states.

ACTION

♦ Thought to reduce monosynaptic and polysynaptic transmission, resulting in decreased excitability of the entire nerve cell ♦ Barbiturates also increase the threshold for electrical stimulation of the motor cortex.

PHARMACOKINETICS

Absorption: Approximately 50% absorbed from the GI tract.
Distribution: Rapidly and widely dis-

tributed. Crosses blood-brain and placental barriers; excreted in breast milk.

Metabolism and Excretion: Metabolized by the liver (75% metabolized to phenobarbital); excreted by the kidneys as metabolites and unchanged drug.

Half-Life: 34 hours.

CONTRAINDICATIONS AND PRECAUTIONS

Contraindicated in: ♦ Hypersensitivity to the drug ♦ Severe hepatic, renal, cardiac, or respiratory disease ♦ Pregnancy and lactation ♦ Individuals with a history of previous addiction ♦ Porphyria.

Use Cautiously in: ♦ Elderly or debilitated patients ♦ Hepatic, renal, or respiratory dysfunction ♦ Depressed/suicidal patients.

ADVERSE REACTIONS AND SIDE EFFECTS*

CNS: drowsiness, headache, lethargy, dizziness, ataxia, residual sedation ("hangover"), confusion, paradoxical excitement.

CV: hypotension, bradycardia.

Derm: skin rashes, urticaria, dermatitis.

GI: nausea/vomiting, constipation, diarrhea, epigastric pain.

Hemat: AGRANULOCYTOSIS, THROMBOCYTOPENIA.

Resp: hypoventilation, RESPIRATORY DEPRESSION.

Other: tolerance, physical and psychological dependence.

INTERACTIONS

Drug-Drug: ♦ Other CNS depressants (including alcohol, benzodiazepines, opiates, tricylic antidepressants): additive CNS depression ♦ Chloramphenicol, MAO inhibitors, valproic acid, disulfiram, cimetidine: increased effects of mephobarbital ♦ Phenytoin: increased or decreased effects of either drug (close monitoring of serum levels required to control seizure activity) ♦ Oral contraceptives: decreased effectiveness of oral contraceptives ♦ Oral anticoagulants: decreased anticoagulant effects ♦ Corticosteroids, digitoxin, doxycycline: decreased effects of these drugs ♦ Furosemide: orthostatic hypotension ♦ Theophyllines, quinidine: decreased effects of these drugs ♦ Methoxyflurane: increased nephrotoxic effects of methoxyflurane ♦ Oral beta-adrenergic blockers: decreased effects of these drugs ♦ Griseofulvin: decreased griseofulvin levels.

Drug-Food: ♦ Vitamin D: increased vitamin D metabolism, possible deficiency ♦ Folic acid: decreased absorption of folic acid, possible deficiency.

ROUTE AND DOSAGE

Tonic-Clonic (Grand Mal) and Absence (Petit Mal) Seizures

♦ **PO (Adults):** 400–600 mg/day.
♦ **PO (Children 5 Years and Older):** 32–64 mg tid or qid.
♦ **PO (Children Under 5):** 16–32 mg tid or qid.
♦ **Combination Therapy:** When used in combination with phenobarbital, dose should be about one-half the amount of each used alone. When used concurrently with phenytoin, a reduced dose of phenytoin is recommended, but full dose of mephobarbital may be given.
♦ **Replacement Therapy:** Gradually increase dose of mephobarbital as dose of medication being replaced is gradually decreased.
♦ **Discontinuation of Therapy:** Withdraw or decrease dose over a period of 4–5 days to prevent precipitation of seizures or status epilepticus.

Anxiety

♦ **PO (Adults):** 32–100 mg tid or qid.
♦ **PO (Children):** 16–32 mg tid or qid.

---

*Underlines indicate most frequent; CAPITALS indicate life-threatening.

PHARMACODYNAMICS

Route	Onset	Peak	Duration
PO	60 min or more	10–12 hr	*

*Varies with dose and duration of administration.

NURSING IMPLICATIONS
Assessment

* Assess occurrence, characteristics, and duration of seizure activity.
* Assess baseline vital signs.
* Assess level of anxiety. Symptoms include: • restlessness • pacing • insomnia • inability to concentrate • increased heart rate • increased respiration • elevated blood pressure • confusion • tremors • rapid speech.
* Assess for suicidal ideation in depressed patients.
* Assess history of allergies, sensitivity to this drug or to other barbiturates.
* Assess date of last menses (possible pregnancy), use of contraceptives.
* Assess whether currently breast-feeding a child.
* Assess current and past alcohol and drug consumption.
* Assess operation of automobile and/or other dangerous machinery.
* Assess for presence of adverse reactions or side effects.
* Assess patient/family knowledge about illness and need for medication.
* In collaboration with physician, assess CBC and renal and liver function tests in patients on prolonged therapy.
* **Lab Test Alterations:** May increase values of bromsulphalein (BSP) retention and protein-bound iodine (PBI).
* **Withdrawal:** Assess for symptoms of withdrawal: • anxiety • tremors • insomnia • nausea/vomiting • weakness • diaphoresis • orthostatic hypotension • delirium • convulsions.
* **Withdrawal Management:** Monitor vital signs.
◊ Place patient in quiet room with low stimuli.

◊ Institute seizure precautions.
◊ Phenytoin may be ordered to prevent seizures.
◊ Some physicians may order oxazepam as needed for objective withdrawal symptoms, gradually decreasing dosage until the drug is discontinued.
* **Toxicity and Overdose:** Assess for symptoms of toxicity: • confusion • drowsiness • dyspnea • slurred speech • staggering.
◊ Assess for symptoms of overdose: • CNS and respiratory depression • hypoventilation • hypothermia • hypotension •oliguria • tachycardia • coma. (May progress to respiratory arrest, circulatory collapse, and death.)
* **Overdose Management:** Monitor vital signs.
◊ Maintain adequate airway.
◊ Induce vomiting in conscious patient.
◊ Initiate gastric lavage in unconscious patient.
◊ Administer activated charcoal to minimize absorption of drug.
◊ Administer IV fluids.
◊ Effect alkalinization of urine to increase renal excretion.
◊ Forced diuresis or hemodialysis may be used in severe intoxication.

Potential Nursing Diagnoses

* Ineffective breathing pattern related to possible side effect of hypoventilation.
* High risk for injury related to seizures; abrupt withdrawal from long-term use; decreased mental alertness cause by side effect of residual sedation; side effects of dizziness and ataxia; effects of overdose.
* High risk for self-directed violence related to depressed mood.
* Anxiety (specify level) related to threats to physical integrity and/or self-concept.
* Sleep pattern disturbance related to situational crises, physical condition, severe level of anxiety.
* High risk for activity intolerance re-

lated to side effects of residual sedation, drowsiness, dizziness.

+ Knowledge deficit related to medication regimen.

Plan/Implementation

+ Monitor vital signs before beginning therapy and at regular intervals (bid) throughout therapy.

+ Observe frequently (every hour) for occurrence of seizure activity.

+ Ensure that patient is protected from injury. Supervise and assist with ambulation if dizziness and drowsiness are problems. Ensure that patient avoids participation in any activity requiring mental alertness (including smoking). Pad siderails and head of bed for patient who experiences seizures during the night.

+ To minimize nausea, medication may be given with food or milk.

+ Ensure that tablet has been swallowed and not "cheeked" to avoid medication or to hoard for later use.

+ Crush tablet and mix with food or fluid for patient who has difficulty swallowing.

+ Store medication in controlled room temperatures between 15° and 30°C (59°–86°F). Protect from heat and moisture.

Patient/Family Education

+ Do not drive or operate dangerous machinery until individual response is determined. Drowsiness and dizziness can occur.

+ Do not stop taking the drug abruptly. To do so can produce serious (even life-threatening) withdrawal symptoms. Could precipitate status epilepticus. If a dose is missed, take it as close as possible to the prescribed time. If it is already close to time for next dose, wait until then; do not double up on dose at the next prescribed time.

+ Do not consume other CNS depressants (including alcohol).

+ Be aware of the risks of taking barbiturates during pregnancy (congeni-

tal malformations may be associated with use during the first trimester). Also, evidence of withdrawal symptoms has been observed in neonates born to mothers who had ingested barbiturates regularly during the last trimester of pregnancy. Notify physician if pregnancy is suspected or planned.

+ To protect patient during a seizure, padding (towels, blankets, pillows) may be used to prevent bumping against hard objects. When convulsion has subsided, turn patient on side to allow secretions to drain and to prevent aspiration. Keep records of occurrence, characteristics, and duration of seizures, so that accurate reports may be given to physician for providing assistance in stabilization and control of seizures. If patient has difficulty breathing or continues to experience subsequent seizures, family should call for emergency assistance immediately.

+ Because barbiturates decrease effectiveness of oral contraceptives, use alternative methods of birth control during mephobarbital therapy.

+ Be aware of potential side effects. Refer to written materials furnished by healthcare providers regarding correct method of self-administration.

+ Report symptoms of sore throat, fever, malaise, unusual bleeding, or easy bruising to physician immediately.

+ Carry card or other identification at all times stating names of medications being taken.

Evaluation

+ Patient demonstrates stabilization of seizure activity with regular administration of mephobarbital.

+ Patient demonstrates a subsiding/resolution of the symptoms of anxiety for which mephobarbital was prescribed.

+ Patient verbalizes understanding of side effects and regimen required for prudent self-administration of mephobarbital.

MEPROBAMATE

(me-proe-ba'mate)
Equanil, Meprospan, Meribam, Miltown, {Mep-Tran}, Neuramate, {Novomepro}

Classification(s):
Antianxiety agent, Propanediol carbamate derivative
Schedule C IV
Pregnancy Category D

INDICATIONS

♦ Anxiety disorders ♦ Anxiety symtpoms (temporary relief).

ACTION

♦ Depresses multiple sites in the central nervous system, including the hypothalamus, thalamus, limbic system, and spinal cord.

PHARMACOKINETICS

Absorption: Rapid absorption from the GI tract.
Distribution: Is widely distributed. Crosses placenta (plasma levels at or near maternal levels); excreted in breast milk (at levels 2–4 times maternal levels).
Metabolism and Excretion: Metabolized by the liver, excreted in urine and feces.
Half-Life: 6–16 hours.

CONTRAINDICATIONS AND PRECAUTIONS

Contraindicated in: ♦ Hypersensitivity to the drug ♦ Combination with other CNS depressants ♦ Children under 6 ♦ Pregnancy and lactation ♦ Acute intermittent porphyria.
Use Cautiously in: ♦ Elderly or debilitated patients ♦ Hepatic or renal dysfunction ♦ Individuals with history of drug abuse/addiction ♦ Patients with a history of seizure disorders ♦ Depressed/suicidal patients.

ADVERSE REACTIONS AND SIDE EFFECTS*

CNS: <u>drowsiness</u>, <u>dizziness</u>, <u>ataxia</u>, headache, vertigo, weakness, <u>slurred speech</u>, paresthesias, depression, anxiety, seizures, euphoria, paradoxical excitement.
CV: tachycardia, hypotension, ECG changes, palpitations, arrhythmias, syncope.
Derm: skin rash, itching, bruising.
GI: dry mouth, nausea/vomiting, diarrhea, anorexia.
GU: oliguria.
Hemat: agranulocytosis.
Other: anaphylaxis, fever, chills, exacerbation of porphyric symptoms, tolerance, physical and psychological dependence.

INTERACTIONS

Drug-Drug: ♦ **Other CNS depressants (including alcohol, barbiturates, opiates), antipsychotics, antidepressants, antihistamines:** additive CNS depressant effects.

ROUTE AND DOSAGE

Anxiety, Anxiety Disorders

♦ **PO (Adults):** 400 mg tid or qid, or 600 mg bid. Maximum daily dose: 2400 mg. Sustained-release: 400–800 mg q a.m. and at H.S.
♦ **PO (Children Ages 6–12):** 100–200 mg bid or tid. Sustained-release: 200 mg q a.m. and at H.S.

PHARMACODYNAMICS

Route	Onset	Peak	Duration
PO	<60 min	1–3 hr	*

*Varies with individual, age, disease state, number of doses.

{} = Only available in Canada.
*<u>Underlines</u> indicate most frequent; CAPITALS indicate life-threatening.

NURSING IMPLICATIONS
Assessment

♦ Assess level of anxiety: • restlessness • pacing • insomnia • inability to concentrate • increased heart rate • increased respiration • elevated blood pressure • confusion • tremors • rapid speech.

♦ Assess for suicidal ideation in depressed patients.

♦ Assess history of allergies, sensitivity to this drug.

♦ Assess date of last menses (possible pregnancy), use of contraceptives.

♦ Assess whether currently breast-feeding a child.

♦ Assess current and past alcohol and drug consumption.

♦ Assess operation of automobile and/or other dangerous machinery.

♦ Assess for presence of adverse reactions or side effects.

♦ Assess patient/family knowledge about illness and need for medication.

♦ In collaboration with physician, assess CBC and renal and liver function tests in patients on long-term therapy.

♦ **Lab Test Alterations:** May cause false increase in urinary steroid values.

♦ **Withdrawal:** Assess for symptoms of withdrawal: • depression • insomnia • increased anxiety • abdominal and muscle cramps • tremors • vomiting • sweating • convulsions • delirium.

♦ **Withdrawal Management:** Monitor vital signs.

◊ Place patient in quiet room with low stimuli.

◊ Institute seizure precautions.

◊ A long-acting barbiturate, such as phenobarbital, may be ordered to suppress withdrawal symptoms.

◊ Phenytoin may be ordered to prevent seizures.

◊ Some physicians may order oxazepam as needed for objective withdrawal symptoms, gradually decreasing dosage until the drug is discontinued.

♦ **Toxicity and Overdose:** Assess serum concentrations of meprobamate. Therapeutic range is 5–20 mcg/mL.

◊ Assess for symptoms of intoxication: • euphoria • relaxation • drowsiness • slurred speech • disorientation • mood lability • incoordination • unsteady gait • disinhibition of sexual and aggressive impulses • judgment and/or memory impairment.

◊ Assess for symptoms of overdose. Serum concentrations of 30–100 mcg/mL may produce symptoms of slurred speech, ataxia, stupor, light coma. At 100–200 mcg/mL, symptoms of respiratory depression, deeper coma, and possibly death can occur. Levels greater than 200 mcg/mL are frequently fatal.

♦ **Overdose Management:** Monitor vital signs.

◊ Maintain adequate airway.

◊ Induce emesis in conscious patient.

◊ Initiate gastric lavage in unconscious patient.

◊ Monitor I&O.

◊ Counteract hypotension with IV fluid therapy, but avoid overhydration, as fatal pulmonary edema has occurred.

◊ Pressor agents may be required.

◊ Forced diuresis or hemodialysis may be instituted.

Potential Nursing Diagnoses

♦ High risk for injury related to seizures; panic anxiety; abrupt withdrawal from long-term meprobamate use; effects of overdose.

♦ High risk for self-directed violence related to depressed mood.

♦ Anxiety (specify level) related to threats to physical integrity and/or self-concept.

♦ High risk for activity intolerance related to meprobamate's side effects of drowsiness, dizziness, muscular weakness, or ataxia.

♦ Knowledge deficit related to medication regimen.

Plan/Implementation

* Monitor vital signs before beginning therapy, and at regular intervals (bid) throughout therapy.
* To minimize nausea, medication may be given with food or milk.
* Ensure that patient practices good oral care. Offer hard, sugarless candy; gum; or frequent sips of water if dry mouth is a problem.
* Ensure that patient is protected from injury. Supervise and assist with ambulation if dizziness and muscular weakness are problems. Pad siderails and headboard for patient who experiences seizures.
* Ensure that tablet or capsule has been swallowed and not "cheeked" to avoid medication or to hoard for later use.
* Tablets and capsules should not be crushed or chewed.
* Store medication at controlled room temperatures between 15° and 30°C (59°–86°F). Protect from heat and moisture.

Patient/Family Education

* Do not drive or operate dangerous machinery. Drowsiness and dizziness can occur.
* Do not stop taking the drug abruptly. Doing so can result in serious withdrawal symptoms.
* Do not consume other CNS depressants (including alcohol).
* Do not take nonprescription medication without approval from physician.
* Do not crush or chew tablets or capsules. Swallow whole.
* Be aware of risks of taking meprobamate during pregnancy (congenital malformations have been associated with use during first trimester). Notify physician of desirability to discontinue drug if pregnancy is suspected or planned.
* Be aware of potential side effects. Refer to written materials furnished by healthcare providers regarding correct method of self-administration.
* Report symptoms of skin rash, sore throat, fever, unusual bleeding, or easy bruising to physician immediately.
* Carry card or piece of paper at all times stating names of medications being taken.

Evaluation

* Patient demonstrates a subsiding/resolution of the symptoms for which meprobamate was prescribed (anxiety symptoms, anxiety disorders).
* Patient verbalizes understanding of side effects and regimen required for prudent self-administration of meprobamate.

MESORIDAZINE

(mez-oh-rid'a-zeen)
Serentil

Classification(s):
Antipsychotic, Neuroleptic, Phenothiazine
Pregnancy Category C

INDICATIONS

* Schizophrenia * Behavioral problems in mental deficiency and chronic brain syndrome * Acute and chronic alcoholism * Manifestations of psychoneurotic and personality disorders.

ACTION

* The exact mechanism of antipsychotic action is not fully understood, but is probably related to the drug's antidopaminergic effects * Antipsychotics may block postsynaptic dopamine receptors in the basal ganglia, hypothalamus, limbic system, brain stem, and medulla * Antipsychotic effects also appear to be related to inhibition of dopamine-mediated neurotransmission at the synapses * Antipsychotic effects may also result from the drug's alpha-adrenergic blocking, muscarinic blocking, and adrenergic activity, as well as effects on other amines (such as GABA) or peptides.

PHARMACOKINETICS

Absorption: Rapidly absorbed in oral tablet dosage forms. Genetic differences in rate of first-pass metabolism results in a wide range of bioavailability from individual to individual. Oral liquid preparations and IM administration result in more consistent absorption.

Distribution: Widely distributed. Highly lipophilic; accumulates in the brain, lungs, and other tissues with high blood supply. Crosses placental barrier. Enters breast milk.

Metabolism and Excretion: Metabolized by the liver and in the kidneys. Excreted through kidneys and enterohepatic circulation. Active metabolites accumulate and are stored in fatty tissue over a prolonged period of time and may be detected in urine up to 3–6 months following discontinuation of the drug.

Half-Life: Not well established.

CONTRAINDICATIONS AND PRECAUTIONS

Contraindicated in: ✦ Hypersensitivity to this drug or to other phenothiazines ✦ Comatose or severely CNS-depressed patients ✦ Presence of large amounts of CNS depressants ✦ Bone marrow depression ✦ Blood dyscrasias ✦ Subcortical brain damage ✦ Parkinson's disease ✦ Hepatic, renal, and/or cardiac insufficiency ✦ Severe hypotension or hypertension ✦ Children under 12 years of age; pregnancy and lactation (safe use not established).

Use Cautiously in: ✦ Patients with a history of seizures ✦ Respiratory, renal, hepatic, thyroid, or cardiovascular disorders (e.g., respiratory infection, COPD, thyrotoxicosis, mitral insufficiency, angina pectoris) ✦ Prostatic hypertrophy ✦ Glaucoma ✦ Diabetes ✦ Elderly or debilitated patients ✦ Patients exposed to high or low environmental temperatures or to organophosphate insecticides ✦ Hypocalcemia ✦ History of severe reactions to insulin or ECT ✦ Pediatric patients with acute illnesses or dehydration.

ADVERSE REACTIONS AND SIDE EFFECTS*

CNS: sedation, headache, seizures, insomnia, dizziness, exacerbation of psychotic symptoms, extrapyramidal symptoms (pseudoparkinsonism, akathisia, akinesia, dystonia, oculogyric crisis), tardive dyskinesia, fatigue, cerebral edema, ataxia, blurred vision, NEUROLEPTIC MALIGNANT SYNDROME, restlessness, anxiety, depression, hyperthermia or hypothermia.

CV: hypotension, orthostatic hypotension, hypertension, tachycardia, bradycardia, CARDIAC ARREST, ECG changes, ARRHYTHMIAS, PULMONARY EDEMA, CIRCULATORY COLLAPSE.

Derm: skin rashes, urticaria, petechiae, seborrhea, photosensitivity, eczema, erythema, hyperpigmentation, contact dermatitis, EXFOLIATIVE DERMATITIS (rare).

Endo: galactorrhea, gynecomastia (men), changes in libido, impotence, hyperglycemia or hypoglycemia, amenorrhea, retrograde ejaculation.

GI: dry mouth, nausea, vomiting, increased appetite and weight gain, anorexia, dyspepsia, constipation, diarrhea, jaundice, polydipsia, PARALYTIC ILEUS.

GU: urinary retention, frequency or incontinence, bladder paralysis, polyuria, enuresis, priapism.

Hemat: AGRANULOCYTOSIS, LEUKOPENIA, ANEMIA, THROMBOCYTOPENIA, PANCYTOPENIA.

Ophth: lens deposition.

Resp: LARYNGEAL EDEMA, LARYNGOSPASM, BRONCHOSPASM, SUPPRESSION OF COUGH REFLEX.

Other: decreased sweating.

INTERACTIONS

Drug-Drug: ✦ **CNS depressants (including alcohol, barbiturates, narcotics, anesthetics):** additive CNS depressant effects ✦ **Anticholinergic**

---

*Underlines indicate most frequent; CAPITALS indicate life-threatening.

agents (e.g., atropine): additive anticholinergic effects, decreased antipsychotic effects ✦ **Barbiturate anesthetics:** increased incidence of excitatory effects and hypotension ✦ **Barbiturates:** possible decreased effects of phenothiazines ✦ **Metyrosine:** potentiation of extrapyramidal side effects ✦ **Levodopa:** decreased efficacy of levodopa ✦ **Quinidine:** additive cardiac depressive effects ✦ **Magnesium- or aluminum-containing antidiarrheal mixtures, antacids:** reduced phenothiazine absorption/effectiveness ✦ **Guanethidine:** decreased antihypertensive action ✦ **Lithium:** decreased plasma levels and effect of antipsychotic drug; severe neurotoxicity reported ✦ **Epinephrine:** reversal of usual pressor action of epinephrine, resulting in decreased blood pressure and tachycardia ✦ **Bromocriptine:** impairment of prolactin-suppressing action ✦ **Angiotensin converting enzyme (ACE) inhibitors:** increased effects of ACE inhibitors ✦ **Phenytoin:** decreased phenytoin metabolism, increased risk of toxicity ✦ **Polypeptide antibiotics:** possible neuromuscular respiratory depression ✦ **Metrizamide:** seizures ✦ **Cimetidine:** decreased effect of phenothiazines ✦ **Clonidine:** possibility of severe hypotension ✦ **Piperazine:** increased seizure potential.
Drug-Food: ✦ **Caffeine-containing beverages (e.g., coffee, tea, colas):** counteracted antipsychotic effect.

ROUTE AND DOSAGE

Schizophrenia
✦ **PO (Adults):** Initial dose: 50 mg tid. Optimal total dosage range: 100–400 mg/day.

Behavior Problems in Mental Deficiency and Chronic Brain Syndrome
✦ **PO (Adults):** Initial dose: 25 mg tid. Optimal total dosage range: 75–300 mg/day.

Acute and Chronic Alcoholism
✦ **PO (Adults):** Initial dose: 25 mg bid. Optimal total dosage range: 50–200 mg/day.

Psychoneurotic Manifestations
✦ **PO (Adults):** Initial dose: 10 mg tid. Optimal total dosage range: 30–150 mg/day.

All Indications
✦ **IM:** For most patients, 25 mg initially. Dosage may be repeated in 30–60 minutes if necessary. Maximum IM dose: 200 mg daily.

PHARMACODYNAMICS

Route	Onset*	Peak†	Duration‡
PO	30–60 min	2–4 hr	4–6 hr
IM	15–30 min	1 hr	4–6 hr

*Full clinical effects may not be observed for 4–8 weeks.
†Steady-state plasma levels are achieved in approximately 4–7 days.
‡Drug may be detected in urine for 3–6 months after last dose.

NURSING IMPLICATIONS

Assessment
✦ Assess mental status daily: • mood • appearance • thought and communication patterns • level of interest in the environment and in activities • level of anxiety or agitation • presence of hallucinations or delusions • suspiciousness • interactions with others • ability to carry out activities of daily living.
✦ Assess for symptoms of blood dyscrasias: • sore throat • fever • malaise • unusual bleeding • easy bruising.
✦ Assess for extrapyramidal symptoms: • pseudoparkinsonism (tremors, shuffling gait, drooling, rigidity) • akinesia (muscular weakness) • akathisia (continuous restlessness and fidgeting) • dystonia (involuntary muscular movements of face, arms, legs, and neck) • oculogyric crisis (uncontrolled rolling back of the eyes) • tardive dyskinesia (bizarre facial and tongue movements) • stiff neck • difficulty swallowing.

- Assess for symptoms of neuroleptic malignant syndrome: • hyperpyrexia up to 107°F (41.6°C) • elevated pulse • increased or decreased blood pressure • severe parkinsonian muscle rigidity • elevated creatinine phosphokinase blood levels • elevated white blood count • altered mental status (including catatonic signs or agitation) • acute renal failure • varying levels of consciousness (including stupor and coma) • pallor • diaphoresis • tachycardia • arrhythmias • rhabdomyolysis.
- Assess vital signs, weight. Record baseline values for comparison.
- Assess history of allergies, sensitivity to this drug or to other phenothiazines.
- Assess for signs and symptoms of cholestatic jaundice: • abdominal pain • nausea • rash • fever • yellow skin • flu-like symptoms • abnormal lab test results (eosinophilia, bile in urine, increased serum transaminases, bilirubin, alkaline phosphatase).
- Assess date of last menses (possible pregnancy), use of contraceptives.
- Assess whether currently breast-feeding a child.
- Assess current and past alcohol and drug consumption.
- Assess operation of automobile and/or other dangerous machinery.
- Assess for presence of adverse reactions or side effects.
- Assess patient/family knowledge about illness and need for medication.
- In collaboration with physician, assess CBC, liver function tests, and ophthalmologic exams in patients on long-term therapy.
- **Lab Test Alterations:** Increased serum alkaline phosphatase, transaminases, bilirubin.
- ◇ Increased protein-bound iodine.
- ◇ False-positive urine pregnancy test, possibly caused by drug metabolite that discolors urine (less likely to occur when serum test is used).
- ◇ Increased urinary glucose.

- ◇ Decreased urinary estrogen, progestin, and gonadotropin.
- ◇ Increased plasma cholesterol level.
- ◇ Increased serum prolactin.
- **Withdrawal:** Assess for symptoms of abrupt withdrawal from long-term therapy: • gastritis • nausea • vomiting • dizziness • headache • tachycardia • insomnia • tremulousness • sweating.
- **Toxicity and Overdose:** No correlation has been established between blood level and therapeutic effect.
- ◇ Assess for symptoms of overdose: • CNS depression, from heavy sedation to deep sleep to coma • hypotension • confusion • excitement • extrapyramidal symptoms • agitation • restlessness • convulsions • fever • autonomic reactions • ECG changes • cardiac arrhythmias • tachycardia • hypothermia • tremor • seizures • cyanosis.
- **Overdose Management:** Monitor vital signs.
- ◇ Ensure maintenance of open airway.
- ◇ Initiate gastric lavage.
- ◇ Do not induce emesis (nuchal rigidity may result in aspiration of vomitus).
- ◇ Antiparkinsonian drugs or diphenhydramine may be given to counteract extrapyramidal symptoms.
- ◇ Administer IV fluids or a vasoconstrictor to maintain adequate blood pressure. **Note:** Epinephrine is not recommended due to its interaction with phenothiazines, which causes further drop in blood pressure.
- ◇ Administer IV phenytoin to control ventricular arrhythmias.
- ◇ Administer phenobarbital or diazepam to control convulsions or hyperactivity.
- ◇ Dialysis does not appear to be a useful intervention.

Potential Nursing Diagnoses

- High risk for violence directed at others related to mistrust and panic anxiety.

♦ High risk for injury related to abrupt withdrawal after prolonged use; overdose; mesoridazine's side effects of sedation, dizziness, ataxia, weakness, lowered seizure threshold.

♦ Sensory-perceptual alteration related to panic anxiety evidenced by hallucinations.

♦ Altered thought processes related to panic anxiety evidenced by delusional thinking.

♦ Social isolation related to inability to trust others.

♦ High risk for activity intolerance related to mesoridazine's side effects of drowsiness, dizziness, ataxia, weakness.

♦ Noncompliance with medication regimen related to suspiciousness and mistrust of others.

♦ Knowledge deficit related to medication regimen.

Plan/Implementation

♦ **General Info:** Monitor vital signs before beginning therapy and at regular intervals (bid or tid) throughout therapy. Take BP lying and standing to monitor for possible hypotensive reaction; elderly are particularly susceptible. Dosage adjustment may be required.

◊ Ensure that patient who is ambulatory is protected from sun when spending time outdoors.

◊ Weigh patient 2–3 times a week, at same time of day, on same scale, if possible. A rapid weight gain or evidence of edema should be reported to physician immediately. Record I&O.

◊ Ensure that patient is protected from injury. Provide supervision and assistance when ambulating if dizziness and drowsiness are problems. Pad siderails and headboard for patient who experiences seizures.

◊ Give patient hard candy, gum, or frequent sips of water if dry mouth is a problem.

◊ Store tablets and injection solution at temperatures below 86°F (30°C). Oral concentrate should be stored below 77°F (25°C). All forms should be protected from light.

♦ **PO:** Medication may be administered with food to minimize GI upset.

◊ Ensure that patient swallows tablet and does not "cheek" to avoid medication or to hoard for later use.

◊ Crush tablet and mix with food or fluid for patient who has difficulty swallowing, or use liquid concentrate.

◊ Just prior to administration, mix concentrate with distilled water, acidified tap water, orange juice, or grape juice. Do not prepare and store bulk dilutions.

◊ If concentrate is accidentally spilled on skin or clothing during preparation or administration, wash area immediately, as contact dermatitis can occur.

♦ **IM:** IM injection may be irritating to tissues; avoid SC injection.

◊ Inject slowly and deeply into upper, outer quadrant of buttock. Massage site thoroughly following injection.

◊ Because of possible hypotensive effects, patient should remain in recumbent position for at least one-half hour following IM injection.

◊ Rotate sites when multiple injections are administered.

◊ Do not mix with other agents in the syringe.

◊ Potency is not altered when solution is slightly yellow in color. Discard if marked discoloration is evident.

Patient/Family Education

♦ Use caution when driving or operating dangerous machinery. Drowsiness and dizziness can occur.

♦ Do not stop taking the drug abruptly. To do so might produce withdrawal symptoms, such as nausea, vomiting, gastritis, headache, tachycardia, insomnia, tremulousness.

♦ Use sunscreens and wear protective clothing when spending time outdoors. Skin is more susceptible to sunburn.

♦ Report occurrence of any of the following symptoms to physician immediately: • sore throat • fever • malaise • unusual bleeding • easy bruising • persistent nausea/vomiting • severe headache • rapid heart rate • difficulty urinating • muscle twitching • tremors • darkly colored urine • pale stools • yellow skin or eyes • muscular incoordination • skin rash.

♦ Drug may turn urine pink to reddish-brown in color. This is not significant nor is it harmful.

♦ Rise slowly from a sitting or lying position to prevent a sudden drop in blood pressure.

♦ If dry mouth is a problem, take frequent sips of water, chew sugarless gum, or suck on hard candy. Good oral care (frequent brushing, flossing) is very important.

♦ If some liquid concentrate is spilled on the skin, wash it off immediately. If not, a rash may appear.

♦ Consult physician regarding smoking while on mesoridazine therapy. Smoking increases metabolism of mesoridazine, requiring adjustment in dosage to achieve therapeutic effect.

♦ Dress warmly in cold weather and avoid extended exposure to very high or low temperatures. Body temperature is harder to maintain while using this medication.

♦ Do not drink alcohol while on mesoridazine therapy. These drugs potentiate each other's effects.

♦ Do not consume other medications (including over-the-counter meds) without physician's approval. Many medications contain substances that interact with mesoridazine in a way that may be harmful.

♦ Be aware of possible risks of taking mesoridazine during pregnancy. Safe use during pregnancy and lactation has not been established. Mesoridazine readily crosses the placental barrier, so a fetus could experience adverse effects of the drug. Inform physician immediately if pregnancy occurs, is suspected, or is planned.

♦ Be aware of side effects of mesoridazine. Refer to written materials furnished by healthcare providers for safe self-administration.

♦ Continue to take medication even if feeling well and as though it is not needed. Symptoms may return if medication is discontinued.

♦ Carry card or other identification at all times describing medications being taken.

Evaluation

♦ Patient demonstrates a subsiding/resolution of the symptoms for which mesoridazine was prescribed (severe to panic anxiety, altered thought processes, altered perceptions, agitation).

♦ Patient verbalizes understanding of side effects and regimen required for prudent self-administration of mesoridazine.

METHADONE HCl

(meth'a-done)
Dolophine

Classification(s):
Narcotic agonist analgesic
Schedule C II
Pregnancy Category C

INDICATIONS

♦ Narcotic addiction (detoxification and maintenance treatment) ♦ Severe pain.

ACTION

♦ Binds to opiate receptors in the central and peripheral nervous systems, resulting in alteration in the patient's perception of and emotional response to pain.

PHARMACOKINETICS

Absorption: Well absorbed from all administration routes (PO, IM, SC).
Distribution: Is widely distributed.

Crosses placental barrier; enters breast milk.

Metabolism and Excretion: Metabolized by the liver. Excreted mainly in urine; small amounts excreted in bile and feces.

Half-Life: 13–47 hours (average 25 hours).

CONTRAINDICATIONS AND PRECAUTIONS

Contraindicated in: ♦ Hypersensitivity to narcotics ♦ Children (safety not established).

Use Cautiously in: ♦Head injury, brain tumor, increased intracranial pressure, or comatose patients ♦ Pregnancy and lactation ♦ Renal, hepatic, cardiac, or respiratory insufficiency ♦ Elderly or debilitated patients ♦ Patients with a history of hypotension ♦ Acute alcoholism ♦ Prostatic hypertrophy or urethral stricture ♦ Addison's disease ♦ Hypothyroidism ♦ Severe CNS depression ♦ Anoxia, hypercapnia ♦ Seizures, delirium tremens, shock, untreated myxedema.

ADVERSE REACTIONS AND SIDE EFFECTS*

CNS: dizziness, sedation, euphoria; dysphoria, weakness, headache, seizures, somnolence, pinpoint pupils, insomnia, agitation, tremor, impairment of mental and physical performance, mood changes, disorientation, confusion, visual disturbances, hallucinations, choreiform movements, COMA.

CV: hypotension; flushing or warmness of face, neck, and upper thorax; orthostatic hypotension; bradycardia; palpitations; sweating; syncope, CIRCULATORY DEPRESSION; SHOCK; CARDIAC ARREST.

Derm: skin rashes, wheals and pain at injection site, local tissue irritation and induration following repeated SC injection, pruritus, urticaria.

GI: nausea, vomiting, constipation, dry mouth, anorexia, biliary tract spasm or colic.

GU: urinary retention, urinary hesitancy, antidiuretic effect, decreased libido, impotence, oliguria.

Resp: RESPIRATORY DEPRESSION, RESPIRATORY ARREST, PULMONARY EDEMA.

Other: tolerance, physical and psychological dependence.

INTERACTIONS

Drug-Drug: ♦ **Other narcotic analgesics, other CNS depressants, antihistamines, sedative-hypnotics, phenothiazines, barbiturates, tricyclic antidepressants:** additive CNS depression ♦ **Cimetidine:** CNS toxicity ♦ **Rifampin, phenytoin:** decreased blood concentration of methadone; may produce withdrawal symptoms ♦ **Pentazocine, butorphanol, nalbuphine:** heroin-addicted patients on methadone therapy may experience withdrawal symptoms ♦ **Barbiturate anesthetics:** increased respiratory and CNS depression.

ROUTE AND DOSAGE

Narcotic Addiction (Detoxification)

♦ **PO (Adults):** 15–40 mg/day. Higher doses may be required in some patients. Continue dosage for 2–3 days, then gradually decrease on a daily or every-other day basis. Should be given in once-daily dosage.

Narcotic Addiction (Maintenance Therapy)

♦ **PO (Adults):** 20–120 mg/day in single dose. Individualize dosage as tolerated and required. Initially, administer 20 mg followed with another 20 mg in 4–8 hr, or administer 40 mg in single dose. Adjust additional doses by patient response. "Light" users or those who have not taken opiates for

---

*Underlines indicate most frequent; CAPITALS indicate life-threatening.

several days may be started with half of above dose.

Severe Pain
* **PO, IM, SC (Adults):** 2.5–10 mg q 3–4 hr as needed.

Severe Chronic Pain
* **PO Solution (Adults):** 5–20 mg q 6–8 hr. Adjust dosage according to pain severity, tolerance, and response.

PHARMACODYNAMICS

Route	Onset	Peak	Duration*
PO	0.5–1 hr	1–2 hr	4–6 hr
IM	10–20 min	1–2 hr	3–4 hr
SC	10–20 min	1–2 hr	3–4 hr

*Duration of action increases with repeated use due to cumulative effects.

NURSING IMPLICATIONS
Assessment
* Assess for symptoms of narcotic withdrawal: • watery eyes • runny nose • yawning • loss of appetite • irritability • tremors • panic • piloerection • excessive sweating • cramps • nausea • vomiting • dilated pupils • diarrhea • insomnia • elevated temperature, pulse, respiration, and blood pressure.
* Assess location, duration, and intensity of pain for which methadone is requested.
* Assess history of allergies, sensitivity to this drug or to other narcotics.
* Assess date of last menses (possible pregnancy), use of contraceptives.
* Assess whether currently breast-feeding a child.
* Assess current and past alcohol and drug consumption.
* Assess for operation of automobile and/or other dangerous machinery.
* Assess for presence of adverse reactions or side effects.
* Assess patient/family knowledge about illness and need for medication.
* In collaboration with physician, assess CBC and renal, liver, and respiratory function tests in patients on prolonged methadone therapy.

* **Lab Test Alterations:** Increased plasma amylase, increased plasma lipase.
* **Withdrawal:** Assess for symptoms of withdrawal. The cumulative effects of methadone delay symptoms of abstinence for 36–72 hours. Symptoms are usually mild and may include: • sweating • hot and cold flashes • anxiety • headache • weakness • insomnia • abdominal discomfort • anorexia.
* **Toxicity and Overdose:** Assess for symptoms of intoxication: • euphoria • dysphoria • apathy • psychomotor retardation • drowsiness • slurred speech • memory impairment • respiratory depression • constricted pupils • nausea • impaired judgment.
◊ Assess for symptoms of overdose: • slow and shallow breathing • clammy skin • convulsions • extreme somnolence (may progress to stupor, coma, or death).
* **Overdose Management:** Ensure maintenance of patent airway.
◊ Monitor vital signs.
◊ In cases of oral overdose, induce emesis in conscious patient or initiate gastric lavage in unconscious patient.
◊ Administer oxygen as required.
◊ Administer IV fluids and vasopressors to control hypotension.
◊ Initiate assisted ventilation if required.
◊ Administer narcotic antagonist (naloxone is drug of choice).

Potential Nursing Diagnoses
* Ineffective breathing pattern related to methadone's side effect of respiratory depression.
* High risk for injury related to abrupt withdrawal from long-term use, decreased mental alertness caused by side effect of sedation; side effects of dizziness, confusion, disorientation; effects of overdose.
* Alteration in comfort related to severe pain.

- Alteration in bowel elimination, constipation, related to side effect of methadone therapy.
- High risk for activity intolerance related to side effects of residual sedation, drowsiness, dizziness, confusion.
- Knowledge deficit related to medication regimen.

Plan/Implementation
- **General Info:** Monitor vital signs before beginning therapy and at regular intervals throughout hospital therapy. Vital signs should be monitored q 15–30 minutes for 2 hours following PO, IM, or SC administration.
- Ensure that patient is protected from injury. Supervise and assist with ambulation if dizziness and drowsiness are problems. Ensure that patient avoids participation in any activity requiring mental alertness (including smoking). Raise siderails when patient is in bed.
- Maintain record of intake and output. Urinary retention and antidiuretic effects can occur.
- Monitor bowel function. Increase fluids and fiber in diet if constipation becomes a problem. Stool softeners may be used.
- Store medication at controlled room temperatures between 15° and 30°C (59°–86°F). Protect from heat, light, and moisture.
- **PO:** To minimize nausea, medication may be given with food or milk.
- Ensure that tablet has been swallowed and not "cheeked" to avoid medication or to hoard for later use.
- Tablet may be crushed and mixed with food or fluid for patient who has difficulty swallowing. Changing to oral solution form may be considered.
- Maintenance dose should be given as oral solution diluted with at least 120 mL of water or acidic fruit beverage to reduce chance of parenteral abuse.
- **IM, SC:** When repeated injections are required, IM administration is preferred to SC, which can cause local tissue irritation and induration.
- To prevent inadvertent IV administration, aspirate carefully before injecting.
- Monitor for respiratory depression. Note changes in rate and rhythm of respiration. Rate that drops below 12 per minute should be reported to physician.
- Ensure availability of artificial ventilation and resuscitation equipment, as well as a narcotic antagonist, when methadone is administered parenterally.

Patient/Family Education
- Use caution in driving or when operating dangerous machinery. Drowsiness and dizziness can occur.
- Do not stop taking the drug abruptly. Doing so can produce withdrawal symptoms, such as nausea, vomiting, abdominal cramping, diarrhea, loss of appetite, insomnia, and increased temperature and blood pressure. Symptoms can be severe.
- Do not consume other CNS depressants (including alcohol).
- Do not take over-the-counter medications without approval from physician.
- Rise slowly from sitting or lying position to prevent a sudden drop in blood pressure.
- Be aware of the risks of taking methadone during pregnancy. Evidence of withdrawal symptoms have been observed in neonates born to mothers who had ingested narcotics regularly during pregnancy. Notify physician if pregnancy is suspected or planned.
- Be aware of potential side effects. Refer to written materials furnished by healthcare providers regarding correct method of self-administration.
- Report to physician symptoms of severe nausea and vomiting, difficulty breathing, persistent constipation, or shortness of breath.

♦ Carry card or other identification at all times stating names of medications being taken.

Evaluation

♦ Patient demonstrates a subsiding/resolution of the symptoms for which methadone was prescribed (symptoms of narcotic withdrawal, severe pain).

♦ Patient verbalizes understanding of side effects and regimen required for prudent self-administration of methadone.

METHAMPHETAMINE HCl

(meth-am-fet′a-meen)
Desoxyn

Classification(s):
CNS stimulant, Amphetamine,
Anorexigenic
Schedule C II
Pregnancy Category C

INDICATIONS

♦ Attention deficit disorder with hyperactivity in children ♦ Exogenous obesity.

ACTION

♦ Exact mechanism of action in CNS not known ♦ Amphetamines are sympathomimetic amines that stimulate the central nervous system, possibly by increasing synaptic release of norepinephrine, dopamine, and, at higher doses, serotonin in the brain. This is also accomplished by blocking reuptake at presynaptic membranes ♦ Central action occurs through cortical stimulation and may also be due to stimulation of the reticular activating system ♦ Action may also be due in part to the inhibition of amine oxidase ♦ Peripheral action is thought to be due to release of norepinephrine from adrenergic nerve stores and to direct effects on alpha- and beta-receptor sites.

PHARMACOKINETICS

Absorption: Rapidly and completely absorbed (within 3 hours) following oral administration.

Distribution: Widely distributed, with high concentrations in the brain and CSF. Crosses placental barrier; enters breast milk.

Metabolism and Excretion: Metabolized by the liver; excreted in urine. Elimination is enhanced by acidic urine, slowed by alkaline urine.

Half-Life: 7–33.6 hours (depending on pH of urine).

CONTRAINDICATIONS AND PRECAUTIONS

Contraindicated in: ♦ Hypersensitivity to sympathomimetic amines or tartrazine (contained in some preparations) ♦ Advanced arteriosclerosis ♦ Symptomatic cardiovascular disease ♦ Moderate to severe hypertension ♦ Hyperthyroidism ♦ Glaucoma ♦ Agitated states ♦ History of drug abuse ♦ Concomitant use or within 14 days of receiving therapy with MAO inhibitors ♦ Children under 3 years of age ♦ Pregnancy and lactation.

Use Cautiously in: ♦ Psychotic children ♦ Tourette's disorder ♦ Mild hypertension ♦ Anorexia ♦ Insomnia ♦ Elderly or debilitated patients.

ADVERSE REACTIONS AND SIDE EFFECTS*

CNS: overstimulation, restlessness, dizziness, insomnia, dyskinesia, euphoria, dysphoria, tremor, headache, symptoms of Tourette's disorder, psychoses (rare), nervousness, irritability, blurred vision, mydriasis.

CV: palpitations, tachycardia, elevation or decrease of blood pressure, arrhythmias.

Derm: urticaria.

Endo: impotence, changes in libido.

GI: dry mouth, unpleasant taste, diar-

---

*Underlines indicate most frequent; CAPITALS indicate life-threatening.

rhea, constipation, anorexia, weight loss, nausea, vomiting, abdominal cramps. **Other:** tolerance, physical and psychological dependence.

INTERACTIONS

Drug-Drug: ♦ **Furazolidone and MAO inhibitors (during or within 14 days of administration):** hypertensive crisis, headache, hyperpyrexia, intracranial hemorrhage, bradycardia ♦ **Insulin:** alteration in requirements ♦ **Guanethidine:** decreased antihypertensive effects ♦ **Phenothiazines:** possible decreased effects of both drugs ♦ **Urinary alkalinizers (e.g., acetazolamide, sodium bicarbonate, potassium citrate, sodium acetate, sodium citrate, sodium lactate, tromethamine):** decreased methamphetamine excretion, increased methamphetamine effects, excess CNS stimulation, excess cardiovascular effects ♦ **Urinary acidifiers (e.g., ammonium chloride, potassium phosphate, sodium acid phosphate):** increased methamphetamine excretion, resulting in decreased methamphetamine effects.

Drug-Food: ♦ **Caffeinated foods and drinks:** increased effects of methamphetamine.

ROUTE AND DOSAGE

Attention Deficit Disorder in Children

♦ **PO (Children):** Initial dosage: 2.5–5 mg daily or bid. May be increased in increments of 5 mg/day at weekly intervals until desired effect is achieved. Usual effective dose is 20–25 mg daily. May be administered in conventional tablets in 2 divided doses, or in long-acting tablets once daily. Long-acting form should not be administered until daily dose with conventional tablets is equal to or greater than the dosage provided in the long-acting tablet.

Exogenous Obesity

♦ **PO (Adults 12 Years and Older):** 2.5–5 mg bid or tid, 30 minutes before meals. Long-acting form: 10–15 mg in the morning before breakfast. Anorexigenic therapy with methamphetamine should not exceed a few weeks.

PHARMACODYNAMICS

Route	Onset	Peak	Duration
PO	30–60 min	1–3 hr*	4–24 hr*

*Varies with individual, dosage form, number of doses, and pH of urine.

NURSING IMPLICATIONS

Assessment

♦ Assess and record baseline temperature, pulse, respiration, blood pressure, and weight for comparison during therapy.

♦ In diabetic patient, assess blood sugar bid–tid. Insulin adjustments may be required due to alteration in eating pattern, as well as possibility of hyperactivity.

♦ Assess knowledge of sound, nutritional, calorie-reduced diet and program of regular exercise for overweight patient using methamphetamine as an anorexigenic.

♦ Assess growth rate of children on methamphetamine therapy carefully. A decrease in rate of development may be observed.

♦ Assess mental status for changes in: • mood • level of activity • degree of stimulation • aggressiveness.

♦ Assess sleeping patterns carefully. Insomnia may occur.

♦ Assess history of allergies, sensitivity to this drug or to other amphetamines.

♦ Assess history of glaucoma.

♦ Assess for presence of adverse reactions or side effects.

♦ Assess date of last menses (possible pregnancy), use of contraceptives.

♦ Assess whether currently breast-feeding a child.

♦ Assess current and past alcohol and drug consumption.

♦ Assess amount of caffeine usually consumed.

♦ Assess for operation of automobile and/or other dangerous machinery.

♦ Assess patient/family knowledge about illness and need for medication.

♦ In collaboration with physician, assess CBC, urinalysis, and liver function tests periodically in patients on methamphetamine therapy.

♦ **Lab Test Alterations:** Elevated serum thyroxine (T_4) levels.

♦ **Withdrawal:** Assess for symptoms of withdrawal: • extreme fatigue • lethargy • increased dreaming • mental depression • suicidal ideations • changes on the sleep EEG.

♦ **Withdrawal Management:** Monitor vital signs.

◊ Place patient in quiet room with low stimuli.

◊ Allow patient to sleep as much as desired.

◊ Observe closely (q 15 min).

◊ Institute suicide precautions.

◊ Some physicians may elect to prescribe antidepressants to counteract feelings of depression and lethargy.

♦ **Toxicity and Overdose:** Assess for symptoms of intoxication: • severe dermatoses • marked insomnia • irritability • hyperactivity • tachycardia • dilated pupils • elevated blood pressure • personality changes • hyperpyrexia • disorganization of thoughts • poor concentration • visual hallucinations • compulsive, stereotyped behavior • psychosis with manifestations similar to paranoid schizophrenia.

◊ Assess for symptoms of overdose: • restlessness • hyperirritability • insomnia • tremor • hyperreflexia • diaphoresis • mydriasis • flushing or pallor • profuse perspiration • hyperactivity • confusion • hypertension • extrasystoles • tachypnea • fever • hallucinations • panic state • paranoid ideations • delirium • marked hypertension • arrhythmias • heart block • convulsions • coma • circulatory collapse • death.

♦ **Overdose Management:** Monitor vital signs.

◊ Maintain adequate airway.

◊ Place patient in cool room.

◊ Induce emesis or initiate gastric lavage.

◊ Administer activated charcoal to minimize absorption.

◊ Administer saline cathartic.

◊ Administer urinary acidifier, such as ammonium chloride, to increase excretion of the drug.

◊ Administer a diuretic.

◊ Administer a short-acting barbiturate to combat hyperactivity.

◊ Administer IV phentolamine to treat severe hypertension.

◊ Use fluid replacement and a vasopressor to counter cardiovascular collapse.

◊ Administer oxygen and employ artificial respiration if necessary.

◊ Hemodialysis or peritoneal dialysis may be effective.

Potential Nursing Diagnoses

♦ High risk for injury related to overstimulation and hyperactivity; abrupt methamphetamine withdrawal; overdose.

♦ High risk for self-directed violence related to suicidal ideations resulting from abrupt methamphetamine withdrawal.

♦ High risk for violence directed at others related to aggressiveness as side effect of methamphetamine.

♦ Alteration in nutrition, more than body requires, related to excessive intake in relation to metabolic needs.

♦ Alteration in nutrition, less than body requires, related to methamphetamine's side effects of anorexia and weight loss.

♦ Sleep pattern disturbance related to overstimulation resulting from methamphetamine use.

* Alteration in thought processes related to adverse methamphetamine effects of overstimulation and difficulty concentrating.
* Knowledge deficit related to medication regimen.

Plan/Implementation

* Monitor medication's effects. Tolerance develops rapidly. If anorexigenic effects begin to diminish, notify physician immediately. Patient should be on reduced-calorie diet and program of regular exercise in addition to the medication.
* Monitor and record vital signs at regular intervals (bid) throughout therapy.
* Encourage use of gum, hard candy, or frequent sips of water for patient who experiences dry mouth. Ensure that patient practices good oral care (frequent brushing, flossing).
* Ensure that patient is protected from injury. Keep stimuli low and environment as quiet as possible to discourage overstimulation.
* Observe patient frequently for signs of impending violence to self or others. Institute suicide precautions if necessary. Assess level of anxiety often to prevent onset of physical aggression as agitation increases.
* In children with behavior disorders, a drug "holiday" should be attempted periodically under direction of physician to determine effectiveness of the medication and need for continuation.
* Ensure that tablet has been swallowed and not "cheeked" to avoid medication or to hoard for later use.
* Tablets may be crushed and mixed with food or fluid for patient who has difficulty swallowing. Do not crush long-acting tablets.
* To prevent insomnia, give last dose at least 6 hours before retiring.
* As an anorexigenic, drug should be administered 30 minutes before meals.

* Store medication at controlled room temperatures between 15° and 30°C (59°–86°F). Protect from heat, light, and moisture.

Patient/Family Education

* Use caution in driving or when operating dangerous machinery. Level of alertness may be diminished due to hyperactivity and stimulation. Dizziness may occur as a side effect.
* Do not stop taking the drug abruptly. Doing so can produce serious withdrawal symptoms.
* Do not take other medications (including over-the-counter drugs) without physician's approval. Many medications contain substances that, in combination with methamphetamine, can be harmful.
* Diabetic patient should monitor blood sugar bid or tid or as instructed by physician. Be aware of need for possible alteration in insulin requirements due to changes in food intake, weight, and activity.
* Avoid consumption of large amounts of caffeinated products (coffee, tea, colas, chocolate), as they may enhance the stimulant effect of methamphetamine.
* Follow reduced-calorie diet provided by dietitian, as well as a program of regular exercise if using methamphetamine for appetite suppressant. Do not exceed recommended dose if appetite suppressant effect diminishes. Contact physician.
* Notify physician if restlessness, insomnia, anorexia, or dry mouth become severe or if rapid and pounding heartbeat becomes evident.
* Be aware of possible risks of taking methamphetamine during pregnancy. Safe use in pregnancy and lactation has not been established. Because methamphetamine crosses placental barrier, it is possible a fetus could experience adverse effects of the drug. Inform physician immediately if preg-

nancy occurs, is suspected, or is planned.
* Be aware of potential side effects of methamphetamine. Refer to written materials furnished by healthcare providers for self-administration.
* Carry card or other identification at all times describing medications being taken.

Evaluation
* Patient demonstrates a subsiding/resolution of the symptoms for which methamphetamine was prescribed (obesity, behavior problems/hyperactivity in children).
* Patient verbalizes understanding of side effects and regimen required for prudent self-administration of methamphetamine.

METHOHEXITAL SODIUM

(meth-oh-hex′i-tal)
Brevital

Classification(s):
Anesthetic Barbiturate
Schedule IV
Pregnancy Category C

INDICATIONS
* Induction of anesthesia * Supplementation of other anesthetic agents * IV anesthesia for short procedures (minor surgery, ECT) with minimal painful stimuli * Induction of a hypnotic state.

ACTION
* Depresses the central nervous system by inhibiting impulse conduction in the ascending reticular activating system * Produces anesthesia, but does not possess analgesic or muscle-relaxant properties.

PHARMACOKINETICS
Distribution: Rapidly crosses blood-brain barrier, then is redistributed to other body tissues, with affinity for highly vascular organs (liver, kidneys, heart) and adipose tissue. Crosses placental barrier; excreted in breast milk.
Metabolism and Excretion: Metabolized in the liver. Excreted in urine.
Half-Life: 3–6 hours.

CONTRAINDICATIONS AND PRECAUTIONS
Contraindicated in: * Latent or manifest porphyria * Hypersensitivity to barbiturates * Absence of suitable veins for IV administration * Status asthmaticus * Pregnancy and lactation (safe use has not been established).

Use Cautiously in: * Severe cardiovascular disease * Hypotension or shock * Condition in which hypnotic effects may be prolonged or potentiated (excessive premedication, Addison's disease, myxedema, increased blood urea, severe anemia) * Increased intracranial pressure * Asthma * Myasthenia gravis * Debilitated patients * Impaired function of respiratory, circulatory, renal, hepatic, or endocrine systems * Patients with a history of drug abuse/dependence.

ADVERSE REACTIONS AND SIDE EFFECTS*
CNS: prolonged somnolence and recovery, headache, emergence delirium, anxiety, restlessness.
CV: hypotension, circulatory depression, thrombophlebitis, MYOCARDIAL DEPRESSION, CARDIAC ARRHYTHMIAS, PERIPHERAL VASCULAR COLLAPSE.
GI: nausea, vomiting, abdominal pain, salivation.
Derm: erythema, pruritus, urticaria, skin rashes, pain or nerve injury at injection site.

---

*Underlines indicate most frequent; CAPITALS indicate life-threatening.

Resp: hiccups, sneezing, coughing, dyspnea, RESPIRATORY DEPRESSION, APNEA, LARYNGOSPASM, BRONCHOSPASM.

Other: tolerance, dependence, skeletal muscle hyperactivity, shivering, rhinitis, ANAPHYLACTIC REACTION.

INTERACTIONS

Drug-Drug: ♦ **CNS depressants (e.g., alcohol, benzodiazepines, other barbiturates, other sedative-hypnotics, opiates):** additive CNS and respiratory depression ♦ **Furosemide:** orthostatic hypotension ♦ **Propranolol, corticosteroids, doxycycline, oral anticoagulants, oral contraceptives, quinidine, theophylline:** decreased effectiveness of these drugs.

ROUTE AND DOSAGE

(To be administered by anesthesiologist or CRNA only.)

Anesthesia for Short Procedures (Minor Surgery or ECT)

♦ **IV (Adults):** Usual range is 5–12 mL of a 1% solution (50–120 mg; average 70 mg). If intermittent injection of a 1% solution is used for maintenance, additional amounts of about 2–4 mL (20–40 mg) will be required, usually every 4–7 minutes. May be administered as a continuous IV drip with a 0.2% solution at an average rate of 3 mL/min.

PHARMACODYNAMICS

Route	Onset	Peak	Duration
IV	30–40 sec	3 min	5–7 min

NURSING IMPLICATIONS
Assessment

♦ In patient receiving ECT, assess: • mood • level of activity • degree of participation in therapies • interaction with others.
♦ Assess for suicidal ideation in depressed patients.
♦ Assess history of allergies, sensitivity to this drug or to other barbiturates, history of porphyria or asthma.
♦ Obtain baseline blood pressure, pulse, respiration, temperature, weight.
♦ Assess level of anxiety regarding impending surgical procedure or electroconvulsive therapy.
♦ Assess status of veins available for IV administration.
♦ Assess date of last menses (possible pregnancy), use of contraceptives.
♦ Assess whether currently breast-feeding a child.
♦ Assess current and past alcohol and drug consumption.
♦ Assess for presence of adverse reactions or side effects.
♦ Assess level of knowledge about condition and need for medication.
♦ In collaboration with physician, assess CBC and renal and liver function tests.
♦ **Toxicity and Overdose:** Assess for symptoms of overdose (may result from too rapid or repeated injections): • profound drop in blood pressure (may progress to shock levels) • apnea • occasional laryngospasm • coughing • other respiratory difficulties.
♦ **Overdose Management:** Discontinue drug.
◊ Maintain patent airway (intubation may be required).
◊ Administer oxygen.
◊ Assist with ventilation if needed.
◊ Administer vasopressors to counteract hypotension.
◊ Administer IV fluids to maintain adequate circulation.
◊ Use diuretics or hemodialysis to promote elimination of the drug.

Potential Nursing Diagnoses

♦ Ineffective breathing pattern related to side effects of respiratory depression, dyspnea, apnea.
♦ High risk for injury related to overdose; extravasation at insertion site.
♦ High risk for self-directed violence related to depressed mood.

- Anxiety (moderate to severe) related to impending surgical procedure or electroconvulsive therapy.
- Knowledge deficit related to medication regimen.

Plan/Implementation

- **General Info:** Drug is administered by anesthesiologist or Certified Registered Nurse Anesthetist (CRNA) only.
- ◇ Ensure immediate availability of resuscitation equipment/drugs to counteract possible respiratory depression or anaphylactic reaction.
- **IV:** Monitor vital signs q 3 minutes during administration and q 5–15 minutes during recovery from anesthesia.
- ◇ Sterile water for injection is the preferred diluent. 5% dextrose injection or 0.9% sodium chloride injection may also be used. Not compatible with lactated Ringer's injection or diluents containing bacteriostatic agents.
- ◇ Methohexital is stable in sterile water for injection at room temperature for at least 6 weeks. Solutions are not stable for more than 24 hours when dextrose injection or sodium chloride injection are the diluents.
- ◇ Solutions may be used within time limits only if they remain clear and colorless.
- ◇ Do not mix with acid solutions or allow contact with parts of disposable syringes that have been treated with silicone.
- ◇ Rate of administration for induction is usually about 1 mL of the 1% solution (10 mg) in 5 seconds.
- ◇ Ensure patency of vein. Extravasation can cause sloughing and necrosis. Intra-arterial injection can cause gangrene.

Patient/Family Education

- Be aware of reasons for drug administration, what to expect in response to drug administration, potential side effects.
- Be aware of potential risks involved

with use of this drug, as well as risks associated with impending procedure.
- Inform physician of response to this or similar drugs in the past.
- Inform physician if pregnancy is suspected or if currently breast-feeding a baby. Safe use of this drug during pregnancy and lactation has not been established.

Evaluation

- Patient verbalizes understanding of need for methohexital (as a short-acting anesthetic for minor surgery or other procedure, such as ECT).
- Patient verbalizes understanding of potential adverse side effects and risks associated with the administration of methohexital.

METHSUXIMIDE

(meth-sux′i-mide)
Celontin

Classification(s):
Anticonvulsant, Succinimide
Pregnancy Category C

INDICATIONS

- Absence (petit mal) seizures refractory to other drugs ◆ Some cases of partial seizures with complex symptomatology (psychomotor seizures).

ACTION

- Depresses motor cortex and elevates central nervous system seizure threshold ◆ Suppresses paroxysmal spike and wave activity common in absence seizures.

PHARMACOKINETICS

Absorption: Well absorbed from the GI tract.
Distribution: Widely distributed. Unknown if drug crosses placental barrier or is excreted in breast milk.
Metabolism and Excretion: Metabolized by the liver; excreted in urine.
Half-Life: 2.6–4 hours.

CONTRAINDICATIONS AND PRECAUTIONS

Contraindicated in: ♦ hypersensitivity to this drug or to other succinimides.
Use Cautiously in: ♦ Severe hepatic and renal disease ♦ Pregnancy and lactation (safety has not been established).

ADVERSE REACTIONS AND SIDE EFFECTS*

CNS: drowsiness, headache, dizziness, ataxia, lethargy, fatigue, irritability, hyperactivity.
Derm: skin rashes, urticaria, pruritus, hirsutism.
GI: nausea/vomiting, anorexia, abdominal cramps, diarrhea, constipation, hiccups.
Hemat: LEUKOPENIA, AGRANULOCYTOSIS, THROMBOCYTOPENIA, APLASTIC ANEMIA.
Other: gingival hypertrophy, swollen tongue, alopecia, vaginal bleeding, RENAL AND HEPATIC DAMAGE, diplopia, sleep disturbances, night terrors, aggressiveness, paranoid psychosis, SLE, myopia.

INTERACTIONS

Drug-Drug: ♦ **Hydantoin anticonvulsants:** decreased metabolism and increased risk of toxic effects of hydantoins ♦ **Oral contraceptives:** decreased effectiveness of oral contraceptives ♦ **CNS depressants (including alcohol, sedative-hypnotics, narcotics, antihistamines):** additive CNS depression ♦ **Carbamazepine:** decreased concentration of methsuximide.

ROUTE AND DOSAGE

Absence (Petit mal) Seizures

♦ **PO (Adults and Children):** 300 mg/day for the first week; dosage may be increased by 300 mg/day at weekly intervals until control is achieved with minimal side effects. Maximum dose: 1.2 g/day in divided doses.

PHARMACODYNAMICS

Route	Onset	Peak	Duration
PO	15–30 min	1–3 hr	4–6 hr

NURSING IMPLICATIONS

Assessment

♦ Assess occurrence, characteristics, and duration of seizure activity.
♦ Assess baseline vital signs.
♦ Assess history of allergies, sensitivity to this drug or to other succinimides.
♦ Assess date of last menses (possible pregnancy), use of contraceptives.
♦ Assess whether currently breast-feeding a child.
♦ Assess current and past alcohol and drug consumption.
♦ Assess operation of automobile and/or other dangerous machinery.
♦ Assess for presence of adverse reactions or side effects.
♦ Assess patient/family knowledge about illness and need for medication.
♦ In collaboration with physician, assess CBC and renal and liver function tests in patients on methsuximide therapy. Periodic urinalysis should be performed.
♦ **Lab Test Alterations:** Increased direct Coombs' test.
♦ **Toxicity and Overdose:** Tentative range of therapeutic serum concentration for the active metabolite NDM is 10–40 mcg/mL.
◊ Assess for symptoms of toxicity/overdose: • bone marrow depression • nausea/vomiting • ataxia • diplopia.
♦ **Overdose Management:** Monitor vital signs.
◊ Maintain adequate airway.
◊ Induce emesis if patient is conscious.
◊ Initiate gastric lavage if patient is unconscious.
◊ Administer activated charcoal to minimize absorption.
◊ Monitor electrolytes.

*Underlines indicate most frequent; CAPITALS indicate life-threatening.

◇ Administer oxygen, vasopressors, and assisted ventilation if required.

Potential Nursing Diagnoses

♦ High risk for injury related to seizures; abrupt withdrawal from long-term methsuximide use; side effects of dizziness, sedation, ataxia.

♦ Social isolation related to fear of experiencing a seizure in the presence of others.

♦ Impaired adjustment related to difficulty accepting diagnosis of epilepsy.

♦ High risk for activity intolerance related to methsuximide's side effects of sedation, drowsiness, dizziness, ataxia.

♦ Knowledge deficit related to medication regimen.

Plan/Implementation

♦ Monitor vital signs at regular intervals (bid) throughout therapy.

♦ Monitor and record lab assessments of serum methsuximide levels. Report presence of skin rash, joint pain, fever, unusual bleeding, easy bruising, dark urine, jaundice to physician immediately.

♦ Observe frequently (every hour) for occurrence of seizure activity.

♦ Ensure that patient is protected from injury. Supervise and assist with ambulation if dizziness and drowsiness are problems. Ensure that patient avoids participation in any activity that requires mental alertness (including smoking). Pad siderails and head of bed with towels or blanket for patient who experiences seizures during the night.

♦ Medication may be administered with food or milk to minimize GI irritation.

♦ Store medication at controlled room temperatures between 15° and 30°C (59°–86°F). Protect from light and moisture.

Patient/Family Education

♦ Do not drive or operate dangerous machinery until individual response is determined. Drowsiness and dizziness can occur.

♦ Do not stop taking drug abruptly. To do so might precipitate absence (petit mal) status.

♦ Avoid alcoholic beverages.

♦ Carry or wear identification informing others of condition and medication usage.

♦ Do not take any other medication without approval from physician. To do so may be harmful and cause loss of seizure control.

♦ Promptly report any of the following symptoms to physician: sore throat • fever • malaise • skin rash • joint pain • unusual bleeding • easy bruising • dark urine • yellow skin or eyes.

♦ Be aware of possible risks of taking methsuximide during pregnancy. Patient who requires the medication to prevent seizures may be maintained on it; however, she must be fully aware of potential risks to unborn child. There is a strong association between the use of anticonvulsant drugs by women with epilepsy and the incidence of birth defects in their children. If pregnancy occurs, is suspected, or is planned, report it to physician immediately.

♦ Due to decreased effectiveness of oral contraceptives, use alternative methods of birth control during therapy.

♦ To protect patient during a tonic-clonic (grand mal) seizure, do not restrain. Padding (towels, blankets, pillows) may be used to prevent bumping against hard objects. When convulsion has subsided, turn patient on side to allow secretions to drain and to prevent aspiration. Keep records of occurrence, characteristics, and duration of seizures, so that accurate reports may be given to physician for providing assistance in stabilization and control of seizures. If patient has difficulty breathing or continues to experience subsequent seizures, family should immediately call for emergency assistance.

♦ Be aware of possible side effects. Refer to written materials furnished by healthcare providers for assistance in self-administration upon discharge.

Evaluation
♦ Patient demonstrates stabilization of seizure activity with regular administration of methsuximide.
♦ Patient verbalizes understanding of necessity for, side effects of, and regimen required for prudent self-administration of methsuximide.

METHYLPHENIDATE

(meth-ill-fen′i-date)
(Methidate); Ritalin, Ritalin-SR

Classification(s):
CNS stimulant, Piperidine derivative
Schedule C II
Pregnancy Category C

INDICATIONS
♦ Narcolepsy ♦ Attention deficit disorder with hyperactivity.

ACTION
♦ Exact mechanism of action not fully understood ♦ Appears to exert a mild CNS stimulation, mainly on the cerebral cortex and subcortical structures ♦ Actions are similar to those of amphetamines.

PHARMACOKINETICS
Absorption: Well absorbed following oral administration.
Distribution: Extent of distribution unknown in humans.
Metabolism and Excretion: Metabolized by the liver; excreted in urine.
Half-Life: 1–2 hours.

CONTRAINDICATIONS AND PRECAUTIONS
Contraindicated in: ♦ Hypersensitivity to this drug ♦ Marked anxiety, tension,

and agitation ♦ Glaucoma ♦ Patients with motor tics or with a family history or diagnosis of Tourette's disorder ♦ Severe depression ♦ Treatment of normal fatigue states ♦ Pregnancy, lactation, children under 6 years of age (safety has not been established).
Use Cautiously in: ♦ Patients with a history of seizure disorder and/or EEG abnormalities ♦ Hypertension ♦ History of drug or alcohol dependence ♦ Emotionally unstable patients.

ADVERSE REACTIONS AND SIDE EFFECTS*
CNS: <u>nervousness</u>, <u>insomnia</u>, dizziness, headache, dyskinesia, chorea, drowsiness, Tourette's disorder, toxic psychosis, akathisia.
CV: <u>palpitations</u>, <u>tachycardia</u>, cardiac arrhythmias, angina, increased or decreased blood pressure, increased or decreased pulse rate.
Derm: skin rash, urticaria, EXFOLIATIVE DERMATITIS, ERYTHEMA MULTIFORME WITH NECROTIZING VASCULITIS, THROMBOCYTOPENIC PURPURA.
GI: <u>anorexia</u>, nausea, abdominal pain, weight loss during prolonged therapy, dry throat.
Hemat: LEUKOPENIA, ANEMIA, THROMBOCYTOPENIA, eosinophilia.
Other: tolerance, physical and psychological dependence, fever, scalp hair loss, arthralgia.

INTERACTIONS
Drug-Drug: ♦ **MAO inhibitors (during or within 14 days of administration), pressor agents:** hypertensive crisis, headache, hyperpyrexia, intracranial hemorrhage, bradycardia ♦ **Coumarin anticoagulants, anticonvulsants (phenobarbital, phenytoin, primidone), phenylbutazone, tricyclic antidepressants:** decreased metabolism and increased activity/toxicity of these drugs ♦ **Bretylium, guanethidine:** decreased antihypertensive effects.

---

*<u>Underlines</u> indicate most frequent; CAPITALS indicate life-threatening.

Drug-Food: ✦ **Caffeinated foods and drinks:** increased effects of methylphenidate.

ROUTE AND DOSAGE

Attention Deficit Disorder with Hyperactivity

✦ **PO (Children 6 and Older):** Initial dosage: 5 mg before breakfast and lunch. Dosage may be increased gradually in increments of 5–10 mg/day at weekly intervals. Maximum daily dosage: 60 mg. If improvement is not observed after dosage adjustment over 1 month, discontinue use. Discontinue use periodically to assess condition and need for continuation of therapy.

Narcolepsy

✦ **PO (Adults):** Dosage is highly individualized. Range is 10–60 mg/day. Average dose is 20–30 mg/day. Administer in 2–3 divided doses, preferably 30–45 minutes before meals.

PHARMACODYNAMICS

Route	Onset	Peak	Duration
PO	30–60 min	1–3 hr	4–6 hr 8 hr (sustained-release)

NURSING IMPLICATIONS

Assessment

✦ Assess and record baseline temperature, pulse, respiration, blood pressure, and weight for comparison during therapy.
✦ In diabetic patient, assess blood sugar bid–tid. Insulin adjustments may be required due to alteration in eating pattern, as well as possibility of hyperactivity.
✦ Assess growth rate of children on methylphenidate therapy carefully. A decrease in rate of development may be observed.
✦ Assess mental status for changes in mood, level of activity, degree of stimulation, aggressiveness.

✦ Assess sleeping patterns carefully. Insomnia may occur.
✦ Assess history of allergies, sensitivity to this drug.
✦ Assess history of glaucoma.
✦ Assess for presence of adverse reactions or side effects.
✦ Assess date of last menses (possible pregnancy), use of contraceptives.
✦ Assess whether currently breast-feeding a child.
✦ Assess current and past alcohol and drug consumption.
✦ Assess amount of caffeine usually consumed.
✦ Assess for operation of automobile and/or other dangerous machinery.
✦ Assess patient/family knowledge about illness and need for medication.
✦ In collaboration with physician, periodically assess CBC and platelet counts, urinalysis, and liver function tests in patients on methylphenidate therapy.
✦ **Lab Test Alterations:** May increase urinary excretion of epinephrine.
✦ **Withdrawal:** Assess for symptoms of withdrawal: • extreme fatigue • lethargy • increased dreaming • mental depression • suicidal ideations • psychotic behavior.
✦ **Withdrawal Management:** Monitor vital signs.
◇ Place patient in quiet room with low stimuli.
◇ Allow patient to sleep as much as desired.
◇ Observe closely (q 15 min).
◇ Institute suicide precautions.
◇ Some physicians may elect to prescribe antidepressants to counteract feelings of depression and lethargy.
✦ **Toxicity and Overdose:** Assess for symptoms of overdose: • vomiting • agitation • tremors • hyperreflexia • muscle twitching • convulsions • coma • euphoria • confusion • hallucinations • delirium • sweating • headache • hyperpyrexia • tachycardia • palpitations • cardiac arrhyth-

mias • hypertension • mydriasis • dry mucous membranes • flushing • toxic psychosis • hyperpyrexia.

♦ **Overdose Management:** Monitor vital signs.
◊ Ensure maintenance of adequate airway.
◊ Induce emesis or initiate gastric lavage.
◊ Maintain adequate circulation and respiratory exchange.
◊ External cooling measures may be required to treat hyperpyrexia.
◊ Efficacy of peritoneal dialysis or hemodialysis has not been established.

Potential Nursing Diagnoses
♦ High risk for injury due to overstimulation and hyperactivity; abrupt methylphenidate withdrawal; overdose.
♦ High risk for self-directed violence related to suicidal ideations resulting from abrupt methylphenidate withdrawal.
♦ Alteration in nutrition, less than body requires, related to methylphenidate's side effects of anorexia and weight loss.
♦ Sleep pattern disturbance related to overstimulation resulting from methylphenidate use.
♦ Alteration in thought processes related to methylphenidate's adverse effects of overstimulation and difficulty concentrating.
♦ Knowledge deficit related to medication regimen.

Plan/Implementation
♦ Monitor and record vital signs at regular intervals (bid) throughout therapy.
♦ Ensure that patient is protected from injury. Keep stimuli low and environment as quiet as possible to discourage overstimulation.
♦ Observe frequently for signs of impending violence to self. Institute suicide precautions, if necessary.
♦ In children with behavior disorders, a drug "holiday" should be attempted

periodically under direction of physician to determine effectiveness of the medication and need for continuation.
♦ Ensure that tablet has been swallowed and not "cheeked" to avoid medication or to hoard for later use.
♦ Tablets may be crushed and mixed with food or fluid for patient who has difficulty swallowing.
♦ Administer medication 30–45 minutes before meals.
♦ To prevent insomnia, give last dose at least 6 hours before retiring.
♦ Store medication at controlled room temperatures between 15° and 30°C (59°–86°F). Protect from heat and moisture.

Patient/Family Education
♦ Use caution in driving or when operating dangerous machinery. Level of alertness may be diminished due to hyperactivity and stimulation. Dizziness may occur as a side effect.
♦ Do not stop taking the drug abruptly. Doing so can produce serious withdrawal symptoms.
♦ Do not take other medications (including over-the-counter drugs) without physician's approval. Many medications contain substances that, in combination with methylphenidate, can be harmful.
♦ Diabetic patient should monitor blood sugar bid or tid or as instructed by physician. Be aware of possible need for alteration in insulin requirements due to changes in food intake, weight, and activity.
♦ Avoid consumption of large amounts of caffeinated products (coffee, tea, colas, chocolate), as they may enhance the stimulant effect of methylphenidate.
♦ Notify physician of nervousness, insomnia, palpitations, vomiting, fever, skin rash, sore throat, unusual bleeding or bruising.
♦ Be aware of possible risks of taking methylphenidate during pregnancy. Safe use in pregnancy and lactation

has not been established. It is unknown if methylphenidate crosses placental barrier. Inform physician immediately if pregnancy occurs, is suspected, or is planned.

♦ Be aware of potential side effects of methylphenidate. Refer to written materials furnished by healthcare providers for safe self-administration.

♦ Carry card or other identification at all times describing medications being taken.

Evaluation

♦ Patient demonstrates a subsiding/resolution of the symptoms for which methylphenidate was prescribed (inability to prevent falling asleep, behavior problems/hyperactivity in children).

♦ Patient verbalizes understanding of side effects and regimen required for prudent self-administration of methylphenidate.

METHYPRYLON

(meth-i-prye′lon)
Noludar

Classification(s):
Sedative-hypnotic, CNS depressant
Schedule C III
Pregnancy Category B

INDICATIONS

♦ Insomnia (short-term [7 days] management).

ACTION

♦ May produce CNS depressant effects by increasing the threshold of the arousal centers in the brain stem.

PHARMACOKINETICS

Absorption: Rapidly absorbed following oral administration.
Distribution: Unknown. Transmission

across placental barrier and excretion in breast milk has not been determined.
Metabolism and Excretion: Metabolized by the liver; excreted by the kidneys.
Half-Life: 3–6 hours.

CONTRAINDICATIONS AND PRECAUTIONS

Contraindicated in: ♦ Hypersensitivity to the drug ♦ Porphyria ♦ Children under age 12; pregnancy and lactation (safety and effectiveness have not been established).
Use Cautiously in: ♦ Elderly or debilitated patients ♦ Hepatic or renal dysfunction ♦ Depressed/suicidal patients ♦ Patients with a history of drug abuse/dependence.

ADVERSE REACTIONS AND SIDE EFFECTS*

CNS: <u>drowsiness</u>, <u>dizziness</u>, headache, <u>hangover</u>, paradoxical excitement, blurred vision, vertigo, depression, nightmares, dreaming.
CV: hypotension.
Derm: skin rashes, pruritus.
GI: nausea, vomiting, diarrhea, constipation, esophagitis.
Hemat: BLOOD DYSCRASIAS (rare), THROMBOCYTOPENIA, NEUTROPENIA, APLASTIC ANEMIA.
Other: tolerance, physical and psychological dependence.

INTERACTIONS

Drug-Drug: ♦ **Other CNS depressants (including alcohol, benzodiazepines, opiates):** additive CNS depression.

ROUTE AND DOSAGE

Insomnia

♦ **PO (Adults):** 200–400 mg 15 minutes before bedtime. Maximum 400 mg daily.
♦ **PO (Children Over 12):** 50 mg at

---

*<u>Underlines</u> indicate most frequent; CAPITALS indicate life-threatening.

bedtime (may be increased to a maximum of 200 mg if required).

PHARMACODYNAMICS

Route	Onset	Peak	Duration
PO	45 min–1 hr	1–2 hr	5–8 hr

NURSING IMPLICATIONS
Assessment

♦ Assess sleep patterns. Keep records for adequate baseline data before the initiation of therapy.
♦ Assess for suicidal ideation in depressed patients.
♦ Assess history of allergies, sensitivity to this drug.
♦ Assess date of last menses (possible pregnancy), use of contraceptives.
♦ Assess whether currently breast-feeding a child.
♦ Assess current and past alcohol and drug consumption.
♦ Assess for operation of automobile and/or other dangerous machinery.
♦ Assess for presence of adverse reactions or side effects.
♦ Assess patient/family knowledge about condition and need for medication.
♦ In collaboration with physician, assess CBC and renal and liver function tests in patients who have been on prolonged therapy.
♦ **Lab Test Alterations:** May interfere with urinary steroid evaluations, including 17-ketosteroids and 17-hydroxycorticosteroids.
♦ **Withdrawal:** Assess for symptoms of withdrawal: • anxiety • tremors • insomnia • nausea/vomiting • weakness • diaphoresis • orthostatic hypotension • confusion • polyuria • hyperreflexia • hallucinations • delirium • convulsions.
♦ **Withdrawal Management:** Monitor vital signs.
◊ Place patient in quiet room with low stimuli.
◊ Institute seizure precautions.
◊ A long-acting barbiturate, such as phe-

nobarbital, may be ordered to suppress withdrawal symptoms.
◊ Phenytoin may be ordered to prevent seizures.
◊ Some physicians may order oxazepam as needed for objective withdrawal symptoms, gradually decreasing dosage until the drug is discontinued.
♦ **Toxicity and Overdose:** Assess for symptoms of toxicity: • confusion • drowsiness • dyspnea • slurred speech • staggering.
◊ Assess for symptoms of overdose: • CNS and respiratory depression • confusion • constricted pupils • hypoventilation • hypothermia or hyperthermia • hypotension • oliguria • coma. (May progress to respiratory arrest, circulatory collapse, and death.)
♦ **Overdose Management:** Monitor vital signs.
◊ Ensure maintenance of adequate airway.
◊ Induce emesis in conscious patient.
◊ Initiate gastric lavage in unconscious patient.
◊ Administer activated charcoal to minimize absorption of drug.
◊ Administer IV fluids.
◊ Use oxygen, vasopressors, and assisted ventilation as required.
◊ For severe intoxication, hemodialysis may be used.

Potential Nursing Diagnoses

♦ High risk for injury related to abrupt withdrawal from long-term use; decreased mental alertness caused by side effects of drowsiness and dizziness; effects of overdose.
♦ High risk for self-directed violence related to depressed mood.
♦ Anxiety (specify level) related to threats to physical integrity and/or self-concept.
♦ Sleep pattern disturbance related to situational crises, physical condition, severe level of anxiety.
♦ High risk for activity intolerance related to side effects of drowsiness, dizziness.

♦ Knowledge deficit related to medication regimen.

Plan/Implementation

♦ Monitor vital signs before beginning therapy and at regular intervals (bid) throughout therapy.
♦ Ensure that patient is protected from injury. Supervise and assist with ambulation if dizziness and drowsiness are problems. Ensure that patient avoids participation in any activity requiring mental alertness (including smoking). Raise siderails and instruct patient to remain in bed following administration.
♦ To minimize nausea, medication may be given with food or milk.
♦ Ensure that tablet/capsule has been swallowed and not "cheeked" to avoid medication or to hoard for later use.
♦ Tablet may be crushed or contents of capsule emptied and mixed with food or fluid for patient who has difficulty swallowing.
♦ Store medication at controlled room temperatures between 15° and 30°C (59°–86°F). Protect from heat, light, and moisture.

Patient/Family Education

♦ Use caution in driving or when operating dangerous machinery. Drowsiness and dizziness can occur.
♦ Do not stop taking the drug abruptly. Doing so can produce serious (even life-threatening) withdrawal symptoms. If a dose is missed, take it as close as possible to the prescribed time. If it is already close to time for next dose, wait until then; do not double up on dose at the next prescribed time.
♦ Do not consume other CNS depressants (including alcohol).
♦ Be aware of the risks of taking methyprylon during pregnancy (safety during pregnancy has not been established). Notify physician if pregnancy is suspected or planned.
♦ Be aware of potential side effects. Refer to written materials furnished by healthcare providers regarding correct method of self-administration.
♦ Report symptoms of sore throat, fever, malaise, unusual bleeding, or easy bruising to physician immediately.
♦ Carry card or other identification at all times stating names of medications being taken.

Evaluation

♦ Patient demonstrates a subsiding/resolution of the symptoms for which methyprylon was prescribed (sleep disturbances).
♦ Patient verbalizes understanding of side effects and regimen required for prudent self-administration of methyprylon.

MOLINDONE

(moe-lin'done)
Moban

Classification(s):
Antipsychotic, Neuroleptic, Dihydroindolone
Pregnancy Category C

INDICATIONS

♦ Manifestations of psychotic disorders.

ACTION

♦ The exact mechanism of antipsychotic action is not fully understood ♦ Molindone is thought to act mainly on the ascending reticular activating system.

PHARMACOKINETICS

Absorption: Rapidly absorbed following oral administration.
Distribution: Thought to be widely distributed. Unknown if drug crosses placental barrier or if it enters breast milk.
Metabolism and Excretion: Rapidly and almost completely metabolized by the liver. Excreted in urine and feces.
Half-Life: 1.5 hours.

CONTRAINDICATIONS AND PRECAUTIONS

Contraindicated in: ♦ Hypersensitivity to this drug, to phenothiazines, or to sulfites (contained in some preparations) ♦ Comatose or severely CNS-depressed patients ♦ Presence of large amounts of CNS depressants ♦ Bone marrow depression ♦ Blood dyscrasias ♦ Brain damage ♦ Parkinson's disease ♦ Liver, renal, and/or cardiac insufficiency ♦ Severe hypotension or hypertension ♦ Children under 12; pregnancy and lactation (safe use has not been established).

Use Cautiously in: ♦ Patients with a history of seizures ♦ Respiratory, renal, hepatic, thyroid, or cardiovascular disorders (e.g., respiratory infection, COPD, thyrotoxicosis, mitral insufficiency, angina pectoris) ♦ Prostatic hypertrophy ♦ Glaucoma ♦ Diabetes ♦ Elderly or debilitated patients.

ADVERSE REACTIONS AND SIDE EFFECTS*

CNS: sedation, headache, seizures, insomnia, dizziness, extrapyramidal symptoms (pseudoparkinsonism, akathisia, akinesia, dystonia, oculogyric crisis) tardive dyskinesia, fatigue, ataxia, blurred vision, tinnitus, hyperactivity, depression, NEUROLEPTIC MALIGNANT SYNDROME.
CV: orthostatic hypotension, hypertension, tachycardia, bradycardia, CARDIAC ARREST, ECG changes, ARRHYTHMIAS, PULMONARY EDEMA, CIRCULATORY COLLAPSE.
Derm: skin rashes, urticaria, petechiae, seborrhea, photosensitivity, eczema, EXFOLIATIVE DERMATITIS (rare).
Endo: galactorrhea, gynecomastia (men), changes in libido, hyperglycemia or hypoglycemia, amenorrhea, retrograde ejaculation, enlarged parotid glands.
GI: dry mouth, nausea, vomiting, increased appetite and weight gain, anorexia, dyspepsia, constipation, diarrhea, jaundice, polydipsia, PARALYTIC ILEUS.
GU: urinary retention, frequency or incontinence, bladder paralysis, polyuria, enuresis, priapism.
Hemat: AGRANULOCYTOSIS, LEUKOPENIA, ANEMIA, THROMBOCYTOPENIA.
Resp: LARYNGOSPASM, BRONCHOSPASM, SUPPRESSION OF COUGH REFLEX.
Other: nasal congestion.

INTERACTIONS

Drug-Drug: ♦ **CNS depressants (including alcohol, barbiturates, narcotics, anesthetics):** additive CNS depressant effects ♦ **Anticholinergic agents (e.g., atropine):** additive anticholinergic effects, decreased antipsychotic effects ♦ **Metyrosine:** potentiation of extrapyramidal side effects ♦ **Levodopa:** decreased efficacy of levodopa ♦ **Quinidine:** additive cardiac depressive effects ♦ **Guanethidine:** decreased antihypertensive action ♦ **Lithium:** decreased plasma levels of antipsychotic drug ♦ **Epinephrine:** reversal of usual pressor action of epinephrine, resulting in decreased blood pressure ♦ **Phenytoin:** decreased phenytoin metabolism and absorption, increased risk of toxicity ♦ **Polypeptide antibiotics:** neuromuscular respiratory depression ♦ **Metrizamide:** seizures ♦ **Tetracyclines:** decreased tetracycline absorption.

Drug-Food: ♦ **Caffeine-containing beverages (e.g., coffee, tea, colas):** counteracted antipsychotic effect.

ROUTE AND DOSAGE

Psychotic Disorders

♦ **PO (Adults):** Initial dosage: 50–75 mg/day, given in 3 or 4 divided doses. Dosage may be increased to 100 mg/day in 3–4 days. Patients with severe symptoms may require up to 225 mg/day initially. Start elderly or debilitated patients on lower dosage.

*Underlines indicate most frequent; CAPITALS indicate life-threatening.

Maintenance

♦ **PO (Adults):** Mild symptoms: 5–15 mg tid or qid. Moderate symptoms: 10–25 mg tid or qid. Severe symptoms: up to 150 mg/day; rarely, up to 225 mg/day. Maintenance dose often can be given in single daily dose.

PHARMACODYNAMICS

Route	Onset*	Peak†	Duration‡
PO	Erratic	1 hr	36 hr

*Full antipsychotic effects may not be observed for 4–8 weeks.
†Steady-state plasma levels are achieved in approximately 4–7 days.
‡Drug may be detected in urine for 3–6 months after last dose.

NURSING IMPLICATIONS

Assessment

♦ Assess mental status daily: • mood • appearance • thought and communication patterns • level of interest in the environment and in activities • level of anxiety or agitation • presence of hallucinations or delusions • suspiciousness • interactions with others • ability to carry out activities of daily living.

♦ Assess for symptoms of blood dyscrasias: • sore throat • fever • malaise • unusual bleeding • easy bruising.

♦ Assess for extrapyramidal symptoms: • pseudoparkinsonism (tremors, shuffling gait, drooling, rigidity) • akinesia (muscular weakness) • akathisia (continuous restlessness and fidgeting) • dystonia (involuntary muscular movements of face, arms, legs, and neck) • oculogyric crisis (uncontrolled rolling back of the eyes) • tardive dyskinesia (bizarre facial and tongue movements, stiff neck, difficulty swallowing).

♦ Assess for symptoms of neuroleptic malignant syndrome: • hyperpyrexia up to 107°F (41.6°C) • elevated pulse • increased or decreased blood pressure • severe parkinsonian muscle rigidity • elevated creatinine phosphokinase blood levels • elevated white blood count • altered mental status (including catatonic signs or agitation) • acute renal failure • varying levels of consciousness (including stupor and coma) • pallor • diaphoresis • tachycardia • arrhythmias • rhabdomyolysis.

♦ Assess vital signs, weight. Record baseline values for comparison.

♦ Assess history of allergies, sensitivity to this drug.

♦ Assess date of last menses (possible pregnancy), use of contraceptives.

♦ Assess whether currently breast-feeding a child.

♦ Assess current and past alcohol and drug consumption.

♦ Assess for operation of automobile and/or other dangerous machinery.

♦ Assess for presence of adverse reactions or side effects.

♦ Assess patient/family knowledge about illness and need for medication.

♦ In collaboration with physician, assess CBC, liver function tests, and ophthalmologic exams in patients on long-term therapy.

♦ **Lab Test Alterations:** Increased serum alkaline phosphatase, transaminases, bilirubin.

◊ Increased protein-bound iodine.

◊ Increased urinary glucose.

◊ Decreased urinary estrogen, progestin, and gonadotropin.

◊ Increased plasma cholesterol level.

◊ Increased serum prolactin.

♦ **Withdrawal:** Assess for symptoms of abrupt withdrawal from long-term therapy: • gastritis • nausea • vomiting • dizziness • headache • tachycardia • insomnia • tremulousness.

♦ **Toxicity and Overdose:** No correlation has been established between blood level and therapeutic effect.

◊ Assess for symptoms of overdose: • CNS depression, from heavy sedation to deep sleep to coma • severe hypotension • shock-like syndrome • severe extrapyramidal symptoms • agitation • restlessness • convulsions •

fever • autonomic reactions • ECG changes • cardiac arrhythmias.

✦ **Overdose Management:** Monitor vital signs.

◊ Ensure maintenance of open airway.

◊ Initiate gastric lavage.

◊ Do not induce emesis (nuchal rigidity may result in aspiration of vomitus).

◊ Antiparkinsonian drugs or diphenhydramine may be administered to counteract extrapyramidal symptoms.

◊ Administer IV fluids or a vasoconstrictor to maintain adequate blood pressure. **Note:** Epinephrine is not recommended due to its interaction with antipsychotics, which causes a further drop in blood pressure.

◊ Administer IV phenytoin to control ventricular arrhythmias.

◊ Administer phenobarbital or diazepam to control convulsions or hyperactivity.

◊ Dialysis does not appear to be a useful intervention.

Potential Nursing Diagnoses

✦ High risk for violence directed at others related to mistrust and panic anxiety.

✦ High risk for injury related to molindone's side effects of sedation, dizziness, ataxia, weakness, lowered seizure threshold; abrupt withdrawal after prolonged use; overdose.

✦ Sensory-perceptual alteration related to panic anxiety evidenced by hallucinations.

✦ Altered thought processes related to panic anxiety evidenced by delusional thinking.

✦ Social isolation related to inability to trust others.

✦ High risk for activity intolerance related to molindone's side effects of drowsiness, dizziness, ataxia, weakness.

✦ Noncompliance with medication regimen related to suspiciousness and mistrust of others.

✦ Knowledge deficit related to medication regimen.

Plan/Implementation

✦ Monitor vital signs before beginning therapy and at regular intervals (bid or tid) throughout therapy. Take BP lying and standing to monitor for possible hypotensive reaction; elderly are particularly susceptible. Dosage adjustment may be required.

✦ Ensure that patient who is ambulatory is protected from sun when spending time outdoors.

✦ Weigh patient 2–3 times a week, at same time of day, on same scale, if possible. A rapid weight gain or evidence of edema should be reported to physician immediately. Record I&O.

✦ Ensure that patient is protected from injury. Provide supervision and assistance when ambulating if dizziness and drowsiness are problems. Pad siderails and headboard for patient who experiences seizures.

✦ Give patient hard candy, gum, or frequent sips of water if dry mouth is a problem.

✦ Ensure that patient swallows tablet and does not "cheek" to avoid medication or to hoard for later use.

✦ Tablet may be crushed and mixed with food or fluid for patient who has difficulty swallowing, or oral concentrate may be used.

✦ Mix concentrate in orange or grapefruit juice before administration.

✦ Store medication at controlled room temperatures between 15° and 30°C (59°–86°F). Protect from heat, light, and moisture.

Patient/Family Education

✦ Use caution when driving or when operating dangerous machinery. Drowsiness and dizziness can occur.

✦ Do not stop taking the drug abruptly. To do so might produce withdrawal symptoms, such as nausea, vomiting, gastritis, headache, tachycardia, insomnia, tremulousness.

✦ Use sunscreens and wear protective clothing when spending time outdoors. Skin is more susceptible to sunburn.

- Report occurrence of any of the following symptoms to physician immediately: sore throat • fever • malaise • unusual bleeding • easy bruising • persistent nausea/vomiting • severe headache • rapid heart rate • difficulty urinating • muscle twitching • tremors • darkly colored urine • pale stools • yellow skin or eyes • muscular inco-ordination • or skin rash.
- Rise slowly from a sitting or lying position to prevent a sudden drop in blood pressure.
- If dry mouth is a problem, take frequent sips of water, chew sugarless gum, or suck on hard candy. Good oral care (frequent brushing, flossing) is very important.
- Do not drink alcohol while on molindone therapy. These drugs potentiate each other's effects.
- Do not consume other medications (including over-the-counter meds) without physician's approval. Many medications contain substances that interact with molindone in a way that may be harmful.
- Be aware of possible risks of taking molindone during pregnancy. Safe use during pregnancy and lactation has not been established. It is unknown if molindone crosses the placental barrier, so adverse effects to a fetus have not been determined. Inform physician immediately if pregnancy occurs, is suspected, or is planned.
- Be aware of side effects of molindone. Refer to written materials furnished by healthcare providers for safe self-administration.
- Continue to take medication even if feeling well and as though it is not needed. Symptoms may return if medication is discontinued.
- Carry card or other identification at all times describing medications being taken.

Evaluation

- Patient demonstrates a subsiding/resolution of the symptoms for which molindone was prescribed (panic anxiety, altered thought processes, altered perceptions).
- Patient verbalizes understanding of side effects and regimen required for prudent self-administration of molindone.

NEOSTIGMINE

(nee-oh-stig′meen)
Prostigmin

Classification(s):
Cholinergic stimulant, Parasympathomimetic, Cholinesterase inhibitor
Pregnancy Category C

INDICATIONS

◆ Postoperative abdominal distention and urinary retention ◆ Myasthenia gravis (diagnosis and control) ◆ Antidote for nondepolarizing neuromuscular blocking agents. **Investigational Uses:** ◆ Urinary retention associated with use of certain drugs, such as antidepressants and antipsychotics ◆ Supraventricular tachycardia in children, resulting from tricyclic antidepressant overdose.

ACTION

◆ Competes with acetylcholine for attachment to acetylcholinesterase at sites of cholinergic transmission. Hydrolysis of acetylcholine is thereby inhibited ◆ Cholinergic action is also enhanced as transmission of impulses across neuromuscular junctions is facilitated ◆ Also effects a direct cholinomimetic response on skeletal muscle and, possibly, on autonomic ganglion cells and neurons of the central nervous system.

PHARMACOKINETICS

Absorption: Poorly absorbed from the GI tract. More rapid and complete absorption following parenteral administration.

Distribution: Not fully understood. Does not cross blood-brain barrier. Unknown if drug crosses placental barrier or enters breast milk.

Metabolism and Excretion: Hydrolyzed by cholinesterases and metabolized by microsomal enzymes in the liver. Excreted by the kidneys.

Half-Life: PO, 40–60 minutes; IM, 50–90 minutes; IV, 47–60 minutes.

CONTRAINDICATIONS AND PRECAUTIONS

Contraindicated in: ✦ Hypersensitivity to this drug or a history of sensitivity to bromides ✦ Peritonitis ✦ Mechanical intestinal or urinary tract obstruction ✦ Questionable bowel viability ✦ Children; pregnancy and lactation (safe use has not been established).

Use Cautiously in: ✦ Epilepsy ✦ Bronchial asthma ✦ Bradycardia ✦ Recent coronary occlusion ✦ Vagotonia ✦ Hyperthyroidism ✦ Cardiac arrhythmias ✦ Peptic ulcers ✦ Megacolon ✦ Decreased GI motility.

ADVERSE REACTIONS AND SIDE EFFECTS*

CNS: dizziness, convulsions, loss of consciousness, drowsiness, headache, weakness, dysarthria, miosis, vision changes.

CV: cardiac arrhythmias (bradycardia, tachycardia, AV block, nodal rhythm), nonspecific ECG changes, syncope, hypotension, CARDIAC ARREST.

Derm: rash, urticaria.

GI: salivation, nausea, vomiting, flatulence, increased peristalsis, abdominal cramps, diarrhea.

GU: urinary frequency.

Resp: increased bronchial secretions, dyspnea, RESPIRATORY DEPRESSION, RESPIRATORY ARREST, BRONCHOSPASM.

Other: muscle cramps, muscle spasms, arthralgia, diaphoresis, flushing, allergic reactions, ANAPHYLAXIS, fasciculation.

INTERACTIONS

Drug-Drug: ✦ **Depolarizing neuromuscular blocking agents (e.g., succinylcholine, decamethonium):** prolonged depolarizing action of these drugs ✦ **Drugs with anticholinergic properties (e.g., atropine, aminoglycosides, phenothiazines, haloperidol, antihistamines, antidepressants, quinidine, disopyramide):** decreased effects of neostigmine ✦ **Corticosteroids:** anticholinesterase effects may be decreased.

ROUTE AND DOSAGE

Urinary Retention

✦ **SC, IM (Adults):** 1 mL of 1:2000 solution (0.5 mg). If urination does not occur within an hour, catheterize the patient, then continue 0.5-mg injections every 3 hours for at least 5 injections.

Postoperative Distention

✦ **SC, IM (Adults):** 1 mL of 1:2000 solution (0.5 mg) as required.

Myasthenia Gravis (Diagnosis)

✦ **IM (Adults):** 0.022 mg/kg. (Administer IM atropine SO_4, 0.011 mg/kg, 30 minutes before neostigmine.)

✦ **IM (Children):** 0.025–0.04 mg/kg. (Administer SC atropine SO_4, 0.011 mg/kg, before neostigmine.)

Myasthenia Gravis (Symptomatic Control)

✦ **PO (Adults):** Initial dose: 15 mg tid. Gradually increase dosage at intervals of 1 or more days. Average dosage is 150 mg given over 24 hours (range is 15–375 mg/day). Individualize interval between doses. May be required day and night. May give larger portions of total daily dose at time of

*Underlines indicate most frequent; CAPITALS indicate life-threatening.

greater fatigue (afternoon, 30 minutes before mealtimes, etc.).

♦ **PO (Children):** 2 mg/kg/day divided and given in doses q 3–4 hours.

♦ **SC, IM, IV (Adults):** 1 mL of 1:2000 solution (0.5 mg). Individualize subsequent doses. Range: 0.5–2.5 mg. Repeat as needed.

♦ **SC, IM, IV (Children):** 0.01–0.04 mg/kg/dose q 2–3 hours as needed.

Reversal of Nondepolarizing Neuromuscular Blocking Agent (Administered by Anesthesiologist)

♦ **IV (Adults):** Administer IV atropine sulfate (0.6–1.2 mg) or IV glycopyrolate (0.2–0.6 mg) several minutes before administering neostigmine, rather than concomitantly. Administer 0.5–2.5 mg neostigmine by slow IV injection and repeat once if required. Maximum dose: 5 mg.

♦ **IV (Children):** 0.07–0.08 mg/kg/dose neostigmine with 0.008–0.025 mg/kg/dose atropine sulfate.

♦ **IV (Neonates and Infants):** 0.04 mg/kg neostigmine with 0.02 mg/kg atropine.

Supraventricular Tachycardia (Tricyclic Antidepressant Overdose)

♦ **IV (Children):** 0.5–1.0 mg slow IV, then 0.25–0.5 mg q 1–3 hours as needed to maintain clinical improvement.

PHARMACODYNAMICS

Route	Onset	Peak	Duration
PO	45–75 min	1–2 hr	2–4 hr
SC, IM	10–30 min	20–30 min	2.5–4 hr
IV	4–8 min	20–30 min	2–4 hr

NURSING IMPLICATIONS

Assessment

♦ Assess I&O and weight daily. Palpate for bladder distention. Observe for urinary incontinence.

♦ Assess mood daily in patient receiving antidepressants and antipsychotics.

Observe behavior changes, level of participation in activities, withdrawal, restlessness, agitation.

♦ Assess vital signs prior to administration. Record baseline values for comparison.

♦ In myasthenic patient, assess for symptoms of myasthenic crisis: extreme muscle weakness and severe respiratory distress. Dosage of neostigmine may have to be increased.

♦ Assess history of allergies, sensitivity to this drug or to other cholinergic drugs.

♦ Assess date of last menses (possible pregnancy), use of contraceptives.

♦ Assess whether currently breast-feeding a child.

♦ Assess current and past alcohol and drug consumption.

♦ Assess for operation of automobile and/or other dangerous machinery.

♦ Assess for presence of adverse reactions or side effects.

♦ Assess patient/family knowledge about illness and need for medication.

♦ **Toxicity and Overdose:** Assess for symptoms of cholinergic crisis (overdose of cholinergic stimulants): • nausea • vomiting • diarrhea • sweating • increased bronchial and salivary secretions • bradycardia or tachycardia • increasing muscle cramps • weakness • miosis • lacrimation • cardiospasm • hypotension • incoordination • blurred vision • fasciculation • paralysis • agitation • fear • restlessness.

♦ **Overdose Management:** Promptly discontinue administration of neostigmine.

◊ Maintain adequate respiratory exchange.

◊ Use suction if required.

◊ Ensure that airway is patent and promote respiration with oxygen.

◊ Tracheostomy may be required.

◊ Atropine is the antidote for neostigmine overdose. Dosage is 1–4 mg IV, with additional doses q 5–30 minutes as required to control symptoms. At-

ropine does not counteract skeletal muscle paralysis or any resulting respiratory paralysis from neostigmine.
◇ Monitor cardiac function.
◇ Institute appropriate precautions if seizures occur.
◇ Monitor for signs of impending shock and intervene to prevent progression.

Potential Nursing Diagnoses
♦ Ineffective breathing pattern related to effects of neuromuscular blocking agents.
♦ Urinary retention related to use of medications that promote adverse effect of urinary retention.
♦ High risk for injury related to neostigmine's side effects of weakness, dizziness, vision changes, convulsions; overdose; muscular weakness secondary to myasthenia gravis.
♦ High risk for activity intolerance related to neostigmine's side effects of drowsiness, dizziness, weakness.
♦ Knowledge deficit related to medication regimen.

Plan/Implementation
♦ **General Info:** Monitor vital signs daily. Report significant changes to physician.
◇ Weigh patient daily and keep strict records of intake and output.
◇ Ensure that patient is protected from injury. Provide supervision and assistance when ambulating if dizziness, drowsiness, or weakness are problems. Observe for seizure activity. May be necessary to pad headboard and siderails if patient experiences seizures during the night.
◇ Check pulse prior to administration. Withhold drug if pulse falls below 80 beats per minute. Notify physician. Atropine may be ordered to increase pulse rate to approximately 80 beats/min prior to administration of neostigmine.
◇ Store medication at controlled room temperatures between 15° and 30°C (59°–86°F). Protect from heat and freezing.

♦ **PO:** Medication may be given with food or milk to minimize GI upset.
◇ If intended to facilitate chewing in myasthenic patient, administer 30 minutes before meals.
◇ Onset of action occurs within 45–75 minutes. Check vital signs q 30 minutes for several hours following oral administration. Monitor for signs of overdose: nausea ● vomiting ● diarrhea ● sweating ● increased bronchial and salivary secretions ● bradycardia ● increasing muscle weakness.
◇ Oral dose is considerably larger than parenteral dose due to poor absorption of the drug via oral route.
♦ **IM, SC:** Rotate sites if multiple injections are administered.
◇ A syringe of atropine containing the appropriate dosage should always be readily available when administering neostigmine should symptoms of cholinergic overstimulation appear.
◇ If atropine and neostigmine are ordered concomitantly, do not mix together. Use separate syringes as well as separate injection sites.
◇ Onset of action occurs within 20 minutes. Check vital signs q 15–30 minutes following SC or IM administration. Monitor for signs and symptoms of cholinergic overstimulation.
◇ Do not mix in syringe with any other drug.
♦ **IV:** Medication may be given undiluted. Do not add to IV solutions. Administer through Y-tube or 3-way stopcock of infusion set.
◇ Administer at rate not exceeding 0.5 mg/min.
◇ IV administration of neostigmine for reversal of nondepolarizing neuromuscular agents is performed by an anesthesiologist.
◇ Ensure availability of atropine sulfate before IV administration of neostigmine. (See Overdose Management for specific dosage and administration of atropine.)

◇ Obtain vital signs q 15 minutes following IV administration for 2–4 hours.

Patient/Family Education

♦ Medication may be taken with food or milk to prevent GI upset.

♦ Use caution when driving or when operating dangerous machinery. Drowsiness, dizziness, weakness, and visual changes can occur.

♦ Report occurrence of any of the following symptoms to physician immediately: nausea • vomiting • diarrhea • sweating • increased salivary secretions • irregular heartbeat • muscle weakness • severe abdominal pain • difficulty in breathing • blurred vision, agitation.

♦ Do not consume other medications (including over-the-counter meds) without physician's approval. Many medications contain substances that may interact with neostigmine in a way that could be harmful.

♦ Be aware of possible risks of taking neostigmine during pregnancy. Safe use during pregnancy and lactation has not been established. It is not known if neostigmine crosses the placental barrier. If it does, a fetus could experience adverse effects of the drug. Inform physician immediately if pregnancy occurs, is suspected, or is planned.

♦ Be aware of side effects of neostigmine. Refer to written materials furnished by healthcare providers for safe self-administration.

♦ Carry card or other identification at all times describing medications being taken.

Evaluation

♦ Patient demonstrates a resolution/subsiding of the symptoms for which neostigmine was prescribed (urinary retention, abdominal distention, muscular weakness, inadequate respiration following use of nondepolarizing neuromuscular blocking agents).

♦ Patient verbalizes understanding of side effects and regimen required for prudent self-administration of neostigmine.

NORTRIPTYLINE

(nor-trip'ti-leen)
Aventyl, Pamelor

Classification(s):
Tricyclic antidepressant
Pregnancy Category C

INDICATIONS

♦ Major depression with melancholia or psychotic symptoms ♦ Depression associated with organic disease, alcoholism, schizophrenia, or mental retardation ♦ Depressive phase of bipolar disorder.

ACTION

♦ Exact mechanism unclear ♦ Blocks reuptake of the neurotransmitters norepinephrine and serotonin, increasing their concentration at the synapse and correcting the deficit that is thought to contribute to the melancholy mood of the depressed person.

PHARMACOKINETICS

Absorption: Not known.
Distribution: Is widely distributed. Crosses blood-brain and placental barriers. Enters breast milk.
Metabolism and Excretion: Metabolized by the liver. Excreted primarily by the kidneys; small amounts excreted in feces.
Half-Life: 16–>90 hours.

CONTRAINDICATIONS AND PRECAUTIONS

Contraindicated in: ♦ Hypersensitivity to this drug or to other tricyclic antidepressants ♦ Concomitant use of MAO inhibitors ♦ Acute recovery period following myocardial infarction ♦ Untreated angle-closure glaucoma ♦ Children; pregnancy and lactation (safety not established).

Use Cautiously in: ♦ Patients with a history of seizures ♦ Urinary retention ♦ Benign prostatic hypertrophy ♦ Glaucoma ♦ Cardiovascular disorders ♦ Respiratory difficulties ♦ Hepatic or renal insufficiency ♦ Psychotic patients ♦ Elderly or debilitated patients.

ADVERSE REACTIONS AND SIDE EFFECTS*

CNS: drowsiness, dizziness, weakness, headache, fatigue, confusion, lethargy, memory deficits, disturbed concentration, tremors, ataxia, tinnitus, extrapyramidal symptoms, paresthesias of extremities, lowered seizure threshold, blurred vision, agitation, excitement, restlessness, insomnia, exacerbation of psychosis, shift to manic behavior.
CV: orthostatic hypotension, tachycardia and other arrhythmias, hypertension, MYOCARDIAL INFARCTION, HEART BLOCK, CONGESTIVE HEART FAILURE, ECG changes, syncope, CARDIOVASCULAR COLLAPSE.
Derm: skin rash, urticaria, photosensitivity, erythema, petechiae.
GI: dry mouth, constipation, nausea, vomiting, anorexia, diarrhea, abdominal cramps, adynamic ileus, esophageal reflux, stomatitis, black tongue.
GU: urinary retention, gynecomastia (men), testicular swelling, menstrual irregularity, breast engorgement and galactorrhea (women), changes in libido, impotence, delayed micturition.
Hemat: AGRANULOCYTOSIS, THROMBOCYTOPENIA, LEUKOPENIA, eosinophilia, purpura.
Hepat: jaundice, hepatitis.
Other: weight gain, nasal congestion, alopecia, hypothermia, peripheral neuropathy.

INTERACTIONS

Drug-Drug: ♦ **MAO inhibitors:** hyperpyretic crisis, hypertensive crisis, severe seizures, tachycardia, death ♦ **Guanethidine, clonidine, (possibly) guanabenz:** decreased effects of these medications ♦ **Cimetidine:** increased nortriptyline serum levels ♦ **Amphetamines, sympathomimetics:** increased hypertensive and cardiac effects of these drugs ♦ **CNS depressants (including alcohol, barbiturates, benzodiazepines):** potentiation of CNS effects ♦ **Thyroid medications:** tachycardia, arrhythmias ♦ **Methylphenidate, phenothiazines, haloperidol:** increased serum nortriptyline levels ♦ **Ethchlorvynol:** transient delirium ♦ **Quinidine, procainamide, disopyramide:** potentiation of adverse cardiovascular effects of nortriptyline ♦ **Oral contraceptives:** decreased effects of nortriptyline ♦ **Smoking:** increased nortriptyline metabolism ♦ **Disulfiram:** decreased nortriptyline metabolism ♦ **Levodopa, phenylbutazone:** delayed or decreased absorption of these drugs ♦ **Dicumarol:** increased plasma dicumarol concentrations.

ROUTE AND DOSAGE
Depression
♦ **PO (Adults):** Initial dose: 25 mg tid or qid. Increase as necessary to 100 mg/day. May be given as single daily dose. For patients who require larger doses (up to 150 mg/day), plasma levels should be monitored. Dosage above 150 mg/day not recommended by manufacturer. Some clinicians consider 300 mg/day to be maximum dose.
♦ **PO (Adolescents, Geriatrics):** 30–50 mg/day in divided doses or single daily dose.
♦ **PO (Maintenance):** Reduce to lowest possible dose from which relief of symptoms is achieved.

---

*Underlines indicate most frequent; CAPITALS indicate life-threatening.

PHARMACODYNAMICS

Route	Onset	Peak	Duration
PO	2–4 wk	7–8.5 hr	Weeks*

*Allow up to 2 weeks following cessation of therapy for complete drug elimination.

NURSING IMPLICATIONS
Assessment

* Assess for suicidal ideation, plan, means. Assess for sudden lifts in mood, which could indicate patient's decision to commit suicide.
* Assess mental status daily: mood • appearance • thought and communication patterns • level of interest in the environment and in activities • suicidal ideation. Improvement in these behavior patterns and level of energy should be expected within 2–4 weeks of initiation of therapy.
* Assess for symptoms of blood dyscrasias: sore throat • fever • malaise • unusual bleeding • easy bruising.
* Assess vital signs, weight.
* Assess history of allergies, sensitivity to this drug or to other tricyclic antidepressants.
* Assess for history of glaucoma.
* Assess date of last menses (possible pregnancy), use of contraceptives.
* Assess whether currently breast-feeding a child.
* Assess current and past alcohol and drug consumption.
* Assess for operation of automobile and/or other dangerous machinery.
* Assess for presence of adverse reactions or side effects.
* Assess patient/family knowledge about illness and need for medication.
* In collaboration with physician, assess CBC and liver function tests in patients on long-term therapy.
* **Lab Test Alterations:** Increased serum bilirubin, alkaline phosphatase, transaminase, and glucose.
◇ Decreased urinary 5-hydroxyindoleacetic acid (HIAA) and vanillylmandelic acid (VMA) excretion.

* **Withdrawal:** Assess for symptoms of abrupt withdrawal from long-term therapy: • nausea • headache • vertigo • malaise • insomnia • nightmares.
* **Toxicity and Overdose:** Range of therapeutic serum concentration is 50–150 ng/mL.
◇ Assess for symptoms of overdose: • confusion • agitation • irritability • hallucinations • seizures • flushing • dry mouth • dilated pupils • delirium • hyperpyrexia • hypotension or hypertension • coma • tachycardia • arrhythmias • respiratory depression • cardiac arrest • renal failure • shock • congestive heart failure • acid-base disturbances.
* **Overdose Management:** Monitor vital signs.
◇ Maintain adequate airway.
◇ Monitor ECG.
◇ Induce emesis in conscious patient.
◇ Initiate gastric lavage in unconscious patient.
◇ Administer activated charcoal to minimize absorption.
◇ Administer IV physostigmine cautiously to reverse anticholinergic effects.
◇ Administer sodium bicarbonate, vasopressors, phenytoin, propranolol, or lidocaine to treat cardiovascular effects.
◇ Administer IV diazepam to control seizures.

Potential Nursing Diagnoses

* High risk for self-directed violence related to depressed mood.
* High risk for injury related to abrupt withdrawal after prolonged use; overdose; nortriptyline's side effects of sedation, dizziness, ataxia, weakness, confusion, lowered seizure threshold.
* Social isolation related to depressed mood.
* High risk for activity intolerance related to nortriptyline's side effects of drowsiness, dizziness, ataxia, weakness, confusion.

- Knowledge deficit related to medication regimen.

Plan/Implementation

- Monitor vital signs before beginning therapy and at regular intervals (bid or tid) throughout therapy. Take BP lying and standing in patients experiencing orthostatic hypotension; elderly are particularly susceptible. Contact physician if tachycardia/arrhythmias are noted.
- Ensure that patient who is ambulatory is protected from sun when spending time outdoors.
- Weigh patient 2–3 times a week, at same time of day, on same scale, if possible. A rapid weight gain or evidence of edema should be reported to physician immediately. Record I&O.
- Ensure that patient is protected from injury. Provide supervision and assistance when ambulating if dizziness and drowsiness are problems. Pad siderails and headboard for patient who experiences seizures.
- Give patient hard candy, gum, or frequent sips of water if dry mouth is a problem.
- Medication may be given with food to minimize GI upset.
- Ensure that patient swallows capsule and does not "cheek" to avoid medication or to hoard for later use.
- Contents of capsule may be emptied and mixed with food or fluid for patient who has difficulty swallowing, or liquid form may be used.
- Liquid form may be mixed with water, fruit juice, or milk.
- Store medication at controlled room temperatures between 15° and 30°C (59°–86°F). Protect from heat and moisture.

Patient/Family Education

- Therapeutic effect may not be seen for as long as 4 weeks. If after this length of time no improvement is noted, physician may prescribe a different medication. Continue to take medication even though symptoms have not subsided.
- Use caution when driving or when operating dangerous machinery. Drowsiness and dizziness can occur. If these side effects become persistent or interfere with activities of daily living, report to physician. Dosage adjustment may be necessary.
- Do not stop taking the drug abruptly. To do so might produce withdrawal symptoms, such as nausea, vertigo, insomnia, headache, malaise, nightmares.
- Use sunscreens and wear protective clothing when spending time outdoors. Skin may be sensitive to sunburn.
- Report occurrence of any of the following symptoms to physician immediately: sore throat • fever • malaise • unusual bleeding • easy bruising • persistent nausea/vomiting • severe headache • rapid heart rate • difficulty urinating.
- Rise slowly from a sitting or lying position to prevent a sudden drop in blood pressure.
- If dry mouth is a problem, take frequent sips of water, chew sugarless gum, or suck on hard candy. Good oral care (frequent brushing, flossing) is very important.
- Do not smoke while on nortriptyline therapy. Smoking increases metabolism of nortriptyline, requiring adjustment in dosage to achieve therapeutic effect.
- Do not drink alcohol while on nortriptyline therapy. These drugs potentiate each other's effects.
- Do not consume other medications (including over-the-counter meds) with nortriptyline without physician's approval. Many medications contain substances that, in combination with tricyclics, could precipitate a life-threatening hypertensive crisis.
- Be aware of possible risks of taking nortriptyline during pregnancy. Safe

use during pregnancy and lactation has not been established. Nortriptyline readily crosses the placental barrier, so a fetus could experience adverse effects of the drug. Inform physician immediately if pregnancy occurs, is suspected, or is planned.

♦ Be aware of side effects of nortriptyline. Refer to written materials furnished by healthcare providers for safe self-administration.

♦ Carry card or other identification at all times describing medications being taken.

Evaluation

♦ Patient demonstrates a subsiding/resolution of the symptoms for which nortriptyline was prescribed (depressed mood, suicidal ideation).

♦ Patient verbalizes understanding of side effects and regimen required for prudent self-administration of nortriptyline.

ORPHENADRINE HYDROCHLORIDE

(or-fen′a-dreen)
Disipal

Classification(s):
Antiparkinsonian agent,
Anticholinergic
Pregnancy Category C

INDICATIONS

♦ Postencephalitic, arteriosclerotic, and idiopathic parkinsonism.

ACTION

♦ Acts to correct an imbalance of dopamine deficiency and acetylcholine excess in the corpus striatum. The acetylcholine receptor is blocked at the synapse to diminish excess cholinergic effect.

PHARMACOKINETICS

Absorption: Rapidly absorbed following oral administration.
Distribution: Not completely understood. May cross placental barrier and may enter breast milk.
Metabolism and Excretion: Metabolized by the liver. Excreted in urine as metabolites and unchanged drug.
Half-Life: ~14 hours.

CONTRAINDICATIONS AND PRECAUTIONS

Contraindicated in: ♦ Hypersensitivity to this drug ♦ Angle-closure glaucoma ♦ Pyloric or duodenal obstruction ♦ Stenosing peptic ulcers ♦ Prostatic hypertrophy or bladder-neck obstructions ♦ Achalasia ♦ Myasthenia gravis ♦ Children less than 12 years old ♦ Ulcerative colitis ♦ Toxic megacolon ♦ Tachycardia secondary to cardiac insufficiency or thyrotoxicosis.

Use Cautiously in: ♦ Narrow-angle glaucoma ♦ Elderly or debilitated patients ♦ Pregnancy and lactation (safety not established) ♦ Hepatic, renal, or cardiac insufficiency ♦ Tendency toward urinary retention ♦ Hyperthyroidism ♦ Hypertension ♦ Autonomic neuropathy ♦ Patients exposed to high environmental temperatures.

ADVERSE REACTIONS AND SIDE EFFECTS*

CNS: drowsiness, dizziness, blurred vision, disorientation, confusion, memory loss, psychoses, agitation, nervousness, delirium, paranoia, depression, hallucinations, mydriasis, cycloplegia, headache, insomnia.
CV: orthostatic hypotension, hypotension, tachycardia, palpitations.
Derm: skin rashes, urticaria, pruritis, ANAPHYLACTIC SHOCK (rare).
GI: dry mouth, nausea, vomiting, epigastric distress, constipation.

---

*Underlines indicate most frequent; CAPITALS indicate life-threatening.

GU: urinary retention, urinary hesitancy. **Other:** muscular cramping, elevated temperature, flushing, decreased sweating, anaphylaxis, increased intraocular pressure.

INTERACTIONS

Drug-Drug: ✦ **Other drugs with anticholinergic properties (e.g., glutethimide, disopyramide, narcotic analgesics, phenothiazines, tricyclic antidepressants, antihistamines, quinidine salts, amantadine):** increased anticholinergic effects ✦ **Levodopa:** possible decreased levodopa absorption ✦ **Slow-dissolving digoxin:** decreased absorption of digoxin ✦ **CNS depressants (e.g., alcohol, barbiturates, narcotics, benzodiazepines):** increased CNS depressant effects ✦ **Phenothiazines, haloperidol:** decreased therapeutic effects of these drugs ✦ **Propoxyphene:** additive CNS depression, mental confusion, anxiety, tremors ✦ **Ketoconazole:** decreased absorption of ketoconazole ✦ **Antacids:** decreased absorption of orphenadrine.

ROUTE AND DOSAGE

Parkinsonism

✦ **PO (Adults):** 50 mg tid. Smaller doses may be sufficient when combined with other agents. Doses as large as 250 mg/day have been used without untoward effects.

PHARMACODYNAMICS

Route	Onset	Peak	Duration
PO	30–60 min	2 hr	4–6 hr

NURSING IMPLICATIONS

Assessment

✦ Assess for symptoms of Parkinson's disease: • tremors • muscular weakness and rigidity • drooling • shuffling gait • disturbances of posture and equilibrium • flat affect • monotone speech.
✦ Assess vital signs, weight. Record baseline values for comparison.
✦ Assess history of allergies, sensitivity to this drug or to other anticholinergics.
✦ Assess date of last menses (possible pregnancy), use of contraceptives.
✦ Assess whether currently breast-feeding a child.
✦ Assess current and past alcohol and drug consumption.
✦ Assess for operation of automobile and/or other dangerous machinery.
✦ Assess for presence of adverse reactions or side effects.
✦ Assess patient/family knowledge about illness and need for medication.
✦ In collaboration with physician, assess CBC, renal and liver function, and intraocular pressure in patients on long-term therapy.
✦ **Toxicity and Overdose:** Assess for symptoms of overdose: • CNS depression preceded or followed by stimulation • intensification of psychotic symptoms • anxiety • ataxia • seizures • incoherence • delusions • paranoia • anhidrosis • hyperpyrexia • hot, dry, flushed skin • dry mucous membranes • decreased bowel sounds • shock • coma • skeletal muscle paralysis • urinary retention • tachycardia • difficulty swallowing • cardiac arrhythmias • circulatory collapse • cardiac arrest • respiratory depression or arrest.
✦ **Overdose Management:** Monitor vital signs.
◊ Maintain adequate airway.
◊ Induce emesis or initiate gastric lavage in conscious patient (contraindicated in precomatose, convulsive, or psychotic states).
◊ Administer activated charcoal to minimize absorption.
◊ Administer pilocarpine, 5 mg PO, to treat peripheral effects.
◊ Administer physostigmine, 1–2 mg SC or slow IV, to reverse anticholinergic effects (use only with availability of advanced life support).
◊ Employ artificial respiration and oxygen for respiratory depression.

◇ Use tepid water sponges, cold packs, or other cooling applications to treat hyperpyrexia.

◇ Darken room to counter photophobia.

◇ Administer IV fluids and a vasopressor to prevent circulatory collapse.

◇ Administer diazepam to control symptoms of acute psychosis.

Potential Nursing Diagnoses

♦ High risk for injury related to confusion, weakness, drowsiness, and dizziness associated with symptoms of parkinsonism and side effects of medication.

♦ Sensory-perceptual alteration related to side effect of orphenadrine evidenced by hallucinations.

♦ Altered thought processes related to side effects of orphenadrine evidenced by memory loss, disorientation, confusion.

♦ Social isolation related to embarrassment by symptoms of Parkinson's disease.

♦ High risk for activity intolerance related to orphenadrine's side effects of drowsiness, dizziness, ataxia, weakness, confusion.

♦ Knowledge deficit related to medication regimen.

Plan/Implementation

♦ Monitor vital signs daily. Be particularly alert for increase in pulse rate or drop in blood pressure.

♦ Weigh patient 2–3 times a week, at same time of day, on same scale, if possible. A rapid weight gain or evidence of edema should be reported to physician immediately. Record I&O.

♦ Monitor for exacerbation of mental symptoms such as psychoses, depression, paranoia.

♦ Ensure that patient is protected from injury. Provide supervision and assistance when ambulating if dizziness and drowsiness are problems.

♦ Give patient hard candy, gum, or frequent sips of water if dry mouth is a problem, or treat with saliva substitute.

♦ Ensure that patient swallows tablet and does not "cheek" to avoid medication or to hoard for later use.

♦ Medication may be administered with food to minimize gastric irritation.

♦ Tablet may be crushed and mixed with food or fluid for patient who has difficulty swallowing.

♦ Monitor vital signs before beginning therapy and at regular intervals (bid or tid) throughout therapy. Take BP lying and standing to monitor for possible hypotensive reaction; elderly are particularly susceptible. Dosage adjustment may be required.

♦ Store medication at controlled room temperatures between 15° and 30°C (59°–86°F). Protect from heat, light, and moisture.

Patient/Family Education

♦ Medication may be taken with food if GI upset occurs.

♦ Use caution when driving or when operating dangerous machinery. Drowsiness and dizziness can occur.

♦ Do not stop taking the drug abruptly. To do so might produce withdrawal symptoms.

♦ Report occurrence of any of the following symptoms to physician immediately: pain or tenderness in area in front of ear, extreme dryness of mouth, difficulty urinating, abdominal pain, constipation, fast and pounding heartbeat, tremors, rash, vision disturbances, mental changes.

♦ Rise slowly from a sitting or lying position to prevent a sudden drop in blood pressure.

♦ If dry mouth is a problem, take frequent sips of water, chew sugarless gum, or suck on hard candy. Good oral care (frequent brushing, flossing) is very important.

♦ Do not drink alcohol while on orphenadrine therapy.

♦ Do not consume other medications (including over-the-counter meds) without physician's approval. Many medications contain substances that interact with orphenadrine in a way that may be harmful.

◆ Be aware of possible risks of taking orphenadrine during pregnancy. Safe use during pregnancy and lactation has not been established. It is thought that orphenadrine crosses the placental barrier; if so, a fetus could experience adverse effects of the drug. Inform physician immediately if pregnancy occurs, is suspected, or is planned.

◆ Be aware of side effects of orphenadrine. Refer to written materials furnished by healthcare providers for safe self-administration.

◆ Continue to take medication even if feeling well and as though it is not needed. Symptoms may return if medication is discontinued.

◆ Carry card or other identification at all times describing medications being taken.

Evaluation

◆ Patient demonstrates a subsiding of the symptoms for which orphenadrine was prescribed (parkinsonism).

◆ Patient verbalizes understanding of side effects and regimen required for prudent self-administration of orphenadrine.

OXAZEPAM

(ox-a'ze-pam)
Serax

Classification(s):
*Antianxiety agent, Benzodiazepine,
Skeletal muscle relaxant,
Anticonvulsant*
Schedule C IV
Pregnancy Category D

INDICATIONS

◆ Anxiety disorders ◆ Anxiety symptoms ◆ Anxiety associated with depression ◆ Acute alcohol withdrawal.

ACTION

◆ Depresses subcortical levels of the central nervous system, particularly the limbic system and reticular formation ◆ May potentiate the effects of the powerful inhibitory neurotransmitter gamma-aminobutyric acid (GABA) in the brain, thereby producing a calmative effect ◆ All levels of CNS depression can be effected, from mild sedation to hypnosis to coma.

PHARMACOKINETICS

Absorption: Rapidly absorbed from the GI tract.
Distribution: Is widely distributed. Crosses blood-brain and placental barriers; excreted in breast milk.
Metabolism and Excretion: Metabolized by the liver; produces inactive metabolites that are excreted for the most part by the kidneys.
Half-Life: 3–21 hours.

CONTRAINDICATIONS AND PRECAUTIONS

Contraindicated in: ◆ Hypersensitivity to this drug or to other benzodiazepines ◆ Hypersensitivity to tartrazine dye (contained in some 100-mg tablets) ◆ Combination with other CNS depressants ◆ Pregnancy and lactation ◆ Narrow-angle glaucoma ◆ Children under 12.
Use Cautiously in: ◆ Elderly or debilitated patients ◆ Hepatic or renal dysfunction ◆ Individuals with a history of drug abuse/addiction ◆ Depressed/suicidal patients.

ADVERSE REACTIONS AND SIDE EFFECTS*

CNS: <u>drowsiness</u>, <u>fatigue</u>, <u>ataxia</u>, <u>dizziness</u>, confusion, headache, syncope, paradoxical excitement.
CV: orthostatic hypotension.
Derm: skin rashes.

---

*<u>Underlines</u> indicate most frequent; CAPITALS indicate life-threatening.

Endo: gynecomastia, galactorrhea.
GI: dry mouth, nausea.
GU: irregular menses, libidinal changes, incontinence.
Hemat: leukopenia, jaundice.
Other: tolerance, physical and psychological dependence.

INTERACTIONS

Drug-Drug: ✦ **Other CNS depressants (including alcohol, barbiturates, narcotics), antipsychotics, antidepressants, antihistamines, anticonvulsants:** additive CNS depression ✦ **Cimetidine:** increased effects of oxazepam ✦ **Cigarette smoking and caffeine:** decreased effects of oxazepam ✦ **Neuromuscular blocking agents:** increased respiratory depression ✦ **Digoxin:** reduced excretion of digoxin, increased potential for toxicity ✦ **Rifampin, valproic acid:** decreased effects of oxazepam ✦ **Levodopa:** decreased effects of levodopa.

ROUTE AND DOSAGE

Anxiety, Anxiety Disorders, Anxiety Associated with Depression

(Efficacy for periods greater than 4 months has not been evaluated.)
✦ **PO (Adults):** 10–30 mg tid or qid.
✦ **PO (Geriatric):** 10 mg tid initially. Dosage may be cautiously increased to 15 mg tid or qid if necessary.

Acute Alcohol Withdrawal
✦ **PO (Adults):** 15–30 mg tid or qid.

PHARMACODYNAMICS

Route	Onset	Peak	Duration
PO	45–90 min	1–2 hr	*

*Varies with individual, age, disease state, number of doses.

NURSING IMPLICATIONS
Assessment
✦ Assess level of anxiety. Symptoms include: • restlessness • pacing • insomnia • inability to concentrate • increased heart rate • increased respiration • elevated blood pressure • confusion • tremors • rapid speech.
✦ Assess for suicidal ideation (CNS depressants aggravate symptoms in depressed patients).
✦ Assess history of allergies, sensitivity to this drug.
✦ Assess history of glaucoma.
✦ Assess date of last menses (possible pregnancy), use of contraceptives.
✦ Assess whether currently breast-feeding a child.
✦ Assess current and past alcohol and drug consumption.
✦ Assess operation of automobile and/ or other dangerous machinery.
✦ Assess for presence of adverse reactions or side effects.
✦ Assess patient/family knowledge about illness and need for medication.
✦ In collaboration with physician, assess CBC and liver function tests in patients on long-term therapy.
✦ **Withdrawal:** Assess for symptoms of withdrawal: • depression • insomnia • increased anxiety • abdominal and muscle cramps • tremors • vomiting • sweating • convulsions • delirium.
✦ **Withdrawal Management:** Monitor vital signs.
◊ Place patient in quiet room with low stimuli.
◊ Institute seizure precautions.
◊ A long-acting barbiturate, such as phenobarbital, may be ordered to suppress withdrawal symptoms.
◊ Phenytoin may be ordered to prevent seizures.
✦ **Toxicity and Overdose:** Assess for symptoms of intoxication: • euphoria • relaxation • drowsiness • slurred speech • disorientation • mood lability • incoordination • unsteady gait • disinhibition of sexual and aggressive impulses • judgment and/or memory impairment.
◊ Assess for symptoms of overdose: • shallow respiration • cold and clammy skin • hypotension • dilated pupils •

weak and rapid pulse • hypnosis • coma • possible death.

♦ **Overdose Management:** Monitor vital signs.

◇ Maintain adequate airway.

◇ Induce vomiting in conscious patient.

◇ Initiate gastric lavage in unconscious patient.

◇ Administer activated charcoal to minimize absorption.

◇ IV fluids and vasopressors may be used to combat hypotension.

◇ Forced diuresis may be used to facilitate elimination of the drug.

Potential Nursing Diagnoses

♦ High risk for injury related to seizures, panic anxiety, abrupt withdrawal from long-term oxazepam use, effects of oxazepam intoxication or overdose.

♦ High risk for self-directed violence related to depressed mood.

♦ Anxiety (specify level) related to threats to physical integrity and/or self-concept.

♦ High risk for activity intolerance related to oxazepam's side effects of lethargy, drowsiness, dizziness, muscular weakness.

♦ Knowledge deficit related to medication regimen.

Plan/Implementation

♦ Monitor vital signs before beginning therapy and at regular intervals (bid) throughout therapy.

♦ Ensure that patient practices good oral care. Offer patient hard, sugarless candy, gum, or frequent sips of water for dry mouth.

♦ Ensure that patient is protected from injury. Supervise and assist with ambulation if dizziness and muscular weakness are problems. Pad siderails and headboard for patient who experiences seizures.

♦ To minimize nausea, medication may be given with food or milk.

♦ If patient has difficulty swallowing, tablet may be crushed or capsule emptied and contents mixed with food or fluid.

♦ Ensure that tablet or capsule has been swallowed and not "cheeked" to avoid medication or to hoard for later use.

♦ Store medication in tightly-closed container at controlled room temperatures between 15° and 30°C (59°–86°F).

Patient/Family Education

♦ Do not drive or operate dangerous machinery. Drowsiness and dizziness can occur.

♦ Do not stop taking the drug abruptly. To do so can produce serious withdrawal symptoms.

♦ Do not consume other CNS depressants (including alcohol).

♦ Do not take nonprescription medication without approval from physician.

♦ Be aware of risks of taking oxazepam during pregnancy (congenital malformations have been associated with use during first trimester). Notify physician of desirability to discontinue drug if pregnancy is suspected or planned.

♦ Be aware of potential side effects. Refer to written materials furnished by healthcare providers regarding correct method of self-administration.

♦ Carry card or other identification at all times stating names of medications being taken.

Evaluation

♦ Patient demonstrates a subsiding/resolution of the symptoms for which oxazepam was prescribed (anxiety symptoms, anxiety disorders).

♦ Patient verbalizes understanding of side effects and regimen required for prudent self-administration of oxazepam.

PARALDEHYDE

(par-al′de-hyde)
Paral

Classification(s):
Anticonvulsant, Sedative-hypnotic
Schedule C IV
Pregnancy Category C

INDICATIONS

♦ Agitation of acute alcohol withdrawal ♦ Seizures associated with emergency situations such as tetanus, eclampsia, status epilepticus, and drug poisoning.

ACTION

♦ Mechanism of action not completely understood ♦ Produces CNS depression similar to the barbiturates and alcohol.

PHARMACOKINETICS

Absorption: Readily absorbed following oral and IM administration.
Distribution: Thought to be widely distributed. Crosses blood-brain and placental barriers; excretion in breast milk unknown.
Metabolism and Excretion: Metabolized by the liver; excreted through the lungs and kidneys.
Half-Life: 3.5–9.5 hours (average 7.5 hours).

CONTRAINDICATIONS AND PRECAUTIONS

Contraindicated in: ♦ Hypersensitivity to the drug ♦ Hepatic insufficiency ♦ Respiratory disease ♦ Gastrointestinal irritation or ulceration.
Use Cautiously in: ♦ Elderly or debilitated patients ♦ Hepatic or renal dysfunction ♦ Individuals with a history of drug abuse/addiction ♦ Depressed/suicidal patients ♦ Pregnancy.

ADVERSE REACTIONS AND SIDE EFFECTS*

CNS: drowsiness, ataxia, dizziness, confusion, headache, hangover, paradoxical excitement.
CV: hypotension; with IV infusion: thrombophlebitis, CIRCULATORY COLLAPSE.
Derm: skin rashes, urticaria, redness at site of IM injection.
GI: nausea/vomiting, unpleasant taste and foul breath, irritation of mucous membranes, TOXIC HEPATITIS.
Other: tolerance, physical and psychological dependence; with IV use: coughing, pulmonary edema, pulmonary hemorrhage, respiratory distress; with IM injection: sterile skin abscesses, muscular irritation, nerve damage.

INTERACTIONS

Drug-Drug: ♦ **Other CNS depressants (including alcohol, barbiturates, opiates):** additive CNS depression ♦ **MAO inhibitors, tricyclic antidepressants, general anesthetics:** increased effects of either paraldehyde or these medications ♦ **Disulfiram:** increased blood levels of paraldehyde ♦ **All drugs for parenteral administration:** paraldehyde is incompatible with all drug substances in solution or syringe.

ROUTE AND DOSAGE
Alcohol Withdrawal

♦ **PO, Rect (Adults):** 5–10 mL every 4–6 hours, not to exceed 60 mL first day, then q 6 hr to maximum 40 mL daily on following days.
♦ **IM (Adults):** 5 mL every 4–6 hours, not to exceed 30 mL for first 24 hours, then q 6 hr to maximum of 30 mL daily on following days.

Seizures (Status Epilepticus)

♦ **IM (Adults):** 5–10 mL.
♦ **IM (Children):** 0.15 mL/kg.
♦ **IV (Adults):** 0.2–0.4 mL/kg diluted

*Underlines indicate most frequent; CAPITALS indicate life-threatening.

in 100 mL 0.9% sodium chloride for injection.

+ **IV (Children):** 0.1–0.15 mL/kg diluted in 100 mL 0.9% sodium chloride for injection.
+ **Rect (Children):** 0.3 mL/kg q 4–6 hr or 1 mL/year of age, not to exceed 5 mL; may repeat in 1 hr prn.

Sedation

+ **PO, Rect (Adults):** 5–10 mL.
+ **IM (Adults):** 2–5 mL.
+ **IV (Adults):** 5 mL diluted with 100 mL 0.9% sodium chloride for injection.
+ **PO, Rect, IM (Children):** 0.15 mL/kg.

Hypnosis

+ **PO, Rect (Adults):** 10–30 mL.
+ **IM (Adults):** 10 mL.
+ **IV (Adults):** 10 mL diluted with at least 200 mL 0.9% sodium chloride for injection.
+ **PO, Rect, IM (Children):** 0.30 mL/kg.

PHARMACODYNAMICS

Route	Onset	Peak	Duration
PO,			
Rect	10–15 min	20–60 min	8–12 hr
IM	30 min	30–60 min	6–8 hr
IV	10–15 min	~immediate	6–8 hr

NURSING IMPLICATIONS

Assessment

+ Assess level of CNS agitation. Symptoms include: • restlessness • pacing • insomnia • inability to concentrate • increased heart rate • increased respiration • elevated blood pressure • confusion • tremors • convulsions • delirium.
+ Assess for suicidal ideation (CNS depressants aggravate symptoms in depressed patients).
+ Assess history of allergies, sensitivity to this drug.
+ Assess for presence of adverse reactions or side effects.
+ Assess date of last menses (possible pregnancy), use of contraceptives.
+ Assess whether currently breast-feeding a child.
+ Assess current and past alcohol and drug consumption.
+ Assess operation of automobile and/or other dangerous machinery.
+ Assess patient/family knowledge about illness and need for medication.
+ Assess for symptoms of withdrawal from long-term use. Could produce: • depression • insomnia • cramping • tremors • vomiting • sweating • convulsions • delirium.
+ In collaboration with physician, assess CBC and liver function tests in patients on long-term therapy.
+ **Lab Test Alterations:** Increased serum and urine ketones.
◊ Altered urinary steroid determinations.
+ **Withdrawal:** Assess for symptoms of abrupt withdrawal after prolonged use. Delirium tremens and vivid hallucinations may occur.
+ **Withdrawal Management:** Monitor vital signs.
◊ Place patient in quiet room with low stimuli.
◊ Institute seizure precautions.
◊ Observe frequently.
◊ Employ supportive measures.
+ **Toxicity and Overdose:** Assess for symptoms of toxicity/overdose: • mental confusion • rapid, labored respiration • nausea/vomiting • rapid, feeble pulse • respiratory depression • hypotension • bleeding gastritis • renal and liver damage • metabolic acidosis • pulmonary edema • right heart failure • cardiovascular collapse • coma.
+ **Overdose Management:** Monitor vital signs.
◊ Ensure maintenance of adequate airway.
◊ Initiate gastric lavage (for oral overdose).
◊ Initiate rectal lavage (for rectal overdose).

◊ Administer IV fluids.

◊ Administer sodium bicarbonate to correct metabolic acidosis.

◊ Hemodialysis or peritoneal dialysis may be required.

Potential Nursing Diagnoses

♦ High risk for injury related to seizures; abrupt withdrawal from long-term paraldehyde use; agitation from acute alcohol withdrawal; effects of paraldehyde overdose.

♦ High risk for self-directed violence related to depressed mood.

♦ Sleep pattern disturbance related to situational crises, physical condition, severe level of anxiety.

♦ High risk for activity intolerance related to paraldehyde's side effects of drowsiness, dizziness, ataxia, hangover.

♦ Knowledge deficit related to medication regimen.

Plan/Implementation

♦ **General Info:** Monitor vital signs before beginning therapy, at regular intervals (bid) throughout therapy, and q 10 min during IV administration.

◊ Ensure that patient is protected from injury. Supervise and assist with ambulation if dizziness and drowsiness are problems. Pad siderails and headboard for patient who experiences seizures.

◊ Store medication at controlled room temperatures between 12° and 25°C (54°–77°F). Do not store in direct sunlight. Keep drug away from heat, open flame, or sparks.

♦ **PO:** Mix with milk or fruit juice to mask odor and taste and to decrease GI irritation. Patient's breath will have strong, unpleasant odor for several hours following administration.

◊ Do not mix, measure, or administer in plastic containers. Paraldehyde decomposes to toxic compounds on contact with plastics.

♦ **Rect:** Dissolve in oil as a retention enema. Mix 10–20 mL with 1 or 2 parts olive oil, cottonseed oil, or isotonic sodium chloride solution to avoid rectal irritation.

♦ **IM:** Do not mix with any other drug solution in vial or syringe.

◊ Administer deeply into large muscle mass and well away from nerve trunk to prevent injury and possible paralysis.

◊ No more than 5 mL should be administered at one time in any one injection site. If more than 5 mL has been ordered, use more than one site. Massage injection site well following administration. Rotate sites.

♦ **IV:** Each 1 mL should be diluted with at least 2 mL of 0.9% sodium chloride for injection.

◊ Administer diluted medication at a rate not exceeding 1 mL/min.

◊ Suction as needed if bronchial secretions increase. May be necessary to keep patient on side to prevent aspiration of secretions.

◊ Ensure availability of emergency respiratory assistance.

◊ Preceding CNS depression, patient may experience brief period of excitement and coughing during IV administration.

Patient/Family Education

♦ Do not drive or operate dangerous machinery until individual response has been determined. Drowsiness and dizziness can occur.

♦ Do not stop taking the drug abruptly. To do so can produce serious withdrawal symptoms.

♦ Do not consume other CNS depressants (including alcohol).

♦ Do not take nonprescription medication without approval from physician.

♦ Carry card or other identification at all times describing condition and medications being taken.

♦ Be aware of risks of taking paraldehyde during pregnancy. Safe use during pregnancy and lactation has not been established. Paralydehyde readily crosses the placental barrier, so a fetus could experience adverse effects of the drug. Notify physician immediately if pregnancy occurs, is suspected, or is planned.

♦ Be aware of possible side effects. Refer to written materials furnished by healthcare providers regarding correct method of self-administration.

Evaluation

♦ Patient demonstrates a subsiding/resolution of the symptoms for which paraldehyde was prescribed (acute agitation, convulsions).

♦ Patient verbalizes understanding of side effects and regimen required for prudent self-administration of paraldehyde.

PARAMETHADIONE

(par-a-meth-a-dye′one)
Paradione

Classification(s):
Antithrombotic, Oxazolidinedione
Pregnancy Category D

INDICATIONS

♦ Absence (petit mal) seizures refractory to other anticonvulsants.

ACTION

♦ Increases seizure threshold in cerebral cortex and basal ganglia ♦ Decreases synaptic response to repetitive low-frequency stimuli.

PHARMACOKINETICS

Absorption: Rapidly absorbed from the GI tract.
Distribution: Is widely distributed. Crosses the blood-brain and placental barriers; unknown if drug is excreted in breast milk.
Metabolism and Excretion: Metab-

olized by the liver; excreted by the kidneys.
Half-Life: First phase: 1.2 hours; second phase: 24 hours.

CONTRAINDICATIONS AND PRECAUTIONS

Contraindicated in: ♦ Hypersensitivity to the drug or to tartrazine dye ♦ Severe hepatic or renal impairment • Pregnancy and lactation (may cause fetal harm) • Severe blood dyscrasias.
Use Cautiously in: ♦ Elderly or debilitated patients ♦ Patients with a history of hepatic or renal disease ♦ Acute intermittent porphyria ♦ Diseases of the retina or optic nerve.

ADVERSE REACTIONS AND SIDE EFFECTS*

CNS: drowsiness, dizziness, headache, fatigue, irritability, ataxia, personality changes.
CV: changes in blood pressure.
Derm: acneiform rash, alopecia, EXFOLIATIVE DERMATITIS, erythema multiforme.
GI: nausea/vomiting, anorexia, hiccups, weight loss, abdominal pain.
GU: POTENTIALLY FATAL NEPHROSIS, proteinuria.
Hemat: BLOOD DYSCRASIAS (aplastic anemia, thrombocytopenia, agranulocytosis, leukopenia, neutropenia, eosinophilia), nosebleed, vaginal bleeding, bleeding gums.
Other: systemic lupus erythematosus, lymphadenopathy, hemeralopia, photophobia, diplopia, lymphoma-like syndrome.

INTERACTIONS

Drug-Drug: ♦ **Drugs with adverse effects similar to those of paramethadione:** increased risk of toxic effects, such as blood dyscrasias and hepatotoxicity.

---

*Underlines indicate most frequent; CAPITALS indicate life-threatening.

ROUTE AND DOSAGE
Absence (Petit Mal) Seizures
* **PO (Adults):** Initial dosage: 900 mg daily divided into 3 equal doses. Increase by 300 mg at weekly intervals until control is achieved with minimal side effects. Maintenance dose: 300–600 mg tid or qid.
* **PO (Children <2 Years Old):** Initial dose: 300 mg/day in divided doses.
* **PO (Children 2–6 Years Old):** Initial dose: 600 mg/day in divided doses.
* **PO (Children >6 Years Old):** Initial dose: 900 mg/day in divided doses.
* **PO (Discontinuation of Therapy):** Withdraw slowly to prevent precipitation of seizures or status epilepticus.

PHARMACODYNAMICS

Route	Onset	Peak	Duration
PO	UK	0.5–2 hr	UK

NURSING IMPLICATIONS
Assessment
* Assess occurrence, characteristics, and duration of seizure activity.
* Assess baseline vital signs.
* Assess history of allergies, sensitivity to this drug.
* Assess date of last menses (possible pregnancy), use of contraceptives.
* Assess whether currently breast-feeding a child.
* Assess current and past alcohol and drug consumption.
* Assess operation of automobile and/or other dangerous machinery.
* Assess for presence of adverse reactions or side effects.
* Assess patient/family knowledge about illness and need for medication.
* In collaboration with physician, assess CBC and renal and liver function tests before initiation of therapy; assess monthly thereafter. Periodic urinalysis should be performed.

* **Toxicity and Overdose:** Assess for symptoms of toxicity/overdose: • nausea • ataxia • drowsiness • dizziness • vision disturbances. Coma may follow massive overdose.
* **Overdose Management:** Monitor vital signs.
◇ Ensure maintenance of adequate airway.
◇ Induce emesis in conscious patient.
◇ Initiate gastric lavage in unconscious patient.
◇ Promote alkalinization of urine to increase renal excretion.
◇ Obtain CBC and lab evaluation of hepatic and renal function following recovery.

Potential Nursing Diagnoses
* High risk for injury related to seizures; abrupt withdrawal from long-term paramethadione use; effects of toxicity or overdose.
* Impaired adjustment related to difficulty accepting diagnosis of epilepsy.
* Social isolation related to fear of experiencing a seizure in the presence of others.
* High risk for activity intolerance related to paramethadione's side effects of drowsiness, dizziness, ataxia.
* Knowledge deficit related to medication regimen.

Plan/Implementation
* Monitor vital signs before beginning therapy and at regular intervals (bid) throughout therapy.
* Observe patient frequently (every hour) for occurrence of seizure activity.
* Ensure that patient is protected from injury. Supervise and assist with ambulation if dizziness and ataxia are problems. Avoid or monitor activities that require mental alertness (including smoking). Pad siderails and headboard for patient who experiences seizures during the night.
* Monitor and report results of CBC, hepatic and renal function tests to phy-

sician. Report presence of: • sore throat • fever • malaise • unusual bleeding • easy bruising • yellowish skin or eyes • vision disturbances • skin rash • excessive drowsiness or dizziness • swollen lymph glands.

• To minimize nausea, medication may be given with food or milk.

• Oral solution has high alcohol content. Dilute with water before administration to small children.

• Ensure capsule has been swallowed and not "cheeked" to avoid medication or to hoard for later use.

• Store medication at controlled room temperatures between 15° and 30°C (59°–86°F). Protect from heat, light, and moisture.

Patient/Family Education

• Do not drive or operate dangerous machinery until individual response has been determined. Drowsiness and dizziness can occur.

• Do not stop taking the drug abruptly. To do so can result in absence (petit mal) status.

• Avoid alcohol intake or nonprescription medication without approval from physician.

• Be aware of risks of taking paramethadione during pregnancy. There is an association between use of anticonvulsant drugs by women with epilepsy and the incidence of birth defects in their children. Fetal defects have occurred when women have taken paramethadione during pregnancy. If pregnancy occurs, is suspected, or is planned, notify physician immediately.

• Report any of the following symptoms to physician promptly: • sore throat • fever • malaise • unusual bleeding • easy bruising • yellow skin or eyes • skin rash • vision disturbances • excessive drowsiness • or dizziness.

• To protect patient during tonic-clonic (grand mal) seizure, do not restrain. Padding (towels, blankets, pillows) may be used to prevent bumping against hard objects. When convulsion has subsided, turn patient on side to allow secretions to drain and to prevent aspiration. Keep records of occurrence, characteristics, and duration of seizures, so that accurate reports may be given to physician for providing assistance in stabilization and control of seizures. If patient has difficulty breathing or continues to experience subsequent seizures, family should immediately call for emergency assistance.

• Be aware of potential side effects. Refer to written materials furnished by healthcare providers regarding correct method of self-administration.

• Carry card or other identification at all times stating illness and names of medications being taken.

Evaluation

• Patient demonstrates stabilization of seizure activity with regular administration of paramethadione.

• Patient verbalizes understanding of necessity for, side effects of, and regimen required for prudent self-administration of paramethadione.

PAROXETINE

(pare-ox′e-teen)
Paxil

Classification(s):
Antidepressant; Serotonin enhancer
Pregnancy Category B

INDICATIONS

• Major depressive disorder.

ACTION

• Inhibits neuronal reuptake of serotonin, thereby potentiating serotonergic activity in the central nervous system.

PHARMACOKINETICS

Absorption: Completely absorbed from the GI tract following oral administration.

Distribution: Is widely distributed throughout the body, including the CNS, with only 1% remaining in the plasma. Unknown if drug crosses placental barrier. Is secreted in breast milk.
Metabolism and Excretion: Extensively metabolized by the liver to metabolites that are essentially inactive. Excreted in urine and feces.
Half-Life: 21 hours.

CONTRAINDICATIONS AND PRECAUTIONS

Contraindicated in: ◆ Hypersensitivity to the drug ◆ Concomitant use with MAO inhibitors ◆ Children and pregnancy (safety not established).
Use Cautiously in: ◆ Patients with hepatic or renal insufficiency ◆ Elderly and debilitated patients ◆ Patients with history of drug abuse ◆ Suicidal patients ◆ Patients with history of mania ◆ Patients with history of seizures.

ADVERSE REACTIONS AND SIDE EFFECTS*

CNS: <u>somnolence</u>, <u>dizziness</u>, <u>insomnia</u>, <u>headache</u>, tremor, nervousness, anxiety, paresthesia, agitation, drugged feeling, myoclonus, CNS stimulation, confusion, manic reaction, psychosis.
CV: palpitation, vasodilation, postural hypotension, hypertension, syncope, tachycardia.
Derm: <u>sweating</u>, pruritus, rash.
GI: <u>nausea</u>, <u>dry mouth</u>, <u>constipation</u>, <u>diarrhea</u>, <u>decreased appetite</u>, <u>flatulence</u>, vomiting, oropharynx disorder, dyspepsia, increased appetite.
GU: <u>ejaculatory disturbance (mostly delay)</u>, <u>impotence</u>, urinary frequency, decreased libido, amenorrhea, cystitis, anorgasmia, urinary disorders.
Hemat: anemia, leukopenia, lymphadenopathy, purpura.
Metab/Nutrit: edema, weight loss or gain, thirst.

MS: myopathy, myalgia, myasthenia, arthritis.
Resp: respiratory infection, yawn, pharyngitis, increased cough, rhinitis, sinusitis.
Special Senses: blurred vision, taste perversion.
Other: <u>asthenia</u>.

INTERACTIONS

Drug-Drug: ◆ **Cimetidine:** increased paroxetine concentration ◆ **MAO inhibitors:** synergistic reaction that may result in hyperthermia, rigidity, myoclonus, autonomic instability with rapid fluctuation of vital signs, and mental status changes that include extreme agitation and coma. Reaction may be fatal. At least 14 days should elapse between discontinuation of one of the drugs (MAOI or paroxetine) and initiation of the other ◆ **Phenobarbital:** decreased effectiveness of paroxetine ◆ **Phenytoin:** decreased effectiveness of either or both drugs ◆ **Alcohol:** possible potentiation of impairment in mental and motor skills ◆ **Digoxin:** possible decrease in digoxin levels ◆ **Procyclidine:** possible increase in procyclidine levels ◆ **Tryptophan:** concurrent use may result in headache, nausea, sweating, and dizziness ◆ **Warfarin:** tendency for increased bleeding.

ROUTE AND DOSAGE

Depression

◆ **PO (Adults):** Initial dosage: 20 mg/day given in the morning. Dosage may be increased in 10-mg/day increments, up to a maximum of 50 mg/day. Dose changes should occur at intervals of at least a week.
◆ **PO (Elderly or Debilitated or Patients with Severe Renal or Hepatic Impairment):** Initial dosage: 10 mg/day. Dosage should not exceed 40 mg/day.

*<u>Underlines</u> indicate most frequent; CAPITALS indicate life-threatening.

PHARMACODYNAMICS

Route	Onset	Peak	Duration
PO	· 1–4 wk	6–8 hr	14 days*

*Allow at least 14 days following cessation of therapy for complete drug elimination before initiating therapy with MAO inhibitors.

NURSING IMPLICATIONS

Assessment

- Assess for suicidal ideation, plan, means. Assess for <u>sudden</u> lifts in mood, which could indicate patient's decision to commit suicide.
- Assess mental status daily: • Assess mood • appearance • thought and communication patterns • level of interest in the environment and in activities • suicidal ideation. Improvement in these behavior patterns and level of energy should be expected in 1–4 weeks following initiation of therapy.
- Assess vital signs, weight.
- Assess history of allergies, sensitivity to this drug.
- Assess date of last menses (possible pregnancy).
- Assess if currently breast-feeding a child.
- Assess current and past alcohol and drug consumption.
- Assess for operation of automobile and/or other dangerous machinery.
- Assess for presence of adverse reactions or side effects, including exacerbation of manic symptoms.
- Assess patient/family knowledge about illness and need for medication.
- In collaboration with physician, assess CBC and liver function tests in patients on long-term therapy.
- **Toxicity and Overdose:** Assess for symptoms of overdose: nausea • vomiting • drowsiness • sinus tachycardia • and dilated pupils.
- **Overdose Management:** Monitor cardiac (ECG) and vital signs.
- Ensure adequate oxygenation and ventilation.
- Initiate gastric evacuation through emesis, lavage, or both.

- Following evacuation, administer 20–30 g of activated charcoal every 4 to 6 hours during the first 24–48 hours after ingestion.
- Provide supportive care with close observation.

Potential Nursing Diagnoses

- High risk for self-directed violence related to depressed mood.
- High risk for injury related to paroxetine overdose or paroxetine's side effects of somnolence, dizziness, paresthesia, and confusion.
- Social isolation related to depressed mood.
- High risk for activity intolerance related to paroxetine's side effects of drowsiness, dizziness, weakness, confusion.
- Knowledge deficit related to medication regimen.

Plan/Implementation

- Monitor vital signs before beginning therapy, and at regular intervals (bid or tid) throughout therapy. Take BP lying and standing in patients experiencing orthostatic hypotension. Elderly are particularly susceptible. Contact physician if tachycardia/arrhythmias are noted.
- Weigh patient 2–3 times a week, at same time of day, on same scale, if possible. A rapid weight gain or evidence of edema should be reported to physician immediately. Record I&O.
- Observe for decrease in appetite and loss of weight.
- Ensure that patient is protected from injury. Provide supervision and assistance when ambulating if dizziness and drowsiness are problems.
- Give hard candy, gum, or frequent sips of water if dry mouth is a problem.
- Administer oral medication with food or milk to minimize GI upset.
- Ensure that patient swallows capsule and does not "cheek" to avoid medication or hoard for later use.

- May crush tablet and mix with food or fluid for patient who has difficulty swallowing.
- Store at controlled room temperatures between 15° and 30°C (59°–86°F). Protect from heat and moisture.

Patient/Family Education

- Therapeutic effect may not be seen for as long as 4 weeks. If after this length of time no improvement is noted, physician may prescribe a different medication. Continue to take medication even though symptoms have not subsided.
- Use caution when driving or operating dangerous machinery. Drowsiness and dizziness can occur. If these side effects become persistent or interfere with activities of daily living, report to physician. Adjustment may be necessary.
- Report occurrence of any of the following symptoms to physician immediately: • rash or hives • sore throat • fever • malaise • unusual bleeding • easy bruising • persistent nausea/vomiting • severe headache • rapid heart rate • difficulty urinating • anorexia/weight loss • rapid weight gain.
- Rise slowly from a sitting or lying position to prevent a sudden drop in blood pressure.
- If dry mouth is a problem, take frequent sips of water, chew sugarless gum, or suck on hard candy. Good oral care (frequent brushing, flossing) is very important.
- Do not drink alcohol while on paroxetine therapy. These drugs may potentiate the effects of each other.
- Do not consume other medications (including over-the-counter meds) with paroxetine without physician's approval. Many medications contain substances that, in combination with paroxetine, could precipitate a potentially life-threatening situation.
- Be aware of possible risks of taking paroxetine during pregnancy. Safe use

during pregnancy and lactation has not been established. Inform physician immediately if pregnancy occurs or is suspected or planned.
- Be aware of side effects of paroxetine. Refer to written materials furnished by healthcare providers for safe self-administration.
- Do not discontinue taking paroxetine abruptly after long-term use. To do so may produce uncomfortable symptoms such as nausea, vomiting, headache, and weakness.
- Carry card or other identification at all times describing medications being taken.

Evaluation

- Patient demonstrates a subsiding/resolution of the symptoms for which paroxetine was prescribed (depressed mood; suicidal ideation).
- Patient verbalizes understanding of side effects and regimen required for prudent self-administration of paroxetine.

PEMOLINE

(pem′oh-leen)
Cylert

Classification(s):
CNS stimulant, Oxazolidinone derivative
Schedule C IV
Pregnancy Category B

INDICATIONS

- Attention deficit disorder with hyperactivity. **Investigational Uses:** • Narcolepsy and excessive daytime sleepiness • Mild stimulant for geriatric patients.

ACTION

- Exact site and mechanism of action unknown • Produces central nervous system stimulation with weak sympathomimetic effects • Thought to act through dopaminergic mechanisms.

PHARMACOKINETICS

Absorption: Rapid absorption following oral administration.
Distribution: Not fully understood. Unknown if drug crosses placental barrier or enters breast milk.
Metabolism and Excretion: More than 50% metabolized by the liver; excreted primarily in the urine.
Half-Life: 9–14 hours (adults); 2–12 hours (children).

CONTRAINDICATIONS AND PRECAUTIONS

Contraindicated in: ♦ Hypersensitivity ♦ History of tics or Tourette's disorder ♦ Pregnancy, lactation, and children under 6 years of age (safety has not been established).
Use Cautiously in: ♦ Renal or hepatic insufficiency ♦ Psychosis ♦ Patients with a history of seizures ♦ History of drug or alcohol dependence.

ADVERSE REACTIONS AND SIDE EFFECTS*

CNS: <u>insomnia</u>, dyskinetic movements of tongue, lips, face, and extremities; Tourette's syndrome; nystagmus and nystagmoid eye movements; seizures; increased irritability; mild mental depression; dizziness; headache; drowsiness; hallucinations; fatigue; malaise.
CV: tachycardia.
Derm: skin rash.
GI: <u>anorexia</u>, <u>weight loss</u>, nausea, abdominal pain, diarrhea.
Hemat: APLASTIC ANEMIA (rare).
Hepat: hepatitis, jaundice, HEPATIC CELLULAR NECROSIS.
Other: <u>tolerance</u>, physical and psychological dependence, prostatic enlargement.

INTERACTIONS

Drug-Drug: Interactions with other drugs have not been studied in humans.

Caution is recommended in administering pemoline concurrently with other agents, particularly those with CNS activity.
Drug-Food: ♦ **Caffeinated foods and drinks:** increased effects of pemoline.

ROUTE AND DOSAGE

Attention Deficit Disorder with Hyperactivity

♦ **PO (Children 6 Years and Older):** Initial dosage: 37.5 mg/day, administered as single dose each morning. Dosage may be gradually increased at 1-week intervals in increments of 18.75 mg/day until desired effect is achieved. Effective dosage usually ranges from 56.25 to 75 mg/day. Maximum recommended dose: 112.5 mg/day.

Narcolepsy and Excessive Daytime Sleepiness

(Investigational use.)

♦ **PO (Adults):** 50–200 mg/day divided into 2 doses, one after breakfast and one after lunch.

Mild Stimulant in Geriatric Patients

(Investigational use.)

♦ **PO (Geriatric):** 25–50 mg daily in divided doses.

PHARMACODYNAMICS

Route	Onset	Peak	Duration
PO	2–4 wk*	2–4 hr†	8 hr–days

*Therapeutic onset in attention deficit disorder may not occur until after 2–4 weeks of therapy.
†Steady-state plasma levels reached in approximately 2–3 days.

NURSING IMPLICATIONS
Assessment

♦ Assess and record baseline temperature, pulse, respiration, blood pressure, and weight for comparison during therapy.

*<u>Underlines</u> indicate most frequent; CAPITALS indicate life-threatening.

* In diabetic patient, assess blood sugar bid–tid. Insulin adjustments may be required due to alteration in eating pattern, as well as possibility of hyperactivity.
* Assess growth rate of children on pemoline therapy carefully. A decrease in rate of development may be observed.
* Assess mental status for changes in mood, level of activity, degree of stimulation, aggressiveness.
* Assess sleeping patterns carefully. Insomnia may occur.
* Assess history of allergies, sensitivity to this drug.
* Assess for presence of adverse reactions or side effects.
* Assess date of last menses (possible pregnancy), use of contraceptives.
* Assess whether currently breast-feeding a child.
* Assess current and past alcohol and drug consumption.
* Assess amount of caffeine usually consumed.
* Assess for operation of automobile and/or other dangerous machinery.
* Assess patient/family knowledge about illness and need for medication.
* In collaboration with physician, assess CBC, urinalysis, and liver function tests periodically in patients on pemoline therapy.
* **Lab Test Alterations:** Increased AST (SGOT), ALT (SGPT), serum LDH, and alkaline phosphatase.
* **Withdrawal:** Assess for symptoms of withdrawal: • mental depression • psychotic behavior • irritability.
* **Withdrawal Management:** Monitor vital signs.
◇ Place patient in quiet room with low stimuli.
◇ Allow patient to sleep as much as desired.
◇ Observe closely (q 15 min).
◇ Institute suicide precautions.
◇ Some physicians may elect to pre-

scribe antidepressants to counteract feelings of depression and lethargy.
* **Toxicity and Overdose:** Assess for symptoms of overdose: • tachycardia • hallucinations • agitation • dyskinetic movements • restlessness • overactivity • irregular respiration • increased salivation • intermittent tongue protrusion and generalized hyperreflexia.
* **Overdose Management:** Monitor vital signs.
◇ Ensure maintenance of adequate airway.
◇ Initiate gastric lavage.
◇ Maintain adequate circulation and respiratory exchange.
◇ Begin cardiac monitoring.
◇ Use external cooling measures for hyperpyrexia.
◇ Haloperidol may be used to counteract agitation, hallucinations, and excitement.
◇ Hemodialysis may be useful; forced diuresis and peritoneal dialysis appear to be of little value.

Potential Nursing Diagnoses
* High risk for injury due to overstimulation and hyperactivity; abrupt pemoline withdrawal; overdose.
* High risk for self-directed violence related to suicidal ideations resulting from abrupt pemoline withdrawal.
* Alteration in nutrition, less than body requires, related to pemoline's side effects of anorexia and weight loss.
* Sleep pattern disturbance related to overstimulation resulting from pemoline use.
* Alteration in thought processes related to pemoline's adverse effects of overstimulation and difficulty concentrating.
* Knowledge deficit related to medication regimen.

Plan/Implementation
* Monitor and record vital signs at regular intervals (bid) throughout therapy.

- Ensure that patient is protected from injury. Keep stimuli low and environment as quiet as possible to discourage overstimulation.
- In patients who are withdrawing from long-term pemoline use, observe frequently for signs of impending violence to self. Institute suicide precautions if necessary.
- In children with behavior disorders, a drug "holiday" should be attempted periodically under direction of physician to determine effectiveness of the medication and need for continuation.
- Ensure that tablet has been swallowed and not "cheeked" to avoid medication or to hoard for later use. Ensure that chewable tablet has been thoroughly chewed and swallowed.
- Tablets may be crushed and mixed with food or fluid for patient who has difficulty swallowing.
- Administer medication in the morning to avoid insomnia and to achieve maximal benefit during waking hours.
- Store at controlled room temperatures between 15° and 30°C (59°–86°F). Protect from heat and moisture.

Patient/Family Education

- Use caution in driving or when operating dangerous machinery. Level of alertness may be diminished due to hyperactivity and stimulation. Dizziness may occur as a side effect.
- Do not stop taking the drug abruptly. To do so can produce serious withdrawal symptoms.
- Do not take other medications (including over-the-counter drugs) without physician's approval. Many medications contain substances that, in combination with pemoline, may be harmful.
- Diabetic patient should monitor blood sugar bid or tid or as instructed by physician. Be aware of need for possible alteration in insulin requirements due to changes in food intake, weight, and activity.
- Avoid consumption of large amounts of caffeinated products (coffee, tea, colas, chocolate), as they may enhance the stimulant effect of pemoline.
- Notify physician of nervousness, insomnia, palpitations, vomiting, or skin rash.
- Be aware of possible risks of taking pemoline during pregnancy. Safe use in pregnancy and lactation has not been established. It is unknown if pemoline crosses placental barrier. Inform physician immediately if pregnancy occurs, is suspected, or is planned.
- Be aware of potential side effects of pemoline. Refer to written materials furnished by healthcare providers for safe self-administration.
- Carry card or other identification at all times describing medications being taken.

Evaluation

- Patient demonstrates a subsiding/resolution of the symptoms for which pemoline was prescribed (inability to prevent falling asleep, behavior problems/hyperactivity in children).
- Patient verbalizes understanding of side effects and regimen required for prudent self-administration of pemoline.

PENTOBARBITAL

(pen-toe-bar'bi-tal)
Nembutal, {Nova-Rectal, Pentogen}

Classification(s):
Sedative-hypnotic, Barbiturate; CNS depressant
Schedule C II (oral, parenteral)
Schedule C III (rectal)
Pregnancy Category D

INDICATIONS

♦ Moderate anxiety states ♦ Insomnia ♦ Acute convulsive conditions ♦ Preoperative sedation. **Investigational Uses:** ♦ Induction of coma for management of increased intracranial pressure and cerebral ischemia in a variety of pathologies.

ACTION

♦ Depresses the central nervous system ♦ Interferes with transmission through the reticular formation, which is concerned with arousal ♦ Causes imbalance in inhibitory and facility mechanisms that influence the cerebral cortex and reticular formation ♦ Action on neurotransmitters is not well defined ♦ All levels of CNS depression can occur, from mild sedation to hypnosis to coma to death.

PHARMACOKINETICS

Absorption: Nearly complete absorption with oral and rectal forms.
Distribution: Rapidly and widely distributed. Crosses blood-brain and placental barriers; excreted in breast milk.
Metabolism and Excretion: Metabolized by the liver; excreted by the kidneys as inactive metabolites.
Half-Life: 15–50 hours.

CONTRAINDICATIONS AND PRECAUTIONS

Contraindicated in: ♦ Hypersensitivity to the drug or other barbiturates ♦ Severe

hepatic, renal, cardiac, or respiratory disease ♦ Lactation ♦ Individuals with a history of previous addiction ♦ Porphyria ♦ Hypersensitivity to tartrazine (contained in some preparations).
Use Cautiously in: ♦ Elderly or debilitated patients ♦ Hepatic, renal, cardiac, or respiratory dysfunction ♦ Depressed/suicidal patients ♦ Pregnancy ♦ Ammonia intoxication.

ADVERSE REACTIONS AND SIDE EFFECTS*

CNS: <u>drowsiness</u>, headache, lethargy, <u>dizziness</u>, mental depression, ataxia, <u>residual sedation</u> ("hangover"), confusion, paradoxical excitement and/or euphoria.
CV: hypotension, bradycardia.
Derm: skin rashes, urticaria, dermatitis (may precede potentially fatal reactions), redness and pain at IM injection site, phlebitis at IV site.
GI: nausea/vomiting, diarrhea/constipation, epigastric pain.
Hemat: AGRANULOCYTOSIS, THROMBOCYTOPENIA.
Resp: hypoventilation, apnea, RESPIRATORY DEPRESSION, LARYNGOSPASM, BRONCHOSPASM.
Other: tolerance, physical and psychological dependence.

INTERACTIONS

Drug-Drug: ♦ **Other CNS depressants (including alcohol, benzodiazepines, antihistamines, opiates):** additive CNS depression ♦ **Chloramphenicol, MAO inhibitors, valproic acid, cimetidine, disulfiram:** increased effects of pentobarbital ♦ **Phenytoin:** increased or decreased effects of either drug (close monitoring of serum levels required to control seizure activity) ♦ **Oral contraceptives:** decreased effectiveness of oral contraceptives ♦ **Oral anticoagulants:** decreased anticoagulant effects ♦ **Corticosteroids, digitoxin, doxycycline:** decreased ef-

{} = Only available in Canada.
*<u>Underlines</u> indicate most frequent; CAPITALS indicate life-threatening.

fects of these drugs ✦ **Furosemide:** orthostatic hypotension ✦ **Griseofulvin:** decreased griseofulvin levels.

Drug-Food: ✦ **Vitamin D:** increased vitamin D metabolism, possible deficiency ✦ **Folic acid:** decreased absorption of folic acid, possible deficiency.

ROUTE AND DOSAGE

Anxiety
- **PO (Adults):** 20–40 mg 2–4 times daily.
- **PO (Children):** 2–6 mg/kg/day in 3 divided doses (depending on age, weight, and degree of sedation desired). Maximum: 100 mg daily.

Insomnia:
(Should not be given for more than 2 weeks.)
- **PO (Adults):** 100–200 mg at bedtime.
- **PO (Children):** Dose judged on basis of individual age and weight.
- **IM (Adults):** 150–200 mg at bedtime.
- **IM (Children):** 2–6 mg/kg at bedtime, not to exceed 100 mg.
- **Rect (Adults):** 120–200 mg at bedtime.
- **Rect (Children 12–14 Years Old):** 60–120 mg at bedtime.
- **Rect (Children 5–12 Years Old):** 60 mg at bedtime.
- **Rect (Children 1–4 Years Old):** 30–60 mg at bedtime.

Preoperative Sedation
- **PO (Children 10–12 Years Old):** 100 mg.
- **Rect (Children under Age 10):** 5 mg/kg, not to exceed 100 mg.
- **IM (Adults):** 150–200 mg.
- **IM (Children):** 2–6 mg/kg, not to exceed 100 mg.

Acute Convulsive Conditions
- **IM (Adults):** 150–200 mg.
- **IM (Children):** 2–6 mg/kg not to exceed 100 mg.
- **IV (Adults):** Initial dose: 100 mg/70 kg. If necessary, additional doses may

be administered in 25–50 mg increments. Maximum total dose for adults: 200–500 mg.
- **IV (Children):** Dosage proportionately reduced from adult dose.

PHARMACODYNAMICS

Route	Onset	Peak	Duration
PO	15–60 min	30–60 min	1–4 hr
Rect	15–60 min	1.5 hr	1–4 hr
IM	10–25 min	30–60 min	1–4 hr
IV	Immediate	1 min	15 min

NURSING IMPLICATIONS

Assessment
- Assess sleep patterns. Keep records for adequate baseline data before the initiation of therapy.
- Assess for suicidal ideation in depressed patients.
- Assess occurrence, characteristics, and duration of seizure activity.
- Assess history of allergies, sensitivity to this drug or other barbiturates.
- Assess date of last menses (possible pregnancy), use of contraceptives.
- Assess whether currently breast-feeding a child.
- Assess current and past alcohol and drug consumption.
- Assess for operation of automobile and/or other dangerous machinery.
- Assess for presence of adverse reactions or side effects.
- Assess patient/family knowledge about illness and need for medication.
- In collaboration with physician, assess CBC and renal and liver function tests in patients on prolonged therapy.
- **Lab Test Alterations:** May increase values of bromsulphalein (BSP) retention and protein-bound iodine (PBI).
- ◊ Elevated blood ammonia.
- **Withdrawal:** Assess for symptoms of withdrawal: • anxiety • tremors • insomnia • nausea/vomiting • weakness • diaphoresis • orthostatic hypotension • delirium • convulsions.

* **Withdrawal Management:** Monitor vital signs.
◇ Place patient in quiet room with low stimuli.
◇ Institute seizure precautions.
◇ A long-acting barbiturate, such as phenobarbital, may be ordered to suppress withdrawal symptoms.
◇ Phenytoin may be ordered to prevent seizures.
◇ Some physicians may order oxazepam as needed for objective withdrawal symptoms, gradually decreasing dosage until the drug is discontinued.
* **Toxicity and Overdose:** Assess for symptoms of toxicity: • confusion • drowsiness • dyspnea • slurred speech • staggering.
◇ Assess for symptoms of overdose: • CNS and respiratory depression • hypoventilation • hypothermia • hypotension • oliguria • tachycardia • coma. (May progress to respiratory arrest, circulatory collapse, and death.)
* **Overdose Management:** Monitor vital signs.
◇ Ensure maintenance of adequate airway.
◇ Induce emesis in conscious patient.
◇ Initiate gastric lavage in unconscious patient.
◇ Administer activated charcoal to minimize absorption of drug.
◇ IV fluids and vasopressors may be used to combat hypotension.
◇ For severe intoxication, forced diuresis or hemodialysis may be used.

Potential Nursing Diagnoses

* Ineffective breathing pattern related to side effects of hypoventilation and respiratory depression.
* High risk for injury related to seizures; abrupt withdrawal from long-term use; decreased mental alertness caused by side effect of residual sedation; side effects of dizziness and ataxia; effects of overdose.
* High risk for self-directed violence related to depressed mood.

* Sleep pattern disturbance related to situational crises, physical condition, severe level of anxiety.
* High risk for activity intolerance related to side effects of residual sedation, drowsiness, dizziness.
* Knowledge deficit related to medication regimen.

Plan/Implementation

* **General Info:** Monitor vital signs before beginning therapy, at regular intervals (bid) throughout therapy, every 3–5 minutes during IV administration, and every 10 minutes for 30 minutes following IM administration.
◇ Ensure that patient is protected from injury. Supervise and assist with ambulation if dizziness and drowsiness are problems. Ensure that patient avoids participation in any activity requiring mental alertness (including smoking). Raise siderails and instruct patient to remain in bed following administration.
* **PO:** To minimize nausea, medication may be given with food or milk.
◇ Ensure that capsule has been swallowed and not "cheeked" to avoid medication or to hoard for later use.
◇ Capsule may be emptied and mixed with food or fluid for patient who has difficulty swallowing. Consider changing medication to elixir form.
◇ Store medication at controlled room temperatures between 15° and 30°C (59°–86°F). Protect from heat and moisture.
* **Rect:** To ensure accurate dose, suppositories should not be divided.
◇ Store suppositories in refrigerator.
* **IM:** Administer deeply into large muscle mass to minimize subcutaneous tissue irritation/necrosis. Use Z-track method.
◇ Volume of injection should not exceed 5 mL or 250 mg at any one site.
◇ Observe closely for oversedation for 20–30 minutes following administration.

• **IV:** Do not use solution if discolored or if precipitate is visible.

◊ Solution may be administered undiluted or may be further diluted in sterile water, sodium chloride, or Ringer's injection.

◊ Do not mix with other medications.

◊ Administer IV solution at no more than 50 mg per minute. Observe closely for potential depression of vital signs.

◊ Solution is highly irritating. Extravasation may result in tissue necrosis. Stop infusion immediately if patient complains of pain. Inadvertent intra-arterial injection may result in gangrene.

◊ Ensure availability of artificial ventilation and resuscitation equipment.

Patient/Family Education

• Use caution in driving or when operating dangerous machinery. Drowsiness and dizziness can occur.

• Do not stop taking the drug abruptly. Doing so can produce serious (even life-threatening) withdrawal symptoms. If you forget a dose, take it as close as possible to the prescribed time. If it is already close to time for next dose, wait until then; do not double up on dose at the next prescribed time.

• Do not consume other CNS depressants (including alcohol).

• Be aware of the risks of taking barbiturates during pregnancy (congenital malformations may be associated with use during the first trimester). Also, evidence of withdrawal symptoms has been observed in neonates born to mothers who had ingested barbiturates regularly during the last trimester of pregnancy. Notify physician if pregnancy is suspected or planned.

• Because barbiturates decrease effectiveness of oral contraceptives, use alternative methods of birth control during pentobarbital therapy.

• Be aware of potential side effects. Refer to written materials furnished by healthcare providers regarding correct method of self-administration.

• Report symptoms of sore throat, fever, malaise, severe headache, conjunctivitis, rhinitis, urethritis, balanitis, easy bruising, petechiae, or epistaxis to physician immediately.

• Carry card or other identification at all times stating names of medications being taken.

Evaluation

• Patient demonstrates a subsiding/resolution of the symptoms for which pentobarbital was prescribed (seizures, sleep disturbances, anxiety).

• Patient verbalizes understanding of side effects and regimen required for prudent self-administration of pentobarbital.

PERPHENAZINE

(per-fen'a-zeen)
{Phenazine}, Trilafon

Classification(s):
Antipsychotic, Neuroleptic,
Antiemetic, Phenothiazine
Pregnancy Category C

INDICATIONS

• Psychotic disorders • Severe nausea and vomiting • Intractable hiccups.

ACTION

• The exact mechanism of antipsychotic action is not fully understood but is probably related to the drug's antidopaminergic effects • Antipsychotics may block postsynaptic dopamine receptors in the basal ganglia, hypothalamus, limbic system, brain stem and medulla • Antipsychotic effects also appear to be related to inhibition of dopamine-mediated neurotransmission at the synapses ♦ Antipsychotic effects may also result from the drug's alpha-adrenergic blocking, muscarinic blocking, and adrenergic activities, as well as effects on other amines (such as GABA) or peptides.

PHARMACOKINETICS

Absorption: Rapid absorption of oral tablet/timed-release capsule dosage forms. Genetic differences in rate of first-pass metabolism result in wide range of bioavailability from individual to individual. Oral liquid preparations and IM administration result in more consistent absorption.

Distribution: Widely distributed. Highly lipophilic; accumulates in brain, lungs, and other tissues with high blood supply. Crosses placental barrier. Enters breast milk.

Metabolism and Excretion: Metabolized by the liver and in the kidneys. Excreted through kidneys and enterohepatic circulation. Active metabolites accumulate and are stored in fatty tissue over a prolonged period of time, and may be detected in urine up to 3–6 months following discontinuation of the drug.

Half-Life: 8–21 hours.

CONTRAINDICATIONS AND PRECAUTIONS

Contraindicated in: ♦ Hypersensitivity to this drug, other phenothiazines, or sulfites or tartrazine (contained in some preparations) ♦ Comatose or severely CNS-depressed patients ♦ Presence of large amounts of CNS depressants ♦ Bone marrow depression ♦ Blood dyscrasias ♦ Subcortical brain damage ♦ Parkinson's disease ♦ Liver, renal, and/or cardiac insufficiency ♦ Severe hypotension or hypertension ♦ Children under 12 years of age; pregnancy and lactation (safe use not established).

Use Cautiously in: ♦ Patients with a history of seizures ♦ Respiratory, renal, hepatic, thyroid, or cardiovascular disorders (e.g., respiratory infection, COPD, thyrotoxicosis, mitral insufficiency, angina pectoris) ♦ Prostatic hypertrophy ♦ Glaucoma ♦ Diabetes ♦ Elderly or debilitated patients ♦ Patients exposed to high or low environmental temperatures or to organophosphate insecticides ♦ Hypocalcemia ♦ History of severe reactions to insulin or ECT ♦ Pediatric patients with acute illnesses or dehydration.

ADVERSE REACTIONS AND SIDE EFFECTS*

CNS: <u>sedation</u>, <u>headache</u>, seizures, insomnia, dizziness, exacerbation of psychotic symptoms, <u>extrapyramidal symptoms</u> (pseudoparkinsonism, akathisia, akinesia, dystonia, oculogyric crisis), tardive dyskinesia, fatigue, cerebral edema, ataxia, <u>blurred vision</u>, NEUROLEPTIC MALIGNANT SYNDROME, restlessness, anxiety, depression, hyperthermia or hypothermia.

CV: hypotension, <u>orthostatic hypotension</u>, hypertension, tachycardia, bradycardia, CARDIAC ARREST, ECG changes, ARRHYTHMIAS, PULMONARY EDEMA, CIRCULATORY COLLAPSE.

Derm: <u>skin rashes</u>, urticaria, petechiae, seborrhea, <u>photosensitivity</u>, eczema, erythema, hyperpigmentation, contact dermatitis, EXFOLIATIVE DERMATITIS (rare).

Endo: galactorrhea, gynecomastia (men), changes in libido, impotence, hyperglycemia or hypoglycemia, amenorrhea, retrograde ejaculation.

GI: <u>dry mouth</u>, nausea, vomiting, increased appetite and weight gain, anorexia, dyspepsia, <u>constipation</u>, diarrhea, jaundice, polydipsia, PARALYTIC ILEUS.

GU: urinary retention, frequency or incontinence, bladder paralysis, polyuria, enuresis, priapism.

Hemat: AGRANULOCYTOSIS, LEUKOPENIA, ANEMIA, THROMBOCYTOPENIA, PANCYTOPENIA.

*<u>Underlines</u> indicate most frequent; CAPITALS indicate life-threatening.

Ophth: lens deposition.
Resp: LARYNGEAL EDEMA, LARYNGOSPASM, BRONCHOSPASM, SUPPRESSION OF COUGH REFLEX.
Other: decreased sweating.

INTERACTIONS

Drug-Drug: ◆ **CNS depressants (including alcohol, barbiturates, narcotics, anesthetics):** additive CNS depressant effects ◆ **Anticholinergic agents (e.g., atropine):** additive anticholinergic effects, decreased antipsychotic effects ◆ **Barbiturate anesthetics:** increased incidence of excitatory effects and hypotension ◆ **Barbiturates:** possible decreased effects of phenothiazines ◆ **Disulfiram:** decreased perphenazine effects ◆ **Metyrosine:** potentiation of extrapyramidal side effects ◆ **Levodopa:** decreased efficacy of levodopa ◆ **Quinidine:** additive cardiac depressive effects ◆ **Magnesium- or aluminum-containing antidiarrheal mixtures, antacids:** reduced phenothiazine absorption/effectiveness ◆ **Guanethidine:** decreased antihypertensive action ◆ **Lithium:** decreased plasma levels and effect of antipsychotic drug, severe neurotoxicity reported ◆ **Epinephrine:** reversal of usual pressor action of epinephrine, resulting in decreased blood pressure and tachycardia ◆ **Bromocriptine:** impairment of prolactin-suppressing action ◆ **Angiotensin converting enzyme (ACE) inhibitors:** increased effects of ACE inhibitors ◆ **Phenytoin:** decreased phenytoin metabolism, increased risk of toxicity ◆ **Polypeptide antibiotics:** possible neuromuscular respiratory depression ◆ **Metrizamide:** seizures ◆ **Cimetidine:** decreased effect of phenothiazines ◆ **Clonidine:** possibility of severe hypotension ◆ **Piperazine:** increased seizure potential.
Drug-Food: ◆ **Caffeine-containing beverages (e.g., coffee, tea, colas):** counteracted antipsychotic effect.

ROUTE AND DOSAGE
Psychotic Disorders
◆ **PO (Adults and Children over 12):** Nonhospitalized patients: 4–8 mg tid (repeat-action tabs 8–16 mg bid). Hospitalized patients: 8–16 mg bid–qid (repeat-action tabs: 8–32 mg bid). Maximum dosage: 64 mg/day.
◆ **IM (Adults and Children over 12):** Initial dose: 5–10 mg q 6 hr. Maximum daily dosage: 15 mg in ambulatory patients or 30 mg in hospitalized patients. Initiate oral therapy as soon as possible.

Severe Nausea and Vomiting, Intractable Hiccups
◆ **PO (Adults):** 8–16 mg/day in divided doses. Some patients may require up to 24 mg.
◆ **IM (Adults):** 5–10 mg.
◆ **IV (Adults):** 1 mg at not less than 1–2 minute intervals to a maximum total dose of 5 mg.

PHARMACODYNAMICS

Route	Onset*	Peak†	Duration‡
PO	30–60 min	2–4 hr	4–6 hr
PO (Repetabs)	30–60 min	—	10–12 hr
IM	10–15 min	1–2 hr	6–24 hr
IV	5 min	5 min	—

*Full clinical effects may not be observed for 4–8 weeks.
†Steady-state plasma levels are achieved in approximately 4–7 days.
‡Drug may be detected in urine for 3–6 months after last dose.

NURSING IMPLICATIONS
Assessment
◆ Assess hydration in patient experiencing severe nausea and vomiting. Note weight, condition of mucous membranes, skin turgor, color, amount and density of urine, and vital signs.
◆ Assess mental status daily: • mood • appearance • thought and communication patterns • level of interest in the environment and in activities • level of anxiety or agitation • presence of hal-

lucinations or delusions • suspiciousness • interactions with others • ability to carry out activities of daily living.

♦ Assess for symptoms of blood dyscrasias: • sore throat • fever • malaise • unusual bleeding • easy bruising.

♦ Assess for extrapyramidal symptoms: • pseudoparkinsonism (tremors, shuffling gait, drooling, rigidity) • akinesia (muscular weakness) • akathisia (continuous restlessness and fidgeting) • dystonia (involuntary muscular movements of face, arms, legs, and neck) • oculogyric crisis (uncontrolled rolling back of the eyes) • tardive dyskinesia (bizarre facial and tongue movements, stiff neck, difficulty swallowing).

♦ Assess for symptoms of neuroleptic malignant syndrome: • hyperpyrexia up to 107°F (41.6°C) • elevated pulse • increased or decreased blood pressure • severe parkinsonian muscle rigidity • elevated creatinine phosphokinase blood levels • elevated white blood count • altered mental status (including catatonic signs or agitation) • acute renal failure • varying levels of consciousness (including stupor and coma) • pallor • diaphoresis • tachycardia • arrhythmias • rhabdomyolysis.

♦ Assess vital signs, weight. Record baseline values for comparison.

♦ Assess history of allergies, sensitivity to this drug or to other phenothiazines.

♦ Assess for signs and symptoms of cholestatic jaundice: • abdominal pain • nausea • rash • fever • yellow skin • flu-like symptoms • abnormal lab test results (eosinophilia, bile in urine, increased serum transaminases, bilirubin, alkaline phosphatase).

♦ Assess date of last menses (possible pregnancy), use of contraceptives.

♦ Assess whether currently breast-feeding a child.

♦ Assess current and past alcohol and drug consumption.

♦ Assess operation of automobile and/ or other dangerous machinery.

♦ Assess for presence of adverse reactions or side effects.

♦ Assess patient/family knowledge about illness and need for medication.

♦ In collaboration with physician, assess CBC, liver function tests, and ophthalmological exams in patients on long-term therapy.

♦ **Lab Test Alterations:** Increased serum alkaline phosphatase, transaminases, bilirubin.

◊ Increased protein-bound iodine.

◊ False-positive urine pregnancy test, possibly caused by drug metabolite that discolors the urine (less likely to occur when serum test is used).

◊ Increased urinary glucose.

◊ Decreased urinary estrogen, progestin, and gonadotropin.

◊ Increased plasma cholesterol level.

◊ Increased serum prolactin.

♦ **Withdrawal:** Assess for symptoms of abrupt withdrawal from long-term therapy: • gastritis • nausea • vomiting • dizziness • headache • tachycardia • insomnia • tremulousness • sweating.

♦ **Toxicity and Overdose:** No correlation has been established between blood level and therapeutic effect.

◊ Assess for symptoms of overdose: • CNS depression, from heavy sedation to deep sleep to coma • hypotension • confusion • excitement • extrapyramidal symptoms • agitation • restlessness • convulsions • fever • autonomic reactions • ECG changes • cardiac arrhythmias • tachycardia • hypothermia • tremor • seizures • cyanosis.

♦ **Overdose Management:** Monitor vital signs.

◊ Ensure maintenance of open airway.

◊ Initiate gastric lavage.

◊ Do not induce emesis (nuchal rigidity may result in aspiration of vomitus).

◊ Antiparkinsonian drugs or diphenhydramine may be administered to counteract extrapyramidal symptoms.

◊ Administer IV fluids or a vasoconstrictor to maintain adequate blood pressure. **Note:** Epinephrine is not recommended due to its interaction with phenothiazines, which causes further drop in blood pressure.

◊ Administer IV phenytoin to control ventricular arrhythmias.

◊ Administer phenobarbital or diazepam to control convulsions or hyperactivity.

◊ Dialysis does not appear to be a useful intervention.

Potential Nursing Diagnoses

♦ High risk for fluid volume deficit related to excessive vomiting.

♦ High risk for violence directed at others related to mistrust and panic anxiety.

♦ High risk for injury related to abrupt withdrawal after prolonged use; overdose; perphenazine's side effects of sedation, dizziness, ataxia, weakness, lowered seizure threshold.

♦ Sensory-perceptual alteration related to panic anxiety evidenced by hallucinations.

♦ Altered thought processes related to panic anxiety evidenced by delusional thinking.

♦ Social isolation related to inability to trust others.

♦ High risk for activity intolerance related to perphenazine's side effects of drowsiness, dizziness, ataxia, weakness.

♦ Noncompliance with medication regimen related to suspiciousness and mistrust of others.

♦ Knowledge deficit related to medication regimen.

Plan/Implementation

♦ **General Info:** Monitor vital signs before beginning therapy and at regular intervals (bid or tid) throughout therapy. Take BP lying and standing to monitor for possible hypotensive reaction; elderly are particularly suscep-

tible. Dosage adjustment may be required.

◊ Ensure that patient who is ambulatory is protected from sun when spending time outdoors.

◊ Weigh patient 2–3 times a week, at same time of day, on same scale, if possible. A rapid weight gain or evidence of edema should be reported to physician immediately. Record I&O.

◊ Ensure that patient is protected from injury. Provide supervision and assistance when ambulating if dizziness and drowsiness are problems. Pad siderails and headboard for patient who experiences seizures.

◊ Give patient hard candy, gum, or frequent sips of water if dry mouth is a problem.

◊ Store all forms of medication in carton until contents are used. Tablets and concentrate should be stored between 2° and 30°C (36°–86°F).

♦ **PO:** Administer oral medication with food to minimize GI upset.

◊ Ensure that patient swallows tablet and does not "cheek" to avoid medication or to hoard for later use.

◊ Crush tablet and mix with food or fluid for patient who has difficulty swallowing, or use oral concentrate. Do not crush repeat-action tabs.

◊ Just prior to administration, mix concentrate with water, milk, carbonated orange drink, or pineapple, apricot, prune, orange, tomato, or grapefruit juice. Do not mix with coffee, tea, colas, or apple juice, as physical incompatibility may result. Use approximately 60 mL diluent for each 16 mg of concentrate.

◊ If concentrate is accidentally spilled on skin or clothing during preparation or administration, wash area immediately, as contact dermatitis can occur.

♦ **IM:** IM injection may be irritating to tissues; avoid SC injection.

◊ Avoid contact with injectable liquid. A contact dermatitis can occur.

◇ Inject slowly and deeply into upper, outer quadrant of buttock. Massage site thoroughly following injection.

◇ Because of possible hypotensive effects, patient should remain in recumbent position for at least one-half hour following IM injection.

◇ Rotate sites when multiple injections are administered.

◇ Do not mix with other agents in the syringe.

◇ Potency is not altered when solution is slightly yellow in color. Discard if marked discoloration is evident.

◇ Avoid injecting undiluted drug into vein. Aspirate carefully before injecting.

✦ **IV:** Because of possible hypotensive effects, drug should be administered with patient in recumbent position.

◇ Monitor blood pressure every 10 minutes during IV administration. Physician may order vasopressor (not epinephrine) if hypotension occurs.

◇ IV solution should be diluted to a concentration of 0.5 mg/mL with normal saline.

◇ Potency is not altered when solution is slightly yellow in color. Discard if marked discoloration is evident.

◇ Administer direct IV at a rate not exceeding each 0.5 mg over 1 minute.

◇ Solution may be diluted further and given as an infusion under observation of anesthesiologist.

Patient/Family Education

✦ Use caution when driving or when operating dangerous machinery. Drowsiness and dizziness can occur.

✦ Do not stop taking the drug abruptly. To do so might produce withdrawal symptoms such as nausea, vomiting, gastritis, headache, tachycardia, insomnia, tremulousness.

✦ Use sunscreens and wear protective clothing when spending time outdoors. Skin is more susceptible to sunburn.

✦ Report occurrence of any of the following symptoms to physician immediately: sore throat ● fever ● malaise ● unusual bleeding ● easy bruising ● persistent nausea/vomiting ● severe headache ● rapid heart rate ● difficulty urinating ● muscle twitching ● tremors ● darkly colored urine ● pale stools ● yellow skin or eyes ● muscular incoordination ● or skin rash.

✦ Drug may turn urine pink to reddish-brown in color. This is not significant nor is it harmful.

✦ Rise slowly from a sitting or lying position to prevent a sudden drop in blood pressure.

✦ If dry mouth is a problem, take frequent sips of water, chew sugarless gum, or suck on hard candy. Good oral care (frequent brushing, flossing) is very important.

✦ If liquid concentrate is spilled on skin, wash it off immediately. If not, a rash may appear on the skin.

✦ Consult physician regarding smoking while on perphenazine therapy. Smoking increases metabolism of perphenazine, requiring adjustment in dosage to achieve therapeutic effect.

✦ Dress warmly in cold weather and avoid extended exposure to very high or low temperatures. Body temperature is harder to maintain while taking this medication.

✦ Do not drink alcohol while on perphenazine therapy. These drugs potentiate each other's effects.

✦ Do not consume other medications (including over-the-counter meds) without physician's approval. Many medications contain substances that interact with perphenazine in a way that may be harmful.

✦ Be aware of possible risks of taking perphenazine during pregnancy. Safe use during pregnancy and lactation has not been established. Perphenazine readily crosses the placental barrier, so a fetus could experience adverse effects of the drug. Inform physician immediately if pregnancy occurs, is suspected, or is planned.

♦ Be aware of side effects of perphenazine. Refer to written materials furnished by healthcare providers for safe self-administration.

♦ Continue to take medication even if feeling well and as though it is not needed. Symptoms may return if medication is discontinued.

♦ Carry card or other identification at all times describing medications being taken.

Evaluation

♦ Patient demonstrates a subsiding/resolution of the symptoms for which perphenazine was prescribed (panic anxiety, altered thought processes, altered perceptions, hiccups, nausea and vomiting).

♦ Patient verbalizes understanding of side effects and regimen required for prudent self-administration of perphenazine.

PHENACEMIDE

(fe-nass'e-mide)
Phenurone

Classification(s):
Anticonvulsant, Hydantoin
Pregnancy Category D

INDICATIONS

♦ Severe epilepsy, particularly partial seizures with complex symptomatology (psychomotor) refractory to other anticonvulsant medications. Because of toxicity, phenacemide should not be used unless all other anticonvulsants are ineffective.

ACTION

♦ Hydantoins act by increasing the seizure threshold in the cerebral cortex ♦ By promoting sodium efflux from neurons in the motor cortex, hydantoins encourage stabilization of the threshold against hyperexcitability ♦ Maximal activity of the brain-stem centers responsible for the tonic phase of grand mal seizures is also reduced.

PHARMACOKINETICS

Absorption: Readily absorbed following oral administration.
Distribution: Not completely understood. Thought to cross placental barrier. Unknown if drug is excreted in breast milk.
Metabolism and Excretion: Metabolized by the liver into inactive metabolites that are excreted by the kidneys.
Half-Life: Unknown.

CONTRAINDICATIONS AND PRECAUTIONS

Contraindicated in: ♦ Hypersensitivity to this drug or to other hydantoins ♦ Hepatic disease ♦ Hematologic disorders ♦ Concomitant use of ethotoin ♦ Lactation; children under 5 years (safe use has not been established).
Use Cautiously in: ♦ Elderly or debilitated patients ♦ Patients with a history of hepatic or renal dysfunction ♦ Combination with other anticonvulsants that produce similar side effects ♦ Patients previously diagnosed with personality disorders.

ADVERSE REACTIONS AND SIDE EFFECTS*

CNS: drowsiness, dizziness, headache, insomnia, fatigue, depression.
Derm: skin rashes.
GI: nausea, vomiting, anorexia, TOXIC HEPATITIS, jaundice, LIVER NECROSIS.
GU: nephritis with marked albuminuria.
Hemat: BLOOD DYSCRASIAS (thrombocytopenia, leukopenia, agranulocytosis, neutropenia), SEVERE BONE MARROW DEPRESSION.

---

*Underlines indicate most frequent; CAPITALS indicate life-threatening.

Psych: SUICIDAL TENDENCIES, aggression, psychoses, personality changes; paranoid symptoms have been noted with concomitant ethotoin use.

Other: fever, muscle pain, palpitations.

INTERACTIONS

Drug-Drug: ♦ **Other anticonvulsants that produce similar side effects (e.g., mephenytoin, trimethadione, paramethadione, phenytoin, ethotoin):** additive effects of phenacemide (increased risk of toxicity).

ROUTE AND DOSAGE

Seizures

♦ **PO (Adults):** Initial dosage: 250–500 mg tid. If seizures are not controlled after 1 week, additional 500 mg may be administered upon arising. Dosage may be further increased in the third week by 500 mg at bedtime. Effective total daily dosage is usually 2–3 g, though some patients may require as much as 5 g or as little as 750 mg daily.

♦ **PO (Children 5–10 Years Old):** Dose is approximately half that of adult dose, given at the same recommended intervals.

♦ **PO (Replacement Therapy):** Dose of phenacemide is gradually increased each week as dose of drug being replaced is gradually decreased.

♦ **PO (Discontinuation of Treatment):** Withdraw slowly to avoid precipitating seizure or status epilepticus.

PHARMACODYNAMICS

Route	Onset	Peak	Duration
PO	—	—	~5 hr

NURSING IMPLICATIONS

Assessment

♦ Assess occurrence, characteristics, and duration of seizure activity.

♦ Assess mood and behavior. Assess for evidence of suicidal ideations.

♦ Assess baseline vital signs.

♦ Assess history of allergies, sensitivity to this drug and/or other drugs.

♦ Assess date of last menses (possible pregnancy), use of contraceptives.

♦ Assess whether currently breast-feeding a child.

♦ Assess current and past alcohol and drug consumption.

♦ Assess for symptoms of possible blood dyscrasias: sore throat ● fever ● malaise ● unusual bleeding ● easy bruising.

♦ Assess for presence of adverse reactions or side effects.

♦ Assess patient's and family's response to diagnosis of epilepsy.

♦ Assess patient/family knowledge about illness and need for medication.

♦ In collaboration with physician, assess CBC and renal and liver function tests in patients on phenacemide therapy. Assess upon initiation of therapy and monthly thereafter.

♦ **Toxicity and Overdose:** Plasma concentrations associated with safety and efficacy have not been established.

◊ Assess for symptoms of toxicity/overdose: excitement or mania, followed by drowsiness, ataxia, and coma.

♦ **Overdose Management:** Monitor vital signs.

◊ Ensure maintenance of airway.

◊ Induce vomiting in conscious patient.

◊ Initiate gastric lavage if patient is unconscious.

◊ Perform hepatic and renal function tests, as well as hematological status and mental status evaluations, when patient is stable.

Potential Nursing Diagnoses

♦ High risk for injury related to seizures, phenacemide's side effects of dizziness, drowsiness and decreased mental alertness, possible toxic serum levels of phenacemide, abrupt withdrawal from phenacemide use.

♦ High risk for violence, self-directed or directed toward others, related to side effects of suicidal tendencies and aggression.

♦ Impaired adjustment related to difficulty accepting diagnosis of epilepsy.

♦ Social isolation related to fear of experiencing a seizure in the presence of others.

♦ High risk for activity intolerance related to phenacemide's side effects of drowsiness, dizziness, decreased mental alertness.

♦ Knowledge deficit related to medication regimen.

Plan/Implementation

♦ Monitor vital signs at regular intervals (bid or tid) throughout therapy.

♦ Observe frequently (every hour) for occurrence of seizure activity.

♦ Provide safe environment for patient who may become aggressive or suicidal.

♦ Ensure that patient is protected from injury. Supervise and assist with ambulation if dizziness and drowsiness are problems. Ensure that patient avoids participation in any activity requiring mental alertness (including smoking). Pad siderails and head of bed with towels or blanket to protect patient who experiences seizures during the night.

♦ Administer medication with food to minimize GI irritation.

♦ For patient who has difficulty swallowing, crush tablet and mix with food or fluid.

♦ Store medication at controlled room temperatures between 15° and 30°C (59°–86°F). Protect from heat and moisture.

Patient/Family Education

♦ Do not drive or operate dangerous machinery until individual response is determined. Drowsiness and decreased mental alertness can occur.

♦ Do not stop taking drug abruptly. To do so could precipitate status epilepticus.

♦ Avoid alcoholic beverages.

♦ Carry or wear at all times identification informing others of illness and medication usage.

♦ Do not take any other medication without approval from physician. Combining drugs may be harmful.

♦ Promptly report any of the following symptoms to physician: • sore throat • fever • malaise • skin rash • severe nausea or vomiting • yellow skin or eyes • pale stools • unusual bleeding • easy bruising • dark urine • marked change in personality • depression • suicidal ideas.

♦ Be aware of possible risks of taking phenacemide during pregnancy. Patient who requires the medication to prevent seizures may be maintained on it; however, she must be fully aware of potential risks to unborn child. There is a strong association between the use of anticonvulsant drugs by women with epilepsy and the incidence of birth defects in their children. A possible association also has been suggested between maternal use of anticonvulsants and a neonatal coagulation defect that poses a threat of serious bleeding during the first 24 hours of life. Notify physician immediately if pregnancy occurs, is suspected, or is planned. (Patient may need to be instructed about available means of birth control.)

♦ To protect patient during a seizure, padding (towels, blankets, pillows) may be used to prevent bumping against hard objects. When convulsion has subsided, turn patient on side to allow secretions to drain and to prevent aspiration. Keep records of occurrence, characteristics, and duration of seizures, so that accurate reports may be given to physician for providing assistance in stabilization and control of seizures. If patient has difficulty breathing or continues to experience subsequent seizures, family should immediately call for emergency assistance.

♦ Be aware of possible side effects of

phenacemide. Refer to written materials furnished by healthcare providers to assist in self-administration.

Evaluation

♦ Patient demonstrates stabilization of seizure activity with regular administration of phenacemide.

♦ Patient verbalizes understanding of necessity for, side effects of, and regimen required for prudent self-administration of phenacemide.

PHENDIMETRAZINE

(fen-dye-me′tra-zeen)
Adphen, Anorex, Bacarate, Bontril, Di-Ap-Trol, Melfiat, Metra, Obalan, Obeval, Phenzine, Plegine, Sprx-1, Statobex, Trimstat, Trimtabs, Weightrol

Classification(s):
Anorexigenic, CNS stimulant, Sympathomimetic amine
Schedule C III
Pregnancy Category C

INDICATIONS

♦ Exogenous obesity (short-term management).

ACTION

♦ Exact mechanism of action is not known ♦ Sympathomimetic amines are thought to produce appetite suppression through direct stimulation of the satiety center in the hypothalamus and limbic system. Pharmacologic effects are similar to those of the amphetamines.

PHARMACOKINETICS

Absorption: Readily absorbed following oral administration.
Distribution/Metabolism and Excretion: Not well established.
Half-Life: 1.9–9.8 hours.

CONTRAINDICATIONS AND PRECAUTIONS

Contraindicated in: ♦ Hypersensitivity to sympathomimetic amines or tartrazine (contained in some preparations) ♦ Advanced arteriosclerosis ♦ Symptomatic cardiovascular disease ♦ Moderate to severe hypertension ♦ Hyperthyroidism ♦ Glaucoma ♦ Agitated states ♦ History of drug abuse ♦ Concomitant therapy with or within 14 days of receiving MAO inhibitors ♦ Concomitant use of other CNS stimulants ♦ Pregnancy and lactation; children under 12 years of age (safe use has not been established).
Use Cautiously in: ♦ Mild hypertension ♦ Diabetes mellitus ♦ Elderly or debilitated patients.

ADVERSE REACTIONS AND SIDE EFFECTS*

CNS: overstimulation, restlessness, dizziness, insomnia, dyskinesia, euphoria, dysphoria, tremor, headache, drowsiness, depression, confusion, incoordination, fatigue, malaise, blurred vision, mydriasis, psychoses (rare).
CV: palpitations, tachycardia, arrhythmias, hypertension or hypotension, fainting.
Derm: urticaria, rash, erythema, burning sensation.
Endo: impotence, changes in libido.
GI: dry mouth, unpleasant taste, nausea, vomiting, diarrhea, constipation, abdominal discomfort.
Other: tolerance, physical and psychological dependence.

INTERACTIONS

Drug-Drug: ♦ **Other CNS stimulants:** additive CNS stimulant effects ♦ **MAO inhibitors (during or within 14 days of administration):** hypertensive crisis, headache, hyperpyrexia, intracranial hemorrhage, bradycardia ♦ **Insulin:** al-

---

*Underlines indicate most frequent; CAPITALS indicate life-threatening.

teration in requirements ◆ **Guanethi-dine:** decreased antihypertensive effects ◆ **Barbiturates, phenothiazines:** decreased phendimetrazine effects ◆ **General anesthetics:** cardiac arrhythmias. **Drug-Food:** ◆ **Caffeinated foods and drinks:** increased effects of phendimetrazine.

ROUTE AND DOSAGE
Exogenous Obesity
◆ **PO (Adults):** 35 mg bid or tid, 1 hour before meals. Dosage range: 17.5 mg bid to 70 mg tid. Sustained-release capsules: 105 mg once daily in the morning.

PHARMACODYNAMICS

Route	Onset	Peak	Duration
PO	30 min	1–2 hr	4 hr
PO (sustained-release)	Variable	—	12 hr

NURSING IMPLICATIONS
Assessment
◆ Assess and record baseline temperature, pulse, respiration, blood pressure, and weight for comparison during therapy.
◆ In diabetic patient, assess blood sugar bid–tid. Insulin adjustments may be required due to alteration in eating pattern, as well as possibility of hyperactivity.
◆ Assess knowledge of sound nutritional, calorie-reduced diet, and importance of regular exercise.
◆ Assess mental status for changes in mood, level of activity, degree of stimulation.
◆ Assess sleeping patterns carefully. Insomnia may occur.
◆ Assess history of allergies, sensitivity to this drug or to other sympathomimetic amines.
◆ Assess history of glaucoma.
◆ Assess for presence of adverse reactions or side effects.
◆ Assess date of last menses (possible pregnancy), use of contraceptives.
◆ Assess whether currently breast-feeding a child.
◆ Assess current and past alcohol and drug consumption.
◆ Assess amount of caffeine usually consumed.
◆ Assess for operation of automobile and/or other dangerous machinery.
◆ Assess patient/family knowledge about illness and need for medication.
◆ In collaboration with physician, periodically assess CBC, urinalysis, and liver function tests.
◆ **Withdrawal:** Assess for symptoms of withdrawal: • nausea • vomiting • abdominal cramping • headache • fatigue • weakness • mental depression • suicidal ideation.
◆ **Withdrawal Management:** Monitor vital signs.
◇ Place patient in quiet room with low stimuli.
◇ Allow patient to sleep as much as desired.
◇ Observe closely (q 15 min).
◇ Institute suicide precautions.
◇ Some physicians may elect to prescribe antidepressants to counteract feelings of depression and lethargy.
◆ **Toxicity and Overdose:** Assess for symptoms of overdose: • restlessness • tremor • hyperreflexia • fever • rapid respiration • disorientation • belligerence • assaultiveness • hallucinations • panic states (stimulation is usually followed by fatigue and depression) • tachycardia • hypertension or hypotension • nausea • vomiting • diarrhea • abdominal cramping • convulsions • coma • circulatory collapse • death.
◆ **Overdose Management:** Initiate gastric lavage.
◇ Maintain adequate airway.
◇ Initiate cardiac monitoring.
◇ Administer barbiturate for sedation.
◇ Administer phentolamine to treat severe acute hypertension.
◇ Administer IV fluids and vasopressor

to treat hypotension secondary to hypovolemia.

◊ Administer urine acidifiers to promote urinary excretion of the drug.

◊ Hemodialysis and peritoneal dialysis are not effective.

Potential Nursing Diagnoses

♦ High risk for injury due to overstimulation and hyperactivity; abrupt phendimetrazine withdrawal; overdose.

♦ High risk for self-directed violence related to suicidal ideations resulting from abrupt phendimetrazine withdrawal.

♦ Alteration in nutrition, more than body requires, related to excessive intake in relation to metabolic needs.

♦ Sleep pattern disturbance related to overstimulation resulting from phendimetrazine use.

♦ Alteration in thought processes related to phendimetrazine's adverse effects of overstimulation and difficulty concentrating.

♦ Knowledge deficit related to medication regimen.

Plan/Implementation

♦ Monitor medication effects. Tolerance develops rapidly. If anorexigenic effects begin to diminish, notify physician immediately. Patient should be on reduced-calorie diet and program of regular exercise in addition to the medication.

♦ Monitor and record vital signs at regular intervals (bid) throughout therapy.

♦ Encourage use of sugarless gum, hard candy, or frequent sips of water for patient who experiences dry mouth. Ensure that patient practices good oral care (frequent brushing, flossing).

♦ Ensure that patient is protected from injury. Keep stimuli low and environment as quiet as possible to discourage overstimulation.

♦ Ensure that tablet/capsule has been swallowed and not "cheeked" to avoid medication or to hoard for later use.

♦ Short-acting tablets may be crushed and mixed with food or fluid for patient who has difficulty swallowing.

♦ Do not open capsules or mix contents with food. Sustained-release capsules must be swallowed whole.

♦ Administer last dose of the day no later than 6 hours before bedtime.

♦ Drug should be administered 1 hour before meals.

♦ Administer sustained-release form at midmorning.

♦ Store medication at controlled room temperatures between 15° and 30°C (59°–86°F). Protect from heat and moisture.

Patient/Family Education

♦ Use caution in driving or when operating dangerous machinery. Drowsiness, dizziness, and blurred vision can occur.

♦ Do not stop taking the drug abruptly. To do so can produce serious withdrawal symptoms.

♦ If insomnia is a problem, avoid taking medication late in the day. Take no later than 6 hours before bedtime.

♦ Do not take other medications (including over-the-counter drugs) without physician's approval. Many medications contain substances that, in combination with phendimetrazine, can be harmful.

♦ Diabetic patient should monitor blood sugar bid or tid or as instructed by physician. Be aware of need for possible alteration in insulin requirements due to changes in food intake, weight, and activity.

♦ Avoid consumption of large amounts of caffeinated products (coffee, tea, colas, chocolate), as they may enhance the stimulant effect of phendimetrazine.

♦ Follow reduced-calorie diet provided by dietitian, as well as a program of regular exercise. Do not exceed recommended dose if appetite suppressant effect diminishes. Contact physician.

* Notify physician if restlessness, insomnia, anorexia, or dry mouth become severe, or if rapid, pounding heartbeat becomes evident.
* Be aware of possible risks of taking phendimetrazine during pregnancy. Safe use during pregnancy and lactation has not been established. Inform physician immediately if pregnancy is suspected or planned.
* Be aware of potential side effects of phendimetrazine. Refer to written materials furnished by healthcare providers for safe self-administration.
* Carry card or other identification at all times describing medications being taken.

Evaluation

* Patient demonstrates a progressive weight loss with the use of phendimetrazine as an adjunct to reduced-caloric intake and a program of regular exercise.
* Patient verbalizes understanding of side effects and regimen required for prudent self-administration of phendimetrazine.

PHENELZINE

(fen'el-zeen)
Nardil

Classification(s):
Antidepressant, Monoamine oxidase inhibitor, Hydrazine
Pregnancy Category C

INDICATIONS

* Atypical, nonendogenous, or neurotic depression * Depression accompanied by anxiety * Patients unresponsive to other antidepressive therapy (tricyclics, serotonin enhancers, ECT); rarely a drug of first choice. **Investigational Uses**: * Bulimia (with characteristics of atypical depression) * Migraine headaches (prophylaxis).

ACTION

* Exact mechanism of action on depression unknown * Inhibits the enzyme monoamine oxidase, which normally inhibits the activity of epinephrine, norepinephrine, dopamine, and serotonin. The concentration of these biogenic amines is then increased in storage sites throughout the nervous system. These increases in biogenic amines are thought to reduce symptoms of depression.

PHARMACOKINETICS

Absorption: Well absorbed from the GI tract following oral administration.
Distribution: Is widely distributed. Thought to cross placental barrier and to enter breast milk.
Metabolism and Excretion: Metabolized by the liver. Excreted in urine as metabolites and unchanged drug.
Half-Life: Not well studied because it has no real relationship to action duration.

CONTRAINDICATIONS AND PRECAUTIONS

Contraindicated in: * Hypersensitivity to this drug or to other MAO inhibitors * Pheochromocytoma * Congestive heart failure * History of liver disease * Severe renal impairment * Cerebrovascular defect * Paranoid schizophrenic disorder * Cardiovascular disease * Hypertension * History of severe or frequent headaches * Patients over 60 * Children less than 16 years of age; pregnancy and lactation (safety not established).
Use Cautiously in: * Patients with a history of seizures * Diabetes mellitus * Renal insufficiency * Suicidal patients * Schizophrenia * Agitated or hypomanic patients * History of angina pectoris or hyperthyroidism.

ADVERSE REACTIONS AND SIDE EFFECTS*

CNS: dizziness, vertigo, headache, overactivity, tremors, muscle twitching, ma-

---

*Underlines indicate most frequent; CAPITALS indicate life-threatening.

nia, confusion, memory impairment, insomnia, <u>drowsiness</u>, <u>blurred vision</u>, restlessness, weakness, agitation.
CV: <u>orthostatic hypotension</u>, disturbances in cardiac rate and rhythm, tachycardia, palpitations, peripheral edema.
Derm: skin rashes.
GI: <u>dry mouth</u>, <u>constipation</u>, anorexia, body weight changes, nausea, vomiting, diarrhea, abdominal pain.
GU: dysuria, incontinence, urinary retention, changes in libido, transient impotence.
Hemat: spider telangiectases.
Other: excessive sweating, arthralgia, neuritis, weight gain, photosensitivity, FATAL PROGRESSIVE NECROTIZING HEPATOCELLULAR DAMAGE (rare).

INTERACTIONS

Drug-Drug: ♦ **Sympathomimetic and catecholamine-releasing drugs (including amphetamines, methyldopa, levodopa, dopamine, tryptophan, epinephrine, norepinephrine):** increased hypertensive effects, headache, hyperpyrexia ♦ **CNS depressants (e.g., alcohol and certain narcotics such as meperidine):** possible hypotension or hypertension, convulsions, coma, death ♦ **Other MAO inhibitors, tricyclic antidepressants, and other dibenzazepines (carbamazepine, cyclobenzaprine):** hypertensive crisis, convulsions, coma, circulatory collapse ♦ **Antihypertensive drugs, thiazide diuretics:** hypotension ♦ **Guanethidine:** decreased antihypertensive effects ♦ **Doxapram:** potentiation of adverse cardiovascular effects ♦ **Insulin, oral hypoglycemics:** increased hypoglycemic effects ♦ **Methylphenidate:** increased effect of methylphenidate ♦ **Anesthetics:** increased hypotensive and CNS depressant effects ♦ **Disulfiram:** increased toxicity ♦ **Metrizamide:** increased risk of seizures.
Drug-Food: ♦ **Foods containing high concentrations of tryptophan, tyramine or other vasopressors, such as** **aged cheeses; other aged, overripe, and fermented foods; broad beans; pickled herring; beef/chicken livers; preserved sausages; beer; wine (especially chianti); yeast products; chocolate; caffeinated drinks; canned figs; sour cream; yogurt; soy sauce; over-the-counter cold medications; diet pills:** hypertensive crisis. **Caution:** Can occur several weeks after MAOI therapy has been discontinued.

ROUTE AND DOSAGE

Depression

♦ **PO (Adults):** Initial dosage: 15 mg tid. Dosage may be increased to at least 60 mg/day at a fairly rapid pace consistent with patient tolerance. It may be necessary to increase dosage up to 90 mg/day to achieve desired response. Many patients do not show a clinical response until treatment at 60 mg has been continued for at least 4 weeks.
♦ **PO:** Maintenance therapy: slowly (over several weeks) reduce dosage as tolerated to as low as 15 mg daily or every other day.

Migraine Headache Prophylaxis

♦ **PO (Adults):** 45–60 mg/day in divided doses.

Bulimia with Characteristics of Atypical Depression

♦ **PO (Adults):** 60–90 mg/day in divided doses. Adjust dosage to patient's response.

PHARMACODYNAMICS

Route	Onset	Peak	Duration
PO	7–10 days*	—	Weeks†

*Maximal clinical response may require 3–4 weeks to achieve.
†Allow up to 2 weeks following cessation of therapy for complete drug elimination.

NURSING IMPLICATIONS

Assessment

♦ Assess for suicidal ideation, plan, means. Assess for sudden lifts in mood, which could indicate patient's decision to commit suicide.

♦ Assess mental status daily: • mood • appearance • thought and communication patterns • level of interest in the environment and in activities • suicidal ideation. Improvement in these behavior patterns and level of energy should be expected within 2–4 weeks following initiation of therapy.

♦ Assess vital signs, weight.

♦ Assess dieting pattern and consult dietitian.

♦ Assess history of allergies, sensitivity to this drug or to other MAO inhibitors.

♦ Assess for history of glaucoma.

♦ Assess date of last menses (possible pregnancy), use of contraceptives.

♦ Assess whether currently breast-feeding a child.

♦ Assess current and past alcohol and drug consumption.

♦ Assess for operation of automobile and/or other dangerous machinery.

♦ Assess for presence of adverse reactions or side effects.

♦ Assess patient/family knowledge about illness and need for medication.

♦ In collaboration with physician, assess CBC and liver and renal function tests in patients on long-term therapy.

♦ **Withdrawal:** Assess for symptoms of abrupt withdrawal from long-term therapy: • headache • excitability • hallucinations • depression.

♦ **Hypertensive Crisis:** Assess for symptoms of hypertensive crisis: • severe occipital headache • palpitations • sharp rise in blood pressure • nuchal rigidity • chest pain • sweating • fever • nausea • vomiting • coma.

♦ **Management of Hypertensive Crisis:** Discontinue drug immediately.

◇ Monitor vital signs.

◇ Institute therapy to lower blood pressure.

◇ Do not use parenteral reserpine.

◇ Administer antihypertensives slowly to avoid producing an excessive hypotensive effect.

◇ Use external cooling measures to control hyperpyrexia.

♦ **Toxicity and Overdose:** Relationship between blood level and therapeutic response has not been established.

◇ Assess for symptoms of overdose: • excitement • irritability • anxiety • flushing • sweating • tachypnea • tachycardia • exaggerated tendon reflexes • hypotension • hypertension • convulsions • coma • cardiorespiratory arrest.

♦ **Overdose Management:** Monitor vital signs.

◇ Ensure maintenance of adequate airway.

◇ Initiate gastric lavage.

◇ Administer activated charcoal to minimize absorption of the drug.

◇ Monitor electrolytes.

◇ Supplemental oxygen and mechanical ventilatory assistance should be provided as needed.

◇ Administer IV diazepam to control convulsions.

◇ Administer IV fluids to treat hypotension and cardiovascular collapse.

◇ Follow up with liver function evaluation.

Potential Nursing Diagnoses

♦ High risk for self-directed violence related to depressed mood.

♦ High risk for injury related to phenelzine's side effects of sedation, dizziness, fatigue, confusion, and lowered seizure threshold; eating foods that contain tyramine or tryptophan; abrupt withdrawal after prolonged use; overdose.

♦ Social isolation related to depressed mood.

♦ High risk for activity intolerance related to phenelzine's side effects of drowsiness, dizziness, fatigue, confusion.

♦ Knowledge deficit related to medication regimen.

Plan/Implementation

♦ Monitor vital signs before beginning therapy and at regular intervals (bid or tid) throughout therapy. Take BP lying and standing in patients experiencing orthostatic hypotension; elderly are particularly susceptible. Contact physician if tachycardia/arrhythmias are noted.

♦ Weigh patient 2–3 times a week, at same time of day, on same scale, if possible. A rapid weight gain or evidence of edema should be reported to physician immediately. Record I&O.

♦ Ensure that patient is protected from injury. Provide supervision and assistance when ambulating if dizziness and drowsiness are problems. Pad siderails and headboard for patient who experiences seizures. Ensure that ambulatory patient is protected when in the sun.

♦ Order low tyramine diet for patient.

♦ Give patient hard candy, gum, or frequent sips of water if dry mouth is a problem.

♦ Administer oral medication with food to minimize GI upset.

♦ Ensure that patient swallows tablet and does not "cheek" to avoid medication or to hoard for later use.

♦ Tablet may be crushed and mixed with food or fluid for patient who has difficulty swallowing.

♦ Store medication at controlled room temperatures between 15° and 30°C (59°–86°F). Protect from heat, light, and moisture.

Patient/Family Education

♦ Therapeutic effect may be seen in 1–2 weeks. However, it may take as long as 6 weeks after upper dose is reached. If after this length of time no improvement is noted, physician may prescribe a different medication. Continue to take medication even though symptoms have not subsided.

♦ Do not consume the following foods/meds while on phenelzine: aged cheese • wine (especially chianti) • beer • chocolate • colas • coffee • tea • sour cream • beef/chicken livers •

canned figs • soy sauce • overripe and fermented foods • pickeled herring • preserved sausages • yogurt • yeast products • broad beans • cold remedies • diet pills.

♦ Use caution when driving or when operating dangerous machinery. Drowsiness and dizziness can occur. If these side effects become persistent or interfere with activities of daily living, report to physician. Dosage adjustment may be necessary.

♦ Do not stop taking the drug abruptly. To do so might produce withdrawal symptoms, such as headache, excitability, hallucinations, and depression.

♦ Report occurrence of any of the following symptoms to physician immediately: persistent nausea/vomiting • severe or frequent headaches • rapid heart rate • difficulty urinating • skin rash • stiff or sore neck • palpitations • chest pain.

♦ Rise slowly from a sitting or lying position to prevent a sudden drop in blood pressure.

♦ Avoid overexertion if you have a history of angina pectoris or coronary artery disease.

♦ Take medication with food to minimize GI upset.

♦ If dry mouth is a problem, take frequent sips of water, chew sugarless gum, or suck on hard candy. Good oral care (frequent brushing, flossing) is very important.

♦ Do not drink alcohol while on phenelzine therapy. Profound CNS depression can be life-threatening.

♦ Do not consume other medications (including over-the-counter meds) with phenelzine without physician's approval. Many medications contain substances that, in combination with MAO inhibitors, could precipitate a life-threatening hypertensive crisis.

♦ Be aware of possible risks of taking phenelzine during pregnancy. Safe use during pregnancy and lactation has not been established. It is thought to enter breast milk, however, so effects on a nursing child should be considered.

♦ Be aware of side effects of phenelzine. Refer to written materials furnished by healthcare providers for safe self-administration.

♦ Carry card or other identification at all times describing medications being taken.

Evaluation

♦ Patient demonstates a subsiding/resolution of the symptoms for which phenelzine was prescribed (depressed mood, suicidal ideation).

♦ Patient verbalizes understanding of side effects and regimen required for prudent self-administration of phenelzine.

PHENMETRAZINE HCl

(fen-met'ra-zeen)
Preludin

Classification(s):
Anorexigenic, CNS stimulant,
Sympathomimetic amine
Schedule C II
Pregnancy Category C

INDICATIONS

♦ Exogenous obesity (short-term management).

ACTION

♦ Exact mechanism of action is not known ♦ Sympathomimetic amines are thought to produce appetite suppression through direct stimulation of the satiety center in the hypothalamus and limbic system. Pharmacologic effects are similar to those of the amphetamines.

PHARMACOKINETICS

Absorption: Readily absorbed following oral administration.
Distribution/Metabolism and Excretion: Not completely understood.
Half-Life: Not well substantiated.

CONTRAINDICATIONS AND PRECAUTIONS

Contraindicated in: ♦ Hypersensitivity to sympathomimetic amines or tartrazine (contained in some preparations) ♦ Advanced arteriosclerosis ♦ Symptomatic cardiovascular disease ♦ Moderate to severe hypertension ♦ Hyperthyroidism ♦ Glaucoma ♦ Agitated states ♦ History of drug abuse ♦ Concomitant therapy with or within 14 days of receiving MAO inhibitors ♦ Concomitant use of other CNS stimulants ♦ Pregnancy and lactation; children under 12 years of age (safe use has not been established).
Use Cautiously in: ♦ Mild hypertension ♦ Diabetes mellitus ♦ Elderly or debilitated patients.

ADVERSE REACTIONS AND SIDE EFFECTS*

CNS: overstimulation, restlessness, dizziness, insomnia, dyskinesia, euphoria, dysphoria, tremor, headache, drowsiness, depression, confusion, incoordination, fatigue, malaise, blurred vision, mydriasis, psychoses (rare).
CV: palpitations, tachycardia, hypertension.
Derm: urticaria, rash, erythema, burning sensation.
Endo: impotence, changes in libido.
GI: dry mouth, unpleasant taste, nausea, vomiting, diarrhea, constipation, abdominal discomfort.
Other: tolerance, physical and psychological dependence, alopecia, chills, fever.

---

*Underlines indicate most frequent; CAPITALS indicate life-threatening.

INTERACTIONS

Drug-Drug: ♦ **Other CNS stimulants:** additive CNS stimulant effects ♦ **MAO inhibitors** (during or within 14 days of administration): hypertensive crisis, headache, hyperpyrexia, intracranial hemorrhage, bradycardia ♦ **Insulin:** alteration in requirements ♦ **Guanethidine:** decreased antihypertensive effects ♦ **Barbiturates, phenothiazines:** decreased phenmetrazine effects ♦ **General anesthetics:** cardiac arrhythmias.

Drug-Food: ♦ **Caffeinated foods and drinks:** increased effects of phenmetrazine.

ROUTE AND DOSAGE

Exogenous Obesity

♦ **PO (Adults):** 25 mg bid or tid given 1 hour before meals. Dosage range: 12.5 mg bid to 25 mg tid maximum. Sustained-release tablets: 75 mg once daily in midmorning.

PHARMACODYNAMICS

Route	Onset	Peak	Duration
PO	30 min	1–2 hr	4 hr
PO (sustained-release)	Variable	—	12 hr

NURSING IMPLICATIONS

Assessment

♦ Assess and record baseline temperature, pulse, respiration, blood pressure, and weight for comparison during therapy.
♦ In diabetic patient, assess blood sugar bid–tid. Insulin adjustments may be required due to alteration in eating pattern, as well as possibility of hyperactivity.
♦ Assess knowledge of sound nutritional, calorie-reduced diet, and importance of regular exercise.
♦ Assess mental status for changes in mood, level of activity, degree of stimulation.
♦ Assess sleeping patterns carefully. Insomnia may occur.
♦ Assess history of allergies, sensitivity to this drug or to other sympathomimetic amines.
♦ Assess history of glaucoma.
♦ Assess for presence of adverse reactions or side effects.
♦ Assess date of last menses (possible pregnancy), use of contraceptives.
♦ Assess whether currently breast-feeding a child.
♦ Assess current and past alcohol and drug consumption.
♦ Assess amount of caffeine usually consumed.
♦ Assess for operation of automobile and/or other dangerous machinery.
♦ Assess patient/family knowledge about condition and need for medication.
♦ In collaboration with physician, periodically assess CBC, urinalysis, and liver function tests.
♦ **Withdrawal:** Assess for symptoms of withdrawal: ● fatigue ● mental depression ● suicidal ideations.
♦ **Withdrawal Management:** Monitor vital signs.
◊ Place patient in quiet room with low stimuli.
◊ Allow patient to sleep as much as desired.
◊ Observe closely (q 15 min).
◊ Institute suicide precautions.
◊ Some physicians may elect to prescribe antidepressants to counteract feelings of depression and lethargy.
♦ **Toxicity and Overdose:** Assess for symptoms of overdose: ● restlessness ● tremor ● hyperreflexia ● fever ● rapid respiration ● disorientation ● belligerence ● assaultiveness ● hallucinations ● panic states (stimulation is usually followed by fatigue and depression) ● tachycardia ● hypertension or hypotension ● nausea ● vomiting ● diarrhea ● abdominal cramping ● convulsions ● coma ● circulatory collapse ● death.
♦ **Overdose Management:** Monitor vital signs.
◊ Maintain adequate airway.

◇ Initiate gastric lavage.

◇ Initiate cardiac monitoring.

◇ Administer barbiturate for sedation.

◇ Administer phentolamine to treat severe acute hypertension.

◇ Administer IV fluids and a vasopressor to treat hypotension secondary to hypovolemia.

◇ Administer urine acidifiers to promote urinary excretion of the drug.

◇ Hemodialysis and peritoneal dialysis are not effective.

Potential Nursing Diagnoses

♦ High risk for injury due to overstimulation and hyperactivity; abrupt phenmetrazine withdrawal; overdose.

♦ High risk for self-directed violence related to suicidal ideations resulting from abrupt phenmetrazine withdrawal.

♦ Alteration in nutrition, more than body requires, related to excessive intake in relation to metabolic needs.

♦ Sleep pattern disturbance related to overstimulation resulting from phenmetrazine use.

♦ Alteration in thought processes related to phenmetrazine's adverse effects of overstimulation and difficulty concentrating.

♦ Knowledge deficit related to medication regimen.

Plan/Implementation

♦ Monitor medication effects. Tolerance develops rapidly. If anorexigenic effects begin to diminish, notify physician immediately. Patient should be on reduced-calorie diet and program of regular exercise in addition to the medication.

♦ Monitor and record vital signs at regular intervals (bid) throughout therapy.

♦ Encourage use of sugarless gum, hard candy, or frequent sips of water for patient who experiences dry mouth. Ensure that patient practices good oral care (frequent brushing, flossing).

♦ Ensure that patient is protected from injury. Keep stimuli low and environment as quiet as possible to discourage overstimulation.

♦ Ensure that tablet has been swallowed and not "cheeked" to avoid medication or to hoard for later use.

♦ Tablets may be crushed and mixed with food or fluid for patient who has difficulty swallowing. Do not crush sustained-release tablets.

♦ Administer last dose of the day no later than 6 hours before bedtime.

♦ Drug should be administered 1 hour before meals.

♦ Administer sustained-release form at midmorning.

♦ Store at controlled room temperatures between 15° and 30°C (59°–86°F). Protect from heat and moisture.

Patient/Family Education

♦ Use caution in driving or when operating dangerous machinery. Drowsiness, dizziness, and blurred vision can occur.

♦ Do not stop taking the drug abruptly. To do so can produce serious withdrawal symptoms.

♦ If insomnia is a problem, avoid taking medication late in the day. Take no later than 6 hours before bedtime.

♦ Do not take other medications (including over-the-counter drugs) without physician's approval. Many medications contain substances that, in combination with phenmetrazine, can be harmful.

♦ Diabetic patient should monitor blood sugar bid or tid or as instructed by physician. Be aware of need for possible alteration in insulin requirements due to changes in food intake, weight, and activity.

♦ Avoid consumption of large amounts of caffeinated products (coffee, tea, colas, chocolate), as they may enhance the stimulant effect of phenmetrazine.

♦ Follow reduced-calorie diet provided by dietitian, as well as a program of regular exercise. Do not exceed recommended dose if appetite suppressant effect diminishes. Contact physician.

* Notify physician if restlessness, insomnia, anorexia, or dry mouth become severe, or if rapid, pounding heartbeat becomes evident.
* Be aware of possible risks of taking phenmetrazine during pregnancy. Safe use during pregnancy and lactation has not been established. Inform physician immediately if pregnancy is suspected or planned.
* Be aware of potential side effects of phenmetrazine. Refer to written materials furnished by healthcare providers for safe self-administration.
* Carry card or other identification at all times describing medications being taken.

Evaluation

* Patient demonstrates a progressive weight loss with the use of phenmetrazine as an adjunct to reduced caloric intake and a program of regular exercise.
* Patient verbalizes understanding of side effects and regimen required for prudent self-administration of phenmetrazine.

PHENOBARBITAL

(fee-noe-bar′bi-tal)
Barbita, Luminal, {Gardenal},
Solfoton

Classification(s):
Sedative-hypnotic, anticonvulsant,
Barbiturate, CNS depressant
Schedule C IV
Pregnancy Category D

INDICATIONS

* Moderate anxiety states * Insomnia * Seizures (long-term management) * Sta-

tus epilepticus * Pre- and postoperative sedation.

ACTION

* Depresses the central nervous system * Interferes with transmission through the reticular formation, which is concerned with arousal * Causes imbalance in inhibitory and facilitatory mechanisms that influence the cerebral cortex and reticular formation * Action on neurotransmitters is not well defined * All levels of CNS depression can occur, from mild sedation to hypnosis to coma to death.

PHARMACOKINETICS

Absorption: Absorbed well, but slowly, following oral, IM, or IV administration.
Distribution: Rapidly and widely distributed. Crosses blood-brain and placental barriers; excreted in breast milk.
Metabolism and Excretion: Metabolized by the liver; excreted by the kidneys (20–25% in unchanged form).
Half-Life: 2–6 days; children, 1.6–2.9 days.

CONTRAINDICATIONS AND PRECAUTIONS

Contraindicated in: * Hypersensitivity to the drug or to other barbiturates * Severe hepatic, renal, cardiac, or respiratory disease * Individuals with a history of previous addiction * History of porphyria.
Use Cautiously in: * Elderly or debilitated patients * Hepatic, renal, cardiac, or respiratory dysfunction * Depressed/suicidal patients * Ammonia intoxication * Pregnancy and lactation.

ADVERSE REACTIONS AND SIDE EFFECTS*

CNS: <u>drowsiness</u>, headache, lethargy, <u>dizziness</u>, mental depression, ataxia, <u>residual sedation</u> ("hangover"), confusion, paradoxical excitement and/or euphoria.

{} = Only available in Canada.
*<u>Underlines</u> indicate most frequent; CAPITALS indicate life-threatening.

CV: hypotension, bradycardia.
Derm: skin rashes, urticaria, dermatitis (may precede potentially fatal reactions), redness and pain at IM injection site, phlebitis at IV site.
GI: nausea/vomiting, diarrhea/constipation, epigastric pain.
Hemat: AGRANULOCYTOSIS, THROMBOCYTOPENIA.
Resp: hypoventilation, apnea, RESPIRATORY DEPRESSION, LARYNGOSPASM, BRONCHOSPASM.
Other: tolerance, physical and psychological dependence.

INTERACTIONS

Drug-Drug: ◆ **Other CNS depressants (including alcohol, benzodiazepines, antihistamines, opiates), ketamine HCl, primidone:** additive CNS depression ◆ **Chloramphenicol, MAO inhibitors, valproic acid, cimetidine, disulfiram:** increased effects of phenobarbital ◆ **Phenytoin:** increased or decreased effects of either drug (close monitoring of serum levels required to control seizure activity) ◆ **Oral contraceptives:** decreased effectiveness of oral contraceptives ◆ **Oral anticoagulants:** decreased anticoagulant effects ◆ **Corticosteroids, digitoxin, doxycycline:** decreased effects of these drugs ◆ **Furosemide:** orthostatic hypotension ◆ **Griseofulvin:** decreased griseofulvin levels.
Drug-Food: ◆ **Vitamin D:** increased vitamin D metabolism, possible deficiency ◆ **Folic acid:** decreased absorption of folic acid, possible deficiency.

ROUTE AND DOSAGE

Anxiety
◆ **PO (Adults):** 15–30 mg bid or tid.
◆ **PO (Children):** 2 mg/kg tid.

Insomnia
(Limit to 2 weeks if given daily.)
◆ **PO (Adults):** 100–320 mg at bedtime.

◆ **PO (Children):** 3–6 mg/kg at bedtime.
◆ **IM (Adults):** 100–320 mg at bedtime.
◆ **IM (Children):** 3–6 mg/kg at bedtime.

Seizures
◆ **PO (Adults):** 100–300 mg/day in 3 divided doses or single dose at bedtime.
◆ **PO (Children):** 3–5 mg/kg/day until blood level of 15 mcg/mL is reached. Dose adjusted to blood levels.

Status Epilepticus
◆ **IM (Adults):** 200–300 mg. Repeat after 6 hours if necessary.
◆ **IM (Children):** 3–5 mg/kg.
◆ **IV (Adults):** 10–20 mg/kg total dose.
◆ **IV (Children):** 5–10 mg/kg. May be repeated q 10–15 min. Maximum 20 mg/kg.

Preoperative Sedation
◆ **PO (Children):** 1–3 mg/kg.
◆ **IM (Children):** 16–100 mg.
◆ **IM (Adults):** 130–200 mg.

Postoperative Sedation
◆ **IM (Adults):** 32–100 mg.
◆ **IM (Children):** 8–30 mg.

PHARMACODYNAMICS

Route	Onset	Peak	Duration
PO	20–60 min	8–12 hr	6–10 hr
IM	10–30 min	20–60 min	4–6 hr
IV	5 min	30 min	4–6 hr

NURSING IMPLICATIONS

Assessment
◆ Assess sleep patterns. Keep records for adequate baseline data before the initiation of therapy.
◆ Assess occurrence, characteristics, and duration of seizure activity.
◆ Assess history of allergies, sensitivity to this drug.
◆ Assess date of last menses (possible pregnancy), use of contraceptives.
◆ Assess whether currently breast-feeding a child.

♦ Assess current and past alcohol and drug consumption.

♦ Assess for suicidal ideation in depressed patients.

♦ Assess for operation of automobile and/or other dangerous machinery.

♦ Assess for presence of adverse reactions or side effects.

♦ Assess patient's and family's response to diagnosis of epilepsy.

♦ Assess patient/family knowledge about illness and need for medication.

♦ In collaboration with physician, assess CBC and renal and liver function tests in patients on prolonged phenobarbital therapy.

♦ **Lab Test Alterations:** May increase values of bromsulphalein (BSP) retention and protein-bound iodine (PBI).

◊ Elevated blood ammonia.

♦ **Withdrawal:** Assess for symptoms of withdrawal: • anxiety • tremors • insomnia • nausea/vomiting • weakness • diaphoresis • orthostatic hypotension • delirium • convulsions.

♦ **Withdrawal Management:** Monitor vital signs.

◊ Place patient in quiet room with low stimuli.

◊ Institute seizure precautions.

◊ Phenytoin may be ordered to prevent seizures.

◊ Some physicians may order oxazepam as needed for objective withdrawal symptoms, gradually decreasing dosage until the drug is discontinued.

♦ **Toxicity and Overdose:** Monitor routine lab values. Range of therapeutic serum concentration is 15–45 mcg/mL.

◊ Assess for symptoms of toxicity: • confusion • drowsiness • dyspnea • slurred speech • staggering.

◊ Assess for symptoms of overdose: • CNS and respiratory depression • hypoventilation • hypothermia • hypotension • oliguria • tachycardia • coma. (May progress to respiratory

arrest, circulatory collapse, and death.)

♦ **Overdose Management:** Monitor vital signs.

◊ Ensure maintenance of adequate airway.

◊ Induce vomiting in conscious patient.

◊ Initiate gastric lavage in unconscious patient.

◊ Administer activated charcoal to minimize absorption of drug.

◊ Administer IV fluids.

◊ Promote urine alkalinization to increase renal excretion.

◊ For severe intoxication, forced diuresis or hemodialysis may be used.

Potential Nursing Diagnoses

♦ Ineffective breathing pattern related to side effects of hypoventilation and respiratory depression.

♦ High risk for injury related to seizures; abrupt withdrawal from long-term use; decreased mental alertness caused by side effect of residual sedation; side effects of dizziness, ataxia; effects of overdose.

♦ High risk for self-directed violence related to depressed mood.

♦ Sleep pattern disturbance related to situational crises, physical condition, severe level of anxiety.

♦ High risk for activity intolerance related to side effects of residual sedation, drowsiness, dizziness.

♦ Knowledge deficit related to medication regimen.

Plan/Implementation

♦ **General Info:** Monitor vital signs before beginning therapy, at regular intervals (bid) throughout therapy, every 3–5 minutes during IV administration, and every 10 minutes for 30 minutes following IM administration.

◊ Ensure that patient is protected from injury. Supervise and assist with ambulation if dizziness and drowsiness are problems. Ensure that patient avoids participation in any activity requiring mental alertness (including smoking). Raise siderails and instruct patient to remain in bed following administration.

◊ Store medication at controlled room temperatures between 15° and 30°C (59°–86°F). Protect from heat and moisture.

♦ **PO:** To minimize nausea, medication may be given with food or milk.

◊ Ensure that tablet/capsule has been swallowed and not "cheeked" to avoid medication or to hoard for later use.

◊ Tablet may be crushed or contents of capsule emptied and mixed with food or fluid for patient who has difficulty swallowing. Consider using elixir form.

♦ **IM:** Administer deeply into large muscle mass to minimize subcutaneous tissue irritation/necrosis. Use Z-tract method.

◊ Volume of injection should not exceed 5 mL at any one site.

♦ **IV:** Solution from powder form should be prepared immediately prior to administration. Use within 30 minutes of preparation.

◊ Dilute sterile powder slowly with 10 mL sterile water for injection. When powder is dissolved, further dilute with 10 mL of sterile water. Do not use if solution is not clear or if precipitate is visible.

◊ Solution is highly alkaline. Extravasation may result in tissue necrosis. Stop infusion immediately if patient complains of pain. Inadvertent intra-arterial injection may result in gangrene.

◊ Administer IV solution at rate not exceeding 60 mg/min. Observe closely for potential depression of vital signs.

◊ Ensure availability of artificial ventilation and resuscitation equipment.

Patient/Family Education

♦ Use caution in driving or operating dangerous machinery. Drowsiness and dizziness can occur.

♦ Do not stop taking the drug abruptly. Doing so can produce serious (even life-threatening) withdrawal symptoms. If a dose is missed, take it as close as possible to the prescribed time. If it is already close to time for next dose, wait until then; do not double up on dose at the next prescribed time.

♦ Do not consume other CNS depressants (including alcohol).

♦ To protect patient during a seizure, do not restrain, but do protect from injury. Padding (towels, blankets, pillows) may be used to prevent bumping against hard objects. When convulsion has subsided, turn patient on side to allow secretions to drain and to prevent aspiration. Keep records of occurrence, characteristics, and duration of seizures, so that accurate reports may be given to physician for providing assistance in stabilization and control of seizures. If patient has difficulty breathing or continues to experience subsequent seizures, call for emergency assistance immediately.

♦ Be aware of the risks of taking barbiturates during pregnancy (congenital malformations have been associated with use during the first trimester). Evidence of withdrawal symptoms also has been observed in neonates born to mothers who had ingested barbiturates regularly during the last trimester of pregnancy. Notify physician if pregnancy is suspected or planned.

♦ Because barbiturates decrease the effectiveness of oral contraceptives, use alternative methods of birth control during phenobarbital therapy.

♦ Be aware of potential side effects. Refer to written materials furnished by healthcare providers regarding correct method of self-administration.

♦ Report symptoms of sore throat, fever, malaise, severe headache, conjunctivitis, rhinitis, urethritis, balanitis, easy bruising, petechiae, or epistaxis to the physician immediately.

+ Carry card or other identification at all times stating names of medications being taken.

Evaluation

+ Patient demonstrates a subsiding/resolution of the symptoms for which phenobarbital was prescribed (seizures, sleep disturbances, anxiety).
+ Patient verbalizes understanding of side effects and regimen required for prudent self-administration of phenobarbital.

PHENSUXIMIDE

(fen-sux'i-mide)
Milontin

Classification(s):
Anticonvulsant, Succinimide
Pregnancy Category C

INDICATIONS

+ Absence (petit mal) seizures.

ACTION

+ Depresses motor cortex and elevates central nervous system seizure threshold
+ Suppresses paroxysmal spike and wave activity common in absence seizures.

PHARMACOKINETICS

Absorption: Rapidly absorbed from the GI tract.
Distribution: Widely distributed. Unknown if drug crosses placental barrier or is excreted in breast milk.
Metabolism and Excretion: Metabolized by the liver; excreted in urine and bile.
Half-Life: 4–12 hours.

CONTRAINDICATIONS AND PRECAUTIONS

Contraindicated in: + Hypersensitivity to this drug or to other succinimides.
Use Cautiously in: + Severe hepatic or renal disease + Acute intermittent porphyria + Pregnancy and lactation (safety has not been established) + **Note:** Sole use of this medication in some patients with mixed type of epilepsy may increase incidence of grand mal seizures.

ADVERSE REACTIONS AND SIDE EFFECTS*

CNS: <u>drowsiness</u>, headache, <u>dizziness</u>, ataxia, <u>lethargy</u>, <u>fatigue</u>, irritability, hyperactivity.
Derm: skin rashes, urticaria, pruritus, hirsuitism.
GI: <u>nausea/vomiting</u>, <u>anorexia</u>, abdominal cramps, diarrhea, constipation, hiccups.
Hemat: LEUKOPENIA, AGRANULOCYTOSIS, THROMBOCYTOPENIA, APLASTIC ANEMIA.
Other: gingival hypertrophy, swollen tongue, alopecia, vaginal bleeding, RENAL AND HEPATIC DAMAGE, diplopia, sleep disturbances, night terrors, aggressiveness, paranoid psychosis, SLE, myopia.

INTERACTIONS

Drug-Drug: + **Hydantoin anticonvulsants:** decreased metabolism and increased risk of toxic effects of hydantoins + **Oral contraceptives:** decreased effectiveness of oral contraceptives + **CNS depressants (including alcohol, sedative-hypnotics, narcotics, antihistamines):** additive CNS depression + **Carbamazepine:** decreased concentration of phensuximide.

ROUTE AND DOSAGE

Absence (Petit Mal) Seizures

+ **PO (Adults and Children):** 500–1000 mg bid or tid. Dosage is highly individualized; total may vary between 1 and 3 g/day.

PHARMACODYNAMICS

Route	Onset	Peak	Duration
PO	Rapid	1–4 hr	UK

---

*<u>Underlines</u> indicate most frequent; CAPITALS indicate life-threatening.

NURSING IMPLICATIONS

Assessment

- Assess occurrence, characteristics, and duration of seizure activity.
- Assess baseline vital signs.
- Assess history of allergies, sensitivity to this drug.
- Assess date of last menses (possible pregnancy), use of contraceptives.
- Assess whether currently breast-feeding a child.
- Assess current and past alcohol and drug consumption.
- Assess operation of automobile and/or other dangerous machinery.
- Assess for presence of adverse reactions or side effects.
- Assess patient/family knowledge about illness and need for medication.
- In collaboration with physician, assess CBC and renal and liver function tests in patients on phensuximide therapy. Periodic urinalysis should be performed.
- **Lab Test Alterations:** Increased direct Coombs' test.
- **Toxicity and Overdose:** Assess for symptoms of toxicity/overdose: • bone marrow depression • nausea/vomiting • ataxia • diplopia.
- **Overdose Management:** Monitor vital signs.
  ◇ Ensure maintenance of adequate airway.
  ◇ Induce emesis if patient is conscious.
  ◇ Initiate gastric lavage if patient is unconscious.
  ◇ Administer activated charcoal to minimize absorption.
  ◇ Monitor electrolytes.
  ◇ Administer IV fluids.
  ◇ Initiate supportive therapy.

Potential Nursing Diagnoses

- High risk for injury related to seizures; abrupt withdrawal from long-term phensuximide use; side effects of dizziness, sedation, and ataxia; overdose.

- Social isolation related to fear of experiencing a seizure in the presence of others.
- Impaired adjustment related to difficulty accepting diagnosis of epilepsy.
- High risk for activity intolerance related to phensuximide's side effects of sedation, drowsiness, dizziness, ataxia.
- Knowledge deficit related to medication regimen.

Plan/Implementation

- Monitor vital signs at regular intervals (bid) throughout therapy.
- Monitor for presence of skin rash, joint pain, fever, unusual bleeding, easy bruising, dark urine, or jaundice; report such symptoms to physician immediately.
- Observe frequently (every hour) for occurrence of seizure activity.
- Ensure that patient is protected from injury. Supervise and assist with ambulation if dizziness and drowsiness are problems. Ensure that patient avoids participation in any activity requiring mental alertness (including smoking). Pad siderails and head of bed with towels or blanket for patient who experiences seizures during the night.
- Administer medication with food or milk to minimize GI irritation.
- Store medication at controlled room temperatures between 15° and 30°C (59°–86°F). Protect from heat, light, and moisture.

Patient/Family Education

- Do not drive or operate dangerous machinery until individual response has been determined. Drowsiness and dizziness can occur.
- Do not stop taking drug abruptly. To do so might precipitate absence (petit mal) status.
- Avoid alcoholic beverages.
- Carry or wear identification informing others of illness and medication usage.

- Urine may appear pink, red, or reddish-brown. This is not significant or harmful.
- Do not take any other medication without approval from physician. To do so may be harmful.
- Promptly report any of the following symptoms to physician: • sore throat • fever • malaise • skin rash • joint pain • unusual bleeding • easy bruising • dark urine • yellow skin or eyes.
- Be aware of possible risks of taking phensuximide during pregnancy. Patient who requires the medication to prevent seizures may be maintained on it; however, she must be fully aware of potential risks to unborn child. There is a strong association between the use of anticonvulsant drugs by women with epilepsy and the incidence of birth defects in their children. If pregnancy occurs, is suspected, or is planned, report it to physician immediately.
- Due to decreased effectiveness of oral contraceptives, use alternative methods of birth control during therapy.
- To protect patient during a grand mal seizure, do not restrain. Padding (towels, blankets, pillows) may be used to prevent bumping against hard objects. When convulsion has subsided, turn patient on side to allow secretions to drain and to prevent aspiration. Keep records of occurrence, characteristics, and duration of seizures, so that accurate reports may be given to physician for providing assistance in stabilization and control of seizures. If patient has difficulty breathing or continues to experience subsequent seizures, family should immediately call for emergency assistance.
- Be aware of possible side effects. Refer to written materials furnished by healthcare providers for assistance during self-administration upon discharge.

Evaluation

- Patient demonstrates stabilization of seizure activity with regular administration of phensuximide.
- Patient verbalizes understanding of necessity for, side effects of, and regimen required for prudent self-administration of phensuximide.

PHENTERMINE HCI

(fen'ter-meen)
Adipex-P, Dapex-37.5, Fastin, Ionamin, Obe-Nix, Obephen, Obermine, Obestin-30, Parmine, Phentamine, Phentrol, Tora, Unifast Unicelles, Wilpowr

Classification(s):
Anorexigenic, CNS stimulant, Sympathomimetic amine
Schedule C IV
Pregnancy Category C

INDICATIONS

- Exogenous obesity (short-term management).

ACTION

- Exact mechanism of action is not known • Sympathomimetic amines are thought to produce appetite suppression through direct stimulation of the satiety center in the hypothalamus and limbic system • Pharmacologic effects are similar to those of the amphetamines.

PHARMACOKINETICS

Absorption: Readily absorbed following oral administration.
Distribution: Is widely distributed. Crosses placental barrier; enters breast milk.
Metabolism and Excretion: Metabolized by the liver and excreted in urine. Renal excretion is enhanced by an acid urine; reabsorption is enhanced by an alkaline urine.
Half-Life: Not well substantiated.

CONTRAINDICATIONS AND PRECAUTIONS

Contraindicated in: ✦ Hypersensitivity to sympathomimetic amines ✦ Advanced arteriosclerosis ✦ Symptomatic cardiovascular disease ✦ Moderate to severe hypertension ✦ Hyperthyroidism ✦ Glaucoma ✦ Agitated states ✦ History of drug abuse ✦ Concomitant therapy with or within 14 days of receiving MAO inhibitors ✦ Concomitant use of other CNS stimulants ✦ Pregnancy and lactation; children under 12 years of age (safe use has not been established).

Use Cautiously in: ✦ Mild hypertension ✦ Diabetes mellitus ✦ Elderly or debilitated patients.

ADVERSE REACTIONS AND SIDE EFFECTS*

CNS: overstimulation, restlessness, dizziness, insomnia, dyskinesia, euphoria, dysphoria, tremor, headache, drowsiness, depression, confusion, incoordination, fatigue, malaise, blurred vision, mydriasis, psychoses (rare).

CV: palpitations, tachycardia, arrhythmias, hypertension or hypotension, fainting.

Derm: urticaria, rash.

Endo: impotence, changes in libido.

GI: dry mouth, unpleasant taste, nausea, vomiting, diarrhea, constipation, abdominal discomfort.

Other: tolerance, physical and psychological dependence, alopecia, chills, fever.

INTERACTIONS

Drug-Drug: ✦ **Other CNS stimulants:** additive CNS stimulant effects ✦ **MAO inhibitors (during or within 14 days of administration):** hypertensive crisis, headache, hyperpyrexia, intracranial hemorrhage, bradycardia ✦ **Insulin:** alteration in requirements ✦ **Guanethidine:** decreased antihypertensive effects

✦ **Barbiturates, phenothiazines:** decreased phentermine effects ✦ **Phenothiazines, haloperidol:** decreased antipsychotic effects ✦ **Acetozolamide, sodium bicarbonate:** increased renal reabsorption of phentermine ✦ **Ammonium chloride, ascorbic acid:** decreased phentermine effects ✦ **General anesthetics:** cardiac arrhythmias.

Drug-Food: ✦ **Caffeinated foods and drinks:** increased effects of phentermine.

ROUTE AND DOSAGE

Exogenous Obesity

✦ **PO (Adults):** 8 mg tid, 30 minutes before meals. Sustained-release forms: 15–37.5 mg as a single daily dose in the morning.

PHARMACODYNAMICS

Route	Onset	Peak	Duration
PO	30 min	1–2 hr	4–6 hr
PO (sustained-release)	Variable	—	10–14 hr

NURSING IMPLICATIONS

Assessment

- ✦ Assess and record baseline temperature, pulse, respiration, blood pressure, and weight for comparison during therapy.
- ✦ In diabetic patient, assess blood sugar bid–tid. Insulin adjustments may be required due to alteration in eating pattern, as well as possibility of hyperactivity.
- ✦ Assess knowledge of sound nutritional, calorie-reduced diet and importance of regular exercise.
- ✦ Assess mental status for changes in mood, level of activity, degree of stimulation.
- ✦ Assess sleeping patterns carefully. Insomnia may occur.
- ✦ Assess history of allergies, sensitivity to

this drug or to other sympathomimetic amines.

- Assess history of glaucoma.
- Assess for presence of adverse reactions or side effects.
- Assess date of last menses (possible pregnancy), use of contraceptives.
- Assess whether currently breast-feeding a child.
- Assess current and past alcohol and drug consumption.
- Assess amount of caffeine usually consumed.
- Assess for operation of automobile and/or other dangerous machinery.
- Assess patient/family knowledge about condition and need for medication.
- In collaboration with physician, periodically assess CBC, urinalysis, and liver function tests.
- **Withdrawal:** Assess for symptoms of withdrawal: • nausea • vomiting • abdominal cramping • headache • fatigue • weakness • mental depression • suicidal ideation.
- **Withdrawal Management:** Monitor vital signs.
◇ Place patient in quiet room with low stimuli.
◇ Allow patient to sleep as much as desired.
◇ Observe closely (q 15 min).
◇ Institute suicide precautions.
◇ Some physicians may elect to prescribe antidepressants to counteract feelings of depression and lethargy.
- **Toxicity and Overdose:** Assess for symptoms of overdose: • restlessness • tremor • hyperreflexia • fever • rapid respirations • disorientation • belligerence • assaultiveness • hallucinations • panic states (stimulation is usually followed by fatigue and depression) • tachycardia • hypertension or hypotension • nausea • vomiting • diarrhea • abdominal cramping • convulsions • coma • circulatory collapse • death.
- **Overdose Management:** Monitor vital signs.

◇ Maintain adequate airway.
◇ Initiate gastric lavage.
◇ Initiate cardiac monitoring.
◇ Administer barbiturate for sedation.
◇ Administer phentolamine for severe acute hypertension.
◇ Administer IV fluids and a vasopressor to treat hypotension secondary to hypovolemia.
◇ Administer urine acidifiers to promote urinary excretion of the drug.
◇ Hemodialysis and peritoneal dialysis are not effective.

Potential Nursing Diagnoses

- High risk for injury due to overstimulation and hyperactivity; abrupt phentermine withdrawal; overdose.
- High risk for self-directed violence related to suicidal ideations resulting from abrupt phentermine withdrawal.
- Alteration in nutrition, more than body requires, related to excessive intake in relation to metabolic needs.
- Sleep pattern disturbance related to overstimulation resulting from phentermine use.
- Alteration in thought processes related to phentermine's adverse effects of overstimulation and difficulty concentrating.
- Knowledge deficit related to medication regimen.

Plan/Implementation

- Monitor medication effects. Tolerance develops rapidly. If anorexigenic effects begin to diminish, notify physician immediately. Patient should be on reduced-calorie diet and program of regular exercise in addition to the medication.
- Monitor and record vital signs at regular intervals (bid) throughout therapy.
- Encourage use of sugarless gum, hard candy, or frequent sips of water for patient who experiences dry mouth. Ensure that patient practices good oral care (frequent brushing, flossing).
- Ensure that patient is protected from

injury. Keep stimuli low and environment as quiet as possible to discourage overstimulation.

♦ Ensure that tablet/capsule has been swallowed and not "cheeked" to avoid medication or to hoard for later use.

♦ Tablets may be crushed and mixed with food or fluid for patient who has difficulty swallowing.

♦ Do not open sustained-release capsules or mix contents with food. Sustained-release capsules must be swallowed whole.

♦ Administer last dose of the day no later than 6 hours before bedtime.

♦ Drug should be administered 30 minutes before meals.

♦ Administer sustained-release form at midmorning.

♦ Store medication at controlled room temperatures between 15° and 30°C (59°–86°F). Protect from heat and moisture.

Patient/Family Education

♦ Use caution in driving or when operating dangerous machinery. Drowsiness, dizziness, and blurred vision can occur.

♦ Do not stop taking the drug abruptly. Doing so can produce serious withdrawal symptoms.

♦ If insomnia is a problem, avoid taking medication late in the day. Take no later than 6 hours before bedtime.

♦ Do not take other medications (including over-the-counter drugs) without physician's approval. Many medications contain substances that, in combination with phentermine, can be harmful.

♦ Diabetic patient should monitor blood sugar bid or tid or as instructed by physician. Be aware of need for possible alteration in insulin requirements due to changes in food intake, weight, and activity.

♦ Avoid consumption of large amounts of caffeinated products (coffee, tea, colas, chocolate), as they may enhance the stimulant effect of phentermine.

♦ Follow reduced-calorie diet provided by dietitian, as well as a program of regular exercise. Do not exceed recommended dose if appetite suppressant effect diminishes. Contact physician.

♦ Notify physician if restlessness, insomnia, anorexia, or dry mouth become severe or if rapid, pounding heartbeat becomes evident.

♦ Be aware of possible risks of taking phentermine during pregnancy. Safe use during pregnancy and lactation has not been established. Inform physician immediately if pregnancy is suspected or planned.

♦ Be aware of potential side effects of phentermine. Refer to written materials furnished by healthcare providers for safe self-administration.

♦ Carry card or other identification at all times describing medications being taken.

Evaluation

♦ Patient demonstrates a progressive weight loss with the use of phentermine as an adjunct to reduced caloric intake and a program of regular exercise.

♦ Patient verbalizes understanding of side effects and regimen required for prudent self-administration of phentermine.

PHENTOLAMINE

(fen-tole′a-meen)
Regitine, {Rogitine}

Classification(s):
Antihypertensive agent, Alpha-adrenergic blocking agent
Pregnancy Category C

INDICATIONS

♦ Prevention and control of hypertensive episodes that may occur as a result of stress or manipulation during preoperative preparation or surgical excision in patients with pheochromocytoma ♦ Dermal necrosis and sloughing following IV administration or extravasation of norepinephrine (prevention and treatment).

Investigational Uses: ♦ Hypertensive crises secondary to MAO inhibitor/sympathomimetic amine interactions ♦ Rebound hypertension on withdrawal of clonidine.

ACTION

♦ Blocks presynaptic and postsynaptic alpha-adrenergic receptors ♦ Acts as a competitive antagonist of endogenous and exogenous alpha-active agents of relatively short duration ♦ Acts on both the arterial tree and venous bed, thus lowering peripheral resistance and diminishing venous return to the heart ♦ Stimulates beta-adrenergic receptors, produces positive inotropic and chronotropic effect on heart, and increases cardiac output.

PHARMACOKINETICS

Absorption: Not well understood.
Distribution: Distribution not completely understood. Unknown if drug crosses placental barrier or enters breast milk.
Metabolism and Excretion: Metab-

olism unknown. Some excretion occurs via the kidneys.
Half-Life: 19 minutes following IV administration.

CONTRAINDICATIONS AND PRECAUTIONS

Contraindicated in: ♦ Myocardial infarction or history of myocardial infarction ♦ Coronary insufficiency ♦ Angina or other evidence suggestive of coronary artery disease ♦ Hypersensitivity to this drug or to related compounds ♦ Pregnancy and lactation (safe use has not been established).

Use Cautiously in: ♦ Gastritis ♦ Peptic ulcer disease ♦ Elderly or debilitated patients.

ADVERSE REACTIONS AND SIDE EFFECTS*

CNS: weakness, dizziness, flushing.
CV: hypotension, tachycardia, arrhythmias, angina, orthostatic hypotension, MYOCARDIAL INFARCTION, CEREBROVASCULAR SPASM, CEREBROVASCULAR OCCLUSION.
GI: nausea, vomiting, diarrhea, abdominal cramping, aggravation of peptic ulcer.
Other: nasal stuffiness.

INTERACTIONS

Drug-Drug: ♦ **Epinephrine, ephedrine:** antagonizes vasoconstricting and hypertensive effects of these drugs.

ROUTE AND DOSAGE

Hypertensive Episodes in Pheochromocytoma (Prevention or Control)

♦ **IM, IV (Adults):** Preoperatively: 5 mg 1–2 hours before surgery. Repeat if necessary. During surgery: 5 mg IV as needed to control episodes of hypertension, tachycardia, respiratory depression, convulsions, or other effects of epinephrine intoxication.

{} = Only available in Canada.
*Underlines indicate most frequent; CAPITALS indicate life-threatening.

IM, IV (Children): Preoperatively: 1 mg (or 0.1 mg/kg) 1–2 hours before surgery. Repeat if necessary. During surgery: 1 mg (or 0.1 mg/kg) IV as needed to control episodes of hypertension, tachycardia, respiratory depression, convulsions, or other effect of epinephrine intoxication.

Dermal Necrosis and Sloughing Following IV Administration or Extravasation of Norepinephrine (Prevention and Treatment)

Prevention: Add 10 mg to each liter of IV solution containing norepinephrine. (Pressor effect of norepinephrine is not affected.)

Treatment: Inject 5–10 mg in 10 mL normal saline into the area of extravasation within 12 hours.

Hypertensive Crises Secondary to MAO Inhibitor/Sympathomimetic Amine Interactions

(Investigational.)

IV (Adults): 5–10 mg slow IV.

PHARMACODYNAMICS

Route	Onset	Peak	Duration
IM	—	20 min	3–4 hr
IV	Immediate	2 min	10–15 min

NURSING IMPLICATIONS

Assessment

- Assess baseline vital signs. Blood pressure should be taken both in lying and standing positions. Measure pulse both radially and apically. Note respiratory rate; auscultate lung sounds.
- Assess history of allergies, sensitivity to this drug or to related drugs.
- Assess date of last menses (possible pregnancy), use of contraceptives.
- Assess whether currently breast-feeding a child.
- Assess patient/family knowledge about illness and need for medication.
- Assess history of cardiovascular disease.
- Assess for symptoms of pheochromocytoma: • headache • sweating • palpitations • apprehension • flushing of the face • nausea and vomiting • tingling of the extremities.

- If extravasation of norepinephrine has occurred, assess and record degree of necrosis or damage to affected area.

- **Toxicity and Overdose:** Assess for symptoms of overdose: • drop in blood pressure to dangerous level • other evidence of impending shock.

- **Overdose Management:** Treat vigorously and promptly with IV infusion of norepinephrine, titrated to maintain normal blood pressure.

◊ Do not use epinephrine, as paradoxic effect of vasodilation results in further drop in blood pressure.

◊ Place patient in Trendelenburg position.

◊ Administer IV fluids.

Potential Nursing Diagnoses

- Decreased cardiac output related to cardiovascular side effects of phentolamine.
- Alteration in tissue perfusion related to arterial vasoconstriction.
- Alteration in comfort, pain, related to tissue damage resulting from extravasation of IV medications.
- High risk for injury related to side effects of phentolamine, such as weakness and dizziness, or to overdose.
- Knowledge deficit related to medication regimen.

Plan/Implementation

- Ensure that patient is protected from injury. Provide supervision and assistance when ambulating if dizziness or weakness are problems.
- Withhold drug and notify physician immediately if significant change in pulse or drop in blood pressure is noted, if chest pain occurs, if dizziness is severe, or if patient experiences severe nausea, vomiting, or diarrhea.
- During IV administration, monitor blood pressure and pulse every 2 minutes until stabilized.

- Each 5 mg should be diluted with 1 mL of sterile water for injection.
- Administer at rate not exceeding 5 mg/min.
- 10 mg of phentolamine may be added to each liter of IV solution containing norepinephrine to prevent dermal necrosis and sloughing.
- To treat dermal necrosis and sloughing due to extravasation of norepinephrine, use very small gauge needle (no larger than 24) and inject phentolamine (5–10 mg in 10 mL normal saline) into and around affected area.
- Store medication at controlled room temperatures between 15° and 30°C (59°–86°F). Protect from heat and freezing.

Patient/Family Education

- Report occurrence of any of the following symptoms to physician or nurse immediately: dizziness • weakness • nausea • vomiting • diarrhea • chest pain • or fast, slow, or irregular heartbeat.
- Arise slowly from a sitting or lying position to prevent a sudden drop in blood pressure. Rapid changes in posture could cause severe dizziness or even fainting. Notify physician or nurse should this occur.
- Do not consume other medications (including over-the-counter meds) without physician's approval. Many medications contain substances that may precipitate hypertensive crisis.
- Be aware of possible risks of taking phentolamine during pregnancy. Safe use during pregnancy and lactation has not been established. Inform physician immediately if pregnancy is suspected.

Evaluation

- Patient verbalizes understanding of need for phentolamine (for hypertensive episodes associated with pheochromocytoma, MAO inhibitor/sympathomimetic amine interactions, withdrawal from antihypertensive agents, prevention/treatment of dermal necrosis and sloughing following IV administration or extravasation of norepinephrine).
- Patient verbalizes understanding of potential adverse side effects and risks associated with the administration of phentolamine.

PHENYTOIN

(fen′i-toy-in)
Dilantin, Diphenylan

Classification(s):
Anticonvulsant, Hydantoin, Antiarrhythmic
Pregnancy Category D

INDICATIONS

- Tonic-clonic (grand mal) and partial seizures with complex symptomatology (psychomotor seizures) ✦ Grand mal seizures associated with status epilepticus or occurring during or following neurosurgery ✦ Autonomic seizures. **Investigational Uses:** ✦ Arrhythmias ✦ Trigeminal neuralgia.

ACTION

- Hydantoins act by increasing the seizure threshold in the cerebral cortex ✦ By promoting sodium efflux from neurons in the motor cortex, hydantoins encourage stabilization of the threshold against hyperexcitability ✦ Maximal activity of the brain-stem centers responsible for the tonic phase of grand mal seizures is also reduced.

PHARMACOKINETICS

Absorption: Rapidly absorbed following oral administration of prompt form; absorption slower with extended-release form. Absorbed slowly and erratically following IM administration.
Distribution: Rapidly and widely distributed, with highest concentrations in liver and adipose tissue. Crosses placental barrier; excreted in breast milk.

Metabolism and Excretion: Metabolized by the liver into inactive metabolites that are excreted in bile and reabsorbed from the GI tract. Final excretion is through the kidneys.

Half-Life: Following oral administration: 7–42 hours; following IV administration: 10–15 hours.

CONTRAINDICATIONS AND PRECAUTIONS

Contraindicated in: ♦ Hypersensitivity to the drug ♦ Lactation ♦ Sinus bradycardia ♦ Heart block ♦ Absence (petit mal) seizures and seizures related to hypoglycemia.

Use Cautiously in: ♦ Hepatic or renal dysfunction ♦ Pregnancy ♦ Elderly or debilitated patients ♦ Diabetes mellitus ♦ Hypotension ♦ Myocardial insufficiency.

ADVERSE REACTIONS AND SIDE EFFECTS*

CNS: nystagmus, ataxia, drowsiness, dizziness, decreased mental alertness, headache, diplopia, confusion, insomnia.

CV: redness and pain at insertion site and along vein of infusion (IV); with rapid IV infusion: HYPOTENSION, ARRHYTHMIAS, CIRCULATORY COLLAPSE, CARDIAC ARREST.

Derm: skin rashes, hypertrichosis, EXFOLIATIVE DERMATITIS.

GI: nausea, vomiting, constipation, anorexia, weight loss, TOXIC HEPATITIS.

Hemat: BLOOD DYSCRASIAS (thrombocytopenia, leukopenia, agranulocytosis).

Misc: gingival hyperplasia, lymphadenopathy, osteomalacia, hyperglycemia, systemic lupus erythematosus.

INTERACTIONS

Drug-Drug: ♦ **Trimethoprim, amiodarone, benzodiazepines, disulfiram, isoniazid, phenylbutazone, chloramphenicol, cimetidine, sulfonamides, salicylates, acute alcohol intake, phenothiazines:** increased effects of phenytoin (increased risk of toxicity) ♦ **Barbiturates, diazoxide, rifampin, antineoplastic agents, chronic alcohol abuse, antacids, calcium gluconate, carbamazepine:** decreased effects of phenytoin ♦ **Phenobarbital, valproic acid, sodium valproate:** increased or decreased effects of either drug ♦ **Coumarin anticoagulants:** increased effects of phenytoin, increased or decreased anticoagulant effects ♦ **Quinidine:** decreased antiarrhythmic effects ♦ **Corticosteroids:** decreased efficacy of corticosteroids ♦ **Oral contraceptives:** decreased efficacy of oral contraceptives ♦ **Digitoxin:** decreased effects of digitoxin ♦ **Furosemide:** decreased effects of furosemide ♦ **Theophylline:** decreased efficacy of both drugs ♦ **Doxycycline:** decreased effects of doxycycline ♦ **Levodopa:** decreased effects of levodopa ♦ **Primidone:** increased primidone effects ♦ **Dopamine:** decreased effects of dopamine.

Drug-Food: ♦ **Vitamin K, vitamin D:** supplemental intake of these nutrients may be needed while on phenytoin ♦ **Folic acid:** alteration in metabolism of either or both (could result in decreased effects of phenytoin or serum folate deficiency).

ROUTE AND DOSAGE

Psychomotor and Grand Mal Seizures

- **PO (Adults):** 100 mg tid or qid (maximum daily dose 600 mg). Dosage should be adjusted according to serum levels (range 10–20 mcg/mL). Total in extended-release form may be administered in one single daily dose.
- **PO (Children):** 4–8 mg/kg/day (maximum dose 300 mg/day) given in 2 or 3 divided doses, or as a single dose. Dosage should be adjusted according to serum levels (range 10–20 mcg/mL).

*Underlines indicate most frequent; CAPITALS indicate life-threatening.

♦ **IM (Adults):** (To be given only when oral administration is not possible and for period of no more than 1 week. If longer time is required, alternative methods of administration should be considered). Dose 50% greater than usual oral dose is required to maintain therapeutic levels. When returning to oral administration, decrease original oral dose by 50% for 1 week. These adjustments must be made to prevent excessive plasma levels due to the slow and erratic absorption of IM phenytoin.

Prophylactic Anticonvulsant During/Following Neurosurgery

♦ **IM (Adults):** 100–200 mg at 4-hour intervals during surgery and postoperative period. (In a patient previously stabilized orally on phenytoin, adjust IM dosages as described above.)

Status Epilepticus

♦ **IV (Adults):** 10–15 mg/kg administered at a rate not to exceed 50 mg per minute.

♦ **IV (Children):** 10–15 mg/kg administered at a rate not to exceed 1–3 mg/kg/min.

PHARMACODYNAMICS

Route	Onset	Peak	Duration
PO (prompt)	0.5–2 hr	1.5–3 hr	6–12 hr
PO (extended-release)	2–3 hr	4–12 hr	12–36 hr
IV	3–5 min	Rapid	12–24 hr
IM	Variable	Erratic	12–14 hr

NURSING IMPLICATIONS

Assessment

♦ Assess occurrence, characteristics, and duration of seizure activity.
♦ Assess baseline vital signs.
♦ Assess history of allergies, sensitivity to this drug and/or to other drugs.
♦ Assess history of past and existing disease states (e.g., diabetes mellitus, cardiac disease).

♦ Assess date of last menses (possible pregnancy), use of contraceptives.
♦ Assess whether currently breast-feeding a child.
♦ Assess current and past alcohol and drug consumption.
♦ Assess for presence of skin rashes.
♦ Assess for presence of adverse reactions or side effects.
♦ Assess patient's and family's response to diagnosis of epilepsy.
♦ Assess patient/family knowledge about illness and need for medication.
♦ In collaboration with physician, assess CBC and renal and liver function tests in patients on prolonged phenytoin therapy.
♦ **Lab Test Alterations:** May increase serum glucose, bromsulphalein, alkaline phosphatase, and gamma-glutamyl transferase (GGT).
◊ May decrease protein-bound iodine, urinary steroid levels, and values for dexamethasone or metapyrone tests.
♦ **Toxicity and Overdose:** Range of therapeutic serum concentration is 10–20 mcg/mL.
◊ Assess for symptoms of toxicity/overdose. At serum levels of 25–30 mcg/mL: • nystagmus • ataxia • diplopia. At serum levels of 30–50 mcg/mL: • confusion • nausea • slurred speech • drowsiness • dizziness • lethargy. Levels above 50 mcg/mL are marked by comatose states. Death may result from respiratory and circulatory depression.
♦ **Overdose Management:** Monitor vital signs.
◊ Ensure maintenance of adequate airway.
◊ Induce vomiting in conscious patient.
◊ Initiate gastric lavage if patient is unconscious.
◊ Administer IV fluids.
◊ Hemodialysis may be considered.

Potential Nursing Diagnoses

♦ High risk for injury related to seizures; phenytoin's side effects of dizziness, drowsiness, and decreased mental alertness; possible toxic serum levels of phenytoin; irritation of tissues resulting from IM or IV injection of phenytoin; abrupt withdrawal from phenytoin use.

♦ Impaired adjustment related to difficulty accepting diagnosis of epilepsy.

♦ Social isolation related to fear of experiencing a seizure in the presence of others.

♦ High risk for activity intolerance related to phenytoin's side effects of drowsiness, dizziness, decreased mental alertness.

♦ Knowledge deficit related to medication regimen.

Plan/Implementation

♦ **General Info:** Monitor vital signs at regular intervals (bid or tid) throughout therapy; every 3–5 minutes during IV administration.

◇ Monitor serum phenytoin levels. Record and report to physician.

◇ Monitor for symptoms of possible blood dyscrasias: sore throat • fever • malaise.

◇ Observe frequently (every hour) for occurrence of seizure activity.

◇ Ensure that patient is protected from injury. Supervise and assist with ambulation if dizziness and drowsiness are problems. Ensure that patient avoids participation in any activity requiring mental alertness (including smoking). Pad siderails and head of bed with towels or blanket to protect patient who experiences seizures during the night.

◇ Perform urine checks daily following initiation of therapy to determine whether hyperglycemia has occurred.

♦ **PO:** Administer medication with food to minimize GI irritation and to enhance absorption.

◇ For patient who has difficulty swallowing, tablet may be crushed or capsule emptied and mixed with food or fluid, or suspension may be given. Do

not empty extended-release capsules, which should be swallowed whole.

◇ Store medication at controlled room temperatures between 15° and 30°C (59°–86°F). Protect from heat and moisture.

♦ **IM:** Administer IM only when other methods of administration are not possible.

◇ Do not mix parenteral preparations with other solutions. Do not use if solution is not clear or if precipitate is visible.

◇ Administer IM for period of no more than 1 week.

◇ Solution is highly alkaline. Extravasation could result in tissue damage.

◇ IM dose should be 50% greater than usual oral dose to maintain therapeutic levels. When returning to oral administration, decrease original oral dose by 50% for 1 week to prevent excessive plasma levels due to slow and erratic absorption of IM phenytoin.

♦ **IV:** Do not mix parenteral preparations with other solutions. Do not use if solution is not clear or if precipitate is visible.

◇ Inject very slowly (no more than 50 mg/min in adults and 1–3 mg/kg/min in children).

◇ Closely monitor patient's response to IV infusion. Too rapid administration could result in life-threatening cardiac arrhythmias, hypotension, bradycardia, cardiovascular collapse, cardiac and respiratory arrest. Ensure availability of artificial ventilation and resuscitation equipment.

◇ Solution is highly alkaline. Extravasation could result in tissue damage.

◇ Follow IV injection with normal saline solution to minimize irritation to vein.

◇ Refrigeration of solution may cause precipitate that should dissolve at room temperature. Solution with faint yellow discoloration is safe to use as long as solution remains clear.

Patient/Family Education

- Do not drive or operate dangerous machinery until individual response is determined. Drowsiness and decreased mental alertness can occur.
- Do not stop taking drug abruptly. To do so could precipitate status epilepticus.
- Avoid alcoholic beverages.
- Maintain good oral care to minimize side effect of gingival hyperplasia.
- Urine may appear pink, red, or reddish-brown. This is not significant or harmful.
- Carry or wear at all times identification informing others of condition and medication usage.
- Do not take any other medication without approval from physician. Combining drugs may be harmful.
- Promptly report any of the following symptoms to physician: • sore throat • fever • malaise • ataxia • slurred speech • nystagmus • skin rash • severe nausea or vomiting • swollen glands • yellow skin or eyes • dark urine.
- Be aware of possible risks of taking phenytoin during pregnancy. Patient who requires the medication to prevent seizures may be maintained on it; however, she must be fully aware of potential risks to unborn child. There is a strong association between the use of anticonvulsant drugs by women with epilepsy and the incidence of birth defects in their children. A possible association also has been suggested between maternal use of anticonvulsants and a neonatal coagulation defect that poses a threat of serious bleeding during the first 24 hours of life. Notify physician immediately if pregnancy occurs, is suspected, or is planned.
- Because phenytoin decreases the effectiveness of oral contraceptives, use alternative method of birth control during phenytoin therapy.
- To protect patient during a seizure, padding (towels, blankets, pillows) may be used to prevent bumping against hard objects. When convulsion has subsided, turn patient on side to allow secretions to drain and to prevent aspiration. Keep records of occurrence, characteristics, and duration of seizures, so that accurate reports may be given to physician for providing assistance in stabilization and control of seizures. If patient has difficulty breathing or continues to experience subsequent seizures, family should call for emergency assistance immediately.
- Be aware of possible side effects of phenytoin. Refer to written materials furnished by healthcare providers to assist in self-administration.

Evaluation

- Patient demonstrates stabilization of seizure activity with regular administration of phenytoin.
- Patient verbalizes understanding of necessity for, side effects of, and regimen required for prudent self-administration of phenytoin.

PIMOZIDE

(pi′moe-zide)
Orap

Classification(s):
Antipsychotic, Neuroleptic,
Diphenylbutylpiperidine
Pregnancy Category C

INDICATIONS

- Severe motor and phonic tics in patients with Tourette's disorder who have failed to respond satisfactorily to conventional treatment.

ACTION

- The exact mechanism of action is not fully understood • Appears to be primarily a result of antidopaminergic effects • Thought to block both postsynaptic and presynaptic dopamine receptor sites.

PHARMACOKINETICS

Absorption: Slowly and variably absorbed. At least 40–50% absorbed following oral administration. Drug is thought to undergo extensive first-pass metabolism.

Distribution: Thought to be widely distributed. Unknown if drug crosses placental barrier or enters breast milk.

Metabolism and Excretion: Metabolized by the liver. Excreted through the kidneys and in feces.

Half-Life: 55 hours.

CONTRAINDICATIONS AND PRECAUTIONS

Contraindicated in: ◆ Hypersensitivity ◆ Tics other than those associated with Tourette's disorder ◆ Drug-induced tics (e.g., pemoline, methylphenidate, amphetamines) ◆ Patients with Tourette's disorder who respond to conventional therapy ◆ History of cardiac arrhythmias or prolonged QT syndrome ◆ Concomitant use of other drugs that prolong QT interval ◆ Severe toxic CNS depression or comatose state ◆ Blood dyscrasias, depressive disorders, parkinsonian syndrome ◆ Children under 12 years of age; pregnancy and lactation (safe use has not been established).

Use Cautiously in: ◆ Hypersensitivity to other antipsychotics (not known if cross-sensitivity exists) ◆ Impaired hepatic or renal function ◆ Seizure disorders ◆ Hypertension ◆ Cardiovascular disorders ◆ Hypokalemia.

ADVERSE REACTIONS AND SIDE EFFECTS*

CNS: <u>sedation</u>, <u>headache</u>, seizures, insomnia, dizziness, <u>extrapyramidal symptoms</u> (pseudoparkinsonism, akathisia, akinesia, dystonia, torticollis, oculogyric crisis), <u>tardive dyskinesia</u>, excitement, agitation, nervousness, adverse behavior effects, blurred vision, lethargy, irritabil-

ity, tension, depression, confusion, nightmares, phobia, NEUROLEPTIC MALIGNANT SYNDROME.

CV: <u>orthostatic hypotension</u>, hypotension, hypertension, <u>tachycardia</u>, palpitations, chest pain, <u>ECG changes</u>, VENTRICULAR ARRHYTHMIAS, CARDIAC ARREST.

Derm: <u>rash</u>, sweating, skin irritation, urticaria.

Endo: weight gain or loss, loss of libido, menstrual disorder, breast secretions, impotence, amenorrhea, dysmenorrhea, galactorrhea.

GI: <u>dry mouth</u>, <u>nausea</u>, <u>vomiting</u>, diarrhea, <u>constipation</u>, thirst, increased appetite, belching, increased salivation, anorexia, GI distress, fecal incontinence, abdominal cramps, altered taste.

GU: nocturia, urinary frequency, urinary incontinence, urinary retention.

Other: facial edema, periorbital edema, cataracts.

INTERACTIONS

Drug-Drug: ◆ **Phenothiazines, tricyclic antidepressants, antiarrhythmic agents:** increased prolongation of QT interval ◆ **CNS depressants (including opiates and other analgesics sedatives, anxiolytics, alcohol):** potentiation of CNS depressant effects of these drugs ◆ **Anticholinergics:** additive anticholinergic effects ◆ **Anticonvulsants:** possible loss of seizure control.

ROUTE AND DOSAGE

Tics Associated with Tourette's Disorder

◆ **PO (Adults):** Initial dose: 1–2 mg/day. Thereafter, dose may be increased every other day. Due to long half-life, can reasonably wait 5–7 days before increasing dose. Increase dose until signs and symptoms decrease by at least 70%, until adverse effects occur without benefit, or until adverse

---

*<u>Underlines</u> indicate most frequent; CAPITALS indicate life-threatening.

effects and benefit occur simultaneously.

♦ **PO (Maintenance):** Lowest effective dose, up to 0.2 mg/kg/day or 10 mg/day, whichever is less (manufacturer recommendation). Occasionally, doses up to 0.3 mg/kg/day or 20 mg/day are given (with increased risk of serious side effects). Gradual withdrawal: Dosage should be reduced periodically (q 6–12 months) to determine if tics persist. Increases in tic frequency and intensity may represent withdrawal symptoms rather than return of disease manifestations. Allow at least 1 or 2 weeks before concluding that increased symptoms are related to the disease process and are not a transient withdrawal response.

PHARMACODYNAMICS

Route	Onset	Peak	Duration
PO	Variable	6–8 hr	24 hr or more

NURSING IMPLICATIONS
Assessment

♦ Assess mental status daily: • mood • appearance • thought and communication patterns • level of interest in the environment and in activities • level of anxiety or agitation • presence of hallucinations or delusions • suspiciousness • interactions with others • ability to carry out activities of daily living.

♦ Assess for presence of spastic facial movement (tics) or unusual vocal utterances.

♦ Assess for extrapyramidal symptoms: • pseudoparkinsonism (tremors, shuffling gait, drooling, rigidity) • akinesia (muscular weakness) • akathisia (continuous restlessness and fidgeting) • dystonia (involuntary muscular movements of face, arms, legs, and neck) • oculogyric crisis (uncontrolled rolling back of the eyes) • tardive dyskinesia (bizarre facial and tongue movements, stiff neck, difficulty swallowing) • torticollis (stiff

neck caused by muscle spasms resulting in head drawing to one side and chin pointing to other side).

♦ Assess for symptoms of neuroleptic malignant syndrome: • hyperpyrexia up to 107°F (41.6°C) • elevated pulse • increased or decreased blood pressure • severe parkinsonian muscle rigidity • elevated creatinine phosphokinase blood levels • elevated white blood count • altered mental status (including catatonic signs or agitation) • acute renal failure • varying levels of consciousness (including stupor and coma) • pallor • diaphoresis • tachycardia • arrhythmias • rhabdomyolysis.

♦ Assess vital signs, weight. Record baseline values for comparison.

♦ Assess history of allergies, sensitivity to this drug.

♦ Assess date of last menses (possible pregnancy), use of contraceptives.

♦ Assess whether currently breast-feeding a child.

♦ Assess current and past alcohol and drug consumption.

♦ Assess for operation of automobile and/or other dangerous machinery.

♦ Assess for presence of adverse reactions or side effects.

♦ Assess patient/family knowledge about illness and need for medication.

♦ In collaboration with physician, assess CBC, liver function tests, and periodic ECG in patients on long-term therapy.

♦ **Withdrawal:** Assess for symptoms of abrupt withdrawal from long-term therapy: • transient dyskinetic signs • motor and phonic tics similar to those manifested by Tourette's disorder.

♦ **Toxicity and Overdose:** No correlation has been established between blood level and therapeutic effect.

◊ Assess for symptoms of overdose: • ECG abnormalities • severe extrapyramidal reactions • hypotension • coma with respiratory depression.

♦ **Overdose Management:** Monitor vital signs.

◇ Ensure maintenance of open airway.

◇ Monitor ECG.

◇ Initiate gastric lavage, followed by activated charcoal.

◇ Do not induce emesis (nuchal rigidity may result in aspiration of vomitus).

◇ May administer antiparkinsonian drugs or diphenhydramine to counteract extrapyramidal symptoms.

◇ Administer IV fluids or a vasoconstrictor to maintain adequate blood pressure. **Note:** Epinephrine is not recommended due to drug interaction, which may cause further drop in blood pressure.

◇ Administer IV phenytoin to control ventricular arrhythmias.

◇ Administer phenobarbital or diazepam to control convulsions or hyperactivity.

◇ Due to drug's long half-life, patients who overdose on pimozide should be observed for at least 4 days.

Potential Nursing Diagnoses

✦ High risk for injury related to pimozide's side effects of sedation, dizziness, ataxia, weakness, lowered seizure threshold; abrupt withdrawal after prolonged use; overdose.

✦ Decreased cardiac output related to pimozide's side effects that alter cardiac rate, rhythm, conduction.

✦ Social isolation related to embarrassment by symptoms of Tourette's disorder.

✦ High risk for activity intolerance related to pimozide's side effects of drowsiness, dizziness, weakness.

✦ Knowledge deficit related to medication regimen.

Plan/Implementation

✦ Ensure that baseline ECG is performed before initiation of therapy and periodically (at least every 6–12 months and with dosage increases) throughout therapy.

✦ Monitor vital signs before beginning therapy and at regular intervals (bid or tid) throughout therapy. Take BP lying and standing to monitor for possible hypotensive reaction; elderly are particularly susceptible. Dosage adjustment may be required.

✦ Ensure that patient is protected from injury. Provide supervision and assistance when ambulating if dizziness and drowsiness are problems. Pad siderails and headboard for patient who experiences seizures.

✦ Give patient hard candy, gum, or frequent sips of water if dry mouth is a problem.

✦ Ensure that patient has adequate fiber and fluid in diet to prevent constipation.

✦ Ensure that patient swallows tablet and does not "cheek" to avoid medication or to hoard for later use.

✦ Crush tablet and mix with food or fluid for patient who has difficulty swallowing.

✦ Store medication at controlled room temperatures between 15° and 30°C (59°–86°F). Protect from heat and moisture.

Patient/Family Education

✦ Use caution when driving or when operating dangerous machinery. Drowsiness and dizziness can occur.

✦ Do not stop taking the drug abruptly. To do so might induce motor and phonic tics of the type associated with Tourette's disorder, as well as other neurological effects, such as extrapyramidal symptoms.

✦ Report occurrence of any of the following symptoms to physician immediately: • fever • muscle rigidity • tremors • weakness • restlessness • stiff neck • loss of control of tic responses • seizures • fast or irregular heart rate • altered mental status.

✦ Rise slowly from a sitting or lying position to prevent a sudden drop in blood pressure.

✦ If dry mouth is a problem, take frequent sips of water, chew sugarless gum, or suck on hard candy. Good oral care (frequent brushing, flossing) is very important.

* Do not drink alcohol while on pimozide therapy. These drugs potentiate each other's effects.
* Do not consume other medications (including over-the-counter meds) without physician's approval. Many medications contain substances that interact with pimozide in a way that may be harmful.
* Be aware of possible risks of taking pimozide during pregnancy. Safe use during pregnancy and lactation has not been established. It is not known if pimozide crosses the placental barrier, so adverse effects on a fetus cannot be determined absolutely. Inform physician immediately if pregnancy occurs, is suspected, or is planned.
* Be aware of side effects of pimozide. Refer to written materials furnished by healthcare providers for safe self-administration.
* Continue to take medication even if feeling well and as though it is not needed. Symptoms may return if medication is discontinued.
* Carry card or other identification at all times describing illness and medications being administered.

Evaluation

* Patient demonstrates a subsiding of the symptoms for which pimozide was prescribed (motor and phonic tics associated with Tourette's disorder).
* Patient verbalizes understanding of side effects and regimen required for prudent self-administration of pimozide.

PRAZEPAM

(pra′ze-pam)
Centrax

Classification(s):
Antianxiety agent, Benzodiazepine,
Skeletal muscle relaxant,
Anticonvulsant
Schedule C IV
Pregnancy Category D

INDICATIONS

* Anxiety disorders * Temporary relief of anxiety symptoms (Efficacy for periods greater than 4 months has not been evaluated).

ACTION

* Depresses subcortical levels of the central nervous system, particularly the limbic system and reticular formation * May potentiate the effects of the powerful inhibitory neurotransmitter gamma-aminobutyric acid (GABA) in the brain, thereby producing a calmative effect * All levels of CNS depression can be effected, from mild sedation to hypnosis to coma.

PHARMACOKINETICS

Absorption: Slowly absorbed from the GI tract.
Distribution: Is widely distributed. Crosses blood-brain and placental barriers; excreted in breast milk.
Metabolism and Excretion: Metabolized by the liver; produces active metabolites that are gradually excreted by the kidneys.
Half-Life: 30–200 hours.

CONTRAINDICATIONS AND PRECAUTIONS

Contraindicated in: * Hypersensitivity to this drug or to other benzodiazepines * Combination with other CNS depressants * Pregnancy and lactation * Narrow-angle glaucoma * Children under 18.

Use Cautiously in: ♦ Elderly or debilitated patients ♦ Hepatic or renal dysfunction ♦ Individuals with a history of drug abuse/addiction ♦ Depressed/suicidal patients.

ADVERSE REACTIONS AND SIDE EFFECTS*

CNS: <u>drowsiness</u>, <u>fatigue</u>, <u>ataxia</u>, <u>dizziness</u>, confusion, headache, syncope, paradoxical excitement, blurred vision.
CV: hypotension, palpitations.
Derm: pruritus, skin rashes.
Endo: gynecomastia, galactorrhea.
GI: dry mouth, nausea/vomiting, diarrhea, constipation, weight gain.
Other: tolerance, physical and psychological dependence.

INTERACTIONS

Drug-Drug: ♦ **Other CNS depressants (including alcohol, barbiturates, narcotics), antipsychotics, antidepressants, antihistamines, anticonvulsants:** additive CNS depression ♦ **Cimetidine:** increased effects of prazepam ♦ **Oral contraceptives:** increased or decreased effects of prazepam ♦ **Cigarette smoking, caffeine:** decreased effects of prazepam ♦ **Neuromuscular blocking agents:** increased respiratory depression ♦ **Digoxin:** reduced excretion of digoxin, increased potential for toxicity ♦ **Disulfiram:** decreased clearance of prazepam.

ROUTE AND DOSAGE
Anxiety, Anxiety Disorders

♦ **PO (Adults):** 10–60 mg/day in divided doses. May be given in single dose at bedtime. Optimum range: 20–40 mg.
♦ **PO (Geriatric or Debilitated Patients):** Initial dosage: 10–15 mg daily in divided doses.

PHARMACODYNAMICS

Route	Onset	Peak	Duration
PO	UK	6 hr	*

*Varies with individual, age, disease state, number of doses.

NURSING IMPLICATIONS
Assessment

♦ Assess level of anxiety. Symptoms include: ● restlessness ● pacing ● insomnia ● inability to concentrate ● increased heart rate ● increased respiration ● elevated blood pressure ● confusion ● tremors ● rapid speech.
♦ Assess for suicidal ideation (CNS depressants aggravate symptoms in depressed patients).
♦ Assess history of allergies, sensitivity to this drug.
♦ Assess history of glaucoma.
♦ Assess date of last menses (possible pregnancy), use of contraceptives.
♦ Assess whether currently breast-feeding a child.
♦ Assess current and past alcohol and drug consumption.
♦ Assess operation of automobile and/or other dangerous machinery.
♦ Assess for presence of adverse reactions or side effects.
♦ Assess patient/family knowledge about illness and need for medication.
♦ In collaboration with physician, assess CBC and liver function tests in patients on long-term therapy.
♦ **Lab Test Alterations:** May increase serum bilirubin, AST, and ALT.
♦ **Withdrawal:** Assess for symptoms of withdrawal: ● depression ● insomnia ● increased anxiety ● abdominal and muscle cramps ● tremors ● vomiting ● sweating ● convulsions ● delirium.
♦ **Withdrawal Management:** Monitor vital signs.
◊ Place patient in quiet room with low stimuli.

---

*<u>Underlines</u> indicate most frequent; CAPITALS indicate life-threatening.

◊ Institute seizure precautions.

◊ A long-acting barbiturate, such as phenobarbital, may be ordered to suppress withdrawal symptoms.

◊ Phenytoin may be ordered to prevent seizures.

◊ Some physicians may order oxazepam as needed for objective withdrawal symptoms, gradually decreasing dosage until the drug is discontinued.

♦ **Toxicity and Overdose:** Assess for symptoms of intoxication: • euphoria • relaxation • drowsiness • slurred speech • disorientation • mood liability • incoordination • unsteady gait • disinhibition of sexual and aggressive impulses • judgment and/or memory impairment.

◊ Assess for symptoms of overdose: • shallow respiration • cold and clammy skin • hypotension • dilated pupils • weak and rapid pulse • hypnosis • coma • possible death.

♦ **Overdose Management:** Monitor vital signs.

◊ Ensure maintenance of adequate airway.

◊ Induce vomiting in conscious patient.

◊ Initiate gastric lavage in unconscious patient.

◊ Administer activated charcoal to minimize absorption.

◊ IV fluids and vasopressors may be used to combat hypotension.

◊ Forced diuresis may be used to facilitate elimination of the drug.

Potential Nursing Diagnoses

♦ High risk for injury related to seizures; panic anxiety; abrupt withdrawal from long-term prazepam use; effects of prazepam intoxication or overdose.

♦ High risk for self-directed violence related to depressed mood.

♦ Anxiety (specify level) related to threats to physical integrity and/or self-concept.

♦ High risk for activity intolerance related to prazepam's side effects of lethargy, drowsiness, dizziness, muscular weakness.

♦ Knowledge deficit related to medication regimen.

Plan/Implementation

♦ Monitor vital signs before beginning therapy and at regular intervals (bid) throughout therapy.

♦ Ensure that patient practices good oral care. Offer hard, sugarless candy; gum; or frequent sips of water for dry mouth.

♦ Ensure that patient is protected from injury. Supervise and assist with ambulation if dizziness and muscular weakness are problems. Pad siderails and headboard for patient who experiences seizures.

♦ To minimize nausea, medication may be given with food or milk.

♦ If patient has difficulty swallowing, tablet may be crushed or capsule emptied and mixed with food or fluid.

♦ Ensure that tablet/capsule has been swallowed and not "cheeked" to avoid medication or to hoard for later use.

♦ Store medication at controlled room temperatures between 15° and 30°C (59°–86°F) in tightly-closed container.

Patient/Family Education

♦ Do not drive or operate dangerous machinery. Drowsiness and dizziness can occur.

♦ Do not stop taking the drug abruptly. To do so can result in serious withdrawal symptoms.

♦ Do not consume other CNS depressants (including alcohol).

♦ Do not take nonprescription medication without approval from physician.

♦ Be aware of risks of taking prazepam during pregnancy (congenital malformations have been associated with use during first trimester). Notify physician of desirability to discontinue drug if pregnancy is suspected or planned.

♦ Be aware of potential side effects. Refer to written materials furnished by healthcare providers regarding correct method of self-administration.

* Carry card or other identification at all times stating names of medications being taken.

Evaluation

* Patient demonstrates a subsiding/resolution of the symptoms for which prazepam was prescribed (anxiety symptoms, anxiety disorders).
* Patient verbalizes understanding of side effects and regimen required for prudent self-administration of prazepam.

PRIMIDONE

(pri'mi-done)
Myidone, Mysoline, {Sertan}

Classification(s):
Anticonvulsant, Barbiturate analog
Pregnancy Category D

INDICATIONS

* Partial seizures with complex symptomatology (psychomotor) * Tonic-clonic (grand mal) seizures * Akinetic seizures * Other partial seizures.

ACTION

* Thought to reduce monosynaptic and polysynaptic transmission, resulting in decreased excitability of the entire nerve cell * Barbiturates also increase the threshold for electrical stimulation of the motor cortex.

PHARMACOKINETICS

Absorption: Readily absorbed (60–80%) following oral administration.
Distribution: Is widely distributed. Crosses blood-brain and placental barriers; excreted in breast milk.
Metabolism and Excretion: Metabolized by the liver to metabolites PEMA and phenobarbital, which are excreted along with unchanged drug in urine.

Half-Life: 10–21 hours (primidone); 24–48 hours (PEMA); 53–118 hours (phenobarbital).

CONTRAINDICATIONS AND PRECAUTIONS

Contraindicated in: * Hypersensitivity to the drug or barbiturates * Pregnancy * Porphyria.
Use Cautiously in: * Elderly or debilitated patients * Patients with hepatic, renal or respiratory dysfunction * Lactation.

ADVERSE REACTIONS AND SIDE EFFECTS*

CNS: ataxia, vertigo, drowsiness, headache, fatigue, hyperirritability, hyperexcitability (children).
Derm: skin rashes, alopecia.
GI: nausea, vomiting, anorexia, decreased serum folate levels.
Hemat: BLOOD DYSCRASIAS (thrombocytopenia, leukopenia, megaloblastic anemia).
Other: sexual impotence, personality deterioration with mood changes and paranoia, diplopia, nystagmus, edema, SLE-like syndrome.

INTERACTIONS

Drug-Drug: * **CNS depressants (including alcohol):** additive CNS depressant effects * **Chloramphenicol, MAO inhibitors, valproic acid, cimetidine, isoniazid:** increased potential for toxic effects of primidone * **Barbiturates, phenytoin:** excessive serum phenobarbital levels, excessive sedation * **Oral contraceptives:** decreased effectiveness of oral contraceptives * **Oral anticoagulants:** decreased effectiveness of anticoagulants * **Corticosteroids, theophyllines, doxycycline, tricyclic antidepressants, phenothiazines, oral beta-adrenergic blockers:**

{} = Only available in Canada.
*Underlines indicate most frequent; CAPITALS indicate life-threatening.

decreased effectiveness of these drugs ♦ **Folic acid:** decreased folate absorption ♦ **Methoxyflurane:** increased nephrotoxic effects of methoxyflurane.

ROUTE AND DOSAGE
Psychomotor, Grand Mal, and Focal Seizures

♦ **PO (Adults, Children over 8 Years Old):** Initial therapy: Days 1–3: 100–125 mg at bedtime. Days 4–6: 100–125 mg bid. Days 7–9: 100–125 mg tid. Day 10—maintenance: 250 mg tid. Usual maintenance dose: 250 mg tid or qid. Dosage may be increased to 250 mg 5–6 times/day. Maximum dose: 500 mg qid.
♦ **PO (Children under 8 Years Old):** Initial therapy: Days 1–3: 50 mg at bedtime. Days 4–6: 50 mg bid. Days 7–9: 100 mg bid. Day 10—maintenance: 125–250 mg tid. Usual maintenance dose: 125–250 mg tid, or 10–25 mg/kg/day in divided doses.
♦ **PO (Replacement Therapy):** Initial dose: 100–125 mg at bedtime; gradually increase to maintenance dose as drug being withdrawn is gradually decreased over a period of at least 2 weeks.
♦ **PO (Discontinuation of Therapy):** Withdraw or decrease dose slowly to prevent status epilepticus or precipitation of seizures.

PHARMACODYNAMICS

Route	Onset	Peak	Duration
PO	UK	4 hr	8–12 hr

NURSING IMPLICATIONS
Assessment

♦ Assess occurrence, characteristics, and duration of seizure activity.
♦ Assess baseline vital signs.
♦ Assess history of allergies, sensitivity to this drug and/or other drugs.
♦ Assess date of last menses (possible pregnancy), use of contraceptives.

♦ Assess whether currently breast-feeding a child.
♦ Assess current and past alcohol and drug consumption.
♦ Assess for symptoms of possible blood dyscrasias: sore throat ● fever ● malaise ● unusual bleeding ● easy bruising.
♦ Assess for presence of adverse reactions or side effects.
♦ Assess patient's and family's response to diagnosis of epilepsy.
♦ Assess patient/family knowledge about illness and need for medication.
♦ In collaboration with physician, assess CBC and renal and liver function tests in patients on prolonged primidone therapy.
♦ **Withdrawal:** Assess for symptoms of abrupt withdrawal: ● anxiety ● tremors ● insomnia ● nausea/vomiting ● weakness ● diaphoresis ● orthostatic hypotension ● delirium ● convulsions (possible status epilepticus).
♦ **Withdrawal Management:** Monitor vital signs.
◊ Place patient in quiet room with low stimuli.
◊ Institute seizure precautions.
◊ Phenytoin may be given to prevent seizures or IV diazepam administered to treat status epilepticus.
♦ **Toxicity and Overdose:** Range of therapeutic serum concentration is thought to be 5–12 mcg/mL (primidone), 15–40 mcg/mL (phenobarbital).
◊ Assess for symptoms of toxicity/overdose: ● lethargy ● vision changes ● confusion ● dyspnea ● hypoventilation ● hypotension ● coma.
♦ **Overdose Management:** Monitor vital signs.
◊ Ensure maintenance of adequate airway.
◊ Induce vomiting in conscious patient.
◊ Initiate gastric lavage in unconscious patient.
◊ Administer IV fluids.
◊ In cases of severe intoxication, forced diuresis or hemodialysis may be used.

Potential Nursing Diagnoses

- High risk for injury related to seizures; primidone's side effects of dizziness, drowsiness, and ataxia; possible toxic serum levels of primidone; abrupt withdrawal from primidone use.
- Impaired adjustment related to difficulty accepting diagnosis of epilepsy.
- Social isolation related to fear of experiencing a seizure in the presence of others.
- High risk for activity intolerance related to primidone's side effects of drowsiness, dizziness, ataxia.
- Knowledge deficit related to medication regimen.

Plan/Implementation

- Monitor vital signs at regular intervals (bid or tid) throughout therapy.
- Monitor serum primidone and phenobarbital levels. Record and report to physician.
- Observe frequently (every hour) for occurrence of seizure activity.
- Ensure that patient is protected from injury. Supervise and assist with ambulation if dizziness and drowsiness are problems. Ensure that patient avoids participation in any activity requiring mental alertness (including smoking). Pad siderails and head of bed with towels or blanket to protect patient who experiences seizures during the night.
- Medication may be administered with food to minimize GI irritation.
- For patient who has difficulty swallowing, crush tablet and mix with food or fluid, or give oral suspension.
- Store medication at controlled room temperatures between 15° and 30°C (59°–86°F). Protect from heat and moisture.

Patient/Family Education

- Do not drive or operate dangerous machinery until individual response has been determined. Drowsiness and dizziness can occur.
- Do not stop taking drug abruptly. To

do so could precipitate status epilepticus.
- Do not drink alcohol while on this medication.
- Carry or wear at all times identification stating illness and medication usage.
- Do not take any other medication without approval from physician. Combining drugs may be harmful.
- Promptly report any of the following symptoms to physician: sore throat • fever • malaise • skin rash • unusual bleeding • easy bruising • changes in vision.
- Be aware of possible risks of taking primidone during pregnancy. Patient who requires the medication to prevent seizures may be maintained on it; however, she must be fully aware of potential risks to unborn child. There is a strong association between the use of anticonvulsant drugs by women with epilepsy and the incidence of birth defects in their children. A possible association has also been suggested between maternal use of anticonvulsants and a neonatal coagulation defect that poses a threat of serious bleeding during the first 24 hours of life. Notify physician immediately if pregnancy occurs, is suspected, or is planned.
- Because primidone decreases the effectiveness of oral contraceptives, use alternative method of birth control during primidone therapy.
- To protect patient during a seizure, padding (towels, blankets, pillows) may be used to prevent bumping against hard objects. When convulsion has subsided, turn patient on side to allow secretions to drain and to prevent aspiration. Keep records of occurrence, characteristics, and duration of seizures, so that accurate reports may be given to physician for providing assistance in stabilization and control of seizures. If patient has difficulty breathing or continues to ex-

perience subsequent seizures, family should call for emergency assistance immediately.
* Be aware of possible side effects of primidone. Refer to written materials furnished by healthcare providers to assist in self-administration.

Evaluation
* Patient demonstrates stabilization of seizure activity with regular administration of primidone.
* Patient verbalizes understanding of necessity for, side effects of, and regimen required for prudent self-administration of primidone.

PROCHLORPERAZINE

(proe-klor-per′a-zeen)
Chlorpazine, Compazine

Classification(s):
Antipsychotic, Neuroleptic,
Antiemetic, Phenothiazine
Pregnancy Category C

INDICATIONS
* Manifestations of psychotic disorders ◆ Moderate to severe anxiety in nonpsychotic patients ◆ Severe nausea and vomiting.

ACTION
* The exact mechanism of antipsychotic action is not fully understood but is probably related to the drug's antidopaminergic effects ◆ Antipsychotics may block postsynaptic dopamine receptors in the basal ganglia, hypothalamus, limbic system, brain stem, and medulla ◆ Antipsychotic effects also appear to be related to inhibition of dopamine-mediated neurotransmission at the synapses ◆ Antipsychotic effects may also result from the drug's alpha-adrenergic blocking, muscarinic blocking, and adrenergic activity, as well as its effects on other amines (such as GABA) or peptides.

PHARMACOKINETICS
Absorption: Rapid absorption of oral tablet/timed-release capsule dosage forms. Genetic differences in rate of first-pass metabolism results in a wide range of bioavailability from individual to individual. Oral liquid preparations and IM administration result in more consistent absorption.
Distribution: Widely distributed. Highly lipophilic; accumulates in brain, lungs, and other tissues with high blood supply. Crosses placental barrier. Enters breast milk.
Metabolism and Excretion: Metabolized by the liver and in the kidneys. Excreted through kidneys and enterohepatic circulation. Active metabolites accumulate and are stored in fatty tissue over a prolonged period of time, and may be detected in urine up to 3–6 months following discontinuation of the drug.
Half-Life: Not well established.

CONTRAINDICATIONS AND PRECAUTIONS
Contraindicated in: ◆ Hypersensitivity to this drug, other phenothiazines, or (contained in some preparations) sulfites or tartrazine ◆ Comatose or severely CNS-depressed patients ◆ Presence of large amounts of CNS depressants ◆ Bone marrow depression ◆ Blood dyscrasias ◆ Subcortical brain damage ◆ Parkinson's disease ◆ Liver, renal, and/or cardiac insufficiency ◆ Severe hypotension or hypertension ◆ Children under 20 pounds or less than 2 years of age; pregnancy and lactation (safe use not established).
Use Cautiously in: ◆ Patients with a history of seizures ◆ Respiratory (e.g., infection; COPD), renal, hepatic, thyroid (e.g., thyrotoxicosis), or cardiovascular (e.g., mitral insufficiency; angina pectoris) disorders ◆ Prostatic hypertrophy ◆ Glaucoma ◆ Diabetes ◆ Elderly or debilitated patients ◆ Patients exposed to high or low environmental temperatures or to organophosphate insecticides ◆ Hypocal-

cemia ✦ History of severe reactions to insulin or ECT ✦ Pediatric patients with acute illnesses or dehydration.

ADVERSE REACTIONS AND SIDE EFFECTS*

CNS: sedation, headache, seizures, insomnia, dizziness, exacerbation of psychotic symptoms, extrapyramidal symptoms (pseudoparkinsonism, akathisia, akanesia, dystonia, oculogyric crisis), tardive dyskinesia, fatigue, cerebral edema, ataxia, blurred vision, NEUROLEPTIC MALIGNANT SYNDROME, restlessness, anxiety, depression, hyperthermia or hypothermia.

CV: hypotension, orthostatic hypotension, hypertension, tachycardia, bradycardia, CARDIAC ARREST, ECG changes, ARRHYTHMIAS, PULMONARY EDEMA, CIRCULATORY COLLAPSE.

Derm: skin rashes, urticaria, petechiae, seborrhea, photosensitivity, eczema, erythema, hyperpigmentation, contact dermatitis, EXFOLIATIVE DERMATITIS (rare).

Endo: galactorrhea, gynecomastia (men), changes in libido, impotence, hyperglycemia or hypoglycemia, amenorrhea, retrograde ejaculation.

GI: dry mouth, nausea, vomiting, increased appetite and weight gain, anorexia, dyspepsia, constipation, diarrhea, jaundice, polydipsia, PARALYTIC ILEUS.

GI: urinary retention, frequency or incontinence, bladder paralysis, polyuria, enuresis, priapism.

Hemat: AGRANULOCYTOSIS, LEUKOPENIA, ANEMIA, THROMBOCYTOPENIA, PANCYTOPENIA.

Ophth: lens deposition.

Resp: LARYNGEAL EDEMA, LARYNGOSPASM, BRONCHOSPASM, SUPPRESSION OF COUGH REFLEX.

Other: decreased sweating.

INTERACTIONS

Drug-Drug: ✦ **CNS depressants (including alcohol, barbiturates, narcotics, anesthetics):** additive CNS depressant effects ✦ **Anticholinergic agents (e.g., atropine):** additive anticholinergic effects, decreased antipsychotic effects ✦ **Barbiturate anesthetics:** increased incidence of excitatory effects and hypotension ✦ **Barbiturates:** possible decreased effects of phenothiazines ✦ **Metyrosine:** potentiation of extrapyramidal side effects ✦ **Levodopa:** decreased efficacy of levodopa ✦ **Quinidine:** additive cardiac depressive effects ✦ **Magnesium- or aluminum-containing antidiarrheal mixtures, antacids:** reduced phenothiazine absorption/effectiveness. ✦ **Guanethidine:** decreased antihypertensive action ✦ **Lithium:** decreased plasma levels and effect of antipsychotic drug; severe neurotoxicity reported ✦ **Epinephrine:** reversal of usual pressor action of epinephrine, resulting in decreased blood pressure and tachycardia ✦ **Bromocriptine:** impairment of prolactin-suppressing action ✦ **Angiotensin converting enzyme (ACE) inhibitors:** increased effects of ACE inhibitors ✦ **Phenytoin:** decreased phenytoin metabolism, increased risk of toxicity ✦ **Polypeptide antibiotics:** possible neuromuscular respiratory depression ✦ **Metrizamide:** seizures ✦ **Cimetidine:** decreased effect of phenothiazines ✦ **Clonidine:** possibility of severe hypotension ✦ **Piperazine:** increased seizure potential.

Drug-Food: ✦ **Caffeine-containing beverages (e.g., coffee, tea, colas):** counteract antipsychotic effect.

ROUTE AND DOSAGE

Psychoses, Acute Anxiety

✦ **PO (Adults):** 5–10 mg tid or qid. Sustained-release: 15 mg on arising, or 10 mg q 12 hr. Increase dosage gradually every 2–3 days until desired effect is achieved or side effects become bothersome. Usual dosage is 50–150 mg/day, depending on severity of symptoms.

*Underlines indicate most frequent; CAPITALS indicate life-threatening.

♦ **Rect (Adults):** 25 mg bid.
♦ **PO, Rect (Children):** 2–12 years: 2.5 mg bid or tid. No more than 10 mg on first day. Increase dosage according to patient response. Maximum daily dosage, ages 2–5: 20 mg; ages 6–12: 25 mg.
♦ **IM (Adults):** Psychosis: Initial dose: 10–20 mg. Repeat every 1–4 hours, if necessary, to achieve control, then switch to oral form at same or higher dosage. If prolonged parenteral therapy is required, give 10–20 mg q 4–6 hr.
♦ **IM (Adults):** Acute anxiety: 5–10 mg. May repeat q 3–4 hr to maximum of 40 mg/day.

Severe Nausea and Vomiting

♦ **PO (Adults):** 5–10 mg tid or qid. Sustained-release: 15 mg upon arising or 10 mg q 12 hr.
♦ **PO, Rect (Children over 2 Years Old):** 20–29 lbs: 2.5 mg daily or bid (maximum 7.5 mg/day). 30–39 lb: 2.5 mg bid or tid (maximum 10 mg/day). 40–85 lb: 2.5 mg tid or 5 mg bid (maximum 15 mg/day).
♦ **Rect (Adults):** 25 mg bid.
♦ **IM (Adults):** Initial dosage: 5–10 mg. Repeat if necessary q 3–4 hr. Maximum daily dose: 40 mg.
♦ **IM (Children over 20 lb or 2 Years Old):** 0.13 mg/kg. Control is usually obtained with one dose.

Pre-, Peri-, and Postoperative Nausea and Vomiting

♦ **IM (Adults):** 5–10 mg 1–2 hr before induction of anesthesia (may be repeated once in 30 minutes), or to control acute symptoms during and after surgery (may be repeated once).
♦ **IV Injection (Adults):** 5–10 mg 15–30 minutes before induction of anesthesia or to control acute symptoms during or after surgery. May be repeated once if necessary.
♦ **IV Infusion (Adults):** 20 mg/L of isotonic solution. Begin infusion 15–30 minutes before induction of anesthesia.

PHARMACODYNAMICS

Route	Onset*	Peak†	Duration‡
PO	30–40 min	2–4 hr	3–4 hr
PO (time-release)	30–60 min	—	10–12 hr
Rect	60 min	—	12 hr
IM	10–20 min	15–30 min	3–4 hr
IV	15 min	15 min	—

*Full clinical effects may not be observed for 4–8 weeks.
†Steady-state plasma levels are achieved in approximately 4–7 days.
‡Drug may be detected in urine for 3–6 months after last dose.

NURSING IMPLICATIONS

Assessment

♦ Assess hydration. **Note:** • weight • condition of mucus membranes • skin turgor • color • amount and density of urine • vital signs.
♦ Assess mental status daily: • mood • appearance • thought and communication patterns • level of interest in the environment and in activities • level of anxiety or agitation • presence of hallucinations or delusions • suspiciousness • interactions with others • ability to carry out activities of daily living.
♦ Assess for symptoms of blood dyscrasias: • sore throat • fever • malaise • unusual bleeding • easy bruising.
♦ Assess for extrapyramidal symptoms: • pseudoparkinsonism (tremors, shuffling gait, drooling, rigidity) • akinesia (muscular weakness) • akathisia (continuous restlessness and fidgeting) • dystonia (involuntary muscular movements of face, arms, legs, and neck) • oculogyric crisis (uncontrolled rolling back of the eyes) • tardive dyskinesia (bizarre facial and tongue movements, stiff neck, difficulty swallowing).
♦ Assess for symptoms of neuroleptic malignant syndrome: • hyperpyrexia up to 107°F (41.6°C), elevated pulse • increased or decreased blood pres-

sure • severe parkinsonian muscle rigidity • elevated creatinine phosphokinase blood levels • elevated white blood count • altered mental status (including catatonic signs or agitation) • acute renal failure • varying levels of consciousness (including stupor and coma) • pallor • diaphoresis • tachycardia • arrhythmias • rhabdomyolysis.

✦ Assess vital signs, weight. Record baseline values for comparison.

✦ Assess history of allergies, sensitivity to this drug or to other phenothiazines.

✦ Assess for signs and symptoms of cholestatic jaundice: • abdominal pain • nausea • rash • fever • yellow skin • flu-like symptoms • abnormal lab test results (eosinophilia, bile in urine, increased serum transaminases, bilirubin, alkaline phosphatase).

✦ Assess date of last menses (possible pregnancy), use of contraceptives.

✦ Assess whether currently breast-feeding a child.

✦ Assess current and past alcohol and drug consumption.

✦ Assess for operation of automobile and/or other dangerous machinery.

✦ Assess for presence of adverse reactions or side effects.

✦ Assess patient/family knowledge about illness and need for medication.

✦ In collaboration with physician, assess CBC, liver function tests, and ophthalmological exams in patients on long-term therapy.

✦ **Lab Test Alterations:** Increased serum alkaline phosphatase, transaminases, bilirubin.

◇ Increased protein-bound iodine.

◇ False-positive urine pregnancy test, possibly caused by drug metabolite that discolors urine (less likely to occur when serum test is used).

◇ Increased urinary glucose.

◇ Decreased urinary estrogen, progestin, and gonadotropin.

◇ Increased plasma cholesterol level.

◇ Increased serum prolactin.

✦ **Withdrawal:** Assess for symptoms of abrupt withdrawal from long-term therapy: • gastritis • nausea • vomiting • dizziness • headache • tachycardia • insomnia • tremulousness • sweating.

✦ **Toxicity and Overdose:** No correlation has been established between blood level and therapeutic effect.

◇ Assess for symptoms of overdose: • CNS depression, from heavy sedation to deep sleep to coma • hypotension • confusion • excitement • extrapyramidal symptoms • agitation • restlessness • convulsions • fever • autonomic reactions • ECG changes • cardiac arrhythmias • tachycardia • hypothermia • tremor • seizures • cyanosis.

✦ **Overdose Management:** Monitor vital signs.

◇ Ensure maintenance of open airway.

◇ Initiate gastric lavage.

◇ Do not induce emesis (nuchal rigidity may result in aspiration of vomitus).

◇ Administer antiparkinsonian drugs or diphenhydramine to counteract extrapyramidal symptoms.

◇ Administer IV fluids or a vasoconstrictor to maintain adequate blood pressure. **Note:** Epinephrine is not recommended due to its interaction with phenothiazines, which causes further drop in blood pressure.

◇ Administer IV phenytoin to control ventricular arrhythmias.

◇ Administer phenobarbital or diazepam to control convulsions or hyperactivity.

◇ Dialysis does not appear to be a useful intervention.

Potential Nursing Diagnoses

✦ High risk for fluid volume deficit related to excessive vomiting.

✦ High risk for violence directed at others related to mistrust and panic anxiety.

✦ High risk for injury related to prochlorperazine's side effects of sedation, dizziness, ataxia, weakness, and lowered seizure threshold; abrupt withdrawal after prolonged use; overdose.

♦ Sensory-perceptual alteration related to panic anxiety evidenced by hallucinations.

♦ Altered thought processes related to panic anxiety evidenced by delusional thinking.

♦ Social isolation related to inability to trust others.

♦ High risk for activity intolerance related to prochlorperazine's side effects of drowsiness, dizziness, ataxia, weakness.

♦ Noncompliance with medication regimen related to suspiciousness and mistrust of others.

♦ Knowledge deficit related to medication regimen.

Plan/Implementation

♦ **General Info:** Monitor vital signs before beginning therapy and at regular intervals (bid or tid) throughout therapy. If nausea and vomiting are severe, monitor VS q 2–4 hr. Take BP lying and standing to monitor for possible hypotensive reaction; elderly are particularly susceptible. Dosage adjustment may be required.

◊ Ensure that patient who is ambulatory is protected from sun when spending time outdoors.

◊ Weigh patient on long-term therapy 2–3 times a week, at same time of day, on same scale, if possible. A rapid weight gain or evidence of edema should be reported to physician immediately. Record I&O. Patient with severe nausea and vomiting should be weighed daily.

◊ Ensure that patient is protected from injury. Provide supervision and assistance when ambulating if dizziness and drowsiness are problems. Pad siderails and headboard for patient who experiences seizures.

◊ Give patient hard candy, gum, or frequent sips of water if dry mouth is a problem.

◊ Store medication at controlled room temperatures between 15° and 30°C (59°–86°F). Protect from heat, light, and freezing.

♦ **PO:** Oral medication may be administered with food to minimize GI upset.

◊ Ensure that patient swallows tablet/capsule and does not "cheek" to avoid medication or to hoard for later use.

◊ Crush tablet and mix with food or fluid for patient who has difficulty swallowing, or use liquid concentrate.

◊ Do not open, crush, or chew capsules. Swallow whole.

◊ Just prior to administration, mix concentrate with juice, water, carbonated beverage, or semisolid food.

◊ If concentrate is accidentally spilled on skin or clothing during preparation or administration, wash area immediately, as contact dermatitis can occur.

♦ **Rect:** To ensure that suppository has been retained, check patient 20–30 minutes following rectal administration.

◊ To ensure accurate dosage, do not divide suppositories.

♦ **IM:** IM injection may be irritating to tissues; avoid SC injection.

◊ Avoid contact with injectable liquid. A contact dermatitis can occur.

◊ Inject slowly and deeply into upper, outer quadrant of buttock. Massage site thoroughly following injection.

◊ Because of possible hypotensive effects, patient should remain in recumbent position for at least one-half hour following IM injection.

◊ Rotate sites when multiple injections are administered.

◊ Do not mix drug with other agents in the syringe.

◊ Potency is not altered when solution is slightly yellow in color. Discard if marked discoloration is evident.

♦ **IV:** Because of possible hypotensive effects, drug should be administered with patient in recumbent position.

◇ Monitor blood pressure every 10 minutes during IV administration. Physician may order vasopressor (not epinephrine) if hypotension occurs.

◇ IV solution should be diluted to a concentration of no more than 0.5 mg/mL with normal saline.

◇ Potency is not altered when solution is slightly yellow in color. Discard if marked discoloration is evident.

◇ Administer direct IV at a rate not exceeding 5 mg/min.

◇ 10–20 mg may be added to 1 liter of isotonic solution and given as an IV infusion. Administer slowly, increasing or decreasing rate as symptoms indicate.

Patient/Family Education

♦ Use caution when driving or operating dangerous machinery. Drowsiness and dizziness can occur.

♦ Do not stop taking the drug abruptly. To do so might produce withdrawal symptoms, such as nausea, vomiting, gastritis, headache, tachycardia, insomnia, tremulousness.

♦ Use sunscreens and wear protective clothing when spending time outdoors. Skin is more susceptible to sunburn.

♦ Report occurrence of any of the following symptoms to physician immediately: sore throat • fever • malaise • unusual bleeding • easy bruising • persistent nausea/vomiting • severe headache • rapid heart rate • difficulty urinating • muscle twitching • tremors • pale stools • yellow skin or eyes • muscular incoordination • or skin rash.

♦ Drug may turn urine pink to reddish-brown in color. This is not significant nor is it harmful.

♦ Rise slowly from a sitting or lying position to prevent a sudden drop in blood pressure.

♦ If dry mouth is a problem, take frequent sips of water, chew sugarless gum, or suck on hard candy. Good oral care (frequent brushing, flossing) is very important.

♦ If some liquid concentrate is spilled on the skin, wash it off immediately. If not, a rash may appear.

♦ Consult physician regarding smoking while on prochlorperazine therapy. Smoking increases metabolism of prochlorperazine, requiring adjustment in dosage to achieve therapeutic effect.

♦ Dress warmly in cold weather and avoid extended exposure to very high or low temperatures. Body temperature is harder to maintain while taking this medication.

♦ Do not drink alcohol while on prochlorperazine therapy. These drugs potentiate the effects of each other.

♦ Do not consume other medications (including over-the-counter meds) without physician's approval. Many medications contain substances that interact with prochlorperazine in a way that may be harmful.

♦ Be aware of possible risks of taking prochlorperazine during pregnancy. Safe use during pregnancy and lactation has not been established. Prochlorperazine readily crosses the placental barrier, so a fetus could experience adverse effects of the drug. Inform physician immediately if pregnancy occurs, is suspected, or is planned.

♦ Be aware of side effects of prochlorperazine. Refer to written materials furnished by healthcare providers for safe self-administration.

♦ Continue to take medication even if feeling well and as though it is not needed. Symptoms may return if medication is discontinued.

♦ Carry card or other identification at all times describing medications being taken.

Evaluation

♦ Patient demonstrates a subsiding/resolution of the symptoms for which prochlorperazine was prescribed (severe panic anxiety, altered thought processes, altered perceptions, nausea and vomiting).

♦ Patient verbalizes understanding of side effects and regimen required for prudent self-administration of prochlorperazine.

PROCYCLIDINE

(proe-sye'kli-deen)
Kemadrin, {Procyclid}

Classification(s):
Antiparkinsonian agent,
Anticholinergic
Pregnancy Category C

INDICATIONS

♦ All forms of parkinsonism ♦ Extrapyramidal symptoms (except tardive dyskinesia) associated with antipsychotic drugs.

ACTION

♦ Acts to correct an imbalance of dopamine deficiency and acetylcholine excess in the corpus striatum. The acetylcholine receptor is blocked at the synapse to diminish excess cholinergic effect.

PHARMACOKINETICS

Absorption: Rapidly absorbed following oral administration.
Distribution: Not completely understood. May cross placental barrier and may enter breast milk.
Metabolism and Excretion: Thought to be at least partially metabolized by the liver. Excreted in urine as metabolites and unchanged drug.
Half-Life: Undetermined.

CONTRAINDICATIONS AND PRECAUTIONS

Contraindicated in: ♦ Hypersensitivity to this drug ♦ Angle-closure glaucoma ♦

Pyloric or duodenal obstruction ♦ Stenosing peptic ulcers ♦ Prostatic hypertrophy or bladder-neck obstructions ♦ Achalasia ♦ Myasthenia gravis ♦ Ulcerative colitis ♦ Toxic megacolon ♦ Tachycardia secondary to cardiac insufficiency or thyrotoxicosis.
Use Cautiously in: ♦ Narrow-angle glaucoma ♦ Elderly or debilitated patients ♦ Children; pregnancy and lactation (safety not established) ♦ Hepatic, renal, or cardiac insufficiency ♦ Tendency toward urinary retention ♦ Hypotension ♦ Hyperthyroidism ♦ Hypertension ♦ Autonomic neuropathy ♦ Patients exposed to high environmental temperatures.

ADVERSE REACTIONS AND SIDE EFFECTS*

CNS: drowsiness, dizziness, blurred vision, disorientation, confusion, memory loss, agitation, nervousness, delirium, weakness, vertigo, mydriasis, cycloplegia, headache, insomnia.
CV: orthostatic hypotension, hypotension, tachycardia, palpitations.
Derm: skin rashes, urticaria, other dermatoses.
GI: dry mouth, nausea, vomiting, epigastric distress, constipation, dilatation of the colon, PARALYTIC ILEUS.
GU: urinary retention, urinary hesitancy, dysuria, difficulty in achieving or maintaining an erection.
Psych: depression, delusions, hallucinations, paranoia.
Other: muscular weakness, muscular cramping, elevated temperature, flushing, decreased sweating, anaphylaxis, increased intraocular pressure.

INTERACTIONS

Drug-Drug: ♦ **Other drugs with anticholinergic properties (e.g., glutethimide, disopyramide, narcotic analgesics, phenothiazines, tricyclic antidepressants, antihistamines,**

{} = Only available in Canada.
*Underlines indicate most frequent; CAPITALS indicate life-threatening.

quinidine salts, amantadine): increased anticholinergic effects, potentially fatal paralytic ileus ♦ **Levodopa:** possible decreased levodopa absorption ♦ **Slow-dissolving digoxin:** decreased absorption of digoxin ♦ **CNS depressants (e.g., alcohol, barbiturates, narcotics, benzodiazepines):** increased CNS depressant effects ♦ **Phenothiazines, haloperidol:** decreased therapeutic effects of these drugs ♦ **Ketoconazole:** decreased absorption of ketoconazole ♦ **Antacids:** decreased absorption of procyclidine ♦ **Phenothiazines, haloperidol:** decreased antipsychotic effect.

ROUTE AND DOSAGE
Parkinsonism
♦ **PO (Adults):** For patients who have received no other therapy, start dosage at 2.5 mg tid pc. Gradually increase dosage to 5 mg tid and, if needed, tid and at H.S. For patients who are being transferred from other therapy, substitute 2.5 mg tid for all or part of the original drug. Increase procyclidine as required, while decreasing other drug until complete replacement is achieved.

Drug-Induced Extrapyramidal Symptoms
♦ **PO (Adults):** Initial dosage: 2.5 mg tid, preferably after meals. Increase in increments of 2.5 mg daily until relief of symptoms is achieved. In most cases, results will be obtained with 10–20 mg daily.

PHARMACODYNAMICS

Route	Onset	Peak	Duration
PO	30–45 min	—	4–6 hr

NURSING IMPLICATIONS
Assessment
♦ Assess for symptoms of Parkinson's disease: • tremors • muscular weakness and rigidity • drooling • shuffling gait • disturbances of posture and equilibrium • flat affect • monotone speech.
♦ Assess for extrapyramidal symptoms: • pseudoparkinsonism (tremors, shuffling gait, drooling, rigidity) • akinesia (muscular weakness) • akathisia (continuous restlessness and fidgeting) • dystonia (involuntary muscular movements of face, arms, legs, and neck) • oculogyric crisis (uncontrolled rolling back of the eyes) • tardive dyskinesia (bizarre facial and tongue movements, stiff neck, difficulty swallowing). **Note:** Procyclidine is not effective in alleviating symptoms of tardive dyskinesia.
♦ Assess for symptoms of paralytic ileus: • constipation • abdominal pain and distention • absence of bowel sounds. Patients taking procyclidine concomitantly with other drugs that produce anticholinergic effects are particularly susceptible.
♦ Assess vital signs, weight. Record baseline values for comparison.
♦ Assess history of allergies, sensitivity to this drug or to other anticholinergics.
♦ Assess date of last menses (possible pregnancy), use of contraceptives.
♦ Assess whether currently breast-feeding a child.
♦ Assess current and past alcohol and drug consumption.
♦ Assess for operation of automobile and/or other dangerous machinery.
♦ Assess for presence of adverse reactions or side effects.
♦ Assess patient/family knowledge about illness and need for medication.
♦ In collaboration with physician, periodically assess CBC, liver function, and intraocular pressure in patients on long-term therapy.
♦ **Toxicity and Overdose:** Assess for symptoms of overdose: • CNS depression preceded or followed by stimulation • intensification of psychotic symptoms • anxiety • ataxia • seizures • incoherence • delusions • paranoia • anhidrosis • hyperpyrexia • hot, dry,

flushed skin • dry mucous membranes • decreased bowel sounds • urinary retention • tachycardia • difficulty swallowing • cardiac arrhythmias • shock • coma • circulatory collapse • skeletal muscle paralysis • cardiac arrest • respiratory depression or arrest.

♦ **Overdose Management:** Monitor vital signs.

◇ Ensure maintenance of adequate airway.

◇ Induce emesis in conscious patient (contraindicated in precomatose, convulsive, or psychotic states).

◇ Initiate gastric lavage.

◇ Administer activated charcoal.

◇ Administer pilocarpine, 5 mg PO, to treat peripheral effects.

◇ Administer physostigmine, 1–2 mg SC or slow IV, to reverse anticholinergic effects (use only with availability of advanced life support).

◇ Use artificial respiration and oxygen to treat respiratory depression.

◇ Use tepid water sponges, cold packs, or other cooling applications to treat hyperpyrexia.

◇ Darken room to counter photophobia.

◇ Administer IV fluids and vasopressor to combat circulatory collapse.

◇ Administer diazepam to control symptoms of acute psychoses.

Potential Nursing Diagnoses

♦ High risk for injury related to symptoms of Parkinson's disease or drug-induced extrapyramidal symptoms.

♦ Hyperthermia related to anticholinergic effect of decreased sweating.

♦ Sensory-perceptual alteration related to side effect of procyclidine evidenced by hallucinations.

♦ Altered thought processes related to side effects of procyclidine evidenced by delusional thinking, disorientation, confusion.

♦ Social isolation related to embarrassment by symptoms of Parkinson's disease.

♦ High risk for activity intolerance re-

lated to procyclidine's side effects of drowsiness, dizziness, ataxia, weakness, confusion.

♦ Knowledge deficit related to medication regimen.

Plan/Implementation

♦ Monitor vital signs daily. Be particularly alert for increase in pulse rate or temperature.

♦ Weigh patient 2–3 times a week, at same time of day, on same scale, if possible. A rapid weight gain or evidence of edema should be reported to physician immediately. Record I&O.

♦ Monitor for exacerbation of mental symptoms in patients who are receiving the drug to counteract extrapyramidal symptoms associated with antipsychotic medications.

♦ Ensure that patient is protected from injury. Provide supervision and assistance when ambulating if dizziness and drowsiness are problems.

♦ Give patient hard candy, gum, or frequent sips of water if dry mouth is a problem, or treat with saliva substitute.

♦ Ensure that patient swallows tablet and does not "cheek" to avoid medication or to hoard for later use.

♦ Medication may be administered after meals to minimize gastric irritation.

♦ Tablet may be crushed and mixed with food or fluid for patient who has difficulty swallowing.

♦ Monitor vital signs before beginning therapy and at regular intervals (bid or tid) throughout therapy. Take BP lying and standing to monitor for possible hypotensive reaction; elderly are particularly susceptible. Dosage adjustment may be required.

♦ Store medication at controlled room temperatures between 15° and 30°C (59°–86°F). Protect from heat and moisture.

Patient/Family Education

♦ Medication may be taken with food if GI upset occurs.

- Use caution when driving or when operating dangerous machinery. Drowsiness and dizziness can occur.
- Do not stop taking the drug abruptly. To do so might produce serious withdrawal symptoms.
- Report occurrence of any of the following symptoms to physician immediately: • pain or tenderness in area in front of ear • extreme dryness of mouth • difficulty urinating • abdominal pain • constipation • fast and pounding heartbeat • rash • vision disturbances • mental changes.
- Rise slowly from a sitting or lying position to prevent a sudden drop in blood pressure.
- Stay inside in air-conditioned room when weather is very hot. Perspiration is decreased by procyclidine, and the body cannot cool itself as well. There is greater susceptibility to heat stroke. Inform physician if air-conditioned housing or work environment is not available.
- If dry mouth is a problem, take frequent sips of water, chew sugarless gum, or suck on hard candy. Good oral care (frequent brushing, flossing) is very important.
- Do not drink alcohol while on procyclidine therapy.
- Do not consume other medications (including over-the-counter meds) without physician's approval. Many medications contain substances that interact with procyclidine in a way that may be harmful.
- Be aware of possible risks of taking procyclidine during pregnancy. Safe use during pregnancy and lactation has not been established. It is thought that procyclidine crosses the placental barrier; if so, a fetus could experience adverse effects of the drug. Inform physician immediately if pregnancy occurs, is suspected, or is planned.
- Be aware of side effects of procyclidine. Refer to written materials furnished by healthcare providers for safe self-administration.
- Continue to take medication even if feeling well and as though it is not needed. Symptoms may return if medication is discontinued.
- Carry card or other identification at all times describing medications being taken.

Evaluation
- Patient demonstrates a subsiding of the symptoms for which procyclidine was prescribed (parkinsonism, drug-induced extrapyramidal symptoms).
- Patient verbalizes understanding of side effects and regimen required for prudent self-administration of procyclidine.

PROMAZINE

(proe'ma-zeen)
{Promanyl}, Prozine, Sparine

Classification(s):
Antipsychotic, Neuroleptic, Phenothiazine
Pregnancy Category C

INDICATIONS

- Psychotic disorders, such as schizophrenia, manic phase of bipolar disorder (until slower-acting lithium takes effect), brief reactive psychoses, schizoaffective disorder • Anxiety and agitation • Symptoms of alcohol withdrawal.

ACTION

- The exact mechanism of antipsychotic action is not fully understood, but is probably related to the drug's antidopaminergic effects • Antipsychotics may block postsynaptic dopamine receptors in the basal ganglia, hypothalamus, limbic system, brain stem, and medulla • Antipsychotic effects also appear to be

{} = Only available in Canada.

related to inhibition of dopamine-mediated neurotransmission at the synapses ♦ Antipsychotic effects may also result from the drug's alpha-adrenergic blocking, muscarinic blocking, and adrenergic activity, as well as its effects on other amines (such as GABA) or peptides.

PHARMACOKINETICS

Absorption: Rapid absorption of oral tablet dosage forms. Genetic differences in rate of first-pass metabolism result in a wide range of bioavailability from individual to individual. IM administration results in more consistent absorption.

Distribution: Widely distributed. Highly lipophilic; accumulates in the brain, lungs, and other tissues with high blood supply. Crosses placental barrier. Enters breast milk.

Metabolism and Excretion: Metabolized by the liver and in the kidneys. Excreted through kidneys and enterohepatic circulation. Active metabolites accumulate and are stored in fatty tissue over a prolonged period of time and may be detected in urine up to 3–6 months following discontinuation of the drug.

Half-Life: Not well established.

CONTRAINDICATIONS AND PRECAUTIONS

Contraindicated in: ♦ Hypersensitivity to this drug, other phenothiazines, or sulfites or tartrazine (contained in some preparations) ♦ Comatose or severely CNS-depressed patients ♦ Presence of large amounts of CNS depressants ♦ Bone marrow depression ♦ Blood dyscrasias ♦ Subcortical brain damage ♦ Parkinson's disease ♦ Liver, renal, and/or cardiac insufficiency ♦ Severe hypotension or hypertension ♦ Children under 12 years of age; pregnancy and lactation (safe use not established).

Use Cautiously in: ♦ Patients with a history of seizures ♦ Respiratory, renal, hepatic, thyroid, or cardiovascular disorders (e.g., respiratory infection, COPD, thyrotoxicosis, mitral insufficiency, angina pectoris) ♦ Prostatic hypertrophy ♦ Glaucoma ♦ Diabetes ♦ Elderly or debilitated patients ♦ Patients exposed to high or low environmental temperatures or to organophosphate insecticides ♦ Hypocalcemia ♦ History of severe reactions to insulin or ECT ♦ Pediatric patients with acute illnesses or dehydration.

ADVERSE REACTIONS AND SIDE EFFECTS*

CNS: sedation, headache, seizures, insomnia, dizziness, exacerbation of psychotic symptoms, extrapyramidal symptoms (pseudoparkinsonism, akathisia, akinesia, dystonia, oculogyric crisis), tardive dyskinesia, fatigue, cerebral edema, ataxia, blurred vision, NEUROLEPTIC MALIGNANT SYNDROME, restlessness, anxiety, depression, hyperthermia or hypothermia.

CV: hypotension, orthostatic hypotension, hypertension, tachycardia, bradycardia, CARDIAC ARREST, ECG changes, ARRHYTHMIAS, PULMONARY EDEMA, CIRCULATORY COLLAPSE.

Derm: skin rashes, urticaria, petechiae, seborrhea, photosensitivity, eczema, erythema, hyperpigmentation, contact dermatitis, EXFOLIATIVE DERMATITIS (rare).

Endo: galactorrhea, gynecomastia (men), changes in libido, impotence, hyperglycemia or hypoglycemia, amenorrhea, retrograde ejaculation.

GI: dry mouth, nausea, vomiting, increased appetite and weight gain, anorexia, dyspepsia, constipation, diarrhea, jaundice, polydipsia, PARALYTIC ILEUS.

GU: urinary retention, frequency or incontinence, bladder paralysis, polyuria, enuresis, priapism.

Hemat: AGRANULOCYTOSIS, LEUKOPENIA, ANEMIA, THROMBOCYTOPENIA, PANCYTOPENIA.

Ophth: lens deposition.

Resp: LARYNGEAL EDEMA, LARYNGOSPASM,

---

*Underlines indicate most frequent; CAPITALS indicate life-threatening.

BRONCHOSPASM, SUPPRESSION OF COUGH REFLEX.
Other: decreased sweating.

INTERACTIONS

Drug-Drug: ◆ **CNS depressants (including alcohol, barbiturates, narcotics, anesthetics):** additive CNS depressant effects ◆ **Anticholinergic agents (e.g., atropine):** additive anticholinergic effects, decreased antipsychotic effects ◆ **Barbiturate anesthetics:** increased incidence of excitatory effects and hypotension ◆ **Barbiturates:** possible decreased effects of phenothiazines ◆ **Metyrosine:** potentiation of extrapyramidal side effects ◆ **Levodopa:** decreased efficacy of levodopa ◆ **Quinidine:** additive cardiac depressive effects ◆ **Magnesium- or aluminum-containing antidiarrheal mixtures, antacids:** reduced phenothiazine absorption/effectiveness ◆ **Guanethidine:** decreased antihypertensive action ◆ **Lithium:** decreased plasma levels and effect of antipsychotic drug; severe neurotoxicity reported ◆ **Epinephrine:** reversal of usual pressor action of epinephrine, resulting in decreased blood pressure and tachycardia ◆ **Bromocriptine:** impairment of prolactin-suppressing action ◆ **Angiotensin converting enzyme (ACE) inhibitors:** increased effects of ACE inhibitors ◆ **Phenytoin:** decreased phenytoin metabolism, increased risk of toxicity ◆ **Polypeptide antibiotics:** possible neuromuscular respiratory depression ◆ **Metrizamide:** seizures ◆ **Cimetidine:** decreased effect of phenothiazines ◆ **Clonidine:** possibility of severe hypotension ◆ **Piperazine:** increased seizure potential.
Drug-Food: ◆ **Caffeine-containing beverages (e.g., coffee, tea, colas):** counteract antipsychotic effect.

ROUTE AND DOSAGE

Psychoses, Acute Agitation

◆ **IM, IV (Adults):** Initial dose: 50–150 mg, depending on degree of agitation.

After 30 minutes, additional dosage up to 300 mg total may be given if desired effect has not been achieved. Once desired effect has been achieved, oral dosage is recommended.

◆ **PO, IM (Adults, Maintenance):** 10–200 mg q 4–6 hr. Maximum daily dose: 1000 mg.
◆ **PO, IM (Children, 12 or over, Maintenance):** 10–25 mg q 4–6 hr.

PHARMACODYNAMICS

Route	Onset*	Peak†	Duration‡
PO	30–60 min	2–4 hr	4–6 hr
IM	15–30 min	1 hr	4–6 hr
IV	5 min	5 min	—

*Full clinical effects may not be observed for 4–8 weeks.
†Steady-state plasma levels are achieved in approximately 4–7 days.
‡Drug may be detected in urine for 3–6 months after last dose.

NURSING IMPLICATIONS

Assessment

◆ Assess mental status daily: • mood • appearance • thought and communication patterns • level of interest in the environment and in activities • level of anxiety or agitation • presence of hallucinations or delusions • suspiciousness • interactions with others • ability to carry out activities of daily living.
◆ Assess for symptoms of blood dyscrasias: • sore throat • fever • malaise • unusual bleeding • easy bruising.
◆ Assess for extrapyramidal symptoms: • pseudoparkinsonism (tremors, shuffling gait, drooling, rigidity) • akinesia (muscular weakness) • akathisia (continuous restlessness and fidgeting) • dystonia (involuntary muscular movements of face, arms, legs, and neck) • oculogyric crisis (uncontrolled rolling back of the eyes) • tardive dyskinesia (bizarre facial and tongue movements, stiff neck, difficulty swallowing).
◆ Assess for symptoms of neuroleptic malignant syndrome: • hyperpyrexia

up to 107°F (41.6°C) • elevated pulse • increased or decreased blood pressure • severe parkinsonian muscle rigidity • elevated creatinine phosphokinase blood levels • elevated white blood count • altered mental status (including catatonic signs or agitation) • acute renal failure • varying levels of consciousness (including stupor and coma) • pallor • diaphoresis • tachycardia • arrhythmias • rhabdomyolysis.

♦ Assess vital signs, weight. Record baseline values for comparison.

♦ Assess history of allergies, sensitivity to this drug or to other phenothiazines.

♦ Assess for signs and symptoms of cholestatic jaundice: • abdominal pain • nausea • rash • fever • yellow skin • flu-like symptoms • abnormal lab test results (eosinophilia, bile in urine, increased serum transaminases, bilirubin, alkaline phosphatase).

♦ Assess date of last menses (possible pregnancy), use of contraceptives.

♦ Assess whether currently breast-feeding a child.

♦ Assess current and past alcohol and drug consumption.

♦ Assess for operation of automobile and/or other dangerous machinery.

♦ Assess for presence of adverse reactions or side effects.

♦ Assess patient/family knowledge about illness and need for medication.

♦ In collaboration with physician, assess CBC, liver function tests, and ophthalmological exams in patients on long-term therapy.

♦ **Lab Test Alterations:** Increased serum alkaline phosphatase, transaminases, bilirubin.

◊ Increased protein-bound iodine.

◊ False-positive urine pregnancy test, possibly caused by drug metabolite that discolors urine (less likely to occur when serum test is used).

◊ Increased urinary glucose.

◊ Decreased urinary estrogen, progestin, and gonadotropin.

◊ Increased plasma cholesterol level.

◊ Increased serum prolactin.

♦ **Withdrawal:** Assess for symptoms of abrupt withdrawal from long-term therapy: • gastritis • nausea • vomiting • dizziness • headache • tachycardia • insomnia • tremulousness • sweating.

♦ **Toxicity and Overdose:** No correlation has been established between blood level and therapeutic effect.

◊ Assess for symptoms of overdose: • CNS depression, from heavy sedation to deep sleep to coma • hypotension • confusion • excitement • extrapyramidal symptoms • agitation • restlessness • convulsions • fever • autonomic reactions • ECG changes • cardiac arrhythmias • tachycardia • hypothermia • tremor • seizures • cyanosis.

♦ **Overdose Management:** Monitor vital signs.

◊ Ensure maintenance of adequate airway.

◊ Initiate gastric lavage.

◊ Do not induce emesis (nuchal rigidity may result in aspiration of vomitus).

◊ Antiparkinsonian drugs or diphenhydramine may be administered to counteract extrapyramidal symptoms.

◊ Administer IV fluids or a vasoconstrictor to maintain adequate blood pressure. **Note:** Epinephrine is not recommended due to its interaction with phenothiazines, which causes further drop in blood pressure.

◊ Administer IV phenytoin to control ventricular arrhythmias.

◊ Administer phenobarbital or diazepam to control convulsions or hyperactivity.

◊ Dialysis does not appear to be a useful intervention.

Potential Nursing Diagnoses

♦ High risk for violence directed at others related to mistrust and panic anxiety.

♦ High risk for injury related to promazine's side effects of sedation, dizziness, ataxia, weakness, lowered seizure threshold; abrupt withdrawal after prolonged use; overdose.

♦ Sensory-perceptual alteration related to panic anxiety evidenced by hallucinations.

♦ Altered thought processes related to panic anxiety evidenced by delusional thinking.

♦ Social isolation related to inability to trust others.

♦ High risk for activity intolerance related to promazine's side effects of drowsiness, dizziness, ataxia, weakness.

♦ Noncompliance with medication regimen related to suspiciousness and mistrust of others.

♦ Knowledge deficit related to medication regimen.

Plan/Implementation

♦ **General Info:** Monitor vital signs before beginning therapy and at regular intervals (bid or tid) throughout therapy. Take BP lying and standing to monitor for possible hypotensive reaction; elderly are particularly susceptible. Dosage adjustment may be required.

◊ Ensure that patient who is ambulatory is protected from sun when spending time outdoors.

◊ Weigh patient 2–3 times a week, at same time of day, on same scale, if possible. A rapid weight gain or evidence of edema should be reported to physician immediately. Record I&O.

◊ Ensure that patient is protected from injury. Provide supervision and assistance when ambulating if dizziness and drowsiness are problems. Pad siderails and headboard for patient who experiences seizures.

◊ Give patient hard candy, gum, or frequent sips of water if dry mouth is a problem.

◊ Store medication at controlled room temperatures between 15° and 30°C

(59°–86°F). Protect from heat, light, and moisture.

♦ **PO:** Administer oral medication with food to minimize GI upset.

◊ Ensure that patient swallows tablet and does not "cheek" to avoid medication or to hoard for later use.

◊ Tablet may be crushed and mixed with food or fluid for patient who has difficulty swallowing.

◊ When tablet form is unsuitable or refused, syrup form may be used. Dilute in citrus- or chocolate-flavored drinks.

♦ **IM:** IM injection may be irritating to tissues; avoid SC injection.

◊ Inject slowly and deeply into upper, outer quadrant of buttock. Massage site thoroughly following injection.

◊ Because of possible hypotensive effects, patient should remain in recumbent position for at least one-half hour following IM injection.

◊ Rotate sites when multiple injections are administered.

◊ Do not mix with other agents in the syringe.

◊ Avoid injecting undiluted drug into vein. Aspirate carefully before injecting.

♦ **IV:** Reserved for hospitalized patients only; not recommended for routine use.

◊ Because of possible hypotensive effects, drug should be administered with patient in recumbent position.

◊ Monitor blood pressure every 10 minutes during IV administration. Physician may order vasopressor (not epinephrine) if hypotension occurs.

◊ IV solution should never exceed a concentration of 25 mg/mL. May be further diluted with normal saline. Improper dilution can result in thrombophlebitis.

◊ Avoid contact with injectable liquid. A contact dermatitis can occur.

◊ Ensure patency of vein. Extravasation or intra-arterial injection can result in gangrene.

◇ Administer at a rate not exceeding 25 mg/min.

Patient/Family Education

♦ Use caution when driving or operating dangerous machinery. Drowsiness and dizziness can occur.

♦ Do not stop taking the drug abruptly. To do so might produce withdrawal symptoms, such as nausea, vomiting, gastritis, headache, tachycardia, insomnia, tremulousness.

♦ Use sunscreens and wear protective clothing when spending time outdoors. Skin is more susceptible to sunburn.

♦ Report occurrence of any of the following symptoms to physician immediately: sore throat • fever • malaise • unusual bleeding • easy bruising • persistent nausea/vomiting • severe headache • rapid heart rate • difficulty urinating • muscle twitching • tremors • pale stools • yellow skin or eyes • muscular incoordination • or skin rash.

♦ Drug may turn urine pink to reddish-brown in color. This is not significant nor is it harmful.

♦ Rise slowly from a sitting or lying position to prevent a sudden drop in blood pressure.

♦ If dry mouth is a problem, take frequent sips of water, chew sugarless gum, or suck on hard candy. Good oral care (frequent brushing, flossing) is very important.

♦ Consult physician regarding smoking while on promazine therapy. Smoking increases metabolism of promazine, requiring adjustment in dosage to achieve therapeutic effect.

♦ Dress warmly in cold weather, and avoid extended exposure to very high or low temperatures. Body temperature is harder to maintain while taking this medication.

♦ Do not drink alcohol while on promazine therapy. These drugs potentiate each other's effects.

♦ Do not consume other medications (including over-the-counter meds) without physician's approval. Many medications contain substances that interact with promazine in a way that may be harmful.

♦ Be aware of possible risks of taking promazine during pregnancy. Safe use during pregnancy and lactation has not been established. Promazine readily crosses the placental barrier, so a fetus could experience adverse effects of the drug. Inform physician immediately if pregnancy occurs, is suspected, or is planned.

♦ Be aware of side effects of promazine. Refer to written materials furnished by healthcare providers for safe self-administration.

♦ Continue to take medication, even if feeling well and as though it is not needed. Symptoms may return if medication is discontinued.

♦ Carry card or other identification at all times describing medications being taken.

Evaluation

♦ Patient demonstrates a subsiding/resolution of the symptoms for which promazine was prescribed (panic anxiety, altered thought processes, altered perceptions, nausea, and vomiting).

♦ Patient verbalizes understanding of side effects and regimen required for prudent self-administration of promazine.

PROPRANOLOL

(proe-pran'oh-lole)
Inderal

Classification(s):
Beta-adrenergic blocking agent,
Antihypertensive, Antiarrhythmic,
Antianginal
Pregnancy Category C

INDICATIONS

♦ Hypertension ♦ Angina pectoris ♦ Cardiac arrhythmias ♦ Migraine headaches (prophylactic treatment) ♦ Essential tremor. **Investigational Uses:** ♦ Acute exacerbation of schizophrenic disorder and anxiety states ♦ Action tremors (e.g., those induced by lithium carbonate and other psychotropic drugs) ♦ Tardive dyskinesia ♦ Acute panic symptoms ♦ Intermittent explosive disorder.

PHARMACOKINETICS

Absorption: Well absorbed following oral administration.
Distribution: Widely distributed. 90% bound to plasma proteins. Crosses blood-brain and placental barriers. Enters breast milk.
Metabolism and Excretion: Metabolized by the liver. Excreted primarily in urine; small amount excreted in feces.
Half-Life: 2–3 hours, single dose; 3.4–6 hours, multiple dosing.

CONTRAINDICATIONS AND PRECAUTIONS

Contraindicated in: ♦ Hypersensitivity to beta-adrenergic blocking agents ♦ Sinus bradycardia ♦ Heart block greater than first degree ♦ Cardiogenic shock ♦ Congestive heart failure (CHF) ♦ Overt cardiac failure ♦ Bronchial asthma ♦ Bronchospasm ♦ Severe COPD ♦ Allergic rhinitis during the pollen season ♦ Raynaud's syndrome ♦ Malignant hypertension ♦ Children; pregnancy and lactation (safe use has not been established).
Use Cautiously in: ♦ Diabetes mellitus ♦ Patients prone to hypoglycemia ♦ Myasthenia gravis ♦ Wolff-Parkinson-White syndrome ♦ Thyrotoxicosis ♦ Impaired hepatic or renal function ♦ Patients undergoing major surgery ♦ Inadequate cardiac function ♦ Patients with well-compensated heart failure ♦ Sinus node dysfunction.

ADVERSE REACTIONS AND SIDE EFFECTS*

CNS: <u>dizziness</u>, vertigo, <u>fatigue</u>, <u>insomnia</u>, <u>weakness</u>, lethargy, nervousness, diminished concentration, nightmares, sedation, short-term memory loss, slurred speech, tinnitus, ataxia, irritability, hearing loss, confusion.
CV: <u>bradycardia</u>, chest pain, worsening of angina, shortness of breath, <u>peripheral arterial insufficiency</u> (cold extremities, paresthesia of hands), intermittent claudication, CONGESTIVE HEART FAILURE, CEREBRAL VASCULAR ACCIDENT, edema, pulmonary edema, vasodilation, syncope, shock, <u>hypotension</u>, tachycardia, arrhythmias, palpitations, worsening of arterial insufficiency, conduction disturbances, FIRST-DEGREE AND THIRD-DEGREE HEART BLOCK, INTENSIFICATION OF AV BLOCK.
Derm: rash, pruritus, skin irritation, sweating, reversible alopecia, dry skin, peripheral skin necrosis, psoriasiform eruption, hyperkeratosis, nail changes.
Endo: hyperglycemia, hypoglycemia, may mask symptoms of hypoglycemia.
GI: gastric pain, flatulence, constipation, <u>nausea</u>, <u>diarrhea</u>, dry mouth, vomiting, anorexia, bloating, abdominal cramping, renal and mesenteric arterial thrombosis, ischemic colitis, retroperitoneal fibrosis, hepatomegaly, acute pancreatitis, discoloration of tongue.
GU: impotence, decreased libido, dysuria, nocturia, urinary frequency.

*<u>Underlines</u> indicate most frequent; CAPITALS indicate life-threatening.

Hemat: AGRANULOCYTOSIS, nonthrombo-cytopenic or thrombocytopenic purpura, transient eosinophilia.

Ophth: eye irritation or discomfort, vision disturbances, dry or burning eyes, blurred vision, conjunctivitis.

Psych: depression, anxiety, bizarre or many dreams, change in behavior, reversible mental depression progressing to catatonia, hallucinations, emotional lability, paranoia (particularly in the elderly).

Resp: rales, wheeziness, nasal stuffiness, rhinitis, pharyngitis, dyspnea, cough, BRONCHIAL OBSTRUCTION, BRONCHOSPASM, LARYNGOSPASM.

Other: joint pain, muscle cramps, back pain, fever combined with aching and sore throat (allergic reaction), lupus erythematosus-like syndrome (extremely rare), Peyronie's disease.

INTERACTIONS

Drug-Drug: ✦ **Catecholamine depleting drugs (e.g., reserpine):** additive reduction in sympathetic tone, resulting in hypotension, bradycardia, vertigo, syncope ✦ **Digitalis glycosides:** additive depression of AV conduction, potentiation of bradycardia ✦ **IV phenytoin, IV verapamil:** additive cardiac depression ✦ **Sympathomimetics (e.g., ritodrine):** decreased effects of sympathomimetics ✦ **Lidocaine, theophylline:** decreased clearance of these drugs ✦ **Antimuscarinics (e.g., atropine), tricyclic antidepressants:** antagonization of propranolol's cardiac effects ✦ **Smoking:** increased clearance of propranolol ✦ **Propylthiouracil, methimazole:** increased effects of propranolol ✦ **Diuretics, other antihypertensives:** increased hypotensive effects ✦ **Other antiarrhythmics:** potential variation of effect of either or both drugs ✦ **Ergot alkaloids:** (high doses): potential increased peripheral vasoconstriction ✦ **Insulin:** prolonged hypoglycemic effects ✦ **Clonidine:** severe rebound hypertension when clonidine is discontinued abruptly

✦ **Chlorpromazine, cimetidine, oral contraceptives, furosemide, hydralazine:** increased effects of these drugs or propranolol ✦ **Succinylcholine, tubocurarine:** increased effects of these drugs ✦ **Indomethacin, salicylates:** decreased antihypertensive effects of propranolol ✦ **Prazosin:** acute postural hypotension ✦ **IV epinephrine:** rapid rise in blood pressure and excessive bradycardia ✦ **Phenytoin, rifampin, phenobarbital, other barbiturates:** decreased serum propranolol levels ✦ **Nifedipine:** increased likelihood of CHF, severe hypotension, or exacerbation of angina ✦ **Thyroid hormones:** decreased effects of propranolol ✦ **Isoproterenol, norepinephrine, dopamine, dobutamine:** reversal of effects of propranolol, antagonism of effects of other drug; protracted severe hypotension ✦ **Aluminum hydroxide gel:** reduced absorption of propranolol ✦ **Ethanol:** slowed rate of absorption of propranolol ✦ **Phenothiazines:** additive hypotensive and pharmacologic effects of both drugs.

ROUTE AND DOSAGE

Cardiac Arrhythmias

✦ **PO (Adults):** 10–30 mg tid–qid.
✦ **IV (Adults):** (Used only for life-threatening arrhythmias or those occurring under anesthesia.) 0.5–3 mg under careful monitoring (e.g., CVP, ECG). Do not exceed 1 mg/min. May be repeated once after 2 minutes if required. Thereafter, do not administer additional drug in less than 4 hours. Transfer to oral therapy as soon as possible.

Hypertension

✦ **PO (Adults):** Initial dosage: 40 mg bid or 80 mg once daily (sustained-release). Usual range: 160–480 mg/day in two or three divided doses, or 120–160 mg once daily (sustained-release). Maximum daily dose: 640 mg. Dosage increases are made at 3- to 7-day intervals.

Angina Pectoris

* **PO (Adults):** Initial dosage: 10–20 mg tid–qid or 80 mg once daily (sustained-release). Gradually increase initial dosage at 3–7 day intervals until optimum response is obtained. Usual range: 160–240 mg/day. Maximum daily dose: 320 mg. When discontinuing, dosage should be slowly reduced over a period of at least 2 weeks.

Migraine Headaches (Prophylaxis)

* **PO (Adults):** Initial dosage: 80 mg/day in divided doses or once daily (sustained-release). Increase dosage gradually to achieve optimum migraine prophylaxis. Usual range: 160–240 mg/day. After 4–6 weeks of maximal dose without adequate response, propranolol should be discontinued slowly over at least 2 weeks.

Essential Tremors

* **PO (Adults):** Initial dosage: 40 mg PO bid. Usual range: 120–320 mg/day divided into three doses.

Acute Exacerbation of Schizophrenic Disorder/Anxiety States

(Investigational.)
* **PO (Adults):** 80–1920 mg/day (average about 500 mg/day).

Action Tremors

(Investigational.)
* **PO (Adults):** 30–160 mg/day.

Tardive Dyskinesia

(Investigational.)
* **PO (Adults):** 30–80 mg/day.

Acute Panic Symptoms

(Investigational.)
* **PO (Adults):** 40–360 mg/day.

Intermittent Explosive Disorder

(Investigational.)
* **PO (Adults):** 60–640 mg/day (most average 180–280 mg/day) in divided doses. Maximum trial recommendation: 640 mg/day for 4 weeks.

PHARMACODYNAMICS

Route	Onset	Peak	Duration
PO	30 min	60–90 min	4–6 hr
PO (sustained-release)	—	6 hr	24 hr
IV	Immediate	1 min	4–6 hr

NURSING IMPLICATIONS

Assessment

* Assess baseline vital signs. Blood pressure should be taken in both lying and standing positions. Measure pulse both radially and apically. Note respiratory rate, auscultate lung sounds.
* Weigh patient for baseline measurement and daily during therapy. Report gain of 5 pounds. Keep strict records of intake and output.
* Assess extremities for coldness, paresthesia.
* Assess history of allergies, sensitivity to this or other beta-blocking drugs.
* Assess date of last menses (possible pregnancy), use of contraceptives.
* Assess whether currently breast-feeding a child.
* Assess current and past alcohol and drug consumption.
* Assess for operation of automobile and/or other dangerous machinery.
* Assess for presence of adverse reactions or side effects.
* Assess patient/family knowledge about illness and need for medication.
* Assess for symptoms of congestive heart failure: • dyspnea on exertion • orthopnea • night cough • pulmonary rales • distended neck veins • edema.
* **Lab Test Alterations:** Elevated serum aminotransferase, alkaline phosphatase, LDH, potassium, uric acid, serum creatinine, and BUN.
◊ Interference with glaucoma screening test.
◊ May produce hypoglycemia and interfere with glucose or insulin tolerance tests.
* **Withdrawal:** Assess for symptoms of

abrupt withdrawal: • tremulousness • sweating • severe headache • malaise • palpitations • rebound hypertension • myocardial infarction • life-threatening arrhythmias (in patients with angina pectoris) • hyperthyroidism (in patients with thyrotoxicosis).

♦ **Withdrawal Management:** When discontinuing chronically administered propranolol, particularly in patients with ischemic heart disease, dosage should be reduced gradually over 1 to 2 weeks while carefully monitoring the patient.

♦ **Toxicity and Overdose:** Assess for symptoms of overdose: • bradycardia • severe hypotension • cardiogenic shock • intraventricular conduction disturbances • AV block • asystole • pulmonary edema • depressed consciousness • delirium to coma • seizures • respiratory depression • bronchospasm • hypoglycemia • hyperkalemia.

♦ **Overdose Management:** Induce emesis or institute gastric lavage.

◊ Administer activated charcoal.

◊ Maintain adequate airway and ventilation.

◊ Administer IV glucose to treat hypoglycemia.

◊ Administer IV diazepam to treat seizures.

◊ Administer IV atropine to control severe bradycardia.

◊ Administer lidocaine to treat ventricular premature contractions.

◊ In the event of cardiac failure, administer a digitalis glycoside, a diuretic, and oxygen.

◊ In refractory cases, IV aminophylline may be used.

◊ Administer IV fluids to treat hypotension.

◊ Place patient in Trendelenburg position.

◊ Vasopressors (e.g., dopamine, dobutamine, norepinephrine) may be administered with blood pressure monitoring.

◊ Administer isoproterenol for 2nd- or 3rd-degree heart block.

◊ A beta-2 adrenergic agonist or theophylline derivative may be administered to treat bronchospasm.

Potential Nursing Diagnoses

♦ Decreased cardiac output related to altered preload, afterload, or inotropic changes in the heart, or to side effects of propranolol.

♦ Ineffective breathing pattern related to side effects of propranolol.

♦ Pain related to migraine headache (indications for propranolol).

♦ High risk for injury related to side effects of propranolol such as weakness, dizziness; vision changes and overdose; abrupt withdrawal.

♦ Anxiety (severe to panic) related to perceived threat to biological integrity or self-concept (indications for propranolol).

♦ High risk for activity intolerance related to propranolol's side effects of drowsiness, dizziness, weakness; tremors (secondary to side effects of psychotropic drugs).

♦ Knowledge deficit related to medication regimen.

Plan/Implementation

♦ **General Info:** Monitor vital signs daily. Report significant changes to physician.

◊ Weigh patient daily and keep strict records of intake and output.

◊ Ensure that patient is protected from injury. Provide supervision and assistance when ambulating if dizziness, drowsiness, or weakness are problems.

◊ Monitor blood pressure and apical/radial pulse just prior to administration of medication. Physician will provide acceptable parameters for administration. Withhold medication and notify physician immediately if a pronounced change in blood pressure or pulse rate or rhythm occurs.

◊ Store medication at controlled room

temperatures between 15° and 30°C (59°–86°F). Protect from heat, light, and moisture.

* **PO:** Medication may be given before meals to enhance absorption.
◊ Tablet may be crushed and given with fluid of choice for patient who has difficulty swallowing, or oral solution may be administered.
◊ Do not crush or empty contents of sustained-release capsules. Take whole.
* **IV:** IV administration of propranolol is reserved for life-threatening arrhythmias or those occurring under anesthesia.
◊ Medication may be given undiluted, or each 1 mg may be diluted in 10 mL of 5% dextrose in water for injection.
◊ Administer medication at rate not exceeding 1 mg/min.
◊ A 1-mg dose may also be diluted for infusion in 50 mL of normal saline and administered over 10–15 minutes.
◊ Continuous ECG and pulmonary wedge or CVP monitoring is mandatory during administration of IV propranolol. Discontinue drug when rhythm change is noted.
◊ Ensure availability of IV atropine or isoproterenol to counteract profound bradycardia should it occur in response to administration of IV propranolol.

Patient/Family Education

* Medication may be taken before meals to minimize GI upset and to enhance absorption. Tablet may be crushed and mixed with fluid of choice if swallowing is difficult, or solution form may be used. Do not crush, chew, or empty contents of sustained-release capsules.
* Use caution when driving or when operating dangerous machinery. Drowsiness, dizziness, weakness, and vision changes can occur.
* Do not discontinue drug abruptly. Serious withdrawal symptoms could occur.

* Report occurrence of any of the following symptoms to physician immediately: • slow pulse rate • dizziness • light-headedness • confusion or depression • skin rash • fever • sore throat • unusual bruising or bleeding • difficulty breathing • night cough • swelling of the extremities.
* Take pulse before each dose. Report significant increase or decrease to physician.
* Avoid smoking while on propranolol therapy. Smoking decreases the effectiveness of this drug.
* Propranolol may have an effect on blood glucose levels. Diabetic patients should adhere strictly to diet as prescribed. Monitor glucose levels daily or as ordered. Report positive results to physician. Be aware of potential for propranolol to mask early signs of hypoglycemia.
* Do not consume other medications (including over-the-counter meds) without physician's approval. Many medications contain substances that may interact with propranolol in a way that could be harmful.
* Be aware of possible risks of taking propranolol during pregnancy. Safe use during pregnancy and lactation has not been established. Propranolol crosses the placental barrier. Therefore, a fetus could experience adverse effects of the drug. Inform physician immediately if pregnancy occurs, is suspected, or is planned.
* Be aware of side effects of propranolol. Refer to written materials furnished by healthcare providers for safe self-administration.
* Carry card or other identification at all times describing medications being taken.

Evaluation

* Patient demonstrates a resolution/subsiding of the symptoms for which propranolol was prescribed (hypertension, angina, cardiac arrhythmias,

prophylaxis for migraine headaches, tremors, anxiety, schizophrenia, tardive dyskinesia, explosive behavior).
* Patient verbalizes understanding of side effects and regimen required for prudent self-administration of propranolol.

PROTRIPTYLINE

(proe-trip'te-leen)
{Triptil}, Vivactil

Classification(s):
Tricyclic antidepressant
Pregnancy Category C

INDICATIONS

* Major depression with melancholia or psychotic symptoms. **Investigational Use:** * Obstructive sleep apnea.

ACTION

* Exact mechanism of action unclear * Blocks the reuptake of the neurotransmitters norepinephrine and serotonin, increasing their concentration at the synapse and correcting the deficit that is thought to contribute to the melancholy mood of the depressed person.

PHARMACOKINETICS

Absorption: Readily absorbed from the GI tract following oral administration.
Distribution: Is widely distributed. Crosses blood-brain and placental barriers. Enters breast milk.
Metabolism and Excretion: Metabolized by the liver. Excreted by the kidneys.
Half-Life: 55–124 hours (avg. 80 hr).

CONTRAINDICATIONS AND PRECAUTIONS

Contraindicated in: * Hypersensitivity to this drug or to other tricyclic antide-

pressants * Concomitant use of MAO inhibitors * Acute recovery period following myocardial infarction * Untreated angle-closure glaucoma * Children; pregnancy and lactation (safety not established).
Use Cautiously in: * Patients with a history of seizures * Urinary retention * Benign prostatic hypertrophy * Glaucoma * Thyroid disease * Cardiovascular disorders * Respiratory difficulties * Hepatic or renal insufficiency * Psychotic patients * Elderly or debilitated patients.

ADVERSE REACTIONS AND SIDE EFFECTS*

CNS: drowsiness, dizziness, weakness, headache, fatigue, confusion, lethargy, memory deficits, disturbed concentration, tremors, ataxia, tinnitus, extrapyramidal symptoms, paresthesias of extremities, lowered seizure threshold, blurred vision, agitation, excitement, restlessness, insomnia, exacerbation of psychosis, shift to manic behavior.
CV: orthostatic hypotension, tachycardia and other arrhythmias, hypertension, MYOCARDIAL INFARCTION, HEART BLOCK, CONGESTIVE HEART FAILURE, ECG changes, syncope, CARDIOVASCULAR COLLAPSE.
Derm: skin rash, urticaria, photosensitivity, erythema, petechiae.
GI: dry mouth, constipation, nausea, vomiting, anorexia, diarrhea, abdominal cramps, adynamic ileus, esophageal reflux, stomatitis, black tongue.
GU: urinary retention, gynecomastia (men), testicular swelling, menstrual irregularity, breast engorgement and galactorrhea (women), changes in libido, impotence, delayed micturation.
Hemat: AGRANULOCYTOSIS, THROMBOCYTOPENIA, LEUKOPENIA, eosinophilia, purpura.
Hepat: jaundice, hepatitis.
Other: weight gain, nasal congestion, al-

{} = Only available in Canada.
*Underlines indicate most frequent; CAPITALS indicate life-threatening.

opecia, hypothermia, peripheral neuropathy.

INTERACTIONS

Drug-Drug: ✦ **MAO inhibitors:** hyperpyretic crisis, hypertensive crisis, severe seizures, tachycardia, death ✦ **Guanethidine, clonidine, (possibly) guanabenz:** decreased effects of these medications ✦ **Cimetidine:** increased protriptyline serum levels ✦ **Amphetamines, sympathomimetics:** increased hypertensive and cardiac effects of these drugs ✦ **CNS depressants (including alcohol, barbiturates, benzodiazepines):** potentiation of CNS effects ✦ **Thyroid medications:** tachycardia, arrhythmias ✦ **Methylphenidate, phenothiazines, haloperidol:** increased serum protriptyline levels ✦ **Ethchlorvynol:** transient delirium ✦ **Quinidine, procainamide, disopyramide:** potentiates adverse cardiovascular effects of protriptyline ✦ **Oral contraceptives:** decreased effects of protriptyline ✦ **Smoking:** increased protriptyline metabolism ✦ **Disulfiram:** decreased protriptyline metabolism ✦ **Levodopa, phenylbutazone:** delayed or decreased absorption of these drugs ✦ **Dicumarol:** increased plasma dicumarol concentrations.

ROUTE AND DOSAGE

Depression

- ✦ **PO (Adults):** 15–40 mg/day divided into 3 or 4 doses. Dosage may be increased to a maximum of 60 mg/day. Increases should be made in the morning dose.
- ✦ **PO (Adolescents, Geriatrics):** Initially, 5 mg tid. Increase gradually, if necessary. Monitor CV system closely in elderly patients if dose exceeds 20 mg/day.
- ✦ **PO (Maintenance):** Reduce to lowest dosage that will provide relief of symptoms.

Obstructive Sleep Apnea

(Investigational.)
- ✦ **PO (Adults):** 10–60 mg/day.

PHARMACODYNAMICS

Route	Onset	Peak	Duration
PO	2–4 wk	24–30 hr	Weeks*

*Allow up to 2 weeks following cessation of therapy for complete drug elimination.

NURSING IMPLICATIONS

Assessment

- ✦ Assess for suicidal ideation, plan, means. Assess for sudden lifts in mood, which could indicate patient's decision to commit suicide.
- ✦ Assess mental status daily: • mood • appearance • thought and communication patterns • level of interest in the environment and in activities • suicidal ideation. Improvement in these behavior patterns and level of energy should be expected within 2–4 weeks following initiation of therapy.
- ✦ Assess for symptoms of blood dyscrasias: • sore throat • fever • malaise • unusual bleeding • easy bruising.
- ✦ Assess vital signs, weight.
- ✦ Assess history of allergies, sensitivity to this drug or to other tricyclic antidepressants.
- ✦ Assess for history of glaucoma.
- ✦ Assess date of last menses (possible pregnancy), use of contraceptives.
- ✦ Assess whether currently breast-feeding a child.
- ✦ Assess current and past alcohol and drug consumption.
- ✦ Assess for operation of automobile and/or other dangerous machinery.
- ✦ Assess for presence of adverse reactions or side effects.
- ✦ Assess patient/family knowledge about illness and need for medication.
- ✦ In collaboration with physician, assess CBC and liver function tests in patients on long-term therapy.
- ✦ **Lab Test Alterations:** Increased se-

rum bilirubin, alkaline phosphatase, transaminase, and glucose.

◇ Decreased urinary 5-hydroxyindole-acetic acid (HIAA) and vanillylmandelic acid (VMA) excretion.

✦ **Withdrawal:** Assess for symptoms of abrupt withdrawal from long-term therapy: ● nausea ● headache ● vertigo ● malaise ● insomnia ● nightmares.

✦ **Toxicity and Overdose:** Range of therapeutic serum concentration not well substantiated.

◇ Assess for symptoms of overdose: ● confusion ● agitation ● irritability ● hallucinations ● seizures ● flushing ● dry mouth ● dilated pupils ● delirium ● hyperpyrexia ● hypotension or hypertension ● coma ● tachycardia ● arrhythmias ● respiratory depression ● cardiac arrest ● renal failure ● shock ● congestive heart failure ● acid-base disturbances.

✦ **Overdose Management:** Monitor vital signs.

◇ Ensure maintenance of adequate airway.

◇ Monitor ECG.

◇ Induce emesis in conscious patient.

◇ Follow emesis with gastric lavage and activated charcoal to minimize absorption.

◇ Initiate gastric lavage in unconscious patient.

◇ Administer IV fluids.

◇ Administer IV physostigmine cautiously to reverse anticholinergic effects.

◇ Administer sodium bicarbonate, vasopressors, phenytoin, propranolol, or lidocaine to treat cardiovascular effects.

◇ Administer IV diazepam to control seizures.

Potential Nursing Diagnoses

✦ High risk for self-directed violence related to depressed mood.

✦ High risk for injury related to protriptyline's side effects of sedation, dizziness, ataxia, weakness, confusion, lowered seizure threshold; abrupt

withdrawal after prolonged use; overdose.

✦ Social isolation related to depressed mood.

✦ High risk for activity intolerance related to protriptyline's side effects of drowsiness, dizziness, ataxia, weakness, and confusion.

✦ Knowledge deficit related to medication regimen.

Plan/Implementation

✦ Monitor vital signs before beginning therapy and at regular intervals (bid or tid) throughout therapy. Take BP lying and standing in patients experiencing orthostatic hypotension; elderly are particularly susceptible. Contact physician if tachycardia/arrhythmias are noted.

✦ Ensure that patient who is ambulatory is protected from sun when spending time outdoors.

✦ Weigh patient 2–3 times a week, at same time of day, on same scale, if possible. A rapid weight gain or evidence of edema should be reported to physician immediately. Record I&O.

✦ Ensure that patient is protected from injury. Provide supervision and assistance when ambulating if dizziness and drowsiness are problems. Pad siderails and headboard for patient who experiences seizures.

✦ Give patient hard candy, gum, or frequent sips of water if dry mouth is a problem.

✦ Medication may be administered with food to minimize GI upset.

✦ Ensure that patient swallows tablet and does not "cheek" to avoid medication or to hoard for later use.

✦ Tablet may be crushed and mixed with food or fluid for patient who has difficulty swallowing.

✦ Store medication in tightly closed container. Avoid storage at temperatures above 40°C (104°F).

Patient/Family Education

✦ Therapeutic effect may not be seen for as long as 4 weeks. If after this length of time no improvement is noted, physician may prescribe a different medication. Continue to take medication even though symptoms have not subsided.

♦ Use caution when driving or when operating dangerous machinery. Drowsiness and dizziness can occur. If these side effects become persistent or interfere with activities of daily living, report to physician. Dosage adjustment may be necessary.

♦ Do not stop taking the drug abruptly. To do so might produce withdrawal symptoms, such as nausea, vertigo, insomnia, headache, malaise, nightmares.

♦ Use sunscreens and wear protective clothing when spending time outdoors. Skin may be sensitive to sunburn.

♦ Report occurrence of any of the following symptoms to physician immediately: • sore throat • fever • malaise • unusual bleeding • easy bruising • persistent nausea/vomiting • severe headache • rapid heart rate • difficulty urinating.

♦ Rise slowly from a sitting or lying position to prevent a sudden drop in blood pressure.

♦ If dry mouth is a problem, take frequent sips of water, chew sugarless gum, or suck on hard candy. Good oral care (frequent brushing, flossing) is very important.

♦ Do not smoke while on protriptyline therapy. Smoking increases metabolism of protriptyline, requiring adjustment in dosage to achieve therapeutic effect.

♦ Do not drink alcohol while on protriptyline therapy. These drugs potentiate each other's effects.

♦ Do not consume other medications (including over-the-counter meds) with protriptyline without physician's approval. Many medications contain substances that, in combination with tricyclics, could precipitate a life-threatening hypertensive crisis.

♦ Be aware of possible risks of taking protriptyline during pregnancy. Safe use during pregnancy and lactation has not been established. Protriptyline readily crosses the placental barrier, so a fetus could experience adverse effects of the drug. Inform physician immediately if pregnancy occurs, is suspected, or is planned.

♦ Be aware of side effects of protriptyline. Refer to written materials furnished by healthcare providers for safe self-administration.

♦ Carry card or other identification at all times describing medications being taken.

Evaluation

♦ Patient demonstrates a subsiding/resolution of the symptoms for which protriptyline was prescribed (depressed mood, suicidal ideation, obstructive sleep apnea).

♦ Patient verbalizes understanding of side effects and regimen required for prudent self-administration of protriptyline.

RISPERIDONE

(ris-per'id-own)
Risperdal

Classification(s):
Antipsychotic; Neuroleptic;
Benzisoxazole derivative
Pregnancy Category C

INDICATIONS

♦ Schizophrenia and related psychoses (short-term use: 6–8 weeks). **Investigational Use:** ♦ Adjunctive therapy of behavioral disturbances in patients with mental retardation.

ACTION

♦ The exact mechanism of antipsychotic action is not fully understood ♦ Risperidone is thought to be a selective monoaminergic antagonist with high affinity for the serotonin type 2 ($5HT_2$) and dopamine type 2 (D_2) receptors.

PHARMACOKINETICS

Absorption: Rapidly absorbed following oral administration.

Distribution: Widely distributed. Approximately 90% protein bound. Unknown if risperidone enters breast milk.

Metabolism and Excretion: Extensively metabolized in the liver to its major active metabolite 9-hydroxyrisperidone. Excreted in the urine.

Half-Life: 3–20 hours (risperidone). 21–30 hours (9-hydroxyrisperidone).

CONTRAINDICATIONS AND PRECAUTIONS

Contraindicated in: ◆ Known hypersensitivity to this drug.

Use Cautiously in: ◆ Patients with cardiovascular disease, cerebrovascular disease, and conditions that would predispose to hypotension ◆ Patients with history of seizures ◆ Patients with previously diagnosed breast cancer ◆ Suicidal patients ◆ Patients with hepatic or renal insufficiency ◆ Elderly and debilitated patients ◆ Safety and efficacy in children, pregnancy, and lactation has not been established.

ADVERSE REACTIONS AND SIDE EFFECTS*

CNS: <u>sedation</u>, <u>drowsiness</u>, <u>insomnia</u>, <u>agitation</u>, <u>anxiety</u>, <u>somnolence</u>, <u>aggression</u>, extrapyramidal symptoms, <u>headache</u>, dizziness, fatigue, impaired concentration, apathy, disinhibition, catatonia, tardive dyskinesia, NEUROLEPTIC MALIGNANT SYNDROME.

CV: <u>tachycardia</u>, <u>orthostatic hypotension</u>, palpitations, hypertension, bradycardia, chest pain, ECG changes.

Derm: rash, dry skin, seborrhea, photosensitivity.

Endo: elevated serum prolactin levels,

gynecomastia, male breast pain, antidiuretic hormone disorder.

GI: <u>constipation</u>, <u>nausea</u>, dyspepsia, vomiting, abdominal pain, increased salivation, toothache, dry mouth, anorexia, increased appetite, weight gain or loss.

GU: urinary retention, erectile dysfunction, ejaculatory dysfunction, orgastic dysfunction, priapism.

Hemat: epistaxis, purpura, ANEMIA, THROMBOCYTOPENIA.

MS: arthralgia, back pain, myalgia.

Ocular: abnormal vision.

Resp: <u>rhinitis</u>, coughing, sinusitis, pharyngitis, dyspnea, upper respiratory infections.

Other: decreased sweating, increased sweating, fever.

INTERACTIONS

Drug-Drug: ◆ **Other CNS active drugs and alcohol:** may have additive CNS effects ◆ **Antihypertensive agents:** increased antihypertensive effects ◆ **Carbamazepine:** increased risperidone clearance ◆ **Clozapine:** decreased risperidone clearance ◆ **Levodopa:** decreased effects of levodopa ◆ **Dopamine agonists:** decreased effects of these drugs.

ROUTE AND DOSAGE

Schizophrenia and Related Psychoses

◆ **PO (Adults):** Initial dose: 1 mg bid. Progressively increase dosage by 1 mg bid on the second and third days, to a target dose of 3 mg bid by the third day. If indicated, further dosage adjustments may occur at intervals of not less than 1 week and in recommended small-dose increments/decrements of 1 mg bid.

Patients with Renal or Hepatic Impairment; Patients at Risk for Hypotension; Elderly or Debilitated Patients

◆ **PO (Adults):** Initial dose: 0.5 mg bid. Dosage increases should occur in in-

---

*<u>Underlines</u> indicate most frequent; CAPITALS indicate life-threatening.

crements of 0.5 mg bid. Dosage increases above 1.5 mg bid should occur at intervals of not less than 1 week.

Reinitiation of Treatment in Patients Previously Discontinued
♦ **PO (Adults):** Follow the 3-day dose titration schedule recommended for initiation of therapy.

Switching from Other Antipsychotics
♦ **PO (Adults):** It is recommended, when medically appropriate, to discontinue the previous antipsychotic treatment upon initiation of risperidone. In all cases, the period of overlapping antipsychotic administration should be minimized. When switching patients from depot antipsychotics, initiate risperidone therapy in place of the next scheduled injection.

PHARMACODYNAMICS

Route	Onset	Peak*	Duration
PO	30–60 min	1–2 hr	10–12 hr

*Steady-state plasma levels are achieved in approximately 1–5 days.

NURSING IMPLICATIONS
Assessment
♦ Assess mental status daily: • mood • appearance • thought and communication patterns • level of interest in the environment and in activities • level of anxiety or agitation • presence of hallucinations or delusions • suspiciousness • interactions with others • ability to carry out activities of daily living.
♦ Assess for symptoms of blood dyscrasias: • sore throat • fever • malaise • unusual bleeding • easy bruising.
♦ Assess for extrapyramidal symptoms: • psuedoparkinsonism (tremors, shuffling gait, drooling, rigidity) • akinesia (muscular weakness) • akathisia (continuous restlessness and fidgeting) • dystonia (involuntary muscular movements of face, arms,

legs, and neck) • oculogyric crisis (uncontrolled rolling back of the eyes) • tardive dyskinesia (bizarre facial and tongue movements, stiff neck, difficulty swallowing).
♦ Assess vital signs, weight. Record baseline values for comparison.
♦ Assess history of allergies and sensitivity to this drug.
♦ Assess date of last menses (possible pregnancy); use of contraceptives.
♦ Assess if currently breast-feeding a child.
♦ Assess patient/family history of breast cancer.
♦ Assess history of seizures.
♦ Assess patient/family history of cardiovascular disease.
♦ Assess current and past alcohol and drug consumption.
♦ Assess operation of automobile and/or other dangerous machinery.
♦ Assess for presence of adverse reactions or side effects.
♦ Assess patient/family knowledge about illness and need for medication.
♦ In collaboration with physician, assess CBC, ECG, liver, and renal function tests in patients on long-term therapy.
♦ Assess for symptoms of neuroleptic malignant syndrome: • hyperpyrexia up to 107°F (41.6°C) • elevated pulse • increased or decreased blood pressure • severe parkinsonian muscle rigidity • elevated creatinine phosphokinase blood levels • elevated white blood count • altered mental status (including catatonic signs or agitation) • acute renal failure • varying levels of consciousness (including stupor and coma) • pallor diaphoresis, tachycardia, arrhythmias, rhabdomyolysis.
♦ **Management of Neuroleptic Malignant Syndrome:** • discontinue risperidone immediately • monitor vital signs, degree of muscle rigidity, I&O, level of consciousness • provide intensive symptomatic treatment and medical monitoring • physician may order

bromocriptine (Parlodel) or dantrolene (Dantrium) to counteract the effects of NMS.

+ **Lab Test Alterations:** • elevated serum AST and ALT • decrease in plasma gammaglutamyl transferase • elevated serum prolactin levels.

+ **Withdrawal:** Assess for symptoms of abrupt withdrawal from long-term therapy: gastritis • nausea • vomiting • dizziness • headache • tachycardia • insomnia • tremulousness • sweating.

+ **Toxicity and Overdose:** No correlation has been established between blood level and therapeutic effect • Assess for symptoms of overdose: drowsiness • sedation • tachycardia • hypotension • exaggerated extrapyramidal symptoms • hyponatremia • hypokalemia • ECG alterations • seizures.

+ **Overdose Management:** • monitor vital signs • ensure maintenance of open airway, adequate oxygenation, and ventilation • initiate gastric lavage (after intubation, if patient is unconscious) and administer activated charcoal • do not induce emesis (possible nuchal rigidity, seizures, or obstruction may result in aspiration of vomitus) • antiparkinsonism drugs or diphenhydramine may be given to counteract extrapyramidal symptoms • IV fluids or administration of a vasoconstrictor to maintain adequate blood pressure • **Note:** epinephrine and dopamine should not be used since beta stimulation may worsen hypotension in the setting of risperidone-induced alpha blockade • cardiac monitoring should commence immediately to detect possible arrhythmias. If antiarrhythmic therapy is administered, avoid use of disopyramide, procainamide, or quinidine, as they could result in additive QT-prolonging effects of risperidone. Similarly, do not use bretylium, as the interaction could result in additive alpha-blocking properties, causing problematic hypotension.

Potential Nursing Diagnoses

+ High risk for violence directed at others related to mistrust and panic anxiety.

+ High risk for injury related to risperidone's side effects of sedation, dizziness, EPS, lowered seizure threshold; abrupt withdrawal after prolonged use; overdose; neuroleptic malignant syndrome.

+ Sensory-perceptual alteration related to panic anxiety evidenced by hallucinations.

+ Altered thought processes related to panic anxiety evidenced by delusional thinking.

+ Social isolation related to inability to trust others.

+ High risk for activity intolerance related to risperidone's side effects of drowsiness, dizziness, ataxia, and weakness.

+ Noncompliance with medication regimen related to suspiciousness and mistrust of others.

+ Knowledge deficit related to medication regimen.

Plan/Implementation

+ Monitor vital signs before beginning therapy and at regular intervals (bid or tid) throughout therapy. Take BP lying and standing to monitor for possible hypotensive reaction. Elderly are particularly susceptible. Dosage adjustment may be required.

+ Ensure that patient who is ambulatory is protected from sun when spending time outdoors.

+ Weigh patient 2–3 times a week, at same time of day, on same scale, if possible. A rapid weight gain, or evidence of edema, should be reported to physician immediately. Record I&O.

+ Ensure that patient is protected from injury. Provide supervision and assistance when ambulating if dizziness and drowsiness are problems. Pad siderails and headboard for patient who experiences seizures.

♦ May administer oral medication with food to patient who experiences GI upset.

♦ Ensure patient swallows tablet and does not "cheek" to avoid medication or hoard for later use.

♦ Crush tablet and mix with food or fluid for patient who has difficulty swallowing.

♦ Store all forms at controlled room temperatures between 15° and 30°C (59°–86°F). Protect from light and moisture.

Patient/Family Education

♦ Use caution when driving or operating dangerous machinery. Drowsiness and dizziness can occur.

♦ Do not stop taking the drug abruptly. To do so might produce withdrawal symptoms, such as nausea, vomiting, gastritis, headache, tachycardia, insomnia, tremulousness.

♦ Use sunscreens and wear protective clothing when spending time outdoors. Skin is more susceptible to sunburn.

♦ Report occurrence of any of the following symptoms to physician immediately: • sore throat • fever • malaise • unusual bleeding • easy bruising • persistent nausea/vomiting • severe headache • rapid heart rate • difficulty urinating • muscle twitching • tremors • darkly colored urine • pale stools • yellow skin or eyes • muscular incoordination • skin rash.

♦ Rise slowly from a sitting or lying position to prevent a sudden drop in blood pressure.

♦ Dress warmly in cold weather, and avoid extended exposure to very high or low temperatures. Body temperature is harder to maintain with this medication.

♦ Do not drink alcohol while on risperidone therapy. These drugs potentiate the effects of each other.

♦ Do not consume other medications (including over-the-counter meds) without physician's approval. Many medications contain substances that may interact with risperidone in a way that could be harmful.

♦ Be aware of possible risks of taking risperidone during pregnancy. Safe use during pregnancy and lactation has not been established. It is not known whether risperidone crosses placental barrier or enters breast milk.

♦ Be aware of side effects of risperidone. Refer to written materials furnished by healthcare providers for safe self-administration.

♦ Continue to take medication, even if feeling well and as though it is not needed. Symptoms may return if medication is discontinued.

♦ Carry card or other identification at all times describing medications being taken.

Evaluation

♦ Patient demonstrates a subsiding/resolution of the symptoms for which risperidone was prescribed (panic anxiety; altered thought processes; altered sensory perceptions; aggressive behavior).

♦ Patient verbalizes understanding of side effects and regimen required for prudent self-administration of risperidone.

SCOPOLAMINE

(skoe-pol′a-meen)
Hyoscine, Transderm-scop, Triptone

Classification(s):
Anticholinergic, Antimuscarinic, Mydriatic, Antispasmodic
Pregnancy Category C

INDICATIONS

♦ Nausea and vomiting associated with motion sickness ♦ Preoperative or preprocedural (including ECT) use to decrease secretions ♦ peptic ulcer and other GI conditions.

ACTION

♦ Competitively inhibits the muscarinic actions of acetylcholine at postganglionic parasympathetic neuroeffector sites, including smooth muscle, secretory glands, and sites within the central nervous system ♦ Specific anticholinergic responses are dose-related ♦ More potent than atropine.

PHARMACOKINETICS

Absorption: Well absorbed from the GI tract, mucous membranes, skin, and eyes.
Distribution: Not well known. Thought to be widely distributed. Crosses blood-brain and placental barriers. Unknown if drug enters breast milk.
Metabolism and Excretion: Metabolized by the liver. Excreted in urine.
Half-Life: 8 hours.

CONTRAINDICATIONS AND PRECAUTIONS

Contraindicated in: ♦ Hypersensitivity to anticholinergic drugs ♦ Angle-closure glaucoma ♦ Adhesions between the iris and lens ♦ Tachycardia ♦ Unstable cardiovascular status in acute hemorrhage ♦ Myocardial ischemia ♦ Obstructive disease of the GI tract ♦ Paralytic ileus ♦ Intestinal atony of the elderly or debilitated patient ♦ Severe ulcerative colitis ♦ Toxic megacolon complicating ulcerative colitis ♦ Obstructive uropathy ♦ Myasthenia gravis ♦ Cardiospasm.
Use Cautiously in: ♦ Autonomic neuropathy ♦ Glaucoma ♦ Hepatic disease ♦ Mild to moderate ulcerative colitis ♦ Esophageal reflux ♦ Hiatal hernia associated with reflux esophagitis ♦ Renal disease ♦ Prostatic hypertrophy ♦ Hyperthyroidism ♦ Coronary heart disease ♦ Congestive heart failure ♦ Cardiac tachy-

arrhythmias ♦ Hypertension ♦ Chronic lung disease ♦ Infants and small children ♦ Down's syndrome ♦ Brain damage ♦ Patients exposed to elevated environmental temperatures ♦ Febrile patients ♦ Geriatric patients ♦ Gastric ulcer ♦ GI infections ♦ Diarrhea ♦ Partial obstructive uropathy.

ADVERSE REACTIONS AND SIDE EFFECTS*

CNS: headache, flushing, nervousness, depression, drowsiness, weakness, dizziness, insomnia, fever, mental confusion, excitement, restlessness, tremor, disorientation, fatigue, delirium, behavioral changes.
CV: palpitations, bradycardia (with low doses), tachycardia (with high doses).
Derm: urticaria and other dermal manifestations.
GI: xerostomia (dry mouth), husky voice, altered taste perception, nausea, vomiting, dysphagia, heartburn, constipation, bloated feeling, PARALYTIC ILEUS, gastroesophageal reflux.
GU: urinary retention, urinary hesitancy, impotence.
Ophth: blurred vision, mydriasis, photophobia, cycloplegia, increased intraocular pressure, dilated pupils.
Resp: DEPRESSED RESPIRATION.
Other: ANAPHYLAXIS, suppression of lactation, nasal congestion, decreased sweating.

INTERACTIONS

Drug-Drug: ♦ **Antihistamines, glutethimide, disopyramide, procainamide, quinidine, antipsychotics, antiparkinsonian agents, buclizine, meperidine, orphenadrine, amantadine, benzodiazepines, tricyclic antidepressants, MAO inhibitors:** enhanced anticholinergic effects ♦ **Nitrates, nitrites, alkalinizing agents, primidone, thioxanthenes, methyl-**

---

*Underlines indicate most frequent; CAPITALS indicate life-threatening.

phenidate: potentiation of adverse effects of scopolamine ◆ **Long-term therapy with corticosteroids or haloperidol:** increased intraocular pressure ◆ **Guanethidine, histamine, reserpine:** decreased effects of scopolamine ◆ **Sympathomimetics, nitrofurantoin, thiazide diuretics:** increased effects of these drugs ◆ **Cholinesterase inhibitors, metoclopramide:** decreased effects of these drugs ◆ **Digitalis, slow-release digoxin tablets, cholinergics, neostigmine:** increased potential for adverse effects ◆ **Antacids:** possible interference with absorption of anticholinergics ◆ **Cyclopropane anesthesia:** possible ventricular arrhythmias.

ROUTE AND DOSAGE

Preoperative or Preprocedural Medication, Obstetric Amnesia/Sedation

◆ **SC, IM, IV (Adults):** 0.32–0.65 mg.
◆ **SC, IM, IV (Children):** 0.006 mg/kg. Maximum dosage: 0.3 mg.

Prevention of Motion Sickness

◆ **PO (Adults):** 0.25 mg 1 hour before anticipated travel. Dosage may be repeated in 4 hours if needed. Maximum dosage: 1 mg/24 hours.
◆ **Transdermal (Adults):** Apply one patch to postauricular skin at least 4 hours before antiemetic effect is required. Delivers 0.5 mg scopolamine over 72 hours. May be replaced with a new patch at a different postauricular site q 72 hours if needed for continuous therapy. System may be removed and site washed thoroughly when antiemetic effect is no longer desired.

PHARMACODYNAMICS

Route	Onset	Peak	Duration
PO, IM, SC	30 min	60–120 min	4–6 hr
IV	10 min	60 min	2–4 hr
Transdermal	4 hr	—	3 days*

*If patch remains intact.

NURSING IMPLICATIONS

Assessment

◆ Assess mood daily in patient receiving ECT: ● appearance ● speech and thought patterns ● behavior ● interaction with others ● somatic complaints ● attendance in activities ● evidence of excitement or agitation.
◆ Assess for symptoms of paralytic ileus: ● constipation ● abdominal pain and distention ● absence of bowel sounds. Patients taking scopolamine concomitantly with other drugs that produce anticholinergic effects are particularly susceptible.
◆ Assess vital signs prior to administration. Record baseline values for comparison.
◆ Assess history of allergies, sensitivity to this drug or to other anticholinergic drugs.
◆ Assess date of last menses (possible pregnancy), use of contraceptives.
◆ Assess whether currently breast-feeding a child.
◆ Assess current and past alcohol and drug consumption.
◆ Assess for operation of automobile and/or other dangerous machinery.
◆ Assess for presence of adverse reactions or side effects.
◆ Assess patient/family knowledge about illness and need for medication.
◆ **Toxicity and Overdose:** Assess for symptoms of overdose: ● dry mouth ● thirst ● dysphagia ● vomiting ● nausea ● abdominal distention ● muscular weakness ● CNS stimulation followed by depression ● delirium ● confusion ● behavioral changes ● drowsiness ● restlessness ● stupor ● fever ● dizziness ● headache ● seizures ● tremor ● hallucinations ● anxiety ● ataxia ● psychotic behavior ● rapid pulse and respiration ● tachycardia with weak pulse ● hypertension ● palpitations ● urinary retention ● blurred vision ● photophobia ● dilated pupils ● leukocytosis ● flushed, hot, dry skin ●

rash over face, neck, and upper trunk • diminished or absent bowel sounds • hypotension • coma • skeletal muscle paralysis • respiratory failure • circulatory failure.

✦ **Overdose Management:** Induce emesis or initiate gastric lavage.
◇ Administer activated charcoal slurry.
◇ Ensure maintenance of adequate airway and ventilation.
◇ Continuously monitor ECG.
◇ Protect patient from injury due to seizures.
◇ Administer physostigmine by slow IV injection to reverse anticholinergic effects.
◇ Administer benzodiazepines or short-acting barbiturates to control excitement.
◇ Initiate fluid therapy and administer levarterenol to control hypotension and circulatory collapse.
◇ Apply cold packs or other cooling measures to treat hyperpyrexia.
◇ Darken room if photophobia occurs.

Potential Nursing Diagnoses
✦ High risk for self-directed violence related to depressed mood.
✦ High risk for injury related to side effects of scopolamine such as weakness, blurred vision, dizziness and delirium, overdose.
✦ Hyperthermia related to anticholinergic effect of decreased sweating.
✦ Altered thought processes related to side effects of scopolamine evidenced by mental confusion.
✦ Anxiety (moderate to severe) related to pending medical procedure (surgery, ECT).
✦ High risk for activity intolerance related to scopolamine's side effects of drowsiness, dizziness, weakness, mental confusion.
✦ Knowledge deficit related to medication regimen.

Plan/Implementation
✦ **General Info:** Monitor vital signs daily. Report any changes to physician.

Withhold dosage if pulse rate is markedly increased or decreased and contact physician immediately.
◇ Weigh patient 2–3 times a week, at same time of day, on same scale, if possible. A rapid weight gain or evidence of edema should be reported to physician immediately. Record I&O.
◇ Ensure that patient is protected from injury. Provide supervision and assistance when ambulating if dizziness and drowsiness are problems.
◇ Give patient hard candy, gum, or frequent sips of water if dry mouth is a problem, or treat with saliva substitute.
◇ Store medication at controlled room temperatures between 15° and 30°C (59°–86°F). Protect from heat, light, and moisture.
✦ **PO:** Medication may be administered prior to or with meals to minimize gastric irritation.
◇ Do not administer medication concurrently with antacids, as they may interfere with absorption of scopolamine.
✦ **SC, IM, IV:** Medication may be administered SC, IM, or IV. Most frequently used SC or IM. Rarely given IV.
◇ SC and IM medication may be given undiluted.
◇ Dilute desired IV dose in at least 10 mL of sterile water for injection.
◇ Administer IV at rate not exceeding 0.6 mg/min.
✦ **Transdermal:** Wash hands before and after applying the patch.
◇ Place on clean, dry, hairless area behind ear.
◇ Apply at least 4 hours before antiemetic effect is required.
◇ If second application is required after 3 days, remove first patch and apply second patch behind other ear.
◇ Remove patch when antiemetic effect is no longer desired.

Patient/Family Education

♦ Medication may be taken with meals to minimize GI upset.

♦ Use caution when driving or when operating dangerous machinery. Drowsiness, dizziness, and blurred vision can occur.

♦ Report occurrence of any of the following symptoms to physician immediately: extreme dryness of mouth, difficulty urinating, constipation, fast and pounding heartbeat, eye pain, rash, vision disturbances, behavioral or mental changes.

♦ Sensitivity to light can be relieved by wearing sunglasses and keeping room darkened.

♦ Stay inside in air-conditioned room when weather is very hot. Perspiration is decreased by scopolamine, and the body cannot cool itself as well. There is greater susceptibility to heat stroke. Inform physician if air-conditioned housing and/or work environment is not available.

♦ If dry mouth is a problem, take frequent sips of water, chew sugarless gum, suck on hard candy, or use a saliva substitute. Good oral care (frequent brushing, flossing) is very important.

♦ Do not consume other medications (including over-the-counter meds) without physician's approval. Many medications contain substances that interact with scopolamine in a way that may be harmful.

♦ Be aware of possible risks of taking scopolamine during pregnancy. Safe use during pregnancy and lactation has not been established. Scopolamine readily crosses the placental barrier, so a fetus could experience adverse effects of the drug. Inform physician immediately if pregnancy occurs, is suspected, or is planned.

♦ Be aware of side effects of scopolamine. Refer to written materials furnished by healthcare providers for safe self-administration.

♦ Carry card or other identification at all times describing medications being taken.

Evaluation

♦ Patient demonstrates a resolution/subsiding of the symptoms for which scopolamine was prescribed (nausea and vomiting associated with motion sickness; to decrease secretions prior to surgery or other procedures).

♦ Patient verbalizes understanding of side effects and regimen required for prudent self-administration of scopolamine.

SECOBARBITAL

(see-koe-bar′bi-tal)
{Secogen Sodium}, Seconal, Seconal Sodium, {Seral}

Classification(s):
Sedative-hypnotic, Barbiturate, CNS depressant
Schedule C II (oral and parenteral)
Schedule C III (rectal)
Pregnancy Category D

INDICATIONS

♦ Insomnia ♦ Anxiety states ♦ Acute convulsive conditions ♦ Preoperative sedation.

ACTION

♦ Depresses the central nervous system ♦ Interferes with transmission through the reticular formation, which is concerned with arousal ♦ Causes imbalance in inhibitory and facilitatory mechanisms that influence the cerebral cortex and reticular formation ♦ Action on neurotransmitters is not well defined ♦ All levels of CNS depression can occur, from mild sedation to hypnosis to coma to death.

{} = Only available in Canada.

PHARMACOKINETICS

Absorption: Readily absorbed following oral and rectal administration.

Distribution: Rapidly and widely distributed. Crosses blood-brain and placental barriers; excreted in breast milk.

Metabolism and Excretion: Metabolized by the liver; excreted by the kidneys as inactive metabolites and unchanged drug.

Half-Life: 30 hours.

CONTRAINDICATIONS AND PRECAUTIONS

Contraindicated in: ✦ Hypersensitivity to the drug ✦ Severe hepatic, renal, cardiac, or respiratory disease ✦ Individuals with a history of previous addiction ✦ Porphyria ✦ Presence of acute or chronic pain ✦ Parturition ✦ History of prophyria ✦ Lactation.

Use Cautiously in: ✦ Elderly or debilitated patients ✦ Hepatic, renal, cardiac, or respiratory dysfunction ✦ Depressed/suicidal patients ✦ Ammonia intoxication ✦ Pregnancy.

ADVERSE REACTIONS AND SIDE EFFECTS*

CNS: <u>drowsiness</u>, headache, lethargy, <u>dizziness</u>, mental depression, ataxia, <u>residual sedation ("hangover")</u>, confusion, paradoxical excitement and/or euphoria.

CV: hypotension, bradycardia.

Derm: skin rashes, urticaria, dermatitis (may precede potentially fatal reactions), redness and pain at IM injection site, phlebitis at IV site.

GI: nausea/vomiting, diarrhea/constipation, epigastric pain.

Hemat: AGRANULOCYTOSIS, THROMBOCYTOPENIA.

Resp: hypoventilation, apnea, RESPIRATORY DEPRESSION, LARYNGOSPASM, BRONCHOSPASM.

Other: tolerance, physical and psychological dependence.

INTERACTIONS:

Drug-Drug: ✦ **Other CNS depressants (including alcohol, benzodiazepines, antihistamines, opiates):** additive CNS depression ✦ **Chloramphenicol, MAO inhibitors, valproic acid, cimetidine, disulfiram:** increased effects of secobarbital ✦ **Phenytoin:** increased or decreased effects of either drug (close monitoring of serum levels required to control seizure activity) ✦ **Oral contraceptives:** decreased effectiveness of oral contraceptives ✦ **Oral anticoagulants:** decreased anticoagulant effects ✦ **Corticosteroids, digitoxin, doxycycline:** decreased effects of these drugs ✦ **Furosemide:** orthostatic hypotension ✦ **Griseofulvin:** decreased griseofulvin levels.

Drug-Food: ✦ **Vitamin D:** increased vitamin D metabolism, possible deficiency ✦ **Folic acid:** decreased absorption of folic acid, possible deficiency.

ROUTE AND DOSAGE

Anxiety

✦ **PO (Adults):** 30–100 mg tid.
✦ **PO (Children):** 6 mg/kg/day in 3 divided doses.
✦ **Rect (Adults):** 30–100 mg tid.
✦ **Rect (Children):** 6 mg/kg/day in 3 divided doses.

Insomnia

(Limit use to 2 weeks.)

✦ **PO (Adults):** 100–200 mg at bedtime.
✦ **Rect (Adults):** 120–200 mg at bedtime.
✦ **IM (Adults):** 100–200 mg at bedtime.
✦ **IM (Children):** 3–5 mg/kg at bedtime; maximum dose: 100 mg.

Acute Convulsive Conditions

✦ **IM (Adults):** 5.5 mg/kg every 3–4 hours.

---

*<u>Underlines</u> indicate most frequent; CAPITALS indicate life-threatening.

- **IM (Children):** 5.5 mg/kg every 3–4 hours.
- **IV (Adults):** 5.5 mg/kg every 3–4 hours.
- **IV (Children):** 5.5 mg/kg every 3–4 hours.

Preoperative Sedation

- **PO (Adults):** 100–300 mg 1–2 hours before surgery.
- **PO (Children):** 50–100 mg 1–2 hours before surgery.
- **Rect (Children):** 4–5 mg/kg 1–2 hours before surgery.
- **IM (Children):** 4–5 mg/kg 1–2 hours before surgery.

PHARMACODYNAMICS

Route	Onset	Peak	Duration
PO	15–30 min	2–4 hr	1–4 hr
Rect	15–30 min	30–60 min	1–4 hr
IM	7–10 min	—	1–4 hr
IV	1–3 min	Immediate	15 min

NURSING IMPLICATIONS

Assessment

- Assess sleep patterns. Keep records for adequate baseline data before the initiation of therapy.
- Assess for suicidal ideation in depressed patients.
- Assess occurrence, characteristics, and duration of seizure activity.
- Assess history of allergies, sensitivity to this drug.
- Assess date of last menses (possible pregnancy), use of contraceptives.
- Assess whether currently breast-feeding a child.
- Assess current and past alcohol and drug consumption.
- Assess for operation of automobile and/or other dangerous machinery.
- Assess for presence of adverse reactions or side effects.
- Assess patient/family knowledge about illness and need for medication.
- In collaboration with physician, assess CBC and renal and liver function tests in patients on prolonged therapy.
- **Lab Test Alterations:** May increase values of bromsulphalein (BSP) retention and protein-bound iodine (PBI).
- ◇ Elevated blood ammonia.
- **Withdrawal:** Assess for symptoms of withdrawal: • anxiety • tremors • insomnia • nausea/vomiting • weakness • diaphoresis • orthostatic hypotension • delirium • convulsions.
- **Withdrawal Management:** Monitor vital signs.
- ◇ Place patient in quiet room with low stimuli.
- ◇ Institute seizure precautions.
- ◇ A long-acting barbiturate, such as phenobarbital, may be ordered to suppress withdrawal symptoms.
- ◇ Phenytoin may be ordered to prevent seizures.
- ◇ Some physicians may order oxazepam as needed for objective withdrawal symptoms, gradually decreasing dosage until the drug is discontinued.
- **Toxicity and Overdose:** Assess for symptoms of toxicity: • confusion • drowsiness • dyspnea • slurred speech • staggering.
- ◇ Assess for symptoms of overdose: • CNS and respiratory depression • hypoventilation • hypothermia • hypotension • oliguria • tachycardia • coma. (May progress to respiratory arrest, circulatory collapse, and death.)
- **Overdose Management:** Monitor vital signs.
- ◇ Ensure maintenance of airway.
- ◇ Induce vomiting in conscious patient.
- ◇ Initiate gastric lavage in unconscious patient.
- ◇ Administer activated charcoal to minimize absorption of drug.
- ◇ Administer IV fluids.
- ◇ In cases of severe intoxication, forced diuresis or hemodialysis may be used.

Potential Nursing Diagnoses

- Ineffective breathing pattern related to

side effects of hypoventilation and respiratory depression.

- High risk for injury related to seizures; abrupt withdrawal from long-term use; decreased mental alertness caused by side effect of residual sedation; side effects of dizziness and ataxia; effects of overdose.
- High risk for self-directed violence related to depressed mood.
- Sleep pattern disturbance related to situational crises, physical condition, severe level of anxiety.
- High risk for activity intolerance related to side effects of residual sedation, drowsiness, dizziness.
- Knowledge deficit related to medication regimen.

Plan/Implementation

- **General Info:** Monitor vital signs before beginning therapy, at regular (bid) intervals throughout therapy, every 3–5 minutes during IV administration, and every 10 minutes for 30 minutes following IM administration.
- ◇ Ensure that patient is protected from injury. Supervise and assist with ambulation if dizziness and drowsiness are problems. Ensure that patient avoids participation in any activity requiring mental alertness (including smoking). Raise siderails and instruct patient to remain in bed following administration.
- **PO:** To minimize nausea, medication may be given with food or milk.
- ◇ Ensure that tablet or capsule has been swallowed and not "cheeked" to avoid medication or to hoard for later use.
- ◇ Tablet may be crushed or capsule emptied and mixed with food or fluid for patient who has difficulty swallowing.
- ◇ Store medication at controlled room temperatures between 15° and 30°C (59°–86°F). Protect from heat and moisture.
- **Rect:** To ensure accurate dose, do not divide suppositories.
- ◇ Store medication in refrigerator.

- **IM:** Powder form should be diluted with sterile water for injection. Use within 30 minutes of preparation. Discard if discolored or if precipitate is visible.
- ◇ Administer deeply into large muscle mass to minimize subcutaneous tissue irritation/necrosis. Use Z-tract method.
- ◇ Volume of injection should not exceed 5 mL at any one site.
- ◇ Observe patient closely for 20–30 minutes following injection for signs of excessive sedation.
- **IV:** Powder form should be diluted with sterile water, normal saline, or Ringer's injection. Use within 30 minutes of preparation.
- ◇ Do not use solution if discolored or if precipitate is visible.
- ◇ Do not mix with other medications.
- ◇ Administer IV solution at no more than 50 mg per 15 seconds. Observe closely for potential depression of vital signs.
- ◇ Solution is highly irritating. Extravasation may result in tissue necrosis. Stop infusion immediately if patient complains of pain.
- ◇ Ensure availability of artificial ventilation and resuscitation equipment.

Patient/Family Education

- Use caution in driving or when operating dangerous machinery. Drowsiness and dizziness can occur.
- Do not stop taking the drug abruptly. To do so can produce serious (even life-threatening) withdrawal symptoms. If a dose is missed, take it as close as possible to the prescribed time. If it is already close to time for next dose, wait until then; do not double up on dose at the next prescribed time.
- Do not consume other CNS depressants (including alcohol).
- Be aware of the risks of taking barbiturates during pregnancy (congenital malformations may be associated

with use during the first trimester). Evidence of withdrawal symptoms also has been observed in neonates born to mothers who had ingested barbiturates regularly during the last trimester of pregnancy. Notify physician if pregnancy is suspected or planned.

♦ Because barbiturates decrease effectiveness of oral contraceptives, use alternative methods of birth control during secobarbital therapy.

♦ Be aware of potential side effects. Refer to written materials furnished by healthcare providers regarding correct method of self-administration.

♦ Report symptoms of sore throat, fever, malaise, severe headache, conjunctivitis, rhinitis, urethritis, balanitis, easy bruising, petechiae, or epistaxis to physician immediately.

♦ Carry card or other identification at all times stating names of medications being taken.

Evaluation

♦ Patient demonstrates a subsiding/resolution of the symptoms for which secobarbital was prescribed (seizures, sleep disturbances, anxiety).

♦ Patient verbalizes understanding of side effects and regimen required for prudent self-administration of secobarbital.

SERTRALINE

(ser′tra-leen)
Zoloft

Classification(s):
Antidepressant; Serotonin enhancer
Pregnancy Category B

INDICATIONS

♦ Major depressive disorder. **Unlabeled Use:** Obsessive compulsive disorder.

ACTION

♦ Inhibits neuronal reuptake of serotonin, thereby potentiating serotonergic activity in the central nervous system. Has only very weak effects on norepinephrine and dopamine neuronal reuptake.

PHARMACOKINETICS

Absorption: Well absorbed following oral administration.

Distribution: Unknown. Highly bound to plasma proteins.

Metabolism and Excretion: Extensively metabolized to N-desmethylsertraline, which is substantially less active than sertraline. Excreted in feces (unchanged sertraline) and urine (metabolite). Unknown if excreted in breast milk.

Half-Life: 26 hours.

CONTRAINDICATIONS AND PRECAUTIONS

Contraindicated in: ♦ Hypersensitivity to the drug ♦ Concomitant use with MAO inhibitors ♦ Children and pregnancy (safety not established).

Use Cautiously in: ♦ Patients with hepatic or renal insufficiency ♦ Elderly and debilitated patients ♦ Patients with history of drug abuse ♦ Suicidal patients ♦ Patients with history of mania ♦ Patients with history of seizures.

ADVERSE REACTIONS AND SIDE EFFECTS*

CNS: <u>headache, dizziness, tremor, insomnia, somnolence, fatigue,</u> agitation, paresthesia, weakness, confusion, yawning, impaired concentration.

CV: palpitations, chest pain, postural hypotension, tachycardia.

Derm: <u>increased sweating,</u> rash, hot flushes.

GI: <u>nausea, dry mouth, diarrhea/loose stools, constipation, dyspepsia,</u> anorexia, vomiting, abdominal pain, increased appetite.

*<u>Underlines</u> indicate most frequent; CAPITALS indicate life-threatening.

GU: <u>male sexual dysfunction (primarily ejaculatory delay)</u>, menstrual disorders, urinary disorders.
Hemat: anemia, leukopenia, lymphadenopathy, purpura.
Metab/Nutrit: edema, weight loss or gain, thirst.
MS: myalgia, arthralgia, back pain.
Resp: rhinitis, pharyngitis.
Special Senses: abnormal vision, taste perversion, tinnitus.
Other: fever.

INTERACTIONS

Drug-Drug: ♦ **MAO inhibitors:** synergistic reaction that may result in hyperthermia, rigidity, myoclonus, autonomic instability with rapid fluctuation of vital signs, and mental status changes that include extreme agitation and coma. Reaction may be fatal. At least 14 days should elapse between discontinuation of one of the drugs (MAOI or sertraline) and initiation of the other ♦ **Alcohol:** possible potentiation of impairment in mental and motor skills ♦ **Cimetidine:** increased sertraline concentration ♦ **Diazepam:** increase in diazepam concentration ♦ **Tolbutamide:** decreased clearance of tolbutamide ♦ **Warfarin:** tendency for increased bleeding.
Drug-Food: ♦ Taking sertraline with food decreases the time to reach peak plasma concentration.

ROUTE AND DOSAGE

Depression

♦ **PO (Adults):** Sertraline should be administered once daily, either in the morning or evening. Initial dose: 50 mg/day. Dosage may be increased at intervals of no less than 1 week, up to a maximum dosage of 200 mg/day.

PHARMACODYNAMICS

Route	Onset	Peak	Duration
PO	1–3 wk	4–8 hr	14 days*

*Allow at least 14 days following cessation of therapy for complete drug elimination before initiating therapy with MAO inhibitors.

NURSING IMPLICATIONS

Assessment:

♦ Assess for suicidal ideation, plan, means. Assess for SUDDEN lifts in mood, which could indicate patient's decision to commit suicide.

♦ Assess mental status daily: • mood • appearance • thought and communication patterns • level of interest in the environment and in activities • suicidal ideation. Improvement in these behavior patterns and level of energy should be expected in 1–4 weeks following initiation of therapy.

♦ Assess vital signs, weight.

♦ Assess history of allergies, sensitivity to this drug or to similar drugs.

♦ Assess date of last menses (possible pregnancy).

♦ Assess if currently breast-feeding a child.

♦ Assess current and past alcohol and drug consumption.

♦ Assess for operation of automobile and/or other dangerous machinery.

♦ Assess for presence of adverse reactions or side effects, including exacerbation of manic symptoms.

♦ Assess patient/family knowledge about illness and need for medication.

♦ In collaboration with physician, assess liver and renal function tests before beginning therapy.

♦ **Lab Test Alterations:**

◊ Possible increase in AST or ALT.

◊ Small increases in total cholesterol and triglycerides.

◊ Small decrease in serum uric acid.

♦ **Toxicity and Overdose:** Assess for symptoms of overdose: • somnolence • nausea • vomiting • tachycardia • ECG changes • anxiety • dilated pupils.

♦ **Overdose Management:** Establish and maintain airway; ensure adequate oxygenation and ventilation.

◊ Monitor cardiac (ECG) and vital signs.

◊ May initiate gastric evacuation through emesis, lavage, or both.

◊ Activated charcoal, which may be used

with sorbitol, may be as or more effective than emesis or lavage.
◇ Provide supportive care with close observation.
◇ It is unlikely that forced diuresis, dialysis, hemoperfusion, or exchange transfusion would be beneficial, given the large volume of sertraline distribution.

Potential Nursing Diagnoses

✦ High risk for self-directed violence related to depressed mood.
✦ High risk for injury related to sertraline overdose or sertraline's side effects of somnolence, dizziness, paresthesia, and confusion.
✦ Social isolation related to depressed mood.
✦ High risk for activity intolerance related to sertraline's side effects of drowsiness, dizziness, weakness, confusion.
✦ Knowledge deficit related to medication regimen.

Plan/Implementation

✦ Monitor vital signs before beginning therapy and at regular intervals (bid or tid) throughout therapy. Take BP lying and standing in patients experiencing orthostatic hypotension. Elderly are particularly susceptible. Contact physician if tachycardia/arrhythmias are noted.
✦ Weigh patient 2–3 times a week, at same time of day, on same scale, if possible. A rapid weight gain or evidence of edema should be reported to physician immediately. Record I&O.
✦ Observe for decrease in appetite and loss of weight.
✦ Ensure that patient is protected from injury. Provide supervision and assistance when ambulating if dizziness and drowsiness are problems.
✦ Give hard candy, gum, or frequent sips of water if dry mouth is a problem.
✦ Administer oral medication with food or milk to minimize GI upset.

✦ Ensure that patient swallows tablet and does not "cheek" to avoid medication or hoard for later use.
✦ May crush tablet and mix with food or fluid for patient who has difficulty swallowing.
✦ Store at controlled room temperatures between 15° and 30°C (59°–86°F). Protect from heat and moisture.

Patient/Family Education

✦ Therapeutic effect may not be seen for as long as 4 weeks. If after this length of time no improvement is noted, physician may prescribe a different medication. Continue to take medication even though symptoms have not subsided.
✦ Use caution when driving or operating dangerous machinery. Drowsiness and dizziness can occur. If these side effects become persistent or interfere with activities of daily living, report to physician. Adjustment may be necessary.
✦ Report occurrence of any of the following symptoms to physician immediately: • rash or hives • sore throat • fever • malaise • unusual bleeding • easy bruising • persistent nausea/vomiting • severe headache • rapid heart rate • difficulty urinating • anorexia/weight loss • rapid weight gain • initiation of hyperactive behavior.
✦ Rise slowly from a sitting or lying position to prevent a sudden drop in blood pressure.
✦ If dry mouth is a problem, take frequent sips of water, chew sugarless gum, or suck on hard candy. Good oral care (frequent brushing, flossing) is very important.
✦ Do not drink alcohol while on sertraline therapy. These drugs may potentiate the effects of each other.
✦ Do not consume other medications (including over-the-counter meds) with sertraline without physician's ap-

proval. Many medications contain substances that, in combination with sertraline, could precipitate a potentially life-threatening situation.
* Be aware of possible risks of taking sertraline during pregnancy. Safe use during pregnancy and lactation has not been established. Inform physician immediately if pregnancy occurs or is suspected or planned.
* Be aware of side effects of sertraline. Refer to written materials furnished by healthcare providers for safe self-administration.
* Carry card or other identification at all times describing medications being taken.

Evaluation
* Patient demonstrates a subsiding/resolution of the symptoms for which sertraline was prescribed (depressed mood; suicidal ideation; obsessive compulsive behavior).
* Patient verbalizes understanding of side effects and regimen required for prudent self-administration of sertraline.

SUCCINYLCHOLINE CHLORIDE

(suk-sin-ill-koe'leen)
Anectine, Quelicin, Sucostrin

Classification(s):
Skeletal muscle relaxant,
Depolarizing neuromuscular
blocking agent
Pregnancy Category C

INDICATIONS

* Adjunct to general anesthesia to facilitate endotracheal intubation, endoscopic examinations, and to induce skeletal muscle relaxation during surgery or mechanical ventilation * Reduction of the intensity of muscle contractions of pharmacologically or electrically induced convulsive therapy (e.g., ECT).

ACTION

* An ultra-short-acting skeletal muscle relaxant that combines with cholinergic receptors of the motor endplate at the myoneural junction to produce depolarization * Initially, twitching or fasciculations are observed, followed by skeletal muscle paralysis * Succinylcholine also has histamine-releasing properties.

PHARMACOKINETICS

Absorption: Not administered orally due to poor absorption from the GI tract. IV is preferred route, but may be given IM.
Distribution: Widely distributed to all skeletal muscles. Small amounts cross placental barrier. Not known if drug is excreted in breast milk.
Metabolism and Excretion: Rapidly hydrolyzed by plasma pseudocholinesterase to succinylmonocholine, then more slowly to succinic acid and choline. Excreted in urine.
Half-Life: Ultrashort.

CONTRAINDICATIONS AND PRECAUTIONS

Contraindicated in: * Hypersensitivity to this drug * Disorders of plasma pseudocholinesterase * Personal or familial history of malignant hyperthermia * Myopathies associated with elevated creatine phosphokinase (CPK) values * Acute narrow-angle glaucoma * Penetrating eye injuries * Pregnancy and lactation (safe use has not been established).

Use Cautiously in: * Patients undergoing delivery by cesarean section * Cardiovascular, hepatic, pulmonary, metabolic, or renal disorders * Extensive or severe burns, electrolyte imbalance, hyperkalemia * Degenerative or dystrophic neuromuscular disease * Spinal cord injury * Eye surgery * Patients taking quinidine or cardiac glycosides, or those with suspected cardiac glycoside toxicity * Paraplegia.

ADVERSE REACTIONS AND SIDE EFFECTS*

CV: bradycardia, tachycardia, hypertension, hypotension, CARDIAC ARREST, arrhythmias.

Derm: rash.

GI: excessive salivation.

GU: myoglobinuria.

Ophth: increased intraocular pressure.

Resp: RESPIRATORY DEPRESSION, APNEA, BRONCHOCONSTRICTION.

Other: ANAPHYLAXIS, myoglobinemia, MALIGNANT HYPERTHERMIA, muscle fasciculation, postoperative muscle pain, hyperkalemia.

INTERACTIONS

Drug-Drug: ◆ **Diazepam:** decreased duration of neuromuscular blockade ◆ **Phenelzine, promazine, oxytocin, gentamicin, kanamycin, neomycin, streptomycins, quinidine, beta-adrenergic blocking agents, procainamide, lidocaine, trimethaphan, lithium carbonate, furosemide, magnesium sulfate, quinidine, chloroquine, acetylcholine, anticholinesterases, procaine-type local anesthetics, isoflurane:** prolonged neuromuscular blocking action ◆ **Nondepolarizing muscle relaxants:** synergistic or antagonistic effect to succinylcholine ◆ **Oral contraceptives, phenothiazines, thiotepa, cyclophosphamide, IV procaine:** prolonged effects of succinylcholine ◆ **Digitalis glycosides:** arrhythmias, increased toxicity of both drugs ◆ **Inhalation anesthetics (e.g., cyclopropane, diethyl ether, halothane, nitrous oxide):** increased incidence of bradycardia, arrhythmias, sinus arrest, apnea, malignant hyperthermia ◆ **Narcotic analgesics:** increased incidence of bradycardia and sinus arrest.

ROUTE AND DOSAGE

(To be administered by anesthesiologist or CRNA only.)

Short Surgical Procedures, Pharmacologically or Electrically Induced Convulsions

◆ **Test Dose (After Anesthesia Induction):** 0.1 mg/kg (about 10 mg).
◆ **IV (Adults):** 0.6 mg/kg given over 10–30 seconds. Range: 0.3–1.1 mg/kg.
◆ **IV (Infants and Small Children):** 2 mg/kg.
◆ **IV (Older Children and Adolescents):** 1 mg/kg.
◆ **IM (Adults):** 2.5–4 mg/kg. Maximum dose: 150 mg.
◆ **IM (Children):** 2.5–4 mg/kg. Maximum dose: 150 mg.

Long Surgical Procedures

◆ **IV (Adults):** Continuous infusion of solution containing 0.1% to 0.2% (1–2 mg/mL). Usual dosage: 2.5 mg/min. Range: 0.5–10 mg/min.

PHARMACODYNAMICS

Route	Onset	Peak	Duration
IM	75 sec–3 min	—	10–30 min
IV	30–60 sec	2–3 min	4–10 min

NURSING IMPLICATIONS

Assessment

◆ Assess mood daily in patient receiving ECT: ● appearance ● speech and thought patterns ● behavior ● interaction with others ● somatic complaints ● attendance in activities ● evidence of excitement or agitation.

◆ Assess history (genetic or disease-related) of disorders of plasma pseudocholinesterase. This is the metabolizing enzyme of succinylcholine, and low levels may result in prolonged paralysis of respiration. Low levels may be found in patients with: ● severe liver disease or cirrhosis ● anemia ●

*Underlines indicate most frequent; CAPITALS indicate life-threatening.

malnutrition • dehydration • burns • cancer • collagen diseases • myxedema • abnormal body temperatures • pregnancy • exposure to neurotoxic insecticides • those receiving antimalarial drugs, anticancer drugs, irradiation, MAO inhibitors, oral contraceptives, pancuronium, chlorpromazine, echothiophate iodide, or neostigmine • those with a recessive hereditary trait.

♦ Assess vital signs prior to administration. Record baseline values for comparison.

♦ Assess baseline serum electrolyte values.

♦ Assess history of allergies, sensitivity to this drug, or history of malignant hyperthermia.

♦ Assess date of last menses (possible pregnancy), use of contraceptives.

♦ Assess history of glaucoma or cardiovascular, hepatic, pulmonary, metabolic, or renal disorders.

♦ Assess whether currently breast-feeding a child.

♦ Assess current and past alcohol and drug consumption.

♦ Assess for operation of automobile and/or other dangerous machinery.

♦ Assess for presence of adverse reactions or side effects.

♦ Assess patient/family knowledge about illness and need for medication.

♦ **Toxicity and Overdose:** Assess for symptoms of malignant hyperthermia: • muscle rigidity, particularly involving jaw muscles • tachycardia and tachypnea unresponsive to increased depth of anesthesia • evidence of increased oxygen requirement and carbon dioxide production • rising temperature • metabolic acidosis.

♦ **Management of Malignant Hyperthermia:** At the first sign, immediately discontinue anesthesia and succinylcholine.

◊ Administer oxygen and sodium bicarbonate.

◊ Apply cooling measures to lower body temperature.

◊ Restore fluid and electrolyte balance.

◊ Promote maintenance of adequate urinary output.

◊ Administer IV dantrolene to reverse symptoms associated with the syndrome.

Potential Nursing Diagnoses

♦ Ineffective breathing pattern related to neuromuscular/musculoskeletal effects of succinylcholine.

♦ Alteration in tissue perfusion related to cardiovascular side effects of succinylcholine.

♦ High risk for self-directed violence related to depressed mood.

♦ High risk for injury related to side effect of malignant hyperthermia.

♦ Anxiety (moderate to severe) related to pending medical procedure (surgery, ECT).

♦ Knowledge deficit related to need for and side effects of succinylcholine.

Plan/Implementation

♦ Drug is administered IM or IV by anesthesiologist or Certified Registered Nurse Anesthetist (CRNA) only.

♦ Drug should be used only when facilities for endotracheal intubation, artificial respiration, and oxygen administration are immediately available.

♦ Small test dose (0.1 mg/kg) may be given to determine patient sensitivity and recovery time.

♦ Drug is administered after unconsciousness is induced to avoid patient distress.

♦ IM injection is given deeply into large muscle mass.

♦ May be given undiluted.

♦ Incompatible with alkaline solutions and will precipitate if mixed or administered simultaneously.

♦ Discard unused solutions after 24 hours.

♦ Administer direct IV for short-term muscle relaxation; single initial dose over 30 seconds.

♦ Rate of administration of intermittent or continuous infusion for prolonged muscular relaxation should never exceed 10 mg/min.

♦ Any of the following symptoms should be reported immediately to the anesthesiologist if they occur in the postanesthesia patient: respiratory difficulties (depression, apnea, bronchospasm), cardiovascular changes (heart rate/rhythm, blood pressure), profound or prolonged skeletal muscle paralysis, hyperthermia, ocular pain.

♦ Follow manufacturer's recommendation for storage of succinylcholine chloride injection and powder prior to and following reconstitution.

Patient/Family Education

♦ Drug is given to relax muscles during medical or surgical procedure. This facilitates surgeon's ability to perform. During ECT procedure, use of succinylcholine prevents fracture of long bones due to intense muscle contractions during convulsion.

♦ Be aware of potential adverse side effects of succinylcholine (as explained by physician or nurse). Emergency equipment will be available to intervene should it be required.

♦ Be aware of possible risks of taking succinylcholine during pregnancy. Safe use during pregnancy and lactation has not been established. It is thought that small amounts of succinylcholine cross the placental barrier, so a fetus could experience adverse effects of the drug. Inform physician prior to procedure if patient is pregnant or if pregnancy is suspected.

♦ If succinylcholine is used during delivery by cesarean section, newborn will be monitored closely for adverse effects of the drug.

Evaluation

♦ Patient verbalizes understanding of need for succinylcholine (to relax skeletal muscles during surgery or to reduce the intensity of muscle contractions during therapeutically induced convulsions).

♦ Patient verbalizes understanding of potential adverse side effects associated with the administration of succinylcholine.

SUMATRIPTAN

(soo-ma-trip′ tan)
Imitrex

Classification(s):
Antimigraine
Pregnancy Category C

INDICATIONS

♦ Treatment of acute migraine attacks with or without aura ♦ **Unlabeled Use:** cluster headache.

ACTION

♦ Acts as a selective agonist at specific vascular serotonin receptor sites (probably a member of the 5- HT_{1D} family) ♦ Binding at these receptor sites results in vasoconstriction of the basilar artery and in the vasculature of the isolated dura mater ♦ This vasoconstriction induces the antimigrainous effects of the drug.

PHARMACOKINETICS

Absorption: Well absorbed (97%) following subcutaneous injection.

Distribution: Has not yet been established. Plasma protein binding is low. Not known if crosses placental barrier or is excreted in breast milk.

Metabolism and Excretion: Metabolized by the liver. Excreted in the urine (approximately 22% as unchanged drug and 38% as the indole acetic acid metabolite).

Half-Life: 2 hours.

CONTRAINDICATIONS AND PRECAUTIONS

Contraindicated in: ◆ IV use ◆ Patients with ischemic heart disease (e.g., angina pectoris, history of myocardial infarction, or documented silent ischemia) ◆ Prinzmetal's angina ◆ Patients with signs or symptoms of ischemic heart disease ◆ Patients with uncontrolled hypertension ◆ Concomitant use with ergotamine-containing preparations ◆ Hypersensitivity to the drug ◆ Patients with basilar or hemiplegic migraine.

Use Cautiously in: ◆ Postmenopausal women ◆ Males over 40 ◆ Patients with risk factors for coronary artery disease (e.g., hypertension, hypercholesterolemia, obesity, diabetes, smokers, and strong family history) ◆ Impaired hepatic or renal function ◆ Pregnancy, lactation, or children (safety not established).

ADVERSE REACTIONS AND SIDE EFFECTS*

CNS: dizziness, vertigo, drowsiness, sedation, headache, anxiety, malaise, feeling strange, confusion, agitation, tight feeling in head.

CV: flushing, tingling, warm/hot sensation, cold sensation, tightness in chest, pressure in chest, hypertension, hypotension, bradycardia, tachycardia, palpitations, angina pectoris, CORONARY VASOSPASM, LIFE-THREATENING ARRHYTHMIAS (atrial fibrillation, ventricular fibrillation, ventricular tachycardia), MYOCARDIAL INFARCTION.

Derm: injection site reaction, burning sensation, sweating.

EENT: throat discomfort, discomfort of nasal cavity/sinuses, vision alterations.

GI: abdominal discomfort, dysphagia, discomfort of mouth and tongue.

MS: weakness, neck pain/stiffness, myalgia, muscle cramps, jaw discomfort.

Neuro: numbness.

INTERACTIONS

Drug-Drug: ◆ **Ergot-containing drugs (e.g., ergotamine):** prolonged vasospastic reactions (avoid use of either drug within 24 hours of each other, as effects may be additive).

ROUTE AND DOSAGE
Acute Migraine Attack

◆ **SC (Adults):** Initial dose: 6 mg SC. May repeat in 1 hour if relief is not achieved, although benefit of a second 6-mg injection is questionable. Maximum dosage: 12 mg in 24 hours (taken in two 6- mg injections at least 1 hour apart).

◆ **Available as:** 6 mg/0.5 mL unit-of-use syringes; 6 mg/0.5 mL single-dose vials; and SELFdose System Kit (which includes unit for self-injection, 2 syringes, and instructions for use).

PHARMACODYNAMICS

Route	Onset	Peak	Duration
SC	5–20 min	1–2 hr	Up to 24 hr

NURSING IMPLICATIONS
Assessment

◆ Assess location, intensity, and duration of pain. Assess presence of nausea and vomiting, photophobia, phonophobia, level of consciousness, blurring of vision, tingling in extremities, and other symptoms associated with migraine headache.

◆ Assess patient/family history of ischemic heart disease: • angina pectoris • myocardial infarction • documented silent ischemia • Prinzmetal's angina.

◆ Assess additional factors that would contraindicate use of sumatriptin: • uncontrolled hypertension • use of ergotamine preparations. Neurological exam may be necessary to differentiate from basilar or hemiplegic migraine.

◆ Assess for risk factors of coronary artery disease (patients for which

*Underlines indicate most frequent; CAPITALS indicate life-threatening.

precautions must be taken in administering sumatriptin): hypertension, hypercholesterolemia, obesity, diabetes, smokers, strong family history, postmenopausal women, and men over 40 years of age.

♦ Assess stress factors in the patient's life. Assess effectiveness of previous OcoOping strategies.
♦ Assess baseline vital signs.
♦ Assess history of allergies, sensitivity to this drug.
♦ Assess date of last menses (possible pregnancy); use of contraceptives.
♦ Assess if currently breast-feeding a child.
♦ Assess current and past alcohol and drug consumption.
♦ Assess operation of automobile and/or other dangerous machinery.
♦ Assess patient/family knowledge about illness and need for medication.
♦ In collaboration with physician, obtain baseline ECG, liver, and renal function studies.
♦ **Lab Test Alterations:** Disturbances of liver function tests.
♦ **Overdose:** No overdoses in clinical practice have been reported. Coronary vasospasm has been observed after IV administration.
◇ Assess for symptoms of overdose (implicated from results of animal studies): • convulsions • tremor • inactivity • erythema of the extremities • reduced respiratory rate • cyanosis • ataxia • mydriasis • injection site reactions (desquamation, hair loss, and scab formation) • paralysis.
♦ **Overdose Management:** Focus on stabilization of vital signs, maintenance of adequate pulmonary ventilation, and control of convulsions. The half-life of sumatriptin is about 2 hours, and therefore monitoring of patients after overdosing should continue for at least 10 hours.

Potential Nursing Diagnoses

♦ Pain related to cerebral vasodilitation.

♦ Altered tissue perfusion (cardiac) related to potential side effect of coronary vasospasm.
♦ High risk for activity intolerance related to potential side effects of dizziness, drowsiness, weakness.
♦ Knowledge deficit related to medication regimen.

Plan/Implementation

♦ Administer single injection subcutaneously.
♦ Administer first dose in physician's office or emergency room for individuals who are at high risk for coronary artery disease (see Assessment section). Monitor blood pressure prior to and for 1 hour following administration. If symptoms of angina occur, assess for ischemic changes through ECG evaluation.
♦ Monitor for side effects and patient's tolerance of the medication.
♦ Monitor for therapeutic effectiveness of the medication.
♦ Provide quiet environment with low external stimuli.
♦ Ensure that patient is protected from injury. Provide supervision and assistance when ambulating if dizziness and drowsiness occur.
♦ Store medication between 2° and 30°C (36° and 86°F). Protect from light.
♦ Explain proper technique for using the auto-injector. Review the pamphlet of instructions with the patient. Allow patient to view videocassette that demonstrates use of the auto-injector (available from manufacturer). Encourage patient to practice with demonstrator model. Observe patient in self-administration technique. Ensure that patient understands proper disposal of syringes.

Patient/Family Education

♦ Be aware that sumatriptin is intended for relief of an acute migraine attack. It cannot be used for migraine prevention.
♦ Administer sumatriptin as soon as

possible after symptoms of migraine appear. It may, however, be given at any time during the attack. If you do not get relief, another injection may be administered after 1 hour. Do not take more than 2 injections in any 24 hours.

♦ Avoid dangerous activity, including driving, immediately after taking sumatriptin. Dizziness and drowsiness can occur.

♦ Do not take any more sumatriptin and notify physician if any of the following symptoms occur: • tightness or pain in chest or throat • wheezing • heart throbbing • swelling of eyelids, face, or lips • skin rash, skin lumps, or hives.

♦ If you develop feelings of tingling, heat, flushing (redness of face lasting a short time), heaviness, pressure, drowsiness, dizziness, tiredness or sickness, tell your doctor about these symptoms at your next visit.

♦ Do not use sumatriptan if you are pregnant, think you might be pregnant, are trying to become pregnant, or are not using adequate contraception. Safe use during pregnancy has not been established.

♦ Do not use sumatriptan if you are breast-feeding an infant. It is not known if sumatriptan is excreted in breast milk. Adverse effects on the infant are possible.

♦ You may experience pain or redness at the site of injection, but this usually disappears within an hour.

♦ Migraine headaches are often triggered by certain foods that are high in the amino acid tyramine. You may want to avoid foods such as aged cheese, alcohol, chocolate, bananas, pickled products, and yogurt. Food additives (such as monosodium glutamate [MSG]) and preservatives (such as nitrites) have also been implicated. Caffeine, as well as certain medications, such as antihyperten-

sives, can trigger migraine in some individuals.

Evaluation

♦ Patient verbalizes relief from pain and associated symptoms attributed to acute migraine attack.

♦ Patient is able to resume previous role responsibilities.

♦ Patient demonstrates ability to self-administer sumatriptin correctly and safely.

♦ Patient verbalizes understanding of possible side effects of sumatriptin and under what conditions to notify physician regarding its use.

TACRINE

(tack′rin)
Cognex

Classification(s):
Cholinesterase inhibitor
Pregnancy Category C

INDICATIONS

♦ For improvement of cognition and functional autonomy in mild to moderate dementia of the Alzheimer type.

ACTION

♦ Acts by elevating acetylcholine concentrations in the cerebral cortex by slowing the degradation of acetylcholine released by still-intact cholinergic neurons ♦ Because the action relies on functionally intact cholinergic neurons, the effects of tacrine may lessen as the disease process advances ♦ There is no evidence that tacrine alters the course of the underlying dementing process.

PHARMACOKINETICS

Absorption: Absolute bioavailability is approximately 17%. Women have a higher bioavailability than men due to different levels of activity of the cytochrome P450 IA2 isozyme, and subsequent serum levels are about 50% higher in women than in men. Bioavailability is reduced by 30% to 40% when tacrine is taken with food.

Distribution: Widely distributed. Protein binding is approximately 55%. Tacrine readily penetrates the blood-brain barrier. Unknown if this drug is excreted in breast milk.

Metabolism and Excretion: Extensive metabolism occurs as a result of hydroxylation by cytochrome P450 IA2 isozymes. At least three biologically active hydroxylated metabolites of tacrine have been identified. Excretion has not been well defined. Less than 3% is recovered in the urine. Biliary or enterohepatic recycling of either tacrine or its metabolites is not well characterized.

Half-Life: 3.5 hours.

CONTRAINDICATIONS AND PRECAUTIONS

Contraindicated in: ♦ Hypersensitivity to the drug or to acridine derivatives ♦ Previous tacrine-induced hepatotoxicity characterized by jaundice and serum bilirubin levels in excess of 3.0 mg/dL ♦ Patients with asthma, hypotension, bradycardia, AV conduction defects, hyperthyroidism, anatomic or functional urinary tract obstruction, peptic ulcer disease, and intestinal obstruction ♦ Pregnancy, lactation, children (safety not known).

Use Cautiously in: ♦ Seizure disorders ♦ Angle-closure glaucoma ♦ History of or current liver disease ♦ Anesthesia with succinylcholine-type muscle relaxants ♦ Concurrent use with nonsteroidal anti-inflammatory agents ♦ Abrupt discontinuation or dosage reductions of 80 mg/day or more may precipitate acute deterioration of cognitive function.

ADVERSE REACTIONS AND SIDE EFFECTS*

CNS: dizziness, agitation, confusion, ataxia, insomnia, somnolence, tremor,

headache, depression, abnormal thinking, anxiety, hostility, hallucinations, seizures, fatigue, asthenia.

CV: hypotension, sinus bradycardia.

Derm: rash, diaphoresis, flushing.

GI: nausea, vomiting, diarrhea, dyspepsia, anorexia, weight loss, abdominal pain, flatulence, constipation.

GU: urinary frequency, urinary tract infection, urinary incontinence.

Hemat: AGRANULOCYTOSIS, purpura.

Hepatic: elevations in liver function tests (e.g., ALT, AST, bilirubin, GGT), jaundice, GRANULOMATOUS HEPATITIS, HEPATOCELLULAR NECROSIS.

MS: myalgia.

Resp: rhinitis, upper respiratory infection, coughing.

INTERACTIONS

Drug-Drug: ♦ **Anticholinergics:** decreased effectiveness of anticholinergics ♦ **Other cholinesterase inhibitors or cholinergic agonists (e.g., bethanechol):** synergistic effect ♦ **Cimetidine:** increased effects of tacrine ♦ **Succinylcholine:** prolongation of the action of succinylcholine ♦ **Theophylline:** increased serum theophylline concentration ♦ **Smoking:** decreased tacrine plasma concentration.

Drug-Food: ♦ When taken with food, the bioavailability of tacrine is reduced by 30% to 40%.

ROUTE AND DOSAGE

Mild to Moderate Dementia of the Alzheimer Type

♦ **PO (Adults):** Initial dosage: 10 mg qid, taken between meals if tolerated. Maintain this dose for at least 6 weeks, monitoring ALT levels weekly. Providing there are no significant ALT elevations and the patient is tolerating treatment, the dose may be increased to 80 mg/day. Patients may be titrated to higher doses (120 and 160 mg/day) at 6-week intervals on the basis

*Underlines indicate most frequent; CAPITALS indicate life-threatening.

of tolerance. Maximum dosage: 160 mg/day. **Note:** Abrupt discontinuation of tacrine or a large reduction in total daily dose (80 mg/day or greater) may cause an acute decline in cognitive function and behavioral disturbances.

♦ **PO (Adults Who Experience Elevations in Alanine Aminotransaminase [ALT] Levels):** ALT ≤ 3 times upper limits of normal: Continue treatment according to recommended titration. ALT > 3 to ≤ 5 times upper limits of normal: Reduce the daily dose by 40 mg/day. Resume dose titration when transaminase returns to within normal limits. ALT > 5 times upper limits of normal: Stop treatment with tacrine. Monitor transaminase levels until within normal limits. Rechallenge may be considered on an individual basis.

♦ **PO (Adults) Rechallenge:** Rechallenge may be undertaken once transaminase levels return to within normal limits. **Exception:** *Patients with clinical jaundice confirmed by a significant elevation in total bilirubin (> 3.0 mg/dL) should permanently discontinue tacrine and not be rechallenged.*
If rechallenged, patients should be given an initial dose of 40 mg/day (10 mg qid), and transaminase levels monitored weekly. If, after 6 weeks on 40 mg/day, the patient is tolerating the dosage with no unacceptable elevations in transaminases, recommended dose titration and transaminase monitoring may be resumed.

PHARMACODYNAMICS

Route	Onset*	Peak	Duration
PO	1–4 wk**	30–90 min	15–24 hr†

*Efficacy is dependent upon the integrity of the cholinergic neuron.
**Onset of therapeutic response.
†Improvement in cognition and functional autonomy on sustained multiple-dose (160 mg/day) tacrine therapy.

NURSING IMPLICATIONS
Assessment

♦ Assess vital signs, weight.
♦ Assess mental status daily: for improvement in memory ● attention ● reason ● language ● and the ability to perform simple tasks.
♦ Assess history of asthma.
♦ Assess history of ulcers, or use of nonsteroidal anti-inflammatory drugs.
♦ Assess history of cardiovascular disease, particularly sick sinus syndrome.
♦ Assess history of urinary tract or intestinal obstruction.
♦ Assess history of seizures.
♦ Assess history of or current liver disease.
♦ Assess history of allergies, sensitivity to this drug, or acridine derivatives.
♦ Assess patient/family knowledge about illness and need for medication.
♦ Assess baseline hepatic and renal function prior to initiation of therapy.
♦ Assess for signs of liver involvement (e.g., jaundice, elevated laboratory values of ALT, AST, bilirubin, and GGT).
♦ **Lab Test Alterations:** Elevations in ALT, AST, bilirubin, and GGT levels. Transaminase levels should be monitored weekly for at least the first 18 weeks of tacrine therapy, after which monitoring may be decreased to every 3 months. Weekly monitoring should be resumed for at least 6 weeks following any increase in dose. Continued weekly monitoring (beyond 18 weeks) may be indicated in patients with modest elevations (>2 times upper limit of normal).
♦ **Toxicity and Overdose:** Therapeutic levels of tacrine in dementia have not been established, although one clinical study has suggested that the therapeutic range is 5–70 ng/mL.
♦ Assess for symptoms of overdose: Cholinergic crisis characterized by symptoms of severe nausea/vomiting, salivation, sweating, bradycardia, hy-

potension, collapse, and convulsions. Increasing muscle weakness is a possibility and may result in death if respiratory muscles are involved.
+ **Overdose Management:** General supportive measures.
+ Continuous cardiovascular monitoring.
+ Tertiary anticholinergics (such as atropine) may be used as an antidote for tacrine overdosage. Initial recommended dosage: 1.0–2.0 mg IV with subsequent doses based upon clinical response.
+ It is not known whether tacrine or its metabolites can be eliminated by hemodialysis, peritoneal dialysis, or hemofiltration.

Potential Nursing Diagnoses
+ High risk for trauma related to potential side effects of confusion, dizziness, seizures; or disorientation and confusion of disease process.
+ High risk for injury related to potential adverse effects on the liver.
+ High risk for activity intolerance related to tacrine's side effects of dizziness, ataxia, weakness, fatigue.
+ Knowledge deficit related to medication regimen.

Plan/Implementation
+ Monitor vital signs before beginning therapy, and at regular intervals (bid or tid) throughout therapy. Contact physician if blood pressure or heart rate drops below parameters established by physician.
+ Observe for decrease in appetite, weight loss.
+ Monitor weekly ALT levels from the initiation of therapy. Report to physician if value increases to 3 times the upper limit of normal.
+ Report the following signs/symptoms to physician: • severe nausea and vomiting • yellow skin or eyes • convulsions • difficulty urinating • sore throat • fever • malaise.
+ Ensure that patient is protected from

injury. Provide supervision and assistance when ambulating if dizziness, weakness, or ataxia are problems.
+ Observe for seizure activity, particularly in patients with a history of seizure disorder.
+ Administer between meals (at least 1 hour before eating) whenever possible. However, if minor GI upset occurs, tacrine may be given with food to improve tolerability. (Taking tacrine with food can be expected to reduce plasma levels by approximately 30% to 40%.)
+ Ensure that patient swallows capsule and does not "cheek" to discard later.

Patient/Family Education
+ Report to lab weekly at specified time to have blood drawn for routine values to test if liver is being affected by the drug.
+ Use caution when in an environment in which injury could result. Dizziness, weakness, and ataxia are common side effects of tacrine.
+ Protect patient from injury should a seizure occur. Report incident to physician.
+ Take medication at regular intervals, exactly as prescribed. The effectiveness of therapy is dependent upon this regularity.
+ Report any of the following adverse effects to physician: • severe and persistent nausea, vomiting, or diarrhea • skin rash • yellow skin or eyes • black or pale stool • seizures • fever • difficulty urinating. Also report the appearance of any new adverse effects, as well as an increase in severity of any existing ones.
+ Do not decrease the dosage or stop taking the drug abruptly without consulting physician. To do so may produce a sudden worsening of the degree of cognitive impairment.
+ Do not consume other medications (including over-the-counter meds) with tacrine without physician's ap-

proval. An interaction that may be physically harmful could occur.

♦ Be aware of side effects of tacrine. Caregivers should refer to written materials furnished by healthcare providers for safe administration.

♦ Patient should carry card or other identification at all times describing medications being taken.

Evaluation

♦ Patient demonstrates an improvement in the symptoms for which tacrine was prescribed (impairment in memory, attention, reason, language, and the ability to perform simple tasks).

♦ Patient/caregivers verbalize understanding of side effects and regimen required for prudent administration of tacrine.

TEMAZEPAM

(te-maz′e-pam)
Razepam, Restoril

Classification(s):
Sedative-hypnotic, Benzodiazepine
Schedule C IV
Pregnancy Category X

INDICATIONS

♦ Insomnia characterized by difficulty in falling asleep, frequent nocturnal awakening, and/or early morning awakening. (For short-term and intermittent use only. Not recommended for administration longer than 5 weeks.)

ACTION

♦ Depresses subcortical levels of the central nervous system, particularly the limbic system and reticular formation ♦ May potentiate the effects of the powerful inhibitory neurotransmitter gamma-aminobutyric acid (GABA) in the brain, thereby producing a calmative effect ♦ All

levels of CNS depression can occur, from mild sedation to hypnosis to coma.

PHARMACOKINETICS

Absorption: Rapidly absorbed from the GI tract.
Distribution: Is widely distributed. Crosses blood-brain and placental barriers; excreted in breast milk.
Metabolism and Excretion: Metabolized by the liver; produces inactive metabolites that are excreted for the most part by the kidneys.
Half-Life: 10–20 hours.

CONTRAINDICATIONS AND PRECAUTIONS

Contraindicated in: ♦ Hypersensitivity to the drug or to other benzodiazepines ♦ Pregnancy and lactation ♦ Narrow-angle glaucoma ♦ Children under 18.
Use Cautiously in: ♦ Elderly or debilitated patients ♦ Hepatic or renal dysfunction ♦ Individuals with a history of drug abuse/addiction ♦ Depressed/suicidal patients ♦ Combination with other CNS depressants ♦ Low serum albumin.

ADVERSE REACTIONS AND SIDE EFFECTS*

CNS: drowsiness, dizziness, confusion, lethargy, weakness, paradoxical excitement.
CV: palpitations.
GI: anorexia, diarrhea.
Other: tolerance, physical and psychological dependence.

INTERACTIONS

Drug-Drug: ♦ **Other CNS depressants (including alcohol, barbiturates, narcotics), antipsychotics, antidepressants, antihistamines, anticonvulsants:** additive CNS depression ♦ **Oral contraceptives:** increased effects of temazepam ♦ **Neuromuscular**

---

*Underlines indicate most frequent; CAPITALS indicate life-threatening.

blocking agents: increased respiratory depression ◆ **Levodopa:** decreased effects of levodopa.

ROUTE AND DOSAGE
Insomnia
◆ **PO (Adults):** 15–30 mg at bedtime.
◆ **PO (Geriatric or Debilitated Patients):** Initially, 15 mg at bedtime. Adjust dosage as response is determined.

PHARMACODYNAMICS

Route	Onset	Peak	Duration
PO	20–40 min	2–3 hr	6–8 hr

NURSING IMPLICATIONS
Assessment
◆ Assess sleep patterns. Keep records for adequate baseline data before the initiation of therapy.
◆ Assess for suicidal ideation (CNS depressants aggravate symptoms in depressed patients).
◆ Assess history of allergies, sensitivity to this drug or to other benzodiazepines.
◆ Assess history of glaucoma.
◆ Assess date of last menses (possible pregnancy), use of contraceptives.
◆ Assess whether currently breast-feeding a child.
◆ Assess current and past alcohol and drug consumption.
◆ Assess operation of automobile and/or other dangerous machinery.
◆ Assess for presence of adverse reactions or side effects.
◆ Assess patient/family knowledge about illness and need for medication.
◆ In collaboration with physician, assess CBC and liver function tests in patients on long-term therapy (not recommended for administration longer than 5 weeks).
◆ **Lab Test Alterations:** May cause increase in total and direct serum bilirubin, AST, and ALT.
◇ Abnormal renal function tests.

◆ **Withdrawal:** Assess for symptoms of withdrawal: ● depression ● insomnia ● increased anxiety ● abdominal and muscle cramps ● tremors ● vomiting ● sweating ● convulsions ● delirium.
◆ **Withdrawal Management:** Monitor vital signs.
◇ Place patient in quiet room with low stimuli.
◇ Institute seizure precautions.
◇ A long-acting barbiturate, such as phenobarbital, may be ordered to suppress withdrawal symptoms.
◇ Phenytoin may be ordered to prevent seizures.
◇ Some physicians may order oxazepam as needed to treat objective withdrawal symptoms, gradually decreasing dosage until the drug is discontinued.
◆ **Toxicity and Overdose:** Assess for symptoms of intoxication: ● euphoria ● excessive drowsiness ● slurred speech ● disorientation ● mood lability ● incoordination ● unsteady gait ● disinhibition of sexual and aggressive impulses ● judgment and/or memory impairment.
◇ Assess for symptoms of overdose: ● shallow respiration ● cold and clammy skin ● hypotension ● dilated pupils ● weak and rapid pulse ● hypnosis ● coma ● possible death.
◆ **Overdose Management:** Monitor vital signs.
◇ Ensure maintenance of adequate airway.
◇ Induce vomiting in conscious patient.
◇ Initiate gastric lavage in unconscious patient.
◇ Administer activated charcoal to minimize absorption.
◇ IV fluids and vasopressors may be used to combat hypotension.
◇ Forced diuresis may be used to facilitate elimination of the drug.

Potential Nursing Diagnoses
◆ High risk for injury related to abrupt withdrawal from long-term use; effects of drug intoxication or overdose; de-

creased mental alertness caused by sedative effect.

♦ High risk for self-directed violence related to depressed mood.

♦ Sleep pattern disturbance related to situational crises, physical condition, severe level of anxiety.

♦ High risk for activity intolerance related to side effects of lethargy, drowsiness, dizziness, weakness.

♦ Knowledge deficit related to medication regimen.

Plan/Implementation

♦ Monitor vital signs before beginning therapy and at regular intervals (bid) throughout therapy.

♦ Ensure that patient is protected from injury. Supervise and assist with ambulation if dizziness and muscular weakness are problems. Pad siderails and headboard for patient who experiences seizures (withdrawal).

♦ Ensure that capsule has been swallowed and not "cheeked" to avoid medication or to hoard for later use.

♦ Raise siderails and ensure that patient remains in bed following administration.

♦ Discourage smoking following administration.

♦ Store medication at controlled room temperatures between 15° and 30°C (59°–86°F). Protect from heat, light, and moisture.

Patient/Family Education

♦ Do not drive or operate dangerous machinery if residual drowsiness and dizziness occur.

♦ Do not stop taking the drug abruptly. To do so can produce serious withdrawal symptoms.

♦ Do not consume other CNS depressants unless prescribed by physician. Do not consume alcohol.

♦ Do not take nonprescription medication without approval from physician.

♦ Be aware of risks of taking temazepam during pregnancy (congenital malformations have been associated with use of benzodiazepines during the first trimester). Notify physician of desirability to discontinue drug if pregnancy is suspected or planned.

♦ Be aware of potential side effects. Refer to written materials furnished by healthcare providers regarding correct method of self-administration.

♦ Carry card or other identification at all times stating names of medications being taken.

Evaluation

♦ Patient demonstrates a subsiding/resolution of the symptoms for which temazepam was prescribed (insomnia, sleep disturbances).

♦ Patient verbalizes understanding of side effects and regimen required for prudent self-administration of temazepam.

THIAMYLAL SODIUM

(thye-am′i-lal)
Surital

Classification(s):
Anesthetic, Barbiturate
Schedule III
Pregnancy Category C

INDICATIONS

♦ Induction of anesthesia ♦ Supplementation of other anesthetic agents ♦ IV anesthesia for short procedures (minor surgery, ECT) with minimal painful stimuli ♦ Induction of a hypnotic state.

ACTION

♦ Depresses the central nervous system by inhibiting impulse conduction in the ascending reticular activating system ♦ Produces anesthesia, but does not possess analgesic properties.

PHARMACOKINETICS

Distribution: Rapidly crosses blood-brain barrier, then is redistributed to other body tissues, with affinity for highly vascular organs (liver, brain, kidneys, heart) and adipose tissue. Crosses placental barrier; excreted in breast milk. **Metabolism and Excretion:** Metabolized in the liver. Excreted in urine. **Half-Life:** 3–8 hours.

CONTRAINDICATIONS AND PRECAUTIONS

Contraindicated in: ♦ Latent or manifest porphyria ♦ Hypersensitivity to barbiturates ♦ Absence of suitable veins for IV administration ♦ Status asthmaticus ♦ Pregnancy and lactation (safe use has not been established).

Use Cautiously in: ♦ Severe cardiovascular disease ♦ Hypotension or shock ♦ Conditions in which hypnotic effects may be prolonged or potentiated (excessive premedication, Addison's disease, hepatic or renal dysfunction, myxedema, increased blood urea, and severe anemia) ♦ Increased intracranial pressure ♦ Asthma ♦ Myasthenia gravis ♦ Debilitated patients ♦ Impaired function of respiratory, circulatory, renal, hepatic, or endocrine systems ♦ Patients with a history of drug abuse/dependence.

ADVERSE REACTIONS AND SIDE EFFECTS*

CNS: prolonged somnolence and recovery, headache, emergence delirium, anxiety, restlessness.
CV: hypotension, circulatory depression, thrombophlebitis, MYOCARDIAL DEPRESSION, CARDIAC ARRHYTHMIAS, PERIPHERAL VASCULAR COLLAPSE.
GI: nausea, vomiting, abdominal pain, salivation.
Derm: erythema, pruritus, urticaria, skin rashes, pain or nerve injury at injection site.
Resp: hiccups, sneezing, coughing, dyspnea, RESPIRATORY DEPRESSION, APNEA, LARYNGOSPASM, BRONCHOSPASM.
Other: tolerance, dependence, skeletal

muscle hyperactivity, shivering, rhinitis, ANAPHYLACTIC REACTION.

INTERACTIONS

Drug-Drug: ♦ **CNS depressants (e.g., alcohol, benzodiazepines, other barbiturates, other sedative-hypnotics, opiates):** additive CNS and respiratory depression ♦ **Furosemide:** orthostatic hypotension ♦ **Propranolol, corticosteroids, doxycycline, oral anticoagulants, oral contraceptives, quinidine, theophylline:** decreased effectiveness of these drugs.

ROUTE AND DOSAGE

(To be administered by anesthesiologist or CRNA only.)

Anesthesia for Short Procedures

(Minor surgery or electroconvulsive therapy.)
♦ **IV (Adults):** Dosage is individualized according to patient response. Manufacturer recommends a 2-mL test dose of a 2.5% solution. A 2.5% solution is recommended for induction and maintenance of anesthesia by intermittent IV injection. Initially, 3–6 mL of a 2.5% solution will usually produce short periods of anesthesia. Rate of administration during induction is about 1 mL every 5 seconds. A dilute solution (0.3%) may be administered by continuous drip for maintenance.

PHARMACODYNAMICS

Route	Onset	Peak	Duration
IV	30–40 sec	—	*

*Ultrashort acting. Duration varies tremendously between patients and with dose given. The more given, the longer the duration.

NURSING IMPLICATIONS
Assessment
♦ In patient receiving ECT, assess mood,

---

*Underlines indicate most frequent; CAPITALS indicate life-threatening.

level of activity, degree of participation in therapies, interaction with others.

♦ Assess for suicidal ideation in depressed patients.

♦ Assess history of allergies, sensitivity to this drug or to other barbiturates, history of porphyria or asthma.

♦ Obtain baseline blood pressure, pulse, respiration, temperature, weight.

♦ Assess level of anxiety regarding impending surgical procedure or electroconvulsive therapy.

♦ Assess status of veins available for IV administration.

♦ Assess date of last menses (possible pregnancy), use of contraceptives.

♦ Assess whether currently breast-feeding a child.

♦ Assess current and past alcohol and drug consumption.

♦ Assess for presence of adverse reactions or side effects.

♦ Assess level of knowledge about illness and need for medication.

♦ In collaboration with physician, ensure performance of CBC and renal and liver function tests.

♦ **Toxicity and Overdose:** Assess for symptoms of overdose (may occur from too rapid or repeated injections): • profound drop in blood pressure (even to shock levels) • apnea • occasional laryngospasm • coughing and other respiratory difficulties.

♦ **Overdose Management:** Discontinue drug.

◇ Maintain patent airway (intubation may be required).

◇ Administer oxygen.

◇ Assist with ventilation if needed.

◇ Administer vasopressors to counteract hypotension.

◇ Administer IV fluids to maintain adequate circulation.

◇ Administer diuretics or hemodialysis to promote elimination of the drug.

Potential Nursing Diagnoses

♦ Ineffective breathing pattern related to side effects of respiratory depression, dyspnea, apnea.

♦ High risk for injury related to overdose; extravasation at insertion site.

♦ High risk for self-directed violence related to depressed mood.

♦ Anxiety (moderate to severe) related to impending surgical procedure or electroconvulsive therapy.

♦ Knowledge deficit related to medication regimen.

Plan/Implementation

♦ Drug is administered by anesthesiologist or Certified Registered Nurse Anesthetist (CRNA) only.

♦ Ensure immediate availability of resuscitation equipment/drugs to counteract possible respiratory depression or anaphylactic reaction.

♦ Monitor vital signs q 3 minutes during administration, q 5–15 minutes during recovery from anesthesia.

♦ Sterile water for injection is the preferred solvent. Do not reconstitute with Ringer's solution or solutions containing bacteriostatic or buffer agents. Precipitation may occur.

♦ In preparing dilute solutions for continuous IV drip, use either 5% dextrose or isotonic sodium chloride. This avoids hypotonicity which can occur with water for injection.

♦ Avoid injection of air into the solution, as this hastens the development of cloudiness.

♦ Rate of administration during induction is usually about 1 mL of 2.5% solution every 5 seconds.

♦ Ensure patency of vein. Extravasation can cause sloughing and necrosis. Intra-arterial injection can cause gangrene.

♦ Refrigerate solutions and use within 6 days (hospital policy may dictate a shorter time period, often less than 48 hours). If kept at room temperature, use within 24 hours.

♦ Use solutions only if clear. Discard

if cloudy or if precipitate is visible. Refrigeration helps maintain clarity.

Patient/Family Education

* Be aware of reasons for drug administration, what to expect in response to drug administration, and potential side effects.
* Be aware of potential risks involved with use of this drug, as well as risks associated with impending procedure.
* Inform physician of response to this or similar drugs in the past.
* Inform physician if pregnancy is suspected or if currently breast-feeding a baby. Safe use of this drug during pregnancy and lactation has not been established.

Evaluation

* Patient verbalizes understanding of need for thiamylal (as a short-acting anesthetic for minor surgery or other procedure, such as ECT).
* Patient verbalizes understanding of potential adverse side effects and risks associated with the administration of thiamylal.

THIOPENTAL SODIUM

(thye-oh-pen′tal)
Pentothal

Classification(s):
Anesthetic, Sedative-hypnotic, Barbiturate
Schedule III
Pregnancy Category C

INDICATIONS

* IV anesthesia for short procedures with minimal painful stimuli (e.g., minor surgical procedures, electroconvulsive therapy) * Basal narcosis * Induction of hypnotic state * Control of convulsive states * Narcoanalysis and narcosynthesis in psychiatric disorders * Supplement to regional anesthesia.

ACTION

* Depresses the central nervous system by inhibiting impulse conduction in the ascending reticular activating system * Produces anesthesia and hypnosis but does not possess analgesic properties.

PHARMACOKINETICS

Absorption: Rectal absorption unpredictable.
Distribution: Rapidly crosses blood-brain barrier, then is redistributed to other body tissues, with affinity for highly vascular organs (liver, kidneys, heart) and adipose tissue. Crosses placental barrier and is excreted in breast milk.
Metabolism and Excretion: Metabolized mainly in the liver, and to a lesser extent in other tissues, especially the kidneys and brain. Excreted in urine.
Half-Life: 3–8 hours.

CONTRAINDICATIONS AND PRECAUTIONS

Contraindicated in: * Latent or manifest porphyria * Hypersensitivity to barbiturates * Absence of suitable veins for IV administration * Status asthmaticus * Rectal suspension form in patients who are to undergo rectal surgery, or in the presence of inflammatory, ulcerative, bleeding or neoplastic lesions of the lower bowel * Pregnancy and lactation (safe use has not been established).
Use Cautiously in: * Severe cardiovascular disease * Hypotension or shock * Conditions in which hypnotic effects may be prolonged or potentiated (excessive premedication, Addison's disease, hepatic or renal dysfunction, myxedema, increased blood urea, and severe anemia) * Increased intracranial pressure * Asthma * Myasthenia gravis * Debilitated patients * Impaired function of respiratory, circulatory, renal, hepatic, or endocrine systems * Patients with a history of drug abuse/dependence.

ADVERSE REACTIONS AND SIDE EFFECTS*

CNS: prolonged somnolence and recovery, headache, emergence delirium, anxiety, restlessness.

CV: hypotension, circulatory depression, thrombophlebitis, MYOCARDIAL DEPRESSION, CARDIAC ARRHYTHMIAS, PERIPHERAL VASCULAR COLLAPSE.

GI: nausea, vomiting, abdominal pain, salivation; rectal administration: rectal irritation, diarrhea, cramping, rectal bleeding.

Derm: erythema, pruritus, urticaria, skin rashes, pain or nerve injury at injection site.

Resp: hiccups, sneezing, coughing, dyspnea, RESPIRATORY DEPRESSION, APNEA, LARYNGOSPASM, BRONCHOSPASM.

Other: tolerance, dependence, skeletal muscle hyperactivity, shivering, rhinitis, ANAPHYLACTIC REACTION.

INTERACTIONS

Drug-Drug: ♦ **CNS depressants (e.g., alcohol, benzodiazepines, other barbiturates, other sedative-hypnotics, opiates):** additive CNS and respiratory depression ♦ **Furosemide:** orthostatic hypotension ♦ **Sulfisoxazole IV:** increased effects of thiopental ♦ **Propranolol, corticosteroids, doxycycline, oral anticoagulants, oral contraceptives, quinidine, theophylline:** decreased effectiveness of these drugs.

ROUTE AND DOSAGE

(To be administered by anesthesiologist or CRNA only.)

Convulsive States
♦ **IV (Adults):** 75–125 mg (3–5 mL of a 2.5% solution) given as soon as possible after the convulsion begins. Convulsions following the use of a local anesthetic may require 125–250 mg given over a 10-minute period.

Anesthesia for Short Procedures

(Minor Surgery, ECT.)
♦ **IV (Adults):** Moderately slow induction may be accomplished by injecting 50–75 mg (2–3 mL of a 2.5% solution) every 20–40 seconds, depending on patient response. Additional doses of 25–50 mg may be given whenever patient moves after anesthesia is established. May be given as continuous IV drip of 0.2% or 0.4% concentration.

Preanesthetic Sedation
♦ **Rect Susp (Adults):** 1 g/75 lb (34 kg) or about 13.5 mg/lb (30 mg/kg).

Basal Narcosis
♦ **Rect Susp (Adults):** up to 1 g/50 lb (22.5 kg) in normally active adults. This is the equivalent to a dose of 20 mg/lb (44 mg/kg), and is the safe upper limit of dosage. In inactive or debilitated patients, use lower dosage. Do not exceed total dosage of 3–4 g for adults weighing 200 lb (90 kg) or more.

♦ **Rect Susp (Children):** up to 1 g/50 lb (22.5 kg) in normally active children. This is the equivalent to a dose of 20 mg/lb (44 mg/kg), and is the safe upper limit of dosage. In inactive or debilitated patients, use lower dosage. Do not exceed total dosage of 1–1.5 g for children weighing 75 lb (34 kg) or more.

PHARMACODYNAMICS

Route	Onset	Peak	Duration
IV	30–40 sec	*	*
Rect	8–10 min	—	60 min

*Ultrashort-acting. Duration varies tremendously between patients and with dose given. The more given, the longer the duration.

NURSING IMPLICATIONS
Assessment
♦ In patient receiving ECT, assess mood, level of activity, degree of participation in therapies, interaction with others.

* Assess for suicidal ideation in depressed patients.
* Assess history of allergies, sensitivity to this drug or to other barbiturates, history of porphyria, asthma.
* Obtain baseline blood pressure, pulse, respiration, temperature, and weight.
* Assess level of anxiety regarding impending surgical procedure or electroconvulsive therapy.
* Assess status of veins available for IV administration.
* Assess date of last menses (possible pregnancy), use of contraceptives.
* Assess whether currently breast-feeding a child.
* Assess current and past alcohol and drug consumption.
* Assess for presence of adverse reactions or side effects.
* Assess patient/family knowledge about illness and need for medication.
* In collaboration with physician, ensure performance of CBC and renal and liver function tests.
* **Toxicity and Overdose:** Assess for symptoms of overdose (may occur from too rapid or repeated injections): • profound drop in blood pressure (even to shock levels) • apnea • occasional laryngospasm • coughing and other respiratory difficulties.
* **Overdose Management:** Discontinue drug.
◇ Maintain patent airway (intubation may be required).
◇ Administer oxygen.
◇ Assist with ventilation if needed.
◇ Administer vasopressors to counteract hypotension.
◇ Administer IV fluids to maintain adequate circulation.
◇ Administer diuretics or hemodialysis to promote elimination of the drug.

Potential Nursing Diagnoses
* Ineffective breathing pattern related to side effects of respiratory depression, dyspnea, apnea.
* High risk for injury related to convul-

sions; overdose; extravasation at insertion site.
* High risk for self-directed violence related to depressed mood.
* Anxiety (moderate to severe) related to impending surgical procedure or electroconvulsive therapy.
* Alteration in bowel elimination related to side effects of rectal suspension administration.
* Knowledge deficit related to medication regimen.

Plan/Implementation
* **General Info:** Drug is administered by anesthesiologist or Certified Registered Nurse Anesthetist (CRNA) only.
◇ Ensure immediate availability of resuscitation equipment/drugs to counteract possible respiratory depression or anaphylactic reaction.
* **IV:** Monitor vital signs q 3 minutes during administration, q 5–15 minutes during recovery from anesthesia.
◇ Each 500 mg sterile thiopental powder is diluted in appropriate amount of sterile water for injection, sodium chloride injection, or 5% dextrose injection to make a 2.5% solution. (Do not use concentrations less than 2% in sterile water for injection—hemolysis can occur.) Final concentration varies from 2% to 5% depending on clinical situation.
◇ Unused portions should be discarded within 24 hours.
◇ Do not use solution if precipitate is visible.
◇ Each 25 mg or fraction thereof is administered over 1 minute and titrated slowly to desired effect.
◇ Ensure patency of vein. Extravasation can cause sloughing and necrosis. Intra-arterial injection can cause gangrene.
* **Rect Susp:** A normal saline enema may be ordered prior to administration of medication.
◇ If evacuation of the instilled rectal dose occurs, assess the effects of any retained portion before administering a repeat dose.

◇ Store medication at controlled room temperatures between 15° and 30°C (59°–86°F). Protect from heat and freezing.

Patient/Family Education

♦ Be aware of reasons for drug administration, what to expect in response to drug administration, and potential side effects.

♦ Be aware of potential risks involved with use of this drug, as well as risks associated with impending procedure.

♦ Inform physician of response to this or similar drugs in the past.

♦ Inform physician if pregnancy is suspected or if currently breast-feeding a baby. Safe use of this drug during pregnancy and lactation has not been established.

Evaluation

♦ Patient verbalizes understanding of need for thiopental (as a short-acting anesthetic for minor surgery or other procedure, or for preanesthetic sedation).

♦ Patient verbalizes understanding of potential adverse side effects and risks associated with the administration of thiopental.

THIORIDAZINE

(thye-or-rid′a-zeen)
Mellaril, {Novoridazine}, SK-Thioridazine

Classification(s):
Antipsychotic, Neuroleptic, Phenothiazine
Pregnancy Category C

INDICATIONS

♦ Psychotic disorders ♦ Moderate to marked depression with variable degrees of anxiety (short-term treatment) ♦ Multiple symptoms such as agitation, anxiety, depression, sleep disturbances, tension, and fears in the geriatric patient ♦ Hyperkinesis, combativeness, and severe behavioral problems in children.

ACTION

♦ The exact mechanism of antipsychotic action is not fully understood but is probably related to the drug's antidopaminergic effects ♦ Antipsychotics may block postsynaptic dopamine receptors in the basal ganglia, hypothalamus, limbic system, brain stem, and medulla ♦ Antipsychotic effects also appear to be related to inhibition of dopamine-mediated neurotransmission at the synapses ♦ Antipsychotic effects may also result from the drug's alpha-adrenergic blocking, muscarinic blocking, and adrenergic activity, as well as effects on other amines (such as GABA) or peptides.

PHARMACOKINETICS

Absorption: Rapid absorption of oral tablet dosage forms. Genetic differences in rate of first-pass metabolism results in a wide range of bioavailability from individual to individual. Oral liquid preparations and IM administration result in more consistent absorption.

Distribution: Widely distributed. Highly lipophilic, accumulates in brain, lungs, and other tissues with high blood supply. Crosses placental barrier. Enters breast milk.

Metabolism and Excretion: Metabolized by the liver and in the kidneys. Excreted through kidneys and enterohepatic circulation. Active metabolites accumulate and are stored in fatty tissue over a prolonged period of time, and may be detected in urine up to 3–6 months following discontinuation of the drug.

Half-Life: 9–30 hours.

CONTRAINDICATIONS AND PRECAUTIONS

Contraindicated in: ♦ Hypersensitivity to this drug, other phenothiazines, or sulfites or tartrazine (contained in some

{} = Only available in Canada.

preparations) ♦ Comatose or severely CNS-depressed patients ♦ Presence of large amounts of CNS depressants ♦ Bone marrow depression ♦ Blood dyscrasias ♦ Subcortical brain damage ♦ Parkinson's disease ♦ Liver, renal, and/or cardiac insufficiency ♦ Severe hypotension or hypertension ♦ Children under 2 years of age; pregnancy and lactation (safe use not established).

Use Cautiously in: ♦ Patients with a history of seizures ♦ Respiratory, renal, hepatic, thyroid, or cardiovascular disorders (e.g., respiratory infection, COPD, thyrotoxicosis, mitral insufficiency, angina pectoris) ♦ Prostatic hypertrophy ♦ Glaucoma ♦ Diabetes ♦ Elderly or debilitated patients ♦ Patients exposed to high or low environmental temperatures or to organophosphate insecticides ♦ Hypocalcemia ♦ History of severe reactions to insulin or ECT ♦ Pediatric patients with acute illnesses or dehydration.

ADVERSE REACTIONS AND SIDE EFFECTS*

CNS: sedation, headache, seizures, insomnia, dizziness, exacerbation of psychotic symptoms, extrapyramidal symptoms (pseudoparkinsonism, akathisia, akinesia, dystonia, oculogyric crisis), tardive dyskinesia, fatigue, cerebral edema, ataxia, blurred vision, NEUROLEPTIC MALIGNANT SYNDROME, restlessness, anxiety, depression, hyperthermia or hypothermia.

CV: hypotension, orthostatic hypotension, hypertension, tachycardia, bradycardia, CARDIAC ARREST, ECG changes, ARRHYTHMIAS, PULMONARY EDEMA, CIRCULATORY COLLAPSE.

Derm: skin rashes, urticaria, petechiae, seborrhea, photosensitivity, eczema, erythema, hyperpigmentation, contact dermatitis, EXFOLIATIVE DERMATITIS (rare).

Endo: galactorrhea, gynecomastia (men), changes in libido, impotence, hyperglycemia or hypoglycemia, amenorrhea, retrograde ejaculation.

GI: dry mouth, nausea, vomiting, increased appetite and weight gain, anorexia, dyspepsia, constipation, diarrhea, jaundice, polydipsia, PARALYTIC ILEUS.

GU: urinary retention, frequency or incontinence, bladder paralysis, polyuria, enuresis, priapism.

Hemat: AGRANULOCYTOSIS, LEUKOPENIA, ANEMIA, THROMBOCYTOPENIA, PANCYTOPENIA.

Ophth: lens deposition.

Resp: LARYNGEAL EDEMA, LARYNGOSPASM, BRONCHOSPASM, SUPPRESSION OF COUGH REFLEX.

Other: decreased sweating.

INTERACTIONS

Drug-Drug: ♦ **CNS depressants (including alcohol, barbiturates, narcotics, anesthetics):** additive CNS depressant effects ♦ **Anticholinergic agents (e.g., atropine):** additive anticholinergic effects, decreased antipsychotic effects ♦ **Barbiturate anesthetics:** increased incidence of excitatory effects and hypotension ♦ **Barbiturates:** possible decreased effects of phenothiazines ♦ **Metyrosine:** potentiation of extrapyramidal side effects ♦ **Levodopa:** decreased efficacy of levodopa ♦ **Quinidine:** additive cardiac depressive effects ♦ **Magnesium- or aluminum-containing antidiarrheal mixtures, antacids:** reduced phenothiazine absorption/effectiveness ♦ **Guanethidine:** decreased antihypertensive action ♦ **Propranolol, metoprolol:** increased plasma levels and effects of both drugs ♦ **Lithium:** decreased plasma levels and effect of antipsychotic drug; severe neurotoxicity reported ♦ **Epinephrine:** reversal of usual pressor action of epinephrine, resulting in decreased blood pressure and tachycardia ♦ **Bromocriptine:** impairment of prolactin-suppressing action ♦ **Angiotensin converting enzyme (ACE) inhibitors:** increased effects of ACE inhibitors ♦ **Phenytoin:** decreased phenytoin metabolism, increased risk of toxicity;

---

*Underlines indicate most frequent; CAPITALS indicate life-threatening.

decreased thioridazine effect ✦ **Poly-peptide antibiotics:** possible neuro-muscular respiratory depression ✦ **Phenylpropanolamine, metriza-mide:** seizures ✦ **Cimetidine:** decreased effect of phenothiazines ✦ **Clonidine:** possibility of severe hypotension ✦ **Pi-perazine:** increased seizure potential. **Drug-Food:** ✦ **Caffeine-containing beverages (e.g., coffee, tea, colas):** counteracted antipsychotic effect.

ROUTE AND DOSAGE
Psychotic Disorders
- ✦ **PO (Adults):** 50–100 mg tid; in-crease gradually to a maximum of 800 mg/day, if necessary, to control symp-toms. When desired effect is achieved, reduce dose gradually to maintenance dose of 200–800 mg daily, divided into 2–4 doses.

Moderate to Marked Depression with Anxiety, Multiple Psychoneurotic Symptoms in the Elderly
- ✦ **PO (Adults):** Initial dosage: 25 mg tid. Dosage ranges from 10 mg bid–qid in milder cases to 50 mg tid–qid for more severely disturbed patients.

✦ Behavioral Disorders of Childhood
- ✦ **PO (Children Age 2–12):** 0.5–3 mg/kg/day. For moderate disorders, the usual starting dose is 10 mg bid or tid. For hospitalized, severely dis-turbed, or psychotic children, the ini-tial daily dose is 25 mg bid or tid. Dosage may be increased to optimal effect. Maximum daily dose: 3 mg/kg.

PHARMACODYNAMICS

Route	Onset*	Peak†	Duration‡
PO	30–60 min	2–4 hr	4–6 hr

*Full clinical effects may not be observed for 4–8 weeks.
†Steady-state plasma levels are achieved in ap-proximately 4–7 days.
‡Drug may be detected in urine for 3–6 months after last dose.

NURSING IMPLICATIONS
Assessment
- ✦ Assess mental status daily: • mood • appearance • thought and communi-cation patterns • level of interest in the environment and in activities • level of anxiety or agitation • presence of hallucinations or delusions • sus-piciousness • interactions with others • ability to carry out activities of daily living.
- ✦ Assess for symptoms of blood dyscra-sias: • sore throat • fever • malaise • unusual bleeding • easy bruising.
- ✦ Assess for extrapyramidal symptoms: • pseudoparkinsonism (tremors, shuffling gait, drooling, rigidity) • aki-nesia (muscular weakness) • akathi-sia (continuous restlessness and fidg-eting) • dystonia (involuntary muscular movements of face, arms, legs, and neck) • oculogyric crisis (uncontrolled rolling back of the eyes) • tardive dyskinesia (bizarre fa-cial and tongue movements, stiff neck, difficulty swallowing).
- ✦ Assess for symptoms of neuroleptic malignant syndrome: • hyperpyrexia up to 107°F (41.6°C) • elevated pulse • increased or decreased blood pres-sure • severe parkinsonian muscle ri-gidity • elevated creatinine phospho-kinase blood levels • elevated white blood count • altered mental status (including catatonic signs or agita-tion) • acute renal failure • varying levels of consciousness (including stu-por and coma, pallor, diaphoresis, tachycardia, arrhythmias, rhabdomy-olysis).
- ✦ Assess vital signs, weight. Record baseline values for comparison.
- ✦ Assess history of allergies, sensitivity to this drug or to other phenothiazines.
- ✦ Assess for signs and symptoms of cho-lestatic jaundice: • abdominal pain • nausea • rash • fever • yellow skin • flu-like symptoms • abnormal lab test results (eosinophilia, bile in urine, in-

creased serum transaminases, bilirubin, alkaline phosphotase).

* Assess date of last menses (possible pregnancy), use of contraceptives.
* Assess whether currently breast-feeding a child.
* Assess current and past alcohol and drug consumption.
* Assess for operation of automobile and/or other dangerous machinery.
* Assess for presence of adverse reactions or side effects.
* Assess patient/family knowledge about illness and need for medication.
* In collaboration with physician, assess CBC, liver function tests, and ophthalmological exams in patients on long-term therapy.
* **Lab Test Alterations:** Increased serum alkaline phosphatase, transaminases, bilirubin.
◊ Increased protein-bound iodine.
◊ False-positive urine pregnancy test, possibly caused by drug metabolite that discolors urine (less likely to occur when serum test is used).
◊ Increased urinary glucose.
◊ Decreased urinary estrogen, progestin, and gonadotropin.
◊ Increased plasma cholesterol level.
◊ Increased serum prolactin.
* **Withdrawal:** Assess for symptoms of abrupt withdrawal from long-term therapy: • gastritis • nausea • vomiting • dizziness • headache • tachycardia • insomnia • tremulousness • sweating.
* **Toxicity and Overdose:** No correlation has been established between blood level and therapeutic effect.
◊ Assess for symptoms of overdose: • CNS depression, from heavy sedation to deep sleep to coma • hypotension • confusion • excitement • extrapyramidal symptoms • agitation • restlessness • convulsions • fever • autonomic reactions • ECG changes • cardiac arrhythmias • tachycardia • hypothermia • tremor • seizures • cyanosis.

* **Overdose Management:** Monitor vital signs.
◊ Ensure maintenance of open airway.
◊ Initiate gastric lavage.
◊ Do not induce emesis (nuchal rigidity may result in aspiration of vomitus).
◊ Administer antiparkinsonian drugs or diphenhydramine to counteract extrapyramidal symptoms.
◊ Administer IV fluids or a vasoconstrictor to maintain adequate blood pressure. **Note:** Epinephrine is not recommended due to its interaction with phenothiazines, which causes further drop in blood pressure.
◊ Administer IV phenytoin to control ventricular arrhythmias.
◊ Administer phenobarbital or diazepam to control convulsions or hyperactivity.
◊ Dialysis does not appear to be a useful intervention.

Potential Nursing Diagnoses

* High risk for violence to self or others related to depressed mood, suspiciousness, and panic anxiety.
* High risk for injury related to thioridazine's side effects of sedation, dizziness, ataxia, weakness, and lowered seizure threshold; abrupt withdrawal after prolonged use; overdose.
* Sensory-perceptual alteration related to panic anxiety evidenced by hallucinations.
* Altered thought processes related to panic anxiety evidenced by delusional thinking.
* Social isolation related to inability to trust others.
* High risk for activity intolerance related to thioridazine's side effects of drowsiness, dizziness, ataxia, weakness.
* Noncompliance with medication regimen related to suspiciousness and mistrust of others.
* Knowledge deficit related to medication regimen.

Plan/Implementation

+ Monitor vital signs before beginning therapy and at regular intervals (bid or tid) throughout therapy. Take BP lying and standing to monitor for possible hypotensive reaction; elderly are particularly susceptible. Dosage adjustment may be required.
+ Ensure that patient who is ambulatory is protected from sun when spending time outdoors.
+ Weigh patient 2–3 times a week, at same time of day, on same scale, if possible. A rapid weight gain or evidence of edema should be reported to physician immediately. Record I&O.
+ Ensure that patient is protected from injury. Provide supervision and assistance when ambulating if dizziness and drowsiness are problems. Pad siderails and headboard for patient who experiences seizures.
+ Give patient hard candy, gum, or frequent sips of water if dry mouth is a problem.
+ Medication may be administered with food to minimize GI upset.
+ Ensure that patient swallows tablet and does not "cheek" to avoid medication or to hoard for later use.
+ Tablet may be crushed and mixed with food or fluid for patient who has difficulty swallowing, or concentrate form may be used.
+ Just prior to administration, mix concentrate with juice, distilled water, or acidified tap water.
+ If concentrate is accidentally spilled on skin or clothing during preparation or administration, wash area immediately, as contact dermatitis can occur.
+ Store medication at controlled room temperatures between 15° and 30°C (59°–86°F). Protect from heat, light, and moisture.

Patient/Family Education

+ Use caution when driving or when operating dangerous machinery. Drowsiness and dizziness can occur.
+ Do not stop taking the drug abruptly. To do so might produce withdrawal symptoms, such as nausea, vomiting, gastritis, headache, tachycardia, insomnia, tremulousness.
+ Use sunscreens and wear protective clothing when spending time outdoors. Skin is more susceptible to sunburn.
+ Report occurrence of any of the following symptoms to physician immediately: • sore throat • fever • malaise • unusual bleeding • easy bruising • persistent nausea/vomiting • severe headache • rapid heart rate • difficulty urinating • muscle twitching • tremors • darkly colored urine • pale stools • yellow skin or eyes • muscular incoordination • skin rash.
+ Drug may turn urine pink to reddish-brown in color. This is not significant nor is it harmful.
+ Rise slowly from a sitting or lying position to prevent a sudden drop in blood pressure.
+ If dry mouth is a problem, take frequent sips of water, chew sugarless gum, or suck on hard candy. Good oral care (frequent brushing, flossing) is very important.
+ If some liquid concentrate is spilled on the skin, wash it off immediately. If not, a rash may appear.
+ Consult physician regarding smoking while on thioridazine therapy. Smoking increases metabolism of thioridazine, requiring adjustment in dosage to achieve therapeutic effect.
+ Dress warmly in cold weather and avoid extended exposure to very high or low temperatures. Body temperature is harder to maintain while taking this medication.
+ Do not drink alcohol while on thioridazine therapy. These drugs potentiate each other's effects.
+ Do not consume other medications (including over-the-counter meds) without physician's approval. Many

medications contain substances that interact with thioridazine in a way that may be harmful.

* Be aware of possible risks of taking thioridazine during pregnancy. Safe use during pregnancy and lactation has not been established. Thioridazine readily crosses the placental barrier, so a fetus could experience adverse effects of the drug. Inform physician immediately if pregnancy occurs, is suspected, or is planned.
* Be aware of side effects of thioridazine. Refer to written materials furnished by healthcare providers for safe self-administration.
* Continue to take medication even if feeling well and as though it is not needed. Symptoms may return if medication is discontinued.
* Carry card or other identification at all times describing medications being taken.

Evaluation

* Patient demonstrates a subsiding/resolution of the symptoms for which thioridazine was prescribed (depression with anxiety, altered thought processes, altered perceptions, behavioral disorders).
* Patient verbalizes understanding of side effects and regimen required for prudent self-administration of thioridazine.

THIOTHIXENE

(thye-oh-thix'een)
Navane

Classification(s):
Antipsychotic, Neuroleptic, Thioxanthene
Pregnancy Category C

INDICATIONS

* Manifestations of psychotic disorders.

ACTION

* The exact mechanism of action is not fully understood ◆ Antipsychotics block postsynaptic dopamine receptors in the hypothalamus, limbic system, and reticular formation ◆ Antipsychotic effects appear to be related to inhibition of dopamine release, increased neuronal cell firing rate in the midbrain, and an increased turnover rate of dopamine in the forebrain ◆ Drug also has autonomic nervous system effects.

PHARMACOKINETICS

Absorption: Slowly but well absorbed following oral or parenteral administration.
Distribution: Widely distributed. Highly lipophilic; accumulates in brain, lungs, and other tissues with high blood supply. Crosses placental barrier. Enters breast milk.
Metabolism and Excretion: Metabolized by the liver. Excreted mainly in feces. Active metabolites accumulate and are stored in fatty tissue over a prolonged period of time, and may be detected in urine up to several weeks following discontinuation of the drug.
Half-Life: 34 hours.

CONTRAINDICATIONS AND PRECAUTIONS

Contraindicated in: ◆ Hypersensitivity to thioxanthenes or phenothiazines ◆ Comatose or severely CNS-depressed patients ◆ Presence of large amounts of CNS depressants ◆ Bone marrow depression ◆ Blood dyscrasias ◆ Subcortical brain damage ◆ Parkinson's disease ◆ Liver, renal, and/or cardiac insufficiency ◆ Severe hypotension or hypertension ◆ Circulatory collapse ◆ Children under age 12 ◆ Pregnancy and lactation (safe use not established).
Use Cautiously in: ◆ Patients with a history of seizures ◆ Respiratory, renal, hepatic, thyroid, or cardiovascular disorders (e.g., respiratory infection, COPD,

thyrotoxicosis, mitral insufficiency, angina pectoris) ◆ Prostatic hypertrophy ◆ Glaucoma ◆ Diabetes ◆ Elderly or debilitated patients ◆ Patients in alcohol withdrawal ◆ Patients exposed to extreme environmental heat ◆ Patients taking atropine or atropine-like drugs.

ADVERSE REACTIONS AND SIDE EFFECTS*

CNS: sedation, headache, seizures, insomnia, dizziness, exacerbation of psychotic symptoms, extrapyramidal symptoms (pseudoparkinsonism, akathisia, akinesia, dystonia, oculogyric crisis), tardive dyskinesia, fatigue, cerebral edema, ataxia, blurred vision, restlessness, agitation, hyperpyrexia.

CV: orthostatic hypotension, hypertension, tachycardia, bradycardia, CARDIAC ARREST, ECG changes, ARRHYTHMIAS, PULMONARY EDEMA, CIRCULATORY COLLAPSE.

Derm: skin rashes, urticaria, petechiae, seborrhea, photosensitivity, eczema, pruritis, contact dermatitis, EXFOLIATIVE DERMATITIS (rare).

Endo: galactorrhea, gynecomastia (men), changes in libido, hyperglycemia or hypoglycemia, amenorrhea, retrograde ejaculation, enlarged parotid glands, glycosuria.

GI: dry mouth, nausea, vomiting, increased appetite and weight gain, anorexia, dyspepsia, constipation, diarrhea, jaundice, polydipsia, PARALYTIC ILEUS.

GU: urinary retention, frequency or incontinence, bladder paralysis, polyuria, enuresis, priapism.

Hemat: AGRANULOCYTOSIS, LEUKOPENIA, ANEMIA, THROMBOCYTOPENIA, PANCYTOPENIA, leukocytosis.

Resp: LARYNGOSPASM, BRONCHOSPASM, SUPPRESSION OF COUGH REFLEX.

Other: NEUROLEPTIC MALIGNANT SYNDROME, increased sweating.

INTERACTIONS

Drug-Drug: ◆ **CNS depressants (including alcohol, barbiturates, narcotics, anesthetics):** additive CNS depressant effects ◆ **Anticholinergic agents (e.g., atropine):** additive anticholinergic effects, decreased antipsychotic effects ◆ **Barbiturate anesthetics:** increased incidence of excitatory effects and hypotension ◆ **Barbiturates:** possible decreased antipsychotic effects ◆ **Metyrosine:** potentiation of extrapyramidal side effects ◆ **Levodopa:** decreased efficacy of levodopa ◆ **Quinidine:** additive cardiac depressive effects ◆ **Guanethidine:** decreased antihypertensive action ◆ **Lithium:** decreased plasma levels of antipsychotic drug ◆ **Epinephrine:** reversal of usual pressor action of epinephrine, resulting in decreased blood pressure and tachycardia ◆ **Bromocriptine:** impairment of prolactin-suppressing action ◆ **Angiotensin converting enzyme (ACE) inhibitors:** increased effects of ACE inhibitors ◆ **Phenytoin:** decreased phenytoin metabolism, increased risk of toxicity ◆ **Polypeptide antibiotics:** neuromuscular respiratory depression ◆ **Metrizamide:** seizures ◆ **Cimetidine:** decreased antipsychotic effect ◆ **Clonidine:** possibility of severe hypotension ◆ **Piperazine:** possible increased seizure potential.

Drug-Food: ◆ Caffeine-containing beverages (e.g., coffee, tea, colas): counteraction of antipsychotic effect.

ROUTE AND DOSAGE

Psychotic Disorders

◆ **PO (Adults):** For mild conditions, initial dose: 2 mg tid. If necessary increase to 15 mg/day. For severe conditions, initial dose: 5 mg bid. Usual optimal dose: 20–30 mg/day. Dosage may be increased to 60 mg/day if needed.

◆ **IM (Adults):** 4 mg bid to qid. Usual daily dosage range: 16–20 mg. Maximum: 30 mg/day.

---

*Underlines indicate most frequent; CAPITALS indicate life-threatening.

PHARMACODYNAMICS

Route	Onset*	Peak†	Duration‡
PO	Slow	2–8 hr	12–24 hr
IM	15–30 min	1–6 hr	up to 12 hr

*Full antipsychotic effects may not be observed for 4–8 weeks.
†Steady-state plasma levels are achieved in approximately 4–7 days.
‡Drug may be detected in urine for 3–6 months after last dose.

NURSING IMPLICATIONS

Assessment

♦ Assess mental status daily: • mood • appearance • thought and communication patterns • level of interest in the environment and in activities • level of anxiety or agitation • presence of hallucinations or delusions • suspiciousness • interactions with others • ability to carry out activities of daily living.

♦ Assess for symptoms of blood dyscrasias: • sore throat • fever • malaise • unusual bleeding • easy bruising.

♦ Assess for extrapyramidal symptoms: • pseudoparkinsonism (tremors, shuffling gait, drooling, rigidity) • akinesia (muscular weakness) • akathisia (continuous restlessness and fidgeting) • dystonia (involuntary muscular movements of face, arms, legs, and neck) • oculogyric crisis (uncontrolled rolling back of the eyes) • tardive dyskinesia (bizarre facial and tongue movements, stiff neck, difficulty swallowing).

♦ Assess for symptoms of neuroleptic malignant syndrome: • hyperpyrexia up to 107°F (41.6°C) • elevated pulse • increased or decreased blood pressure • severe parkinsonian muscle rigidity • elevated creatinine phosphokinase blood levels • elevated white blood count • altered mental status (including catatonic signs or agitation) • acute renal failure • varying levels of consciousness (including stupor and coma) • pallor • diaphoresis • tachycardia • arrhythmias • rhabdomyolysis.

♦ Assess vital signs, weight. Record baseline values for comparison.

♦ Assess history of allergies, sensitivity to this drug or to other thioxanthenes or phenothiazines.

♦ Assess for signs and symptoms of cholestatic jaundice: • abdominal pain • nausea • rash • fever • yellow skin • flu-like symptoms • abnormal lab test results (eosinophilia, bile in urine, increased serum transaminases, bilirubin, alkaline phosphotase).

♦ Assess date of last menses (possible pregnancy), use of contraceptives.

♦ Assess whether currently breast-feeding a child.

♦ Assess current and past alcohol and drug consumption.

♦ Assess for operation of automobile and/or other dangerous machinery.

♦ Assess for presence of adverse reactions or side effects.

♦ Assess patient/family knowledge about illness and need for medication.

♦ In collaboration with physician, assess CBC, liver function tests, and ophthalmological exams in patients on long-term therapy.

♦ **Lab Test Alterations:** Increased serum alkaline phosphatase, transaminases, bilirubin.

◊ Increased protein-bound iodine.

◊ False-positive urine pregnancy test, possibly caused by drug metabolite that discolors urine (less likely to occur when serum test is used).

◊ Increased urinary glucose.

◊ Decreased urinary estrogen, progestin, and gonadotropin.

◊ Increased plasma cholesterol level.

◊ Increased serum prolactin.

♦ **Withdrawal:** Assess for symptoms of abrupt withdrawal from long-term therapy: • gastritis • nausea • vomiting • dizziness • headache • tachycardia • insomnia • tremulousness • sweating.

♦ **Toxicity and Overdose:** No correlation has been established between blood level and therapeutic effect.

◊ Assess for symptoms of overdose: •

CNS depression, from heavy sedation to deep sleep to coma • hypotension • confusion • excitement • extrapyramidal symptoms • agitation • restlessness • convulsions • fever • autonomic reactions • ECG changes • cardiac arrhythmias • tachycardia • hypothermia • tremor • seizures • cyanosis.

• **Overdose Management:** Monitor vital signs.

◊ Ensure maintenance of adequate airway.

◊ Initiate gastric lavage.

◊ Do not induce emesis (nuchal rigidity may result in aspiration of vomitus).

◊ Administer antiparkinsonian drugs or diphenhydramine to counteract extrapyramidal symptoms.

◊ Administer IV fluids or a vasoconstrictor to maintain adequate blood pressure. **Note:** Epinephrine is not recommended due to its interaction with antipsychotics, which causes further drop in blood pressure.

◊ Administer IV phenytoin to control ventricular arrhythmias.

◊ Administer phenobarbital or diazepam to control convulsions or hyperactivity.

◊ Dialysis does not appear to be a useful intervention.

Potential Nursing Diagnoses

• High risk for violence directed at others related to mistrust and panic anxiety.

• High risk for injury related to thiothixene's side effects of sedation, dizziness, ataxia, weakness, and lowered seizure threshold; abrupt withdrawal after prolonged use; overdose.

• Sensory-perceptual alteration related to panic anxiety evidenced by hallucinations.

• Altered thought processes related to panic anxiety evidenced by delusional thinking.

• Social isolation related to inability to trust others.

• High risk for activity intolerance related to thiothixene's side effects of drowsiness, dizziness, ataxia, weakness.

• Noncompliance with medication regimen related to suspiciousness and mistrust of others.

• Knowledge deficit related to medication regimen.

Plan/Implementation

• **General Info:** Monitor vital signs before beginning therapy and at regular intervals (bid or tid) throughout therapy. Take BP lying and standing to monitor for possible hypotensive reaction; elderly are particularly susceptible. Dosage adjustment may be required.

◊ Ensure that patient who is ambulatory is protected from sun when spending time outdoors.

◊ Weigh patient 2–3 times a week, at same time of day, on same scale, if possible. A rapid weight gain or evidence of edema should be reported to physician immediately. Record I&O.

◊ Ensure that patient is protected from injury. Provide supervision and assistance when ambulating if dizziness and drowsiness are problems. Pad siderails and headboard for patient who experiences seizures.

◊ Give patient hard candy, gum, or frequent sips of water if dry mouth is a problem.

◊ Store medication at controlled room temperatures between 15° and 30°C (59°–86°F). Protect from heat, light, and moisture.

• **PO:** Medication may be administered with food to minimize GI upset.

◊ Ensure that patient swallows capsule and does not "cheek" to avoid medication or to hoard for later use.

◊ Capsule may be emptied and mixed with food or fluid for patient who has difficulty swallowing, or liquid concentrate may be used.

◊ Just prior to administration, dilute

concentrate with milk, water, fruit juice, soup, or carbonated beverage.

◊ If concentrate is accidentally spilled on skin or clothing during preparation or administration, wash area immediately, as contact dermatitis can occur.

✦ **IM:** Avoid contact with injectable liquid. A contact dermatitis can occur.

◊ Inject slowly and deeply into upper, outer quadrant of buttock or other large muscle mass, such as midlateral thigh.

◊ Because of possible hypotensive effects, patient should remain in recumbent position for at least 1 hour following IM injection. Monitor blood pressure every 10 minutes during this time.

◊ Rotate sites when multiple injections are administered.

◊ Aspirate carefully to avoid injection directly into blood vessel.

◊ Reconstitute the powder for injection with 2.2 mL of sterile water for injection. Reconstituted solution may be stored at room temperature for 48 hours before discarding.

Patient/Family Education

✦ Use caution when driving or when operating dangerous machinery. Drowsiness and dizziness can occur.

✦ Do not stop taking the drug abruptly. To do so might produce withdrawal symptoms, such as nausea, vomiting, gastritis, headache, tachycardia, insomnia, tremulousness.

✦ Use sunscreens and wear protective clothing when spending time outdoors. Skin is more susceptible to sunburn.

✦ Report occurrence of any of the following symptoms to physician immediately: • sore throat • fever • malaise • unusual bleeding • easy bruising • persistent nausea/vomiting • severe headache • rapid heart rate • difficulty urinating • muscle twitching • tremors

• darkly colored urine • pale stools • yellow skin or eyes • muscular incoordination • skin rash.

✦ Rise slowly from a sitting or lying position to prevent a sudden drop in blood pressure.

✦ If dry mouth is a problem, take frequent sips of water, chew sugarless gum, or suck on hard candy. Good oral care (frequent brushing, flossing) is very important.

✦ If some liquid concentrate is spilled on the skin, wash it off immediately. If not, a rash may appear.

✦ Consult physician regarding smoking while on thiothixene therapy. Smoking increases metabolism of thiothixene, requiring adjustment in dosage to achieve therapeutic effect.

✦ Dress warmly in cold weather and avoid extended exposure to very high or low temperatures. Body temperature is harder to maintain while taking this medication.

✦ Do not drink alcohol while on thiothixene therapy. These drugs potentiate each other's effects.

✦ Do not consume other medications (including over-the-counter meds) without physician's approval. Many medications contain substances that interact with thiothixene in a way that may be harmful.

✦ Be aware of possible risks of taking thiothixene during pregnancy. Safe use during pregnancy and lactation has not been established. Thiothixene readily crosses the placental barrier, so a fetus could experience adverse effects of the drug. Inform physician immediately if pregnancy occurs, is suspected, or is planned.

✦ Be aware of side effects of thiothixene. Refer to written materials furnished by healthcare providers for safe self-administration.

✦ Continue to take medication even if feeling well and as though it is not needed. Symptoms may return if medication is discontinued.

✦ Carry card or other identification at all

times describing medications being taken.

Evaluation

♦ Patient demonstrates a subsiding/resolution of the symptoms for which thiothixene was prescribed (panic anxiety, altered thought processes, altered perceptions).

♦ Patient verbalizes understanding of side effects and regimen required for prudent self-administration of thiothixene.

TRANYLCYPROMINE

(tran-ill-sip'roe-meen)
Parnate

Classification(s):
Antidepressant, Monoamine oxidase inhibitor
Pregnancy Category C

INDICATIONS

♦ Major depression without melancholia in closely supervised patients unresponsive to other antidepressive therapy (e.g., tricyclics, ECT). Rarely drug of first choice. **Investigational Use:** ♦ Bulimia with characteristics of atypical depression.

ACTION

♦ Exact mechanism of action on depression unknown ♦ Inhibits the enzyme monoamine oxidase, which normally inhibits the activity of epinephrine, norepinephrine, dopamine, and serotonin. The concentration of these biogenic amines is then increased in storage sites throughout the nervous system. These increases in biogenic amines are thought to reduce symptoms of depression.

PHARMACOKINETICS

Absorption: Well absorbed from the GI tract following oral administration.

Distribution: Widely distributed. It is thought to cross placental barrier and to enter breast milk.

Metabolism and Excretion: Metabolized by the liver. Excreted in urine as metabolites and unchanged drug.

Half-Life: 1.5–3.2 hours (average 2.5 hours).

CONTRAINDICATIONS AND PRECAUTIONS

Contraindicated in: ♦ Hypersensitivity to this drug or to other MAO inhibitors ♦ Pheochromocytoma ♦ Congestive heart failure ♦ History of liver disease ♦ Severe renal impairment ♦ Cerebrovascular defect ♦ Paranoid schizophrenic disorder ♦ Cardiovascular disease ♦ Hypertension ♦ History of severe or frequent headaches ♦ Patients over 60 ♦ Children less than 16 years of age; pregnancy and lactation (safety not established).

Use Cautiously in: ♦ Patients with a history of seizures ♦ Diabetes mellitus ♦ Renal insufficiency ♦ Suicidal patients ♦ Schizophrenia ♦ Agitated or hypomanic patients ♦ History of angina pectoris or hyperthyroidism.

ADVERSE REACTIONS AND SIDE EFFECTS*

CNS: dizziness, vertigo, headache, overactivity, tremors, muscle twitching, mania, confusion, memory impairment, insomnia, drowsiness, blurred vision, restlessness, weakness, agitation.

CV: orthostatic hypotension, disturbances in cardiac rate and rhythm, tachycardia, palpitations, peripheral edema.

Derm: skin rashes.

GI: dry mouth, constipation, anorexia, body weight changes, nausea, vomiting, diarrhea, abdominal pain.

GU: dysuria, incontinence, neuritis, urinary retention, changes in libido, transient impotence.

Hemat: spider telangiectases.

---

*Underlines indicate most frequent; CAPITALS indicate life-threatening.

Other: excessive sweating, arthralgia, weight gain, FATAL PROGRESSIVE NECROTIZING HEPATOCELLULAR DAMAGE (rare).

INTERACTIONS

Drug-Drug: ♦ **Sympathomimetic and catecholamine-releasing drugs (including amphetamines, methyldopa, levodopa, dopamine, tryptophan, epinephrine, norepinephrine):** increased hypertensive effects, headache, hyperpyrexia ♦ **CNS depressants (e.g., alcohol and certain narcotics such as meperidine):** possible hypo/hypertension, convulsions, coma, death ♦ **Other MAO inhibitors, tricylic antidepressants, other dibenzazepines (carbamazepine, cyclobenzaprine):** hypertensive crisis, convulsions, coma, circulatory collapse ♦ **Antihypertensive drugs, thiazide diuretics:** hypotension ♦ **Guanethidine:** decreased antihypertensive effects ♦ **Doxapram:** potentiation of adverse cardiovascular effects ♦ **Insulin, oral hypoglycemics:** increased hypoglycemic effects ♦ **Methylphenidate:** increased effect of methylphenidate ♦ **Anesthetics:** increased hypotensive and CNS depressant effects ♦ **Disulfiram:** increased toxicity ♦ **Metrizamide:** increased risk of seizures.
Drug-Food: ♦ **Foods containing high concentrations of tryptophan, tyramine, or other vasopressors** (examples include aged cheeses, other aged, overripe, and fermented foods, broad beans, pickled herring, beef/chicken livers, preserved sausages, beer, wine, [especially chianti], yeast products, chocolate, caffeinated drinks, canned figs, sour cream, yogurt, soy sauce, OTC cold medications, diet pills): hypertensive crisis.
Caution: Can occur several weeks after MAOI therapy has been discontinued.

ROUTE AND DOSAGE

Depression
♦ **PO (Adults):** Start at 30 mg/day in 2 divided doses (morning and afternoon). After 2–3 weeks, dosage may be increased by 10 mg/day at 1–3 week intervals until desired response is achieved or maximum of 60 mg/day is reached.
♦ **PO, Maintenance (Adults):** Start maintenance dose when desired effect has been achieved. Reduce dose to 10–20 mg/day for maintenance.

Bulimia with Characteristics of Atypical Depression
(Investigational)
♦ **PO (Adults):** 30–40 mg/day.

PHARMACODYNAMICS

Route	Onst	Peak	Duration
PO	2–21 days	1–3 hr	1 week*

*Allow up to 1 week following cessation of therapy for complete drug elimination, although it appears tranylcypromine's activity may terminate in as little as 22–120 hours.

NURSING IMPLICATIONS

Assessment
♦ Assess for suicidal ideation, plan, means. Assess for sudden lifts in mood, which could indicate patient's decision to commit suicide. ♦ mood ♦
♦ Assess mental status daily: ♦ mood ♦ appearance ♦ thought and communication patterns ♦ level of interest in the environment and in activities ♦ suicidal ideation. Improvement in these behavior patterns and level of energy should be expected within 2 days–3 weeks following initiation of therapy.
♦ Assess vital signs, weight.
♦ Assess dieting pattern and consult dietitian.
♦ Assess history of allergies, sensitivity to this drug or to other MAO inhibitors.
♦ Assess for history of glaucoma.
♦ Assess date of last menses (possible pregnancy), use of contraceptives.
♦ Assess whether currently breast-feeding a child.
♦ Assess current and past alcohol and drug consumption.
♦ Assess for operation of automobile and/or other dangerous machinery.

◆ Assess for presence of adverse reactions or side effects.

◆ Assess patient/family knowledge about illness and need for medication.

◆ In collaboration with physician, assess CBC and liver and renal function tests in patients on long-term therapy.

◆ **Withdrawal:** Assess for symptoms of abrupt withdrawal from long-term therapy: • headache • excitability • hallucinations • depression.

◆ **Hypertensive Crisis:** Assess for symptoms of hypertensive crisis: • severe occipital headache • palpitations • sharp rise in blood pressure • nuchal rigidity • chest pain • sweating • fever • nausea • vomiting • coma.

◆ **Management of Hypertensive Crisis:** Discontinue drug immediately.

◇ Monitor vital signs.

◇ Institute therapy to lower blood pressure.

◇ Do not use parenteral reserpine.

◇ Administer antihypertensives slowly to avoid producing an excessive hypotensive effect.

◇ Use external cooling measures to control hyperpyrexia.

◆ **Toxicity and Overdose:** Relationship between blood level and therapeutic response has not been established.

◇ Assess for symptoms of overdose: • excitement • irritability • anxiety • flushing • sweating • tachypnea • tachycardia • exaggerated tendon reflexes • hypotension • hypertension • convulsions • coma • cardiorespiratory arrest.

◆ **Overdose Management:** Monitor vital signs.

◇ Ensure maintenance of adequate airway.

◇ Initiate gastric lavage.

◇ Administer activated charcoal to minimize absorption of the drug.

◇ Monitor electrolytes.

◇ Supplemental oxygen and mechanical ventilatory assistance should be provided as needed.

◇ Administer IV diazepam to control convulsions.

◇ Administer IV fluids to treat hypotension and cardiovascular collapse.

◇ Follow up with liver function evaluation.

Potential Nursing Diagnoses

◆ High risk for self-directed violence related to depressed mood.

◆ High risk for injury related to tranylcypromine's side effects of sedation, dizziness, fatigue, confusion, and lowered seizure threshold; eating foods that contain tyramine or tryptophan; abrupt withdrawal after prolonged use; overdose.

◆ Social isolation related to depressed mood.

◆ High risk for activity intolerance related to tranylcypromine's side effects of drowsiness, dizziness, fatigue, confusion.

◆ Knowledge deficit related to medication regimen.

Plan/Implementation

◆ Monitor vital signs before beginning therapy and at regular intervals (bid or tid) throughout therapy. Take BP lying and standing in patients experiencing orthostatic hypotension, elderly are particularly susceptible. Contact physician if tachycardia/arrhythmias are noted.

◆ Weigh patient 2–3 times a week, at same time of day, on same scale, if possible. A rapid weight gain or evidence of edema should be reported to physician immediately. Record I&O.

◆ Ensure that patient is protected from injury. Provide supervision and assistance when ambulating if dizziness and drowsiness are problems. Pad siderails and headboard for patient who experiences seizures. Ensure that ambulatory patient is protected when in the sun.

◆ Order low tyramine diet for patient.

- Give patient hard candy, gum, or frequent sips of water if dry mouth is a problem.
- Medication may be administered with food to minimize GI upset.
- Ensure that patient swallows tablet and does not "cheek" to avoid medication or to hoard for later use.
- Tablet may be crushed and mixed with food or fluid for patient who has difficulty swallowing.
- Store medication at controlled room temperatures between 15° and 30°C (59°–86°F). Protect from heat and moisture.

Patient/Family Education

- Therapeutic effect may be seen as early as 2 days. However, it may take as long as 3 weeks at a given dosage. If after this length of time no improvement is noted, physician may prescribe a different medication. Continue to take medication even though symptoms have not subsided.
- Do not consume the following foods/meds while on tranylcypromine: • aged cheese • wine (especially chianti) • beer • chocolate • colas • coffee, tea • sour cream • beef/chicken livers • canned figs • soy sauce • overripe or fermented foods • pickled herring • preserved sausages • yogurt • yeast products • broad beans • cold remedies • diet pills.
- Use caution when driving or when operating dangerous machinery. Drowsiness and dizziness can occur. If these side effects become persistent or interfere with activities of daily living, report to physician. Dosage adjustment may be necessary.
- Do not stop taking the drug abruptly. To do so might produce withdrawal symptoms, such as headache, excitability, hallucinations, and depression.
- Report occurrence of any of the following symptoms to physician immediately: • persistent nausea/vomiting • severe or frequent headaches • rapid heart rate • difficulty urinating • skin rash • stiff or sore neck • palpitations • chest pain.
- Rise slowly from a sitting or lying position to prevent a sudden drop in blood pressure.
- Avoid overexertion if you have a history of angina pectoris or coronary artery disease.
- Take medication with food to minimize GI upset.
- If dry mouth is a problem, take frequent sips of water, chew sugarless gum, or suck on hard candy. Good oral care (frequent brushing, flossing) is very important.
- Do not drink alcohol while on tranylcypromine therapy. Profound CNS depression can be life-threatening.
- Do not consume other medications (including over-the-counter meds) with tranylcypromine without physician's approval. Many medications contain substances that, in combination with MAO inhibitors, could precipitate a life-threatening hypertensive crisis.
- Be aware of possible risks of taking tranylcypromine during pregnancy. Safe use during pregnancy and lactation has not been established. Drug is thought to enter breast milk, so effect on nursing child should be considered.
- Be aware of side effects of tranylcypromine. Refer to written materials furnished by healthcare providers for safe self-administration.
- Carry card or other identification at all times describing medications being taken.

Evaluation

- Patient demonstrates a subsiding/resolution of the symptoms for which tranylcypromine was prescribed (depressed mood, suicidal ideation).
- Patient verbalizes understanding of side effects and regimen required for prudent self-administration of tranylcypromine.

TRAZODONE

(tray′zoe-done)
Desyrel

Classification(s):
Antidepressant, Triazolopyridine
derivative
Pregnancy Category C

INDICATIONS

♦ Major depression with or without symptoms of anxiety (efficacy has been demonstrated in both inpatient and outpatient settings). **Investigational Uses:** ♦ Schizophrenic disorder ♦ Alcohol dependence ♦ Anxiety states ♦ Drug-induced dyskinesias.

ACTION

♦ Mechanism of action not fully understood ♦ Blocks the reuptake of serotonin, increasing its concentration at the synapse and potentiating its effects.

PHARMACOKINETICS

Absorption: Rapidly and completely absorbed from the GI tract following oral administration.
Distribution: Widely distributed. Unknown if drug crosses placental barrier. It is thought to enter breast milk.
Metabolism and Excretion: Metabolized by the liver. Excreted in urine and feces.
Half-Life: 5–9 hours.

CONTRAINDICATIONS AND PRECAUTIONS

Contraindicated in: ♦ Hypersensitivity to the drug ♦ acute recovery period following myocardial infarction ♦ Children less than 18 years of age; pregnancy (safety not established).
Use Cautiously in: ♦ Patients with existing cardiac disease ♦ Suicidal patients ♦ Lactation.

ADVERSE REACTIONS AND SIDE EFFECTS*

CNS: drowsiness, dizziness, weakness, headache, fatigue, confusion, memory deficits, agitation, nervousness, insomnia, impaired speech; less frequently: tremors, seizures, paresthesias, blurred vision, tinnitus.
CV: hypotension (including orthostatic), hypertension, tachycardia, arrhythmias, palpitations, chest pain, syncope, shortness of breath, MYOCARDIAL INFARCTION.
Derm: skin rashes, pruritis, urticaria.
GI: dry mouth, constipation, nausea, vomiting, bad taste, diarrhea, flatulance, hypersalivation (rare).
GU: urinary retention, priapism, hematuria, delayed urine flow, urinary frequency, impotence, menstrual irregularity, increased or decreased libido, retrograde ejaculation.
Hemat: ANEMIA, LEUKOPENIA
Other: weight gain or loss, nasal/sinus congestion.

INTERACTIONS

Drug-Drug: ♦ **Digoxin, phenytoin:** increased serum levels of these drugs ♦ **CNS depressants (including alcohol, barbiturates, opiates):** enhanced depressant effects ♦ **Antihypertensives:** increased hypotensive effect ♦ **MAO inhibitors:** interaction unknown; use concomitantly with caution ♦ **General anesthetics:** interaction unknown; discontinuation of trazodone for as long as clinically feasible prior to elective surgery is recommended ♦ **Oral anticoagulants:** decreased anticoagulant effect ♦ **Hydantoins (phenytoin, mephenytoin, ethotoin):** increased effects, toxicity of hydantoins.
Drug-Food: ♦ Taken with or shortly after food: ♦ Short term: trazodone takes longer to reach peak, peak is lower, slightly more drug is absorbed (as much

---

*Underlines indicate most frequent; CAPITALS indicate life-threatening.

as 20% more) ♦ Long term: decreased incidence of dizziness from trazodone.

ROUTE AND DOSAGE
Depression
♦ **PO (Adults):** Initial dose: 150 mg/day in divided doses. Dosage may be increased by 50 mg/day every 3–4 days. Maximum dose for outpatients not to exceed 400 mg/day in divided doses. Inpatients or more severely depressed patients may be given up to, but not exceeding, 600 mg/day in divided doses.
♦ **PO, Maintenance (Adults):** Lowest effective dose. Adjust dosage to achieve desired response.

Schizophrenic Disorder
(Investigational)
♦ **PO (Adults):** Usual dose: 300 mg/day. Range: 150–600 mg/day.

Alcohol Dependence
(Investigational)
♦ **PO (Adults):** 50–75 mg/day.

Anxiety States
(Investigational)
♦ **PO (Adults):** 25–150 mg/day.

Drug-Induced Dyskinesias
(Investigational)
♦ **PO (Adults):** 60–120 mg/day.

PHARMACODYNAMICS

Route	Onset	Peak	Duration
PO	1–2 wk*	1–2 hr	Weeks†

*1–2 weeks may be required to achieve clinical response. Approximately 25% of patients require 2–4 weeks.
†Allow up to 2 weeks following cessation of therapy for complete drug elimination.

NURSING IMPLICATIONS
Assessment
♦ Assess for suicidal ideation, plan, means. Assess for sudden lifts in mood, which could indicate patient's decision to commit suicide.
♦ Assess mental status daily: • mood • appearance • thought and communication patterns • level of interest in the environment and in activities • suicidal ideation. Improvement in these behavior patterns and level of energy should be expected within 2–4 weeks following initiation of therapy.
♦ Assess for symptoms of blood dyscrasias: • sore throat • fever • malaise.
♦ Assess for symptoms of prolonged or inappropriate penile erection in men.
♦ Assess vital signs, weight.
♦ Assess history of allergies, sensitivity to this drug.
♦ Assess for history of glaucoma.
♦ Assess date of last menses (possible pregnancy), use of contraceptives.
♦ Assess whether currently breast-feeding a child.
♦ Assess current and past alcohol and drug consumption.
♦ Assess for operation of automobile and/or other dangerous machinery.
♦ Assess for presence of adverse reactions or side effects.
♦ Assess patient/family knowledge about illness and need for medication.
♦ In collaboration with physician, assess CBC and liver function tests in patients on long-term therapy.
♦ **Lab Test Alterations:** Increased alkaline phosphatase, AST, and ALT.
♦ **Withdrawal:** Assess for symptoms of abrupt withdrawal from long-term therapy: • nausea • headache • vomiting • muscle pain • weakness.
♦ **Toxicity and Overdose:** Relationship between blood level and therapeutic response has not been established.
◊ Assess for symptoms of overdose: • increased incidence or severity of adverse reactions. Death has occurred in patients who ingested an overdose of trazodone mixed with other CNS depressants. Severe reactions that have occurred due to overdose of trazodone alone include priapism, respiratory arrest, seizures, and ECG changes.
♦ **Overdose Management:** No specific antidote.

◇ Treatment is symptomatic and supportive.

◇ Monitor vital signs.

◇ Ensure maintenance of adequate airway.

◇ Monitor ECG.

◇ Induce emesis in conscious patient.

◇ Initiate gastric lavage in unconscious patient.

◇ Administer activated charcoal to minimize absorptions of the drug.

◇ Protect patient from injury if seizures occur (anticonvulsant may be ordered).

◇ Administer IV fluids to counteract hypotension.

◇ Elimination of the drug may be facilitated by forced diuresis.

Potential Nursing Diagnoses

✦ High risk for self-directed violence related to depressed mood.

✦ High risk for injury related to trazodone's side effects of sedation, dizziness, fatigue, confusion, and lowered seizure threshold; abrupt withdrawal after prolonged use; overdose.

✦ High risk for sexual dysfunction related to trazodone's side effect of priapism.

✦ Social isolation related to depressed mood.

✦ High risk for activity intolerance related to trazodone's side effects of drowsiness, dizziness, fatigue, confusion.

✦ Knowledge deficit related to medication regimen.

Plan/Implementation

✦ Monitor vital signs before beginning therapy and at regular intervals (bid or tid) throughout therapy. Take BP lying and standing in patients experiencing orthostatic hypotension; elderly are particularly susceptible. Contact physician if tachycardia/arrhythmias are noted.

✦ Weigh patient 2–3 times a week, at same time of day, on same scale, if possible. A rapid weight gain or evidence of edema should be reported to physician immediately. Record I&O.

✦ Ensure that patient is protected from injury. Provide supervision and assistance when ambulating if dizziness and drowsiness are problems. Pad siderails and headboard for patient who experiences seizures.

✦ If patient complains of prolonged or inappropriate penile erection, withhold medication dosage and notify physician immediately.

✦ Give patient hard candy, gum, or frequent sips of water if dry mouth is a problem.

✦ Medication may be administered with food to minimize GI upset and enhance absorption.

✦ Ensure that patient swallows tablet and does not "cheek" to avoid medication or to hoard for later use.

✦ Tablet may be crushed and mixed with food or fluid for patient who has difficulty swallowing.

✦ Store medication at room temperature. Protect from temperatures above 40°C (104°F).

Patient/Family Education

✦ Therapeutic effect may be seen in 1–2 weeks. However, it may take as long as 4 weeks. If after this length of time no improvement is noted, physician may prescribe a different medication. Continue to take medication even though symptoms have not subsided.

✦ Use caution when driving or when operating dangerous machinery. Drowsiness and dizziness can occur. If these side effects become persistent or interfere with activities of daily living, report to physician. Dosage adjustment may be necessary.

✦ Do not stop taking the drug abruptly. To do so might produce withdrawal symptoms, such as: • nausea • vomiting • headache • muscle pain • weakness.

✦ Report occurrence of any of the following symptoms to physician immediately: • sore throat • fever • malaise • unusual bleeding • easy bruising • persistent nausea/vomiting • severe headache • rapid heart rate • difficulty urinating • blood in urine.

• Should inappropriate or prolonged penile erections occur, stop taking the medication and notify physician immediately. If the erection persists longer than 1 hour, seek emergency room treatment. This condition is rare but has occurred in some men who have taken trazodone. If measures are not instituted immediately, impotence can result.

• Rise slowly from a sitting or lying position to prevent a sudden drop in blood pressure.

• Take medication with food to enhance absorption and to decrease effects of dizziness/lightheadedness.

• If dry mouth is a problem, take frequent sips of water, chew sugarless gum, or suck on hard candy. Good oral care (frequent brushing, flossing) is very important.

• Do not drink alcohol while on trazodone therapy. These drugs potentiate each other's effects.

• Do not consume other medications (including over-the-counter meds) with trazodone without physician's approval. Many medications contain substances that, in combination with tricyclics, could precipitate a life-threatening hypertensive crisis.

• Be aware of possible risks of taking trazodone during pregnancy. Safe use during pregnancy and lactation has not been established. The drug is thought to enter breast milk, so effect on nursing child should be considered.

• Be aware of side effects of trazodone. Refer to written materials furnished by healthcare providers for safe self-administration.

• Carry card or other identification at all times describing medications being taken.

Evaluation

♦ Patient demonstrates a subsiding/resolution of the symptoms for which trazodone was prescribed (depressed mood; suicidal ideation, anxiety states, drug-induced dyskinesias).

♦ Patient verbalizes understanding of side effects and regimen required for prudent self-administration of trazodone.

TRIAZOLAM

(trye-ay′zoe-lam)
Halcion

Classification(s):
Sedative-hypnotic, Benzodiazepine
Schedule C IV
Pregnancy Category X

INDICATIONS

♦ Insomnia characterized by difficulty in falling asleep, frequent nocturnal awakening, and/or early morning awakening. (For short-term and intermittent use only. Not recommended for administration beyond 6 weeks.)

ACTION

♦ Depresses subcortical levels of the central nervous system, particularly the limbic system and reticular formation ♦ May potentiate the effects of the powerful inhibitory neurotransmitter gamma-aminobutyric acid (GABA) in the brain, thereby producing a calmative effect ♦ All levels of CNS depression can occur, from mild sedation to hypnosis to coma.

PHARMACOKINETICS

Absorption: Rapid absorption from the GI tract.
Distribution: Is widely distributed. Crosses blood-brain and placental barriers; excreted in breast milk.
Metabolism and Excretion: Metabolized by the liver; produces inactive me-

tabolites that are excreted primarily by the kidneys.
Half-Life: 1.6–5.4 hours.

CONTRAINDICATIONS AND PRECAUTIONS

Contraindicated in: ✦ Hypersensitivity to this drug or to other benzodiazepines ✦ Pregnancy and lactation ✦ Children under 18.

Use Cautiously in: ✦ Elderly or debilitated patients ✦ Hepatic or renal dysfunction ✦ Individuals with a history of drug abuse/addiction ✦ Depressed/suicidal patients ✦ Combination with other CNS depressants.

ADVERSE REACTIONS AND SIDE EFFECTS*

CNS: <u>residual sedation</u>, <u>dizziness</u>, <u>headache</u>, nervousness, ataxia, depression, vision disturbances.
CV: tachycardia.
GI: nausea/vomiting, anorexia, constipation, diarrhea.
Other: tolerance, physical and psychological dependence.

INTERACTIONS

Drug-Drug: ✦ **Other CNS depressants (including alcohol, barbiturates, narcotics), antipsychotics, antidepressants, antihistamines, anticonvulsants:** additive CNS depression ✦ **Smoking and caffeine:** decreased effects of triazolam ✦ **Neuromuscular blocking agents:** increased respiratory depression ✦ **Disulfiram, cimetidine:** increased length of action of triazolam ✦ **Erythromycin:** increased triazolam activity, often requiring dosage reduction.

ROUTE AND DOSAGE
Insomnia
✦ **PO (Adults):** 0.125–0.5 mg at bedtime.
✦ **PO (Geriatric or Debilitated Patients):** 0.125–0.25 mg at bedtime.

Initiate dose at 0.125 mg and adjust as response is determined.

PHARMACODYNAMICS

Route	Onset	Peak	Duration
PO	15–30 min	1.3 hr	6–8 hr

NURSING IMPLICATIONS
Assessment

✦ Assess sleep patterns. Keep records for adequate baseline data before the initiation of therapy.
✦ Assess for suicidal ideation (CNS depressants aggravate symptoms in depressed patients).
✦ Assess history of allergies, sensitivity to this drug or to other benzodiazepines.
✦ Assess history of glaucoma.
✦ Assess date of last menses (possible pregnancy), use of contraceptives.
✦ Assess whether currently breast-feeding a child.
✦ Assess current and past alcohol and drug consumption.
✦ Assess operation of automobile and/or other dangerous machinery.
✦ Assess for presence of adverse reactions or side effects.
✦ Assess patient/family knowledge about illness and need for medication.
✦ In collaboration with physician, assess CBC and liver function tests in patients on long-term therapy.
✦ **Lab Test Alterations:** May cause increase in total and direct serum bilirubin, AST, and ALT.
◇ Abnormal renal function tests.
✦ **Withdrawal:** Assess for symptoms of withdrawal: ● depression ● insomnia ● increased anxiety ● abdominal and muscle cramps ● tremors ● vomiting ● sweating ● convulsions ● delirium.
✦ **Withdrawal Management:** Monitor vital signs.
◇ Place patient in quiet room with low stimuli.
◇ Institute seizure precautions.

---

*<u>Underlines</u> indicate most frequent; CAPITALS indicate life-threatening.

◊ A long-acting barbiturate, such as phenobarbital, may be ordered to suppress withdrawal symptoms.

◊ Phenytoin may be ordered to prevent seizures.

◊ Some physicians may order oxazepam as needed to treat objective withdrawal symptoms, gradually decreasing dosage until the drug is discontinued.

♦ **Toxicity and Overdose:** Assess for symptoms of intoxication: • euphoria • excessive drowsiness • slurred speech • disorientation • mood lability • incoordination • unsteady gait • disinhibition of sexual and aggressive impulses • judgment and/or memory impairment.

◊ Assess for symptoms of overdose: • shallow respiration • cold and clammy skin • hypotension • dilated pupils • weak and rapid pulse • hypnosis • coma • possible death.

♦ **Overdose Management:** Monitor vital signs.

◊ Ensure maintenance of adequate airway.

◊ Induce vomiting if patient is conscious.

◊ Initiate gastric lavage in unconscious patient.

◊ Administer activated charcoal to minimize absorption.

◊ IV fluids and vasopressors may be used to combat hypotension.

◊ Forced diuresis may be used to facilitate elimination of the drug.

Potential Nursing Diagnoses

♦ High risk for injury related to abrupt withdrawal from long-term use; effects of drug intoxication or overdose; decreased mental alertness caused by sedative effect.

♦ High risk for self-directed violence related to depressed mood.

♦ Sleep pattern disturbance related to situational crises, physical condition, severe level of anxiety.

♦ High risk for activity intolerance related to side effects of lethargy, drowsiness, dizziness, and weakness.

♦ Knowledge deficit related to medication regimen.

Plan/Implementation

♦ Monitor vital signs before beginning therapy and at regular intervals (bid) throughout therapy.

♦ Ensure that patient is protected from injury. Supervise and assist with ambulation if dizziness and muscular weakness are problems. Pad siderails and headboard for patient who experiences seizures (withdrawal).

♦ Ensure that tablet has been swallowed and not "cheeked" to avoid medication or to hoard for later use.

♦ Raise siderails and ensure patient remains in bed following administration.

♦ Discourage smoking during triazolam therapy.

♦ Store medication at controlled room temperatures between 15° and 30°C (59°–86°F). Protect from heat and moisture.

Patient/Family Education

♦ Do not drive or operate other dangerous machinery if residual drowsiness and dizziness occur.

♦ Do not stop taking the drug abruptly. Doing so can produce serious withdrawal symptoms.

♦ Do not consume other CNS depressants unless prescribed by physician. Do not consume alcohol.

♦ Do not take nonprescription medication without approval from physician.

♦ Be aware of risks of taking triazolam during pregnancy (congenital malformations have been associated with use of benzodiazepines during first trimester). Notify physician of desirability to discontinue drug if pregnancy is suspected or planned.

♦ Be aware of potential side effects. Refer to written materials furnished by healthcare providers regarding correct method of self-administration.

♦ Carry card or other identification at all

times stating names of medications being taken.

Evaluation

♦ Patient demonstrates a subsiding/resolution of the symptoms for which triazolam was prescribed (insomnia, sleep disturbances).

♦ Patient verbalizes understanding of side effects and regimen required for prudent self-administration of triazolam.

TRIFLUOPERAZINE

(trye-floo-oh-per′a-zeen)
{Novoflurazine, Solazine}, Stelazine, Suprazine, {Terfluzine, Triflurin}

Classification(s):
Antipsychotic, Neuroleptic,
Phenothiazine
Pregnancy Category C

INDICATIONS

♦ Manifestations of psychotic disorders
♦ Moderate to severe anxiety in nonpsychotic patients.

ACTION

♦ The exact mechanism of antipsychotic action is not fully understood, but is probably related to the drug's antidopaminergic effects ♦ Antipsychotics may block postsynaptic dopamine receptors in the basal ganglia, hypothalamus, limbic system, brain stem, and medulla ♦ Antipsychotic effects also appear to be related to inhibition of dopamine-mediated neurotransmission at the synapses ♦ Antipsychotic effects may also result from the drug's alpha-adrenergic blocking, muscarinic blocking, and adrenergic activity, as well as its effects on other amines (such as GABA) or peptides.

PHARMACOKINETICS

Absorption: Rapid absorption of oral tablet dosage forms. Genetic differences in rate of first-pass metabolism result in a wide range of bioavailability from individual to individual. Oral liquid preparations and IM administration result in more consistent absorption.

Distribution: Widely distributed. Highly lipophilic; accumulates in brain, lungs, and other tissues with high blood supply. Crosses placental barrier. Enters breast milk.

Metabolism and Excretion: Metabolized by the liver and in the kidneys. Excreted through kidneys and enterohepatic circulation. Active metabolites accumulate and are stored in fatty tissue over a prolonged period of time, and may be detected in urine up to 3–6 months following discontinuation of the drug.

Half-Life: Not well established.

CONTRAINDICATIONS AND PRECAUTIONS

Contraindicated in: ♦ Hypersensitivity to this drug, other phenothiazines, or (contained in some preparations) sulfites or tartrazine ♦ Comatose or severely CNS-depressed patients ♦ Presence of large amounts of CNS depressants ♦ Bone marrow depression ♦ Blood dyscrasias ♦ Subcortical brain damage ♦ Parkinson's disease ♦ Liver, renal, and/or cardiac insufficiency ♦ Severe hypotension or hypertension ♦ Children under 6 years of age; pregnancy and lactation (safe use not established).

Use Cautiously in: ♦ Patients with a history of seizures ♦ Respiratory, renal, hepatic, thyroid, or cardiovascular disorders (e.g., respiratory infection, COPD, thyrotoxicosis, mitral insufficiency, angina pectoris) ♦ Prostatic hypertrophy ♦ Glaucoma ♦ Diabetes ♦ Elderly or debilitated patients ♦ Patients exposed to high

---

{ } = Only available in Canada.

or low environmental temperatures or to organophosphate insecticides ✦ Hypocalcemia ✦ History of severe reactions to insulin or ECT ✦ Pediatric patients with acute illnesses or dehydration.

ADVERSE REACTIONS AND SIDE EFFECTS*

CNS: sedation, headache, seizures, insomnia, dizziness, exacerbation of psychotic symptoms, extrapyramidal symptoms (pseudoparkinsonism, akathisia, akinesia, dystonia, oculogyric crisis), tardive dyskinesia, fatigue, cerebral edema, ataxia, blurred vision, NEUROLEPTIC MALIGNANT SYNDROME, restlessness, anxiety, depression, hyperthermia or hypothermia. **CV:** hypotension, orthostatic hypotension, hypertension, tachycardia, bradycardia, CARDIAC ARREST, ECG changes, ARRHYTHMIAS, PULMONARY EDEMA, CIRCULATORY COLLAPSE.
Derm: skin rashes, urticaria, petechiae, seborrhea, photosensitivity, eczema, erythema, hyperpigmentation, contact dermatitis, EXFOLIATIVE DERMATITIS (rare).
Endo: galactorrhea, gynecomastia (men), changes in libido, impotence, hyperglycemia or hypoglycemia, amenorrhea, retrograde ejaculation.
GI: dry mouth, nausea, vomiting, increased appetite and weight gain, anorexia, dyspepsia, constipation, diarrhea, jaundice, polydipsia, PARALYTIC ILEUS.
GU: urinary retention, frequency or incontinence, bladder paralysis, polyuria, enuresis, priapism.
Hemat: AGRANULOCYTOSIS, LEUKOPENIA, ANEMIA, THROMBOCYTOPENIA, PANCYTOPENIA.
Ophth: lens deposition.
Resp: LARYNGEAL EDEMA, LARYNGOSPASM, BRONCHOSPASM, SUPPRESSION OF COUGH REFLEX.
Other: decreased sweating.

INTERACTIONS

Drug-Drug: ✦ **CNS depressants (including alcohol, barbiturates, nar-** cotics, anesthetics):** additive CNS depressant effects ✦ **Anticholinergic agents (e.g., atropine):** additive anticholinergic effects, decreased antipsychotic effects ✦ **Barbiturate anesthetics:** increased incidence of excitatory effects and hypotension ✦ **Barbiturates:** possible decreased effects of phenothiazines ✦ **Metyrosine:** potentiation of extrapyramidal side effects ✦ **Levodopa:** decreased efficacy of levodopa ✦ **Quinidine:** additive cardiac depressive effects ✦ **Magnesium- or aluminum-containing antidiarrheal mixtures, antacids:** reduced phenothiazine absorption/effectiveness ✦ **Guanethidine:** decreased antihypertensive action ✦ **Lithium:** decreased plasma levels and effect of antipsychotic drug; severe neurotoxicity reported ✦ **Epinephrine:** reversal of usual pressor action of epinephrine, resulting in decreased blood pressure and tachycardia ✦ **Bromocriptine:** impairment of prolactin-suppressing action ✦ **Angiotensin converting enzyme (ACE) inhibitors:** increased effects of ACE inhibitors ✦ **Phenytoin:** decreased phenytoin metabolism, increased risk of toxicity ✦ **Polypeptide antibiotics:** possible neuromuscular respiratory depression ✦ **Metrizamide:** seizures ✦ **Cimetidine:** decreased effect of phenothiazines ✦ **Clonidine:** possibility of severe hypotension ✦ **Piperazine:** increased seizure potential.
Drug-Food: ✦ **Caffeine-containing beverages (e.g., coffee, tea, colas):** counteraction of antipsychotic effect.

ROUTE AND DOSAGE
Psychotic Disorders
✦ **PO (Adults):** Initial dosage: 2–5 mg bid. Usual dosage 15–20 mg/day, although a few may require 40 mg/day or more. Optimum therapeutic dosage levels should be reached within 2–3 weeks.

*Underlines indicate most frequent; CAPITALS indicate life-threatening.

♦ **PO (Children 6–12 Years Old):** Initial dose: 1 mg daily or bid. Usual dosage up to 15 mg/day, although some older children with severe symptoms may require higher doses.

♦ **IM (Adults):** for prompt control of severe symptoms: 1–2 mg q 4–6 hr as needed. More than 6 mg/24 hr is rarely necessary. Only in very exceptional cases should IM dosage exceed 10 mg/24 hr. Switch to oral dosage once control is achieved.

♦ **IM (Children 6–12 Years Old):** if necessary to achieve rapid control of severe symptoms, administer 1 mg once or twice a day.

Nonpsychotic Anxiety

♦ **PO, IM (Adults):** 1–2 mg bid. Maximum dosage: 6 mg/day. Do not administer for longer than 12 weeks.

PHARMACODYNAMICS

Route	Onset*	Peak†	Duration‡
PO	30–40 min	2–4 hr	4–6 hr
IM	10–20 min	15–30 min	12 hr

*Full clinical effects may not be observed for 4–8 weeks.
†Steady-state plasma levels are achieved in approximately 4–7 days.
‡Drug may be detected in urine for 3–6 months after last dose.

NURSING IMPLICATIONS

Assessment

♦ Assess mental status daily: • mood • appearance • thought and communication patterns • level of interest in the environment and in activities • level of anxiety or agitation • presence of hallucinations or delusions • suspiciousness • interactions with others • ability to carry out activities of daily living.

♦ Assess for symptoms of blood dyscrasias: • sore throat • fever • malaise • unusual bleeding • easy bruising.

♦ Assess for extrapyramidal symptoms: • pseudoparkinsonism (tremors, shuffling gait, drooling, rigidity) • akinesia (muscular weakness) • akathisia (continuous restlessness and fidgeting) • dystonia (involuntary muscular movements of face, arms, legs, and neck) • oculogyric crisis (uncontrolled rolling back of the eyes), tardive dyskinesia (bizarre facial and tongue movements, stiff neck, difficulty swallowing).

♦ Assess for symptoms of neuroleptic malignant syndrome: • hyperpyrexia up to 107°F (41.6°C) • elevated pulse • increased or decreased blood pressure • severe parkinsonian muscle rigidity • elevated creatinine phosphokinase blood levels • elevated white blood count • altered mental status (including catatonic signs or agitation) • acute renal failure • varying levels of consciousness (including stupor and coma), pallor, diaphoresis, tachycardia, arrhythmias, rhabdomyolysis.

♦ Assess vital signs, weight. Record baseline values for comparison.

♦ Assess history of allergies, sensitivity to this drug or to other phenothiazines.

♦ Assess for signs and symptoms of cholestatic jaundice: • abdominal pain • nausea • rash • fever • yellow skin • flu-like symptoms • abnormal lab test results (eosinophilia, bile in urine, increased serum transaminases, bilirubin, alkaline phosphatase).

♦ Assess date of last menses (possible pregnancy), use of contraceptives.

♦ Assess whether currently breast-feeding a child.

♦ Assess current and past alcohol and drug consumption.

♦ Assess for operation of automobile and/or other dangerous machinery.

♦ Assess for presence of adverse reactions or side effects.

♦ Assess patient/family knowledge about illness and need for medication.

♦ In collaboration with physician, assess CBC, liver function tests, and ophthalmological exams in patients on long-term therapy.

♦ **Lab Test Alterations:** Increased serum alkaline phosphatase, transaminases, bilirubin.

◇ Increased protein-bound iodine.

◇ False-positive urine pregnancy test, possibly caused by drug metabolite that discolors urine (less likely to occur when serum test is used).

◇ Increased urinary glucose.

◇ Decreased urinary estrogen, progestin, and gonadotropin.

◇ Increased plasma cholesterol level.

◇ Increased serum prolactin.

✦ **Withdrawal:** Assess for symptoms of abrupt withdrawal from long-term therapy: • gastritis • nausea • vomiting • dizziness • headache • tachycardia • insomnia • tremulousness • sweating.

✦ **Toxicity and Overdose:** No correlation has been established between blood level and therapeutic effect.

◇ Assess for symptoms of overdose: • CNS depression, from heavy sedation to deep sleep to coma • hypotension • confusion • excitement • extrapyramidal symptoms • agitation • restlessness • convulsions • fever • autonomic reactions • ECG changes • cardiac arrhythmias • tachycardia • hypothermia • tremor • seizures • cyanosis.

✦ **Overdose Management:** Monitor vital signs.

◇ Ensure maintenance of open airway.

◇ Initiate gastric lavage.

◇ Do not induce emesis (nuchal rigidity may result in aspiration of vomitus).

◇ Antiparkinsonian drugs or diphenhydramine may be given to counteract extrapyramidal symptoms.

◇ Administer IV fluids or a vasoconstrictor to maintain adequate blood pressure. **Note:** Epinephrine is not recommended due to its interaction with phenothiazines, which causes further drop in blood pressure.

◇ Administer IV phenytoin to control ventricular arrhythmias.

◇ Administer phenobarbital or diazepam to control convulsions or hyperactivity.

◇ Dialysis does not appear to be a useful intervention.

Potential Nursing Diagnoses

✦ High risk for violence directed at others related to mistrust and panic anxiety.

✦ High risk for injury related to trifluoperazine's side effects of sedation, dizziness, ataxia, weakness, and lowered seizure threshold; abrupt withdrawal after prolonged use; overdose.

✦ Sensory-perceptual alteration related to panic anxiety evidenced by hallucinations.

✦ Altered thought processes related to panic anxiety evidenced by delusional thinking.

✦ Social isolation related to inability to trust others.

✦ High risk for activity intolerance related to trifluoperazine's side effects of drowsiness, dizziness, ataxia, weakness.

✦ Noncompliance with medication regimen related to suspiciousness and mistrust of others.

✦ Knowledge deficit related to medication regimen.

Plan/Implementation

✦ **General info:** Monitor vital signs before beginning therapy and at regular intervals (bid or tid) throughout therapy. Take BP lying and standing to monitor for possible hypotensive reaction; elderly are particularly susceptible. Dosage adjustment may be required.

◇ Ensure that patient who is ambulatory is protected from sun when spending time outdoors.

◇ Weigh patient 2–3 times a week, at same time of day, on same scale, if possible. A rapid weight gain or evidence of edema should be reported to physician immediately. Record I&O.

◊ Ensure that patient is protected from injury. Provide supervision and assistance when ambulating if dizziness and drowsiness are problems. Pad siderails and headboard for patient who experiences seizures.

◊ Give patient hard candy, gum, or frequent sips of water if dry mouth is a problem.

◊ Store medication at controlled room temperatures between 15° and 30°C (59°–86°F). Protect from heat, light, and moisture.

♦ **PO:** Oral medication may be administered with food to minimize GI upset.

◊ Ensure that patient swallows tablet and does not "cheek" to avoid medication or to hoard for later use.

◊ Crush tablet and mix with food or fluid for patient who has difficulty swallowing, or use liquid concentrate form.

◊ Just prior to administration, mix concentrate with at least 60 mL of juice, milk, water, simple syrup, orange syrup, coffee, tea, or carbonated beverage, or with semisolid food.

◊ If concentrate is accidentally spilled on skin or clothing during preparation or administration, wash area immediately, as contact dermatitis can occur.

♦ **IM:** Avoid contact with injectable liquid. A contact dermatitis can occur.

◊ Inject slowly and deeply into upper, outer quadrant of buttock. Massage site thoroughly following injection.

◊ Because of possible hypotensive effects, patient should remain in recumbent position for at least one-half hour following IM injection.

◊ Do not give injections at intervals less than 4 hours because of a possible cumulative effect.

◊ Rotate sites when multiple injections are administered.

◊ Do not mix with other agents in the syringe.

◊ Potency is not altered when solution is slightly yellow in color. Discard if marked discoloration is evident.

Patient/Family Education

♦ Use caution when driving or when operating dangerous machinery. Drowsiness and dizziness can occur.

♦ Do not stop taking the drug abruptly. To do so might produce withdrawal symptoms, such as nausea, vomiting, gastritis, headache, tachycardia, insomnia, tremulousness.

♦ Use sunscreens and wear protective clothing when spending time outdoors. Skin is more susceptible to sunburn.

♦ Report occurrence of any of the following symptoms to physician immediately: • sore throat • fever • malaise • unusual bleeding • easy bruising • persistent nausea/vomiting • severe headache • rapid heart rate • difficulty urinating • muscle twitching • tremors • darkly colored urine • pale stools • yellow skin or eyes • muscular incoordination • skin rash.

♦ Drug may turn urine pink to reddish-brown in color. This is not significant nor is it harmful.

♦ Rise slowly from a sitting or lying position to prevent a sudden drop in blood pressure.

♦ If dry mouth is a problem, take frequent sips of water, chew sugarless gum, or suck on hard candy. Good oral care (frequent brushing, flossing) is very important.

♦ If some liquid concentrate is spilled on the skin, wash it off immediately. If not, a rash may appear.

♦ Consult physician regarding smoking while on trifluoperazine therapy. Smoking increases metabolism of trifluoperazine, requiring adjustment in dosage to achieve therapeutic effect.

♦ Dress warmly in cold weather and avoid extended exposure to very high or low temperatures. Body temperature is harder to maintain while taking this medication.

♦ Do not drink alcohol while on trifluoperazine therapy. These drugs potentiate each other's effects.

- Do not consume other medications (including over-the-counter meds) without physician's approval. Many medications contain substances that interact with trifluoperazine in a way that may be harmful.
- Be aware of possible risks of taking trifluoperazine during pregnancy. Safe use during pregnancy and lactation has not been established. Trifluoperazine readily crosses the placental barrier, so a fetus could experience adverse effects of the drug. Inform physician immediately if pregnancy occurs, is suspected, or is planned.
- Be aware of side effects of trifluoperazine. Refer to written materials furnished by healthcare providers for safe self-administration.
- Continue to take medication even if feeling well and as though it is not needed. Symptoms may return if medication is discontinued.
- Carry card or other identification at all times describing medications being taken.

Evaluation

- Patient demonstrates a subsiding/resolution of the symptoms for which trifluoperazine was prescribed (severe to panic anxiety, altered thought processes, altered perceptions).
- Patient verbalizes understanding of side effects and regimen required for prudent self-administration of trifluoperazine.

TRIFLUPROMAZINE

(trye-floo-proe′ma-zeen)
Vesprin

Classification(s):
Antipsychotic, Neuroleptic,
Antiemetic, Phenothiazine
Pregnancy Category C

INDICATIONS

- Psychotic disorders, such as schizophrenia, manic phase of bipolar disorder (until slower-acting lithium takes effect), brief reactive psychoses, and schizoaffective disorder ◆ Severe nausea and vomiting.

ACTION

◆ The exact mechanism of antipsychotic action is not fully understood but is probably related to the drug's antidopaminergic effects ◆ Antipsychotics may block postsynaptic dopamine receptors in the basal ganglia, hypothalamus, limbic system, brain stem, and medulla ◆ Antipsychotic effects also appear to be related to inhibition of dopamine-mediated neurotransmission at the synapses ◆ Antipsychotic effects may also result from the drug's alpha-adrenergic blocking, muscarinic blocking, and adrenergic activity, as well as its effects on other amines (such as GABA) or peptides.

PHARMACOKINETICS

Absorption: Well absorbed following IM administration.

Distribution: Widely distributed. Highly lipophilic; accumulates in brain, lungs, and other tissues with high blood supply. Crosses placental barrier. Enters breast milk.

Metabolism and Excretion: Metabolized by the liver and in the kidneys. Excreted through kidneys and enterohepatic circulation. Active metabolites accumulate and are stored in fatty tissue over a prolonged period of time, and may be detected in urine up to 3–6 months following discontinuation of the drug.

Half-Life: Not well established.

CONTRAINDICATIONS AND PRECAUTIONS

Contraindicated in: ◆ Hypersensitivity to this drug, other phenothiazines, or tartrazine (contained in some preparations) ◆ Comatose or severely CNS-depressed patients ◆ Presence of large amounts of CNS depressants ◆ Bone marrow depression ◆ Blood dyscrasias ◆ Subcortical brain damage ✦ Parkinson's disease ✦ Liver, renal, and/or cardiac insufficiency ✦ Severe hypotension or hypertension ✦ Children under 2.5 years of age; pregnancy and lactation (safe use not established).

Use Cautiously in: ✦ Patients with a history of seizures ✦ Respiratory, renal, thyroid, or cardiovascular disorders (e.g., respiratory infection, COPD, thyrotoxicosis, mitral insufficiency, angina pectoris ✦ Prostatic hypertrophy ✦ Glaucoma ✦ Diabetes ✦ Elderly or debilitated patients ✦ Patients exposed to high or low environmental temperatures or to organophosphate insecticides ✦ Hypocalcemia ✦ History of severe reactions to insulin or ECT ✦ Pediatric patients with acute illnesses or dehydration.

ADVERSE REACTIONS AND SIDE EFFECTS*

CNS: <u>sedation</u>, <u>headache</u>, seizures, insomnia, dizziness, exacerbation of psychotic symptoms, <u>extrapyramidal symptoms</u> (pseudoparkinsonism, akathisia, akinesia, dystonia, oculogyric crisis), tardive dyskinesia, fatigue, cerebral edema, ataxia, <u>blurred vision</u>, NEUROLEPTIC MALIGNANT SYNDROME, restlessness, anxiety, depression, hyperthermia or hypothermia.

CV: hypotension, <u>orthostatic hypotension</u>, hypertension, tachycardia, bradycardia, CARDIAC ARREST, ECG changes, ARRHYTHMIAS, PULMONARY EDEMA, CIRCULATORY COLLAPSE.

Derm: <u>skin rashes</u>, urticaria, petechiae, seborrhea, <u>photosensitivity</u>, eczema, erythema, hyperpigmentation, contact dermatitis, EXFOLIATIVE DERMATITIS (rare).

Endo: galactorrhea, gynecomastia (men), changes in libido, impotence, hyperglycemia or hypoglycemia, amenorrhea, retrograde ejaculation.

GI: <u>dry mouth</u>, nausea, vomiting, increased appetite and weight gain, anorexia, dyspepsia, <u>constipation</u>, diarrhea, jaundice, polydipsia, PARALYTIC ILEUS.

GU: urinary retention, frequency or in-

continence, bladder paralysis, polyuria, enuresis, priapism.

Hemat: AGRANULOCYTOSIS, LEUKOPENIA, ANEMIA, THROMBOCYTOPENIA, PANCYTOPENIA.

Ophth: lens deposition.

Resp: LARYNGEAL EDEMA, LARYNGOSPASM, BRONCHOSPASM, SUPPRESSION OF COUGH REFLEX.

Other: decreased sweating.

INTERACTIONS

Drug-Drug: ✦ **CNS depressants (including alcohol, barbiturates, narcotics, anesthetics):** additive CNS depressant effects ✦ **Anticholinergic agents (e.g., atropine):** additive anticholinergic effects, decreased antipsychotic effects ✦ **Barbiturate anesthetics:** increased incidence of excitatory effects and hypotension ✦ **Barbiturates:** possible decreased effects of phenothiazines ✦ **Metyrosine:** potentiation of extrapyramidal side effects ✦ **Levodopa:** decreased efficacy of levodopa ✦ **Quinidine:** additive cardiac depressive effects ✦ **Magnesium- or aluminum-containing antidiarrheal mixtures, antacids:** reduced phenothiazine absorption/effectiveness ✦ **Guanethidine:** decreased antihypertensive action ✦ **Lithium:** decreased plasma levels and effect of antipsychotic drug; severe neurotoxicity reported ✦ **Epinephrine:** reversal of usual pressor action of epinephrine, resulting in decreased blood pressure and tachycardia ✦ **Bromocriptine:** impairment of prolactin-suppressing action ✦ **Angiotensin converting enzyme (ACE) inhibitors:** increased effects of ACE inhibitors ✦ **Phenytoin:** decreased phenytoin metabolism, increased risk of toxicity ✦ **Polypeptide antibiotics:** possible neuromuscular respiratory depression ✦ **Metrizamide:** seizures ✦ **Cimetidine:** decreased effect of phenothiazines ✦ **Clonidine:** possibility of severe hypotension ✦ **Piperazine:** increased seizure potential.

Drug-Food: ✦ **Caffeine-containing**

*<u>Underlines</u> indicate most frequent; CAPITALS indicate life-threatening.

beverages (e.g., coffee, tea, colas): counteraction of antipsychotic effects.

ROUTE AND DOSAGE

Psychotic Disorders

* **IM (Adults):** 60 mg/day in divided doses. Maximum daily dosage: 150 mg.
* **IM (Children over 2.5 Years Old):** 0.2–0.25 mg/kg/day. Maximum total daily dosage: 10 mg.

Severe Nausea and Vomiting

* **IM (Adults):** 5–15 mg repeated q 4 hr, up to 60 mg maximum daily dosage.
* **IM (Elderly or Debilitated Patients):** 2.5 mg. Maximum daily dosage: 15 mg.
* **IM (Children over 2.5 Years Old):** 0.2–0.25 mg/kg. Maximum daily dosage: 10 mg.
* **IV (Adults):** 1 mg. May be repeated up to maximum total daily dosage of 3 mg.

PHARMACODYNAMICS

Route	Onset*	Peak†	Duration‡
IM	15–30 min	1 hr	12 hr
IV	5 min	5 min	—

*Full clinical effects may not be observed for 4–8 weeks.
†Steady-state plasma levels are achieved in approximately 4–7 days.
‡Drug may be detected in urine for 3–6 months after last dose.

NURSING IMPLICATIONS

Assessment

* Assess mental status daily: • mood • appearance • thought and communication patterns • level of interest in the environment and in activities • level of anxiety or agitation • presence of hallucinations or delusions • suspiciousness • interactions with others • ability to carry out activities of daily living.
* Assess for symptoms of blood dyscrasias: • sore throat • fever • malaise • unusual bleeding • easy bruising.
* Assess for extrapyramidal symptoms:

• pseudoparkinsonism (tremors, shuffling gait, drooling, rigidity) • akinesia (muscular weakness) • akathisia (continuous restlessness and fidgeting) • dystonia (involuntary muscular movements of face, arms, legs, and neck) • oculogyric crisis (uncontrolled rolling back of the eyes) • tardive dyskinesia (bizarre facial and tongue movements, stiff neck, difficulty swallowing.

* Assess for symptoms of neuroleptic malignant syndrome: • hyperpyrexia up to 107°F (41.6°C) • elevated pulse • increased or decreased blood pressure • severe parkinsonism muscle rigidity • elevated creatinine phosphokinase blood levels • elevated white blood count • altered mental status (including catatonic signs or agitation) • acute renal failure • varying levels of consciousness (including stupor and coma) • pallor • diaphoresis • tachycardia • arrhythmias • rhabdomyolysis.
* Assess vital signs, weight. Record baseline values for comparison.
* Assess history of allergies, sensitivity to this drug, other phenothiazines, or tartrazine.
* Assess for signs and symptoms of cholestatic jaundice: • abdominal pain • nausea • rash • fever • yellow skin • flu-like symptoms • abnormal lab test results (eosinophilia, bile in urine, increased serum transaminases, bilirubin, alkaline phosphatase).
* Assess date of last menses (possible pregnancy), use of contraceptives.
* Assess whether currently breast-feeding a child.
* Assess current and past alcohol and drug consumption.
* Assess for operation of automobile and/or other dangerous machinery.
* Assess for presence of adverse reactions or side effects.
* Assess patient/family knowledge about illness and need for medication.
* In collaboration with physician, assess

CBC, liver function tests, and ophthalmological exams in patients on long-term therapy.

✦ **Lab Test Alterations:** Increased serum alkaline phosphatase, transaminases, bilirubin.

◇ Increased protein-bound iodine.

◇ False-positive urine pregnancy test, possibly caused by drug metabolite that discolors urine (less likely to occur when serum test is used).

◇ Increased urinary glucose.

◇ Decreased urinary estrogen, progestin, and gonadotropin.

◇ Increased plasma cholesterol level.

◇ Increased serum prolactin.

✦ **Withdrawal:** Assess for symptoms of abrupt withdrawal from long-term therapy: ● gastritis ● nausea ● vomiting ● dizziness ● headache ● tachycardia ● insomnia ● tremulousness ● sweating.

✦ **Toxicity and Overdose:** No correlation has been established between blood level and therapeutic effect.

◇ Assess for symptoms of overdose: ● CNS depression, from heavy sedation to deep sleep to coma ● hypotension ● confusion ● excitement ● extrapyramidal symptoms ● agitation ● restlessness ● convulsions ● fever ● autonomic reactions ● ECG changes ● cardiac arrhythmias ● tachycardia ● hypothermia ● tremor ● seizures ● cyanosis.

✦ **Overdose Management:** Monitor vital signs.

◇ Ensure maintenance of open airway.

◇ Initiate gastric lavage.

◇ Do not induce emesis (nuchal rigidity may result in aspiration of vomitus.)

◇ Administer antiparkinsonian drugs or diphenhydramine to counteract extrapyramidal symptoms.

◇ Administer IV fluids or a vasoconstrictor to maintain adequate blood pressure. **Note:** Epinephrine is not recommended due to its interaction with phenothiazines, which causes further drop in blood pressure.

◇ Administer IV phenytoin to control ventricular arrhythmias.

◇ Administer phenobarbital or diazepam to control convulsions or hyperactivity.

◇ Dialysis does not appear to be a useful intervention.

Potential Nursing Diagnoses

✦ High risk for violence directed at others related to mistrust and panic anxiety.

✦ High risk for injury related to triflupromazine's side effects of sedation, dizziness, ataxia, weakness, and lowered seizure threshold; abrupt withdrawal after prolonged use; overdose.

✦ Sensory-perceptual alteration related to panic anxiety evidenced by hallucinations.

✦ Altered thought processes related to panic anxiety evidenced by delusional thinking.

✦ Social isolation related to inability to trust others.

✦ High risk for activity intolerance related to triflupromazine's side effects of drowsiness, dizziness, ataxia, weakness.

✦ Noncompliance with medication regimen related to suspiciousness and mistrust of others.

✦ Knowledge deficit related to medication regimen.

Plan/Implementation

✦ **General Info:** Monitor vital signs before beginning therapy and at regular intervals (bid or tid) throughout therapy. Take BP lying and standing to monitor for possible hypotensive reaction; elderly are particularly susceptible. Dosage adjustment may be required.

◇ Ensure that patient who is ambulatory is protected from sun when spending time outdoors.

◇ Weigh patient 2–3 times a week, at same time of day, on same scale, if possible. A rapid weight gain or evidence of edema should be reported to physician immediately. Record I&O.

◇ Ensure that patient is protected from injury. Provide supervision and assistance when ambulating if dizziness and drowsiness are problems. Pad siderails and headboard for patient who experiences seizures.

◇ Give patient hard candy, gum, or frequent sips of water if dry mouth is a problem.

◇ Store medication at controlled room temperatures between 15° and 30°C (59°–86°F). Protect from heat and light.

✦ **IM:** IM injection may be irritating to tissues; avoid SC injection.

◇ Avoid contact with injectable liquid. A contact dermatitis can occur.

◇ Inject slowly and deeply into upper, outer quadrant of buttock. Massage site thoroughly following injection.

◇ Because of possible hypotensive effects, patient should remain in recumbent position for at least one-half hour following IM injection.

◇ Rotate sites when multiple injections are administered.

◇ Do not mix with other agents in the syringe.

◇ Solution that is darker than light amber in color should be discarded.

✦ **IV:** Because of possible hypotensive effects, drug should be administered with patient in recumbent position.

◇ Monitor blood pressure every 10 minutes during IV administration. Physician may order vasopressor (not epinephrine) if hypotension occurs.

◇ Administer each 8 mg or fraction thereof over at least 1 minute.

◇ Handle solution carefully; may cause contact dermatitis.

◇ Solution that is darker than light amber in color should be discarded.

Patient/Family Education

✦ Use caution when driving or when operating dangerous machinery. Drowsiness and dizziness can occur.

✦ Do not stop using the drug abruptly.

To do so might produce withdrawal symptoms, such as: • nausea • vomiting • gastritis • headache • tachycardia • insomnia • tremulousness.

✦ Use sunscreens and wear protective clothing when spending time outdoors. Skin is more susceptible to sunburn.

✦ Report occurrence of any of the following symptoms to physician immediately: • sore throat • fever • malaise • unusual bleeding • easy bruising • persistent nausea/vomiting • severe headache • rapid heart rate • difficulty urinating • muscle twitching • tremors • darkly colored urine • pale stools • yellow skin or eyes • muscular incoordination • skin rash.

✦ Drug may turn urine pink to reddish-brown in color. This is not significant nor is it harmful.

✦ Rise slowly from a sitting or lying position to prevent a sudden drop in blood pressure.

✦ If dry mouth is a problem, take frequent sips of water, chew sugarless gum, or suck on hard candy. Good oral care (frequent brushing, flossing) is very important.

✦ Consult physician regarding smoking while on triflupromazine therapy. Smoking increases metabolism of triflupromazine, requiring adjustment in dosage to achieve therapeutic effect.

✦ Dress warmly in cold weather, and avoid extended exposure to very high or low temperatures. Body temperature is harder to maintain while taking this medication.

✦ Do not drink alcohol while on triflupromazine therapy. These drugs potentiate each other's effects.

✦ Do not consume other medications (including over-the-counter meds) without physician's approval. Many medications contain substances that interact with triflupromazine in a way that may be harmful.

✦ Be aware of possible risks of using triflupromazine during pregnancy.

Safe use during pregnancy and lactation has not been established. Triflupromazine readily crosses the placental barrier, so a fetus could experience adverse effects of the drug. Inform physician immediately if pregnancy occurs, is suspected, or is planned.
* Be aware of side effects of triflupromazine. Refer to written materials furnished by healthcare providers for safe self-administration.
* Continue to use medication even if feeling well and as though it is not needed. Symptoms may return if medication is discontinued.
* Carry card or other identification at all times describing medications being taken.

Evaluation
* Patient demonstrates a subsiding/resolution of the symptoms for which triflupromazine was prescribed: ● panic anxiety ● altered thought processes ● altered perceptions ● severe agitation ● nausea ● vomiting.
* Patient verbalizes understanding of side effects and regimen required for prudent self-administration of triflupromazine.

TRIHEXYPHENIDYL

(trye-hex-ee-fen′i-dill)
{Aparkane}, Aphen, Artane, {Novohexidyl}, Tremin, Trihexane, Trihexidyl, Trihexy

Classification(s):
Antiparkinsonian agent,
Anticholinergic
Pregnancy Category C

INDICATIONS
* All forms of parkinsonism (adjunctive therapy) ● Extrapyramidal symptoms

(except tardive dyskinesia) associated with antipsychotic drugs.

ACTION
* Acts to correct an imbalance of dopamine deficiency and acetylcholine excess in the corpus striatum ● The acetylcholine receptor is blocked at the synapse to diminish excess cholinergic effect.

PHARMACOKINETICS
Absorption: Rapidly absorbed following oral administration.
Distribution: Not completely understood. May cross placental barrier and may enter breast milk.
Metabolism and Excretion: Thought to be at least partially metabolized by the liver. Excreted in urine primarily as unchanged drug.
Half-Life: 1.3–8.7 hr (average 3.7 hr).

CONTRAINDICATIONS AND PRECAUTIONS
Contraindicated in: ● Hypersensitivity to this drug or to other anticholinergics ● Angle-closure glaucoma ● Pyloric or duodenal obstruction ● Stenosing peptic ulcers ● Prostatic hypertrophy or bladderneck obstructions ● Achalasia ● Myasthenia gravis ● Children under 3 years of age ● Ulcerative colitis ● Toxic megacolon ● Tachycardia secondary to cardiac insufficiency or thyrotoxicosis.
Use Cautiously in: ● Narrow-angle glaucoma ● Elderly or debilitated patients ● Children; pregnancy and lactation (safety not established) ● Hepatic, renal, or cardiac insufficiency ● Hyperthyroidism ● Hypertension ● Autonomic neuropathy ● Tendency toward urinary retention ● Older children ● Patients exposed to high environmental temperature.

{} = Only available in Canada.

ADVERSE REACTIONS AND SIDE EFFECTS*

CNS: drowsiness, dizziness, blurred vision, disorientation, confusion, memory loss, agitation, nervousness, delirium, weakness, amnesia (rare), mydriasis, cycloplegia, headache, insomnia.

CV: orthostatic hypotension, hypotension, tachycardia, palpitations.

Derm: skin rashes, urticaria, other dermatoses.

GI: dry mouth, nausea, vomiting, epigastric distress, constipation, dilatation of the colon, PARALYTIC ILEUS, suppurative parotitis.

GU: urinary retention, urinary hesitancy, dysuria, difficulty in achieving or maintaining an erection.

Psych: depression, delusions, hallucinations, paranoia.

Other: muscular weakness, muscular cramping, elevated temperature, flushing, decreased sweating, anaphylaxis, increased intraocular pressure.

INTERACTIONS

Drug-Drug: ◆ **Other drugs with anticholinergic properties (e.g., glutethimide, disopyramide, narcotic analgesics, phenothiazines, tricyclic antidepressants, antihistamines, quinidine salts, amantadine):** increased anticholinergic effects; potentially fatal paralytic ileus ◆ **Levodopa:** possible decreased levodopa absorption ◆ **Slow-dissolving digoxin:** decreased absorption of digoxin ◆ **CNS depressants (e.g., alcohol, barbiturates, narcotics, benzodiazepines):** increased CNS depressant effects ◆ **Chlorpromazine, phenothiazines, haloperidol:** decreased therapeutic effects of these drugs ◆ **MAO inhibitors:** increased effects of trihexyphenidyl ◆ **Ketoconazole:** decreased absorption of ketoconazole ◆ **Antacids:** decreased absorption of trihexyphenidyl.

ROUTE AND DOSAGE

Parkinsonism

◆ **PO (Adults):** Initial dosage: 1–2 mg first day. Dosage may be increased by 2 mg q 3–5 days until a total of 6–10 mg is given daily. Some patients with postencephalitic parkinsonism syndrome may require as much as 12–15 mg/day. Best tolerated if given tid with meals. Higher doses may be given qid with meals and at bedtime.

Concomitant Use with Levodopa

◆ **PO (Adults):** Usual dose of each drug may need to be reduced. Trihexyphenidyl dosage of 3–6 mg/day in divided doses is usually adequate.

Concomitant Use with Other Anticholinergics

◆ **PO (Adults):** To substitute in whole or part for other anticholinergics, the usual procedure is gradual progressive reduction in the other medication as the dose of trihexyphenidyl is increased.

Sustained-Release

◆ **PO (Adults):** Do not use until patient has been stabilized on tablet or elixir form. Medication may then be switched to sustained-release form at same total daily dose, administered as a single dose after breakfast or in 2 divided doses 12 hours apart.

Drug-Induced Extrapyramidal Symptoms

◆ **PO (Adults):** Usual daily dosage range: 5–15 mg. Initial dose: 1 mg. If reactions are not controlled in a few hours, gradually increase dose until control of symptoms is achieved. More rapid control of symptoms may occur by temporarily reducing antipsychotic dose when instituting trihexyphenidyl therapy, and then adjusting both drugs until desired effect is retained.

*Underlines indicate most frequent; CAPITALS indicate life-threatening.

PHARMACODYNAMICS

Route	Onset	Peak	Duration
PO	1 hr	1.5 hr	6–12 hr
PO (sus- tained-release)	—	—	12–24 hr

NURSING IMPLICATIONS

Assessment

* Assess for symptoms of Parkinson's disease: • tremors • muscular weakness and rigidity • drooling • shuffling gait • disturbances of posture and equilibrium • flat affect • monotone speech.
* Assess for extrapyramidal symptoms: • pseudoparkinsonism (tremors, shuffling gait, drooling, rigidity) • akinesia (muscular weakness) • akathisia (continuous restlessness and fidgeting) • dystonia (involuntary muscular movements of face, arms, legs, and neck) • oculogyric crisis (uncontrolled rolling back of the eyes) • tardive dyskinesia (bizarre facial and tongue movements, stiff neck, difficulty swallowing). **Note:** Trihexyphenidyl is not effective in alleviating symptoms of tardive dyskinesia.
* Assess for symptoms of paralytic ileus: • constipation • abdominal pain and distention • absence of bowel sounds. Patients taking trihexyphenidyl concomitantly with other drugs that produce anticholinergic effects are particularly susceptible.
* Assess vital signs, weight. Record baseline values for comparison.
* Assess history of allergies, sensitivity to this drug or to other anticholinergics.
* Assess date of last menses (possible pregnancy), use of contraceptives.
* Assess whether currently breast-feeding a child.
* Assess current and past alcohol and drug consumption.
* Assess for operation of automobile and/or other dangerous machinery.

* Assess for presence of adverse reactions or side effects.
* Assess patient/family knowledge about illness and need for medication.
* In collaboration with physician, periodically assess CBC, liver function, and intraocular pressure in patients on long-term therapy.
* **Toxicity and Overdose:** Assess for symptoms of overdose: • CNS depression preceded or followed by stimulation • intensification of psychotic symptoms • anxiety • ataxia • seizures • incoherence • delusions • paranoia • anhidrosis • hyperpyrexia • hot, dry, flushed skin • dry mucous membranes • decreased bowel sounds • urinary retention • tachycardia • difficulty swallowing • cardiac arrhythmias • shock • coma • circulatory collapse • skeletal muscle paralysis • cardiac arrest • respiratory depression or arrest.
* **Overdose Management:** Monitor vital signs.
◊ Ensure maintenance of adequate airway.
◊ Induce emesis in conscious patient (contraindicated in precomatose, convulsive, or psychotic states).
◊ Initiate gastric lavage in unconscious patient.
◊ Administer activated charcoal to minimize absorption of the drug.
◊ Administer pilocarpine, 5 mg PO, to treat peripheral effects.
◊ Administer physostigmine, 1–2 mg SQ or slow IV, to reverse anticholinergic effects (use only with availability of advanced life support).
◊ Employ artificial respiration and oxygen to treat respiratory depression.
◊ Apply tepid water sponges, cold packs, or other cooling applications to treat hyperpyrexia.
◊ Darken room to counter photophobia.
◊ Administer fluids and vasopressor to control circulatory collapse.
◊ Administer diazepam to control symptoms of acute psychosis.

Potential Nursing Diagnoses

* High risk for injury related to symptoms of Parkinson's disease or drug-induced extrapyramidal symptoms.
* Hyperthermia related to anticholinergic effect of decreased sweating.
* Sensory-perceptual alteration related to side effect of trihexyphenidyl evidenced by hallucinations.
* Altered thought processes related to side effects of trihexyphenidyl evidenced by delusional thinking, disorientation, confusion.
* Social isolation related to embarrassment by symptoms of Parkinson's disease.
* High risk for activity intolerance related to trihexyphenidyl's side effects of drowsiness, dizziness, ataxia, weakness, confusion.
* Knowledge deficit related to medication regimen.

Plan/Implementation

* Monitor vital signs daily. Be particularly alert for increase in pulse rate or temperature.
* Weigh patient 2–3 times a week, at same time of day, on same scale, if possible. A rapid weight gain or evidence of edema should be reported to physician immediately. Record I&O.
* Monitor for exacerbation of mental symptoms in patients who are receiving the drug to counteract extrapyramidal symptoms associated with antipsychotic medications.
* Ensure that patient is protected from injury. Provide supervision and assistance when ambulating if dizziness and drowsiness are problems.
* Give patient hard candy, gum, or frequent sips of water if dry mouth is a problem, or treat with saliva substitute.
* Ensure that patient swallows tablet/capsule and does not "cheek" to avoid medication or to hoard for later use.

* Medication may be administered with food to minimize gastric irritation.
* Tablet may be crushed and mixed with food or fluid for patient who has difficulty swallowing, or elixir form may be used.
* Sustained-release capsules should not be emptied. Contents should remain intact and capsule should be taken whole.
* Monitor vital signs before beginning therapy and at regular intervals (bid or tid) throughout therapy. Take BP lying and standing to monitor for possible hypotensive reaction; elderly are particularly susceptible. Dosage adjustment may be required.
* Store medication at controlled room temperatures between 15° and 30°C (59°–86°F). Protect from heat and moisture.

Patient/Family Education

* Medication may be taken with food if GI upset occurs.
* Use caution when driving or when operating dangerous machinery. Drowsiness and dizziness can occur.
* Do not stop taking the drug abruptly. To do so might produce serious withdrawal symptoms.
* Report occurrence of any of the following symptoms to physician immediately: • pain or tenderness in area in front of ear • extreme dryness of mouth • difficulty urinating • abdominal pain • constipation • fast and pounding heartbeat • rash • vision disturbances • mental changes.
* Rise slowly from a sitting or lying position to prevent a sudden drop in blood pressure.
* Stay inside in air-conditioned room when weather is very hot. Perspiration is decreased by trihexyphenidyl and the body cannot cool itself as well. There is greater susceptibility to heat stroke. Inform physician if air-conditioned housing is not available.

♦ If dry mouth is a problem, take frequent sips of water, chew sugarless gum, or suck on hard candy. Good oral care (frequent brushing, flossing) is very important.

♦ Do not drink alcohol while on trihexyphenidyl therapy.

♦ Do not consume other medications (including over-the-counter meds) without physician's approval. Many medications contain substances that interact with trihexyphenidyl in a way that may be harmful.

♦ Be aware of possible risks of taking trihexyphenidyl during pregnancy. Safe use during pregnancy and lactation has not been established. It is thought that trihexyphenidyl crosses the placental barrier; if so, a fetus could experience adverse effects of the drug. Inform physician immediately if pregnancy occurs, is suspected, or is planned.

♦ Be aware of side effects of trihexyphenidyl. Refer to written materials furnished by healthcare providers for safe self-administration.

♦ Continue to take medication even if feeling well and as though it is not needed. Symptoms may return if medication is discontinued.

♦ Carry card or other identification at all times describing medications being taken.

Evaluation

♦ Patient demonstrates a subsiding of the symptoms for which trihexyphenidyl was prescribed (parkinsonism, drug-induced extrapyramidal symptoms).

♦ Patient verbalizes understanding of side effects and regimen required for prudent self-administration of trihexyphenidyl.

TRIMETHADIONE

(trye-meth-a-dye′own)
Tridione

Classification(s):
Anticonvulsant, Oxazolidinedione
Pregnancy Category D

INDICATIONS

♦ Absence (petit mal) seizures refractory to other anticonvulsants.

ACTION

♦ Increases seizure threshold in cerebral cortex and basal ganglia ♦ Decreases synaptic response to repetitive low-frequency stimuli.

PHARMACOKINETICS

Absorption: Rapidly absorbed from the GI tract.

Distribution: Is widely distributed. Crosses the blood-brain and placental barriers; unknown if excreted in breast milk.

Metabolism and Excretion: Metabolized by the liver; excreted by the kidneys.

Half-Life: 5–10 days (metabolite dimethadione).

CONTRAINDICATIONS AND PRECAUTIONS

Contraindicated in: ♦ Hypersensitivity to this drug or to other oxazolidinediones ♦ Severe hepatic or renal impairment ♦ Pregnancy and lactation (safety not established; may cause fetal harm) ♦ Severe blood dyscrasias.

Use Cautiously in: ♦ Elderly or debilitated patients ♦ Patients with a history of hepatic or renal disease ♦ Acute intermittent porphyria ♦ Diseases of the retina or optic nerve.

ADVERSE REACTIONS AND SIDE EFFECTS*

CNS: <u>drowsiness</u>, dizziness, headache, fatigue, irritability, ataxia, personality changes.

CV: changes in blood pressure.

Derm: acneiform rash, alopecia, EXFO-LIATIVE DERMATITIS, erythema multiforme.

GI: <u>nausea/vomiting</u>, anorexia, hiccups, weight loss, abdominal pain.

GU: POTENTIALLY FATAL NEPHROSIS, protein-uria.

Hemat: BLOOD DYSCRASIAS (aplastic anemia, thrombocytopenia, agranulocytosis, leukopenia, neutropenia, eosinophilia), nosebleed, vaginal bleeding, bleeding gums.

Other: systemic lupus erythematosus, lymphadenopathy, hemeralopia, photophobia, diplopia, lymphoma-like syndrome.

INTERACTIONS

Drug-Drug: ♦ **Drugs that cause adverse effects similar to those caused by trimethadione:** increased risk of toxic effects, such as blood dyscrasias and hepatoxicity.

ROUTE AND DOSAGE

Absence (Petit Mal) Seizures

♦ **PO (Adults):** Initial dosage: 900 mg daily divided into 3 equal doses. Increase by 300 mg at weekly intervals until control is achieved with minimal side effects. Maintenance dose: 300–600 mg tid or qid.

♦ **PO (Children under 2 Years Old):** Initial dosage: 300 mg daily in divided doses.

♦ **PO (Children 2–6 Years Old):** Initial dosage: 600 mg daily in divided doses.

♦ **PO (Children over 6 Years Old):** Initial dosage: 900 mg daily in divided doses.

♦ **PO (Discontinuation of Therapy):** Withdraw gradually to prevent precipitation of seizures or status epilepticus.

PHARMACODYNAMICS

Route	Onset	Peak	Duration
PO	UK	30 min–2 hr	UK

NURSING IMPLICATIONS

Assessment

♦ Assess occurrence, characteristics, and duration of seizure activity.

♦ Assess baseline vital signs.

♦ Assess history of allergies, sensitivity to this drug.

♦ Assess date of last menses (possible pregnancy), use of contraceptives.

♦ Assess whether currently breast-feeding a child.

♦ Assess current and past alcohol and drug consumption.

♦ Assess operation of automobile and/or other dangerous machinery.

♦ Assess for presence of adverse reactions or side effects.

♦ Assess patient/family knowledge about illness and need for medication.

♦ In collaboration with physician, assess CBC and renal and liver function tests before initiation of therapy; assess monthly thereafter. Periodic urinalysis should be performed.

♦ **Toxicity and Overdose:** Therapeutic serum concentration level of dimethadione is thought to be 700–800 mcg/mL.

◊ Assess for symptoms of toxicity/overdose: • nausea • ataxia • drowsiness • dizziness • vision disturbances. Coma may follow massive overdose.

♦ **Overdose Management:** Monitor vital signs.

◊ Ensure maintenance of adequate airway.

◊ Induce emesis in conscious patient.

◊ Initiate gastric lavage in unconscious patient.

◊ Alkalinization of urine increases renal excretion.

*<u>Underlines</u> indicate most frequent; CAPITALS indicate life-threatening.

◇ Obtain CBC and lab evaluation of hepatic and renal function following recovery.

Potential Nursing Diagnoses

♦ High risk for injury related to seizures; abrupt withdrawal from long-term trimethadione use; effects of toxicity or overdose.

♦ Impaired adjustment related to difficulty accepting diagnosis of epilepsy.

♦ Social isolation related to fear of experiencing a seizure in the presence of others.

♦ High risk for activity intolerance related to trimethadione's side effects of drowsiness, dizziness, ataxia.

♦ Knowledge deficit related to medication regimen.

Plan/Implementation

♦ Monitor vital signs before beginning therapy and at regular intervals (bid) throughout therapy.

♦ Observe patient frequently (every hour) for occurrence of seizure activity.

♦ Ensure that patient is protected from injury. Supervise and assist with ambulation if dizziness and ataxia are problems. Avoid or monitor activities that require mental alertness (including smoking). Pad siderails and headboard for patient who experiences seizures during the night.

♦ Monitor and record lab assessments of serum trimethadione levels. Report results of CBC and hepatic and renal function tests to physician. Report presence of: • sore throat • fever • malaise • unusual bleeding • easy bruising • yellowish skin or eyes • vision disturbances • skin rash • excessive drowsiness or dizziness • swollen lymph glands.

♦ To minimize nausea, give medication with food or milk.

♦ Ensure that capsule has been swallowed or that tablet has been chewed and swallowed and not "cheeked" to avoid medication or to hoard for later use.

♦ Protect medication from heat; avoid storing at temperatures above 25°C (77°F). Protect from light and moisture.

Patient/Family Education

♦ Do not drive or operate dangerous machinery until individual response has been determined. Drowsiness and dizziness can occur.

♦ Do not stop taking the drug abruptly. To do so can result in absence (petit mal) status.

♦ Avoid alcohol intake or nonprescription medication without approval from physician.

♦ Be aware of risks of taking trimethadione during pregnancy. There is an association between use of anticonvulsant drugs by women with epilepsy and the incidence of birth defects in their children. Fetal defects have occurred when women take this medication during pregnancy. If pregnancy occurs, is suspected, or is planned, notify physician immediately.

♦ Report any of the following symptoms to physician promptly: • sore throat • fever • malaise • unusual bleeding • easy bruising • yellow skin or eyes • skin rash • vision disturbances • excessive drowsiness or dizziness.

♦ To protect patient during tonic-clonic (grand mal) seizure, do not restrain. Padding (towels, blankets, pillows) may be used to prevent bumping against hard objects. When convulsion has subsided, turn patient on side to allow secretions to drain and to prevent aspiration. Keep records of occurrence, characteristics, and duration of seizures, so that accurate reports may be given to physician for providing assistance in stabilization and control of seizures. If patient has difficulty breathing or continues to experience subsequent seizures, family should immediately call for emergency assistance.

♦ Be aware of potential side effects of trimethadione. Refer to written materials furnished by healthcare providers regarding correct method of self-administration.

♦ Carry card or other identification at all times stating illness and names of medications being taken.

Evaluation

♦ Patient demonstrates stabilization of seizure activity with regular administration of trimethadione.

♦ Patient verbalizes understanding of necessity for, side effects of, and regimen required for prudent self-administration of trimethadione.

TRIMIPRAMINE

(tri-mip′ra-meen)
Surmontil

Classification(s):
Tricyclic antidepressant
Pregnancy Category C

INDICATIONS

♦ Major depression with melancholia or psychotic symptoms.

ACTION

♦ Exact mechanism of action unclear ♦ Blocks the reuptake of the neurotransmitters norepinephrine and serotonin, increasing their concentration at the synapse and correcting the deficit that is thought to contribute to the melancholy mood of the depressed person.

PHARMACOKINETICS

Absorption: Readily absorbed from the GI tract following oral administration.
Distribution: Is widely distributed. Crosses blood-brain and placental barriers. Enters breast milk.
Metabolism and Excretion: Metabolized by the liver. Excreted in urine, possibly in feces.

Half-Life: 9.1 hours.

CONTRAINDICATIONS AND PRECAUTIONS

Contraindicated in: ♦ Hypersensitivity to this drug or to other tricyclic antidepressants ♦ Concomitant use of MAO inhibitors ♦ Acute recovery period following myocardial infarction ♦ Untreated angle-closure glaucoma ♦ Children; pregnancy and lactation (safety not established).
Use Cautiously in: ♦ Patients with a history of seizures ♦ Urinary retention ♦ Benign prostatic hypertrophy ♦ Glaucoma ♦ Thyroid disease ♦ Cardiovascular disorders ♦ Respiratory difficulties ♦ Hepatic or renal insufficiency ♦ Psychotic patients ♦ Elderly or debilitated patients.

ADVERSE REACTIONS AND SIDE EFFECTS*

CNS: drowsiness, dizziness, weakness, headache, fatigue, confusion, lethargy, memory deficits, disturbed concentration, tremors, ataxia, tinnitus, extrapyramidal symptoms, paresthesias of extremities, lowered seizure threshold, blurred vision, agitation, excitement, restlessness, insomnia, exacerbation of psychosis, shift to manic behavior.
CV: orthostatic hypotension, tachycardia and other arrhythmias, hypertension, MYOCARDIAL INFARCTION, HEART BLOCK, CONGESTIVE HEART FAILURE, ECG changes, syncope, CARDIOVASCULAR COLLAPSE.
Derm: skin rash, urticaria, photosensitivity, erythema, petechiae.
GI: dry mouth, constipation, nausea, vomiting, anorexia, diarrhea, abdominal cramps, adynamic ileus, esophageal reflux, stomatitis, black tongue.
GU: urinary retention, gynecomastia (men), testicular swelling, menstrual irregularity, breast engorgement and galactorrhea (women), changes in libido, impotence, delayed micturation.

---

*Underlines indicate most frequent; CAPITALS indicate life-threatening.

Hemat: AGRANULOCYTOSIS, THROMBOCYTO-PENIA, LEUKOPENIA, eosinophilia, purpura. **Hepat:** jaundice, hepatitis. **Other:** weight gain, nasal congestion, alopecia, hypothermia, peripheral neuropathy.

INTERACTIONS

Drug-Drug: ♦ **MAO inhibitors:** hyperpyretic crisis, hypertensive crisis, severe seizures, tachycardia, death ♦ **Guanethidine, clonidine, (possibly) guanabenz:** decreased effects of these medications ♦ **Cimetidine:** increased trimipramine serum levels ♦ **Amphetamines, sympathomimetics:** increased hypertensive and cardiac effects of these drugs ♦ **CNS depressants (including alcohol, barbiturates, benzodiazepines):** potentiation of CNS effects ♦ **Thyroid medications:** tachycardia, arrhythmias ♦ **Methylphenidate, phenothiazines, haloperidol:** increased serum trimipramine levels ♦ **Ethchlorvynol:** transient delirium ♦ **Quinidine, procainamide, disopyramide:** potentiation of adverse cardiovascular effects of trimipramine ♦ **Oral contraceptives:** decreased effects of trimipramine ♦ **Smoking:** increased trimipramine metabolism ♦ **Disulfiram:** decreased trimipramine metabolism ♦ **Levodopa, phenylbutazone:** delayed or decreased absorption of these drugs ♦ **Dicumarol:** increased plasma dicumarol concentrations.

ROUTE AND DOSAGE

Depression

♦ **PO (Adults, Outpatient):** Initially, 75 mg/day in divided doses; increase to maximum of 200 mg/day. Total dosage requirement may be given at bedtime.

♦ **PO (Adults, Hospitalized):** Initially, 100 mg/day in divided doses, increased gradually in a few days to 200 mg/day depending upon individual response and tolerance. If improvement does not occur in 2–3 weeks, increase to a maximum dose of 250 to 300 mg/day.

♦ **PO (Adolescent and Geriatric Patients):** Initially, 50 mg/day, increased in gradual increments up to 100 mg/day.

♦ **PO (Maintenance):** Lowest dose that will maintain remission (range 50–150 mg/day). Administer as single bedtime dose. To minimize relapse, continue maintenance therapy for about 3 months.

PHARMACODYNAMICS

Route	Onset	Peak	Duration
PO	2–4 wk	2 hr	Weeks*

*Allow up to 2 weeks following cessation of therapy for complete drug elimination.

NURSING IMPLICATIONS

Assessment

♦ Assess for suicidal ideation, plan, means. Assess for sudden lifts in mood, which could indicate patient's decision to commit suicide.

♦ Assess mental status daily: • mood • appearance • thought and communication patterns • level of interest in the environment and in activities • suicidal ideation. Improvement in these behavior patterns and level of energy should be expected within 2–4 weeks following initiation of therapy.

♦ Assess for symptoms of blood dyscrasias: • sore throat • fever • malaise • unusual bleeding • easy bruising.

♦ Assess vital signs, weight.

♦ Assess history of allergies, sensitivity to this drug or to other tricyclic antidepressants.

♦ Assess for history of glaucoma.

♦ Assess date of last menses (possible pregnancy), use of contraceptives.

♦ Assess whether currently breast-feeding a child.

♦ Assess current and past alcohol and drug consumption.

♦ Assess for operation of automobile

and/or other dangerous machinery.
* Assess for presence of adverse reactions or side effects.
* Assess patient/family knowledge about illness and need for medication.
* In collaboration with physician, assess CBC and liver function tests in patients on long-term therapy.
* **Lab Test Alterations:** Increased serum bilirubin, alkaline phosphatase, and glucose.
◊ Decreased urinary 5-hydroxyindole-acetic acid (HIAA) and vanilmandelic acid (VMA) excretion.
* **Withdrawal:** Assess for symptoms of abrupt withdrawal from long-term therapy: • nausea • headache • vertigo • malaise • insomnia • nightmares.
* **Toxicity and Overdose:** Level of therapeutic serum concentration not well substantiated.
◊ Assess for symptoms of overdose: • confusion • agitation • irritability • hallucinations • seizures • flushing • dry mouth • dilated pupils • delirium • hyperpyrexia • hypotension or hypertension • coma • tachycardia • arrhythmias • respiratory depression • cardiac arrest • renal failure • shock • congestive heart failure • acid-base disturbances.
* **Overdose Management:** Monitor vital signs.
◊ Ensure maintenance of adequate airway.
◊ Monitor ECG.
◊ Induce emesis in conscious patient.
◊ Initiate gastric lavage in unconscious patient.
◊ Administer activated charcoal to minimize absorption.
◊ Administer IV physostigmine cautiously to reverse anticholinergic effects.
◊ Administer sodium bicarbonate, vasopressors, phenytoin, propranolol, or lidocaine to treat cardiovascular effects.
◊ Administer IV diazepam to control seizures.

Potential Nursing Diagnoses
* High risk for self-directed violence related to depressed mood.
* High risk for injury related to trimipramine's side effects of sedation, dizziness, ataxia, weakness, confusion, and lowered seizure threshold; abrupt withdrawal after prolonged use; overdose.
* Social isolation related to depressed mood.
* High risk for activity intolerance related to trimipramine's side effects of drowsiness, dizziness, ataxia, weakness, confusion.
* Knowledge deficit related to medication regimen.

Plan/Implementation
* Monitor vital signs before beginning therapy and at regular intervals (bid or tid) throughout therapy. Take BP lying and standing in patients experiencing orthostatic hypotension; elderly are particularly susceptible. Contact physician if tachycardia/arrhythmias are noted.
* Ensure that patient who is ambulatory is protected from sun when spending time outdoors.
* Weigh patient 2–3 times a week, at same time of day, on same scale, if possible. A rapid weight gain or evidence of edema should be reported to physician immediately. Record I&O.
* Ensure that patient is protected from injury. Provide supervision and assistance when ambulating if dizziness and drowsiness are problems. Pad siderails and headboard for patient who experiences seizures.
* Give patient hard candy, gum, or frequent sips of water if dry mouth is a problem.
* Administer oral medication with food to minimize GI upset.
* Ensure that patient swallows capsule and does not "cheek" to avoid medication or to hoard for later use.
* Empty contents of capsule and mix

with food or fluid for patient who has difficulty swallowing.

♦ Store medication at controlled room temperatures between 15° and 30°C (59°–86°F). Protect from heat and moisture.

Patient/Family Education

♦ Therapeutic effect may not be seen for as long as 4 weeks. If after this length of time no improvement is noted, physician may prescribe a different medication. Continue to take medication even though symptoms have not subsided.

♦ Use caution when driving or when operating dangerous machinery. Drowsiness and dizziness can occur. If these side effects become persistent or interfere with activities of daily living, report to physician. Dosage adjustment may be necessary.

♦ Do not stop taking the drug abruptly. To do so might produce withdrawal symptoms, such as nausea, vertigo, insomnia, headache, malaise, nightmares.

♦ Use sunscreens and wear protective clothing when spending time outdoors. Skin may be sensitive to sunburn.

♦ Report occurrence of any of the following symptoms to physician immediately: • sore throat • fever, malaise • unusual bleeding • easy bruising • persistent nausea/vomiting • severe headache • rapid heart rate • difficulty urinating.

♦ Rise slowly from a sitting or lying position to prevent a sudden drop in blood pressure.

♦ If dry mouth is a problem, take frequent sips of water, chew sugarless gum, or suck on hard candy. Good oral care (frequent brushing, flossing) is very important.

♦ Do not smoke while on trimipramine therapy. Smoking increases metabolism of trimipramine, requiring adjustment in dosage to achieve therapeutic effect.

♦ Do not drink alcohol while on trimipramine therapy. These drugs potentiate each other's effects.

♦ Do not consume other medications (including over-the-counter meds) with trimipramine without physician's approval. Many medications contain substances that, in combination with tricylics, could precipitate a life-threatening hypertensive crisis.

♦ Be aware of possible risks of taking trimipramine during pregnancy. Safe use during pregnancy and lactation has not been established. Trimipramine readily crosses the placental barrier, so a fetus could experience adverse effects of the drug. Inform physician immediately if pregnancy occurs, is suspected, or is planned.

♦ Be aware of side effects of trimipramine. Refer to written materials furnished by healthcare providers for safe self-administration.

♦ Carry card or other identification at all times describing medications being taken.

Evaluation

♦ Patient demonstrates a subsiding/resolution of the symptoms for which trimipramine was prescribed (depressed mood, suicidal ideation).

♦ Patient verbalizes understanding of side effects and regimen required for prudent self-administration of trimipramine.

VALPROIC ACID

(val-proe'ic)
Depakene, Depakote, Myproic Acid

Classification(s):
Anticonvulsant
Pregnancy Category D

INDICATIONS

♦ Simple and complex absence (petit mal) seizures. **Investigational Use:** ♦

Atypical absence, myoclonic, tonic-clonic (grand mal), atonic, akinetic, complex partial, elementary partial, infantile spasm, and recurrent febrile seizures in children ✦ Bipolar disorder ✦ Tardive dyskinesia in patients on long-term antipsychotic therapy.

ACTION

✦ Mechanism of action not fully established ✦ May increase brain levels of the inhibitory neurotransmitter gamma-aminobutyric acid (GABA).

PHARMACOKINETICS

Absorption: Rapidly and almost completely absorbed from the GI tract.
Distribution: Is widely distributed. Crosses the blood-brain and placental barriers; excreted in breast milk.
Metabolism and Excretion: Metabolized by the liver; excreted by the kidneys. Small amounts excreted in feces and expired air.
Half-Life: 5–20 hours (average 10.6 hours).

CONTRAINDICATIONS AND PRECAUTIONS

Contraindicated in: ✦ Hypersensitivity to the drug ✦ Hepatic disease or substantial hepatic dysfunction.
Use Cautiously in: ✦ Elderly or debilitated patients ✦ Renal or cardiac disease ✦ Pregnancy and lactation ✦ Concomitant use of other anticonvulsants.

ADVERSE REACTIONS AND SIDE EFFECTS*

CNS: drowsiness, dizziness, headache, ataxia, tremors, muscle weakness, decreased alertness, fatigue, personality changes, nystagmus, diplopia, anxiety, mental depression, acute psychosis.
Derm: skin rash, alopecia.
Endo: irregular menses, amenorrhea.
GI: nausea/vomiting, indigestion, an-

orexia, weight loss, abdominal cramps, diarrhea, constipation, weight gain, HEPATIC FAILURE, ACUTE PANCREATITIS, HEPATOTOXICITY.
Hemat: BLOOD DYSCRASIAS (anemia, thrombocytopenia, agranulocytosis, leukopenia, eosinophilia), petechiae, bone marrow suppression, prolonged bleeding time, inhibition of platelet aggregation, epistaxis, lymphocytosis.
Other: hyperammonemia, edema of extremities, hyperglycinemia, muscular weakness.

INTERACTIONS

Drug-Drug: ✦ **CNS depressants (including alcohol, barbituates, opiates):** potentiation of CNS depression ✦ **Phenobarbital, primidone:** decreased renal clearance of these drugs may result in severe CNS depression ✦ **Phenytoin:** breakthrough seizures ✦ **Clonazepam:** absence (petit mal) seizures or status ✦ **Aspirin, warfarin:** prolonged bleeding time ✦ **Salicylates:** increased valproic acid serum levels ✦ **MAO inhibitors:** increased MAOI effects.

ROUTE AND DOSAGE

Simple and Complex Absence Seizures

✦ **PO (Adults and Children):** Initial dosage: 15 mg/kg/day. Increase dosage by 5–10 mg/kg/day at weekly intervals until control is achieved with minimal side effects. Maximum dosage: 60 mg/kg/day. If total dosage exceeds 250 mg/day, give in divided doses to prevent adverse GI effects.

PHARMACODYNAMICS

Route	Onset	Peak	Duration
PO	15–30 min*	1–4 hr	4–6 hr

*Onset of therapeutic effect is several days to more than 1 week.

---

*Underlines indicate most frequent; CAPITALS indicate life-threatening.

NURSING IMPLICATIONS
Assessment

- Assess occurrence, characteristics, and duration of seizure activity.
- Assess baseline vital signs.
- Assess history of allergies, sensitivity to this drug.
- Assess date of last menses (possible pregnancy), use of contraceptives.
- Assess whether currently breast-feeding a child.
- Assess current and past alcohol and drug consumption.
- Assess operation of automobile and/or other dangerous machinery.
- Assess for presence of adverse reactions or side effects.
- Assess patient/family knowledge about illness and need for medication.
- In collaboration with physician, assess CBC, renal and liver function tests, platelet counts, and bleeding times.
- **Lab Test Interferences:** Increased ALT/AST and LDH.
- False-positive test for urinary ketones.
- Altered thyroid function tests.
- **Toxicity and Overdose:** Therapeutic serum concentration level is thought to be 50–100 mcg/mL.
- Assess for symptoms of toxicity/overdose: • motor restlessness • visual hallucinations • asterixis • somnolence • pulmonary edema • coma.
- **Overdose Management:** Monitor vital signs.
- Ensure maintenance of adequate airway and adequate urinary output.
- Initiate gastric lavage.
- Naloxone may be administered for reversal of CNS depressant effects but should be given cautiously since it may reverse anticonvulsant activity.
- Hemodialysis and hemoperfusion may be employed.

Potential Nursing Diagnoses

- High risk for injury related to seizures; abrupt withdrawal from long-term valproic acid use; effects of toxicity or overdose.
- Impaired adjustment related to difficulty accepting diagnosis of epilepsy.
- Social isolation related to fear of experiencing a seizure in the presence of others.
- High risk for activity intolerance related to valproic acid's side effects of drowsiness, dizziness, ataxia.
- Knowledge deficit related to medication regimen.

Plan/Implementation

- Monitor vital signs before beginning therapy and at regular intervals (bid) throughout therapy.
- Observe patient frequently (every hour) for occurrence of seizure activity.
- Ensure that patient is protected from injury. Supervise and assist with ambulation if dizziness and ataxia are problems. Avoid or monitor activities that require mental alertness (including smoking). Pad siderails and headboard for patient who experiences seizures during the night.
- Monitor and report results of CBC and hepatic and renal function tests to physician. Report presence of: • sore throat • fever • malaise • unusual bleeding • easy bruising • yellowish skin or eyes • vision disturbances • skin rash • excessive drowsiness or dizziness • swollen lymph glands.
- To minimize nausea, give medication with food or milk.
- Capsules should be swallowed whole to prevent oral irritation.
- Ensure that capsule has been swallowed and not "cheeked" to avoid medication or to hoard for later use.
- Store medication at controlled room temperatures between 15° and 30°C (59°–86°F). Protect from heat and moisture.

Patient/Family Education

- Do not drive or operate dangerous machinery until individual response has been determined. Drowsiness and dizziness can occur.

♦ Do not stop taking the drug abruptly. To do so can result in status epilepticus.

♦ Do not take nonprescription medication without approval from physician.

♦ Do not consume alcohol or other CNS depressants.

♦ Be aware of risks of taking valproic acid during pregnancy. Patient who requires the medication to prevent seizures may be maintained on it; however, she must be fully aware of potential risks to unborn child. There is an association between use of anticonvulsant drugs by women with epilepsy and the incidence of birth defects in their children. If pregnancy occurs, is suspected, or is planned, notify physician immediately.

♦ Report any of the following symptoms to physician promptly: • sore throat • fever • malaise • unusual bleeding • easy bruising • yellow skin or eyes • increase in frequency or severity of seizures.

♦ To protect patient during tonic-clonic (grand mal) seizure, do not restrain. Padding (towels, blankets, pillows) may be used to prevent bumping against hard objects. When convulsion has subsided, turn patient on side to allow secretions to drain and to prevent aspiration. Keep records of occurrence, characteristics, and duration of seizures, so that accurate reports may be given to physician for providing assistance in stabilization and control of seizures. If patient has difficulty breathing or continues to experience subsequent seizures, family should immediately call for emergency assistance.

♦ Be aware of potential side effects of valproic acid. Refer to written materials furnished by healthcare providers regarding correct method of self-administration.

♦ Carry card or other identification at all times stating illness and names of medications being taken.

Evaluation

♦ Patient demonstrates stabilization of seizure activity with regular administration of valproic acid.

♦ Patient demonstrates stabilization of mood when valproic acid is administered for symptoms of bipolar disorder.

♦ Patient verbalizes understanding of necessity for, side effects of, and regimen required for prudent self-administration of valproic acid.

VENLAFAXINE

(ven-la-fax′een)
Effexor

Classification(s):
Phenethylamine bicyclic antidepressant; Serotonin enhancer
Pregnancy Category C

INDICATIONS

♦ Major depressive disorder. **Investigational Use:** ♦ Obsessive compulsive disorder.

ACTION

♦ Selectively inhibits neuronal uptake of serotonin, norepinephrine, and dopamine in order of decreasing potency.

PHARMACOKINETICS

Absorption: Well absorbed following oral administration.

Distribution: Exact distribution is unclear. The drug is 30% protein-bound and extensively tissue-bound. It is not known if venlafaxine or its metabolites are excreted in breast milk.

Metabolism and Excretion: Extensively metabolized to its major active metabolite, O-desmethylvenlafaxine, which maintains similar activity to the parent compound, and two other metabolites which exhibit minimal activity. Approximately 5% to 10% is excreted in the urine as unchanged drug, 55% as O-desmethylvenlafaxine, and 27% as the less active metabolites.

Half-Life: 3–4 hours (velafaxine). 10 hours (O-desmethylvenlafaxine).

CONTRAINDICATIONS AND PRECAUTIONS

Contraindicated in: ♦ Hypersensitivity to the drug ♦ Children and pregnancy (safety not established) ♦ Concomitant use with MAO inhibitors.

Use Cautiously in: ♦ Patients with hepatic or renal insufficiency ♦ Elderly and debilitated patients ♦ Patients with history of drug abuse ♦ Suicidal patients ♦ Patients with history of or existing cardiovascular disease or hyperlipidemia ♦ Patients with history of mania ♦ Patients with history of seizures.

ADVERSE REACTIONS AND SIDE EFFECTS*

CNS: dizziness, somnolence, nervousness, fatigue, headache, anxiety, insomnia.

CV: palpitations, increases in blood pressure, increases in heart rate.

Derm: increased sweating.

Endo/Metab: increases in serum cholesterol, weight loss.

GI: nausea and vomiting, dry mouth, constipation, anorexia.

GU: sexual dysfunction (including erectile failure, delayed orgasm, anorgasmia, impotence, and abnormal ejaculation).

MS: asthenia.

Ocular: blurred vision.

INTERACTIONS

Drug-Drug: ♦ **Cimetidine:** slight increase in venlafaxine concentration ♦ **MAO inhibitors:** synergistic reaction that may result in hyperthermia, rigidity, myoclonus, autonomic instability with rapid fluctuation of vital signs, and mental status changes that include extreme agitation and coma. Reaction may be fatal. At least 14 days should elapse between discontinuation of one of the drugs (MAOI or venlafaxine) and initiation of the other.

ROUTE AND DOSAGE

Depression

♦ **PO (Adults):** 75–375 mg/day in three divided doses.

Obsessive Compulsive Disorder

♦ **PO (Adults):** 25 mg/day increasing to 375 mg/day over a period of 5 weeks.

PHARMACODYNAMICS

Route	Onset	Peak	Duration
PO	2 wk	1–2 hr (venlafaxine) 3–4 hr (O-desmethyl-venlafaxine)	UK

NURSING IMPLICATIONS

Assessment

♦ Assess for suicidal ideation, plan, means. Assess for sudden lifts in mood, which could indicate patient's decision to commit suicide.

♦ Assess mental status daily: • mood • appearance • thought and communication patterns • level of interest in the environment and in activities • suicidal ideation. Improvement in these behavior patterns and level of energy should be expected in approximately 2 weeks following initiation of therapy.

♦ Assess vital signs, weight.

♦ Assess history of cardiovascular disease or hyperlipidemia.

♦ Assess history of allergies, sensitivity to this drug or to similar drugs.

♦ Assess date of last menses (possible pregnancy).

♦ Assess if currently breast-feeding a child.

♦ Assess current and past alcohol and drug consumption.

♦ Assess for operation of automobile and/or other dangerous machinery.

*Underlines indicate most frequent; CAPITALS indicate life-threatening.

* Assess patient/family knowledge about illness and need for medication.
* In collaboration with physician, assess liver and renal function tests before beginning therapy.
* **Lab Test Alterations:** Possible increase in serum cholesterol.
* **Toxicity and Overdose:** Therapeutic serum levels of venlafaxine have not been defined.
* Assess for symptoms of overdose: • somnolence • nausea • vomiting • tachycardia • ECG changes • anxiety • convulsions.
* **Overdose Management:** Establish and maintain airway; ensure adequate oxygenation and ventilation.
* Monitor cardiac (ECG) and vital signs; medications to stabilize pulse and blood pressure may be required.
* May initiate gastric evacuation through emesis, lavage, or both.
* Activated charcoal, which may be used with sorbitol, may be effective.
* Protection from injury should convulsions occur.
* Provide supportive care with close observation.

Potential Nursing Diagnoses

* High risk for self-directed violence related to depressed mood.
* High risk for injury related to venlafaxine overdose or venlafaxine's side effects of somnolence, dizziness, or asthenia.
* Social isolation related to depressed mood.
* High risk for activity intolerance related to venlafaxine's side effects of drowsiness, dizziness, or weakness.
* Knowledge deficit related to medication regimen.

Plan/Implementation

* Monitor vital signs before beginning therapy and at regular intervals (bid or tid) throughout therapy. Contact physician if pulse or blood pressure

rise above parameters established by physician.
* Observe for decrease in appetite and loss of weight.
* Ensure that patient is protected from injury. Provide supervision and assistance when ambulating if dizziness, drowsiness, or weakness are problems. Institute precautions according to institutional policy for patient who experiences seizures.
* Give hard candy, gum, or frequent sips of water if dry mouth is a problem.
* Administer with food or milk to minimize GI upset if necessary.
* Ensure that patient swallows tablet and does not "cheek" to avoid medication or hoard for later use.
* May crush tablet and mix with food or fluid for patient who has difficulty swallowing.
* Store at controlled room temperatures between 15° and 30°C (59°–86°F). Protect from heat and moisture.

Patient/Family Education

* A subsiding of symptoms may be observed in as little as 2 weeks. Given this length of time (or perhaps somewhat longer), if no improvement is noted, physician may prescribe a different medication. Continue to take this medication even though symptoms have not subsided until directed by physician to do otherwise.
* Use caution when driving or operating dangerous machinery. Drowsiness and dizziness can occur. If these side effects become persistent or interfere with activities of daily living, report to physician. Adjustment may be necessary.
* Report occurrence of any of the following symptoms to physician immediately: • rash or hives • persistent nausea/vomiting • severe headache • rapid heart rate • anorexia/weight loss.
* If dry mouth is a problem, take frequent sips of water, chew sugarless gum, or suck on hard candy. Good

oral care (frequent brushing, flossing) is very important.

* Do not drink alcohol while on venlafaxine therapy. These drugs may potentiate the effects of each other.
* Do not consume other medications (including over-the-counter meds) with venlafaxine without physician's approval. Many medications contain substances that, in combination with venlafaxine, could precipitate a potentially life-threatening situation.
* Be aware of possible risks of taking venlafaxine during pregnancy. Safe use during pregnancy and lactation has not been established. Inform physician immediately if pregnancy occurs or is suspected or planned.
* Be aware of side effects of venlafaxine. Refer to written materials furnished by healthcare providers for safe self-administration.
* Carry card or other identification at all times describing medications being taken.

Evaluation

* Patient demonstrates a subsiding/resolution of the symptoms for which venlafaxine was prescribed (depressed mood; suicidal ideation; obsessive-compulsive behavior).
* Patient verbalizes understanding of side effects and regimen required for prudent self-administration of venlafaxine.

VERAPAMIL HCI

(ver-ap'a-mill)
Calan, Isoptin

Classification(s):
Calcium channel blocking agent,
Antihypertensive, Antiarrhythmic,
Antianginal
Pregnancy Category C

INDICATIONS

* Angina pectoris ◆ Essential hypertension ◆ Supraventricular tachyarrhythmias. **Investigational Uses:** ◆ Migraine headache prophylaxis ◆ Bipolar disorder.

ACTION

◆ Inhibits movement of calcium ions across the membrane of myocardial and vascular smooth muscle cells, resulting in inhibition of muscle contraction, vasoconstriction, and cardiac conduction ◆ Mechanism of action in the treatment of bipolar disorder is unknown.

PHARMACOKINETICS

Absorption: Well absorbed following oral administration.
Distribution: Widely distributed. 90% bound to plasma proteins. Crosses into CNS. Crosses placental barrier. Excreted in breast milk.
Metabolism and Excretion: Metabolized by the liver. Excreted in urine and feces.
Half-Life: 2–8 hours initially; 4.5–12 hours with multiple dosing.

CONTRAINDICATIONS AND PRECAUTIONS

Contraindicated in: ◆ Hypersensitivity to this drug or to other calcium channel blockers ◆ Sick sinus syndrome (except with a functioning ventricular pacemaker) ◆ Second- or third-degree AV block ◆ Severe hypotension (less than 90 mmHg systolic) ◆ Cardiogenic shock ◆ Severe CHF (unless secondary to a supraventricular tachycardia amenable to verapamil therapy) ◆ Concomitant use of IV beta-adrenergic blocking agents and IV verapamil ◆ Ventricular tachycardia ◆ Severe left ventricular dysfunction ◆ Children; pregnancy and lactation (safe use has not been established).
Use Cautiously in: Duchenne's muscular dystrophy ◆ Patients with supratentorial tumors undergoing anesthesia induction ◆ Increased intracranial pressure ◆ Impaired hepatic or renal function ◆ Elderly or debilitated patients ◆ Moderately severe to severe ventricular dys-

function or heart failure ♦ Hypertrophic cardiomyopathy.

ADVERSE REACTIONS AND SIDE EFFECTS*

CNS: <u>dizziness</u>, <u>headache</u>, <u>fatigue</u>, sleep disturbances, blurred vision, rotary nystagmus, mental depression, seizures, confusion, psychotic symptoms.

CV: <u>hypotension</u>, <u>peripheral edema</u>, <small>CONGESTIVE HEART FAILURE</small>, <u>pulmonary edema</u>, <u>bradycardia</u>, first-, second-, and third-degree AV block, syncope tachycardia (with IV use), AV dissociation, bundle branch block, arrhythmias.

Derm: alopecia, rash.

GI: <u>constipation</u>, <u>nausea</u>, abdominal discomfort/cramps (with IV use), dry mouth, gingival hyperplasia, diarrhea.

GU: urinary frequency, impotence.

Hepat: hepatitis, <small>HEPATOTOXICITY</small>.

Other: muscle cramps, dyspnea, arthralgia, gynecomastia, diaphoresis, <small>BRONCHOSPASM</small>, <small>LARYNGOSPASM</small>, hyperprolactinemia.

INTERACTIONS

Drug-Drug: ♦ **Beta-adrenergic blockers (e.g., propranolol, metoprolol):** additive depression of myocardial contractility and AV conduction ♦ **Carbamazepine, theophylline:** increased toxic effects of these drugs ♦ **Cimetidine:** possible increased effects of verapamil ♦ **Digoxin, digitoxin:** increased plasma levels of these drugs, possibly resulting in toxicity ♦ **Lithium:** decreased plasma levels of lithium ♦ **Antihypertensive agents (e.g., diuretics, vasodilators, ACE inhibitors):** increased hypotensive effects ♦ **Disopyramide:** additive effects, impairment of left ventricular function ♦ **Neuromuscular blocking agents:** possible increased neuromuscular blocking effects ♦ **Prazosin, methyldopa, quinidine:** acute hypotensive effects ♦ **Rifampin:** decreased effects of verapamil ♦ **Other highly protein-bound drugs (e.g., warfarin, oralhypoglycemics, hydantoins, sulfonamides, salicylates):** increased or decreased plasma levels of these drugs or verapamil.

Drug-Food: ♦ **Calcium salts, vitamin D:** decreased pharmacologic effects of verapamil.

ROUTE AND DOSAGE

Angina Pectoris, Essential Hypertension

♦ **PO, Short-Acting (Adults):** Initial dosage: 80 mg q 6–8 hours. Individualize dose by titration. Increase dosage daily or weekly until optimal clinical response is achieved. Optimal daily dosage range: 240–480 mg, given in 3 or 4 divided doses.

Essential Hypertension

♦ **PO, Sustained-Release (Adults):** 240 mg daily, given in the morning. One-half caplet (120 mg) may be sufficient for individuals with increased response to verapamil (e.g., small or elderly patients). After 24 hours, dosage may be increased if required to 240 mg each morning and 120 mg each evening; then, if needed, to 240 mg q 12 hr.

Supraventricular Tachyarrhythmias (Management)

♦ **IV (Adults):** Initial dose: 5–10 mg (0.075–0.15 mg/kg). May give repeat dose of 10 mg (0.15 mg/kg) 15–30 minutes after first dose if initial response is not adequate but tolerated by patient.

♦ **IV (Children up to 1 Year):** 0.1–0.2 mg/kg (usual single dose range is 0.75–2 mg) as an IV bolus over 2 minutes (under continuous ECG monitoring). May be repeated 30 minutes after first dose if initial response is not adequate.

♦ **IV (Children 1–15 Years):** 0.1–0.3 mg/kg (usual single dose range is 2–

*<u>Underlines</u> indicate most frequent; <small>CAPITALS</small> indicate life-threatening.

5 mg) IV bolus over 2 minutes. Do not exceed 5 mg. May be repeated 30 minutes after first dose if initial response is not adequate.

Paroxysmal Supraventricular Tachycardia (Prevention)
* **PO (Adults):** 240–480 mg/day in 3–4 divided doses.

Bipolar Disorder
(Investigational.)
* **PO (Adults):** 80 mg tid or qid.

Migraine Headache Prophylaxis
(Investigational.)
* **PO (Adults):** Initial dosage: 80 mg tid. Dosage may be increased gradually to a maximum of 480 mg/day. Continue at least 8 weeks before concluding therapy is ineffective.

PHARMACODYNAMICS

Route	Onset	Peak	Duration
PO	30 min	1–2.2 hr	6–8 hr
PO (sustained-release)	—	4–8 hr	12–24 hr
IV	Rapid	5–15 min	0.5–6 hr

NURSING IMPLICATIONS
Assessment
* Assess baseline blood pressure, pulse, respiration.
* Weigh patient for baseline measurement and daily during therapy. Report gain of 5 pounds. Keep strict records of intake and output.
* Assess baseline hepatic and renal function.
* Assess frequency, intensity, and duration of anginal pain.
* Assess history of allergies, sensitivity to this drug or to other drugs.
* Assess date of last menses (possible pregnancy), use of contraceptives.
* Assess whether currently breast-feeding a child.
* Assess current and past alcohol and drug consumption.

* Assess for operation of automobile and/or other dangerous machinery.
* Assess for presence of adverse reactions or side effects.
* Assess patient/family knowledge about illness and need for medication.
* In patient receiving drug for bipolar disorder, assess: • mood • level of activity • interest in the environment • nutritional needs • rapid mood swings.
* Assess for symptoms of abrupt withdrawal: increased frequency and duration of chest pain.
* Assess for symptoms of congestive heart failure: • dyspnea on exertion • orthopnea • night cough • pulmonary rales • distended neck veins • edema.
* **Lab Test Alterations:** Elevated serum AST, ALT, alkaline phosphatase, and bilirubin.
* **Toxicity and Overdose:** Therapeutic plasma level range: 80–300 ng/mL.
◊ Assess for symptoms of overdose: marked and prolonged hypotension and bradycardia, both of which may result in decreased cardiac output. Junctional rhythms and second- or third-degree AV block may also occur.
* **Overdose Management:** If patient is seen shortly after oral ingestion, induce emesis or employ gastric lavage.
◊ Administer beta-adrenergic agonists and IV calcium to reverse effects of inhibited calcium flow (except in patients with hypertrophic cardiomyopathy).
◊ Monitor cardiac and respiratory function.
◊ Administer vasopressor and IV fluids and place patient in Trendelenburg position to maintain blood pressure.
◊ Dialysis is not useful.

Potential Nursing Diagnoses
* Decreased cardiac output related to altered preload, afterload, or inotropic changes in the heart or to side effects of verapamil.

♦ Alteration in tissue perfusion (cardio-pulmonary) related to interruption of arterial flow.

♦ Pain related to decreased arterial flow to cardiac muscle or to migraine headaches.

♦ High risk for injury related to verapamil's side effects of dizziness, blurred vision; and fatigue; overdose; abrupt withdrawal; hyperactivity, (manic episode).

♦ High risk for self-directed violence related to depressed mood (bipolar disorder).

♦ Constipation related to side effect of verapamil.

♦ High risk for activity intolerance related to verapamil's side effects of dizziness, fatigue.

♦ Knowledge deficit related to medication regimen.

Plan/Implementation

♦ **General Info:** Weigh patient daily and keep strict records of intake and output.

◊ Ensure that patient is protected from injury. Provide supervision and assistance when ambulating if dizziness is a problem.

◊ Monitor blood pressure, pulse, and respiration just prior to administration. Physician will provide acceptable parameters for administration. Withhold medication and notify physician immediately if a pronounced change occurs.

◊ Store medication at controlled room temperatures between 15° and 30°C (59°–86°F). Protect from heat, light, and moisture.

♦ **PO:** Medication may be given with food to minimize GI upset.

◊ Short-acting tablet may be crushed and given with fluid of choice for patient who has difficulty swallowing.

◊ Do not crush sustained-release tablet. Should be taken whole.

◊ Encourage increased fluid (if indicated) and fiber in diet for patient who experiences constipation.

♦ **IV:** Patient should be on ECG monitor while receiving IV verapamil.

◊ Emergency resuscitation equipment should be immediately available.

◊ Medication may be given slowly, undiluted, through Y-tube or 3-way stopcock of tubing containing dextrose 5%, sodium chloride 0.9%, or Ringer's solution for infusion.

◊ Administer a single dose over 2 minutes for adults and children; over 3 minutes in the elderly.

◊ Patient should be in recumbent position when dose is given IV, and should remain recumbent for 1 hour following administration.

◊ Monitor blood pressure and pulse every 10 minutes for 1 hour after dose is given. Report symptomatic hypotension or bradycardia immediately. Pharmacologic intervention may be required. Drugs for treatment of acute response (e.g., isoproterenol, atropine, norepinephrine) should be readily available for use if needed.

◊ Solution should be protected from light. Discard if discolored or if a precipitate is visible.

Patient/Family Education

♦ Medication may be taken with meals to minimize GI upset.

♦ Short-acting tablet may be crushed and mixed with fluid of choice if swallowing is difficult. Do not crush or chew sustained-release tablets.

♦ Use caution when driving or when operating dangerous machinery. Dizziness, fatigue, and blurred vision can occur.

♦ Do not abruptly discontinue taking drug. To do so may precipitate an increase in frequency and duration of chest pain.

♦ Report occurrence of any of the following symptoms to physician immediately: ● irregular heartbeat ● shortness of breath • swelling of the hands and feet • pronounced dizziness • constipation • nausea • chest pain that does not subside or begins to occur more frequently • profound mood swings • severe and persistent headache.

♦ Take radial pulse as instructed before each dose. Report significant increase or decrease from baseline normal to physician.

♦ Rise slowly from lying or sitting position to prevent a sudden drop in blood pressure.

♦ Do not consume other medications (including over-the-counter meds) without physician's approval. Many medications contain substances that may interact with verapamil in a way that could be harmful.

♦ Be aware of possible risks of taking verapamil during pregnancy. Safe use during pregnancy and lactation has not been established. Verapamil crosses the placental barrier. Therefore, a fetus could experience adverse effects of the drug. Inform physician immediately if pregnancy occurs, is suspected, or is planned.

♦ Be aware of side effects of verapamil. Refer to written materials furnished by healthcare providers for safe self-administration.

♦ Carry card or other identification at all times describing medications being taken.

Evaluation

♦ Patient demonstrates a resolution/subsiding of the symptoms for which verapamil was prescribed (hypertension, angina, cardiac arrhythmias, migraine headaches, bipolar disorder).

♦ Patient verbalizes understanding of side effects and regimen required for prudent self-administration of verapamil.

ZOLPIDEM

(zole'pi-dem)
Ambien

Classification(s):
Sedative-hypnotic;
Nonbenzodiazepine; CNS
depressant; Imidazopyridine
Schedule C IV
Pregnancy Category B

INDICATIONS

♦ Short-term treatment of insomnia. (Therapy should not exceed 7–10 days without reevaluation of the patient.)

ACTION

♦ Zolpidem possesses sedative, anticonvulsant, anxiolytic, and myorelaxant properties which are thought to be the result of binding to gamma-aminobutyric acid (GABA) receptors in the central nervous system. It appears to be selective for the $omega_1$-receptor subtype.

PHARMACOKINETICS

Absorption: Rapidly absorbed following oral administration.

Distribution: Widely distributed. Highest concentrations are noted in glandular and adipose tissues, while distribution to the brain is low but homogeneous. Plasma protein binding averages 90%. Zolpidem is excreted in breast milk.

Metabolism and Excretion: Metabolized by the liver; converted to inactive metabolites that are excreted primarily by the kidneys.

Half-Life: 2.6 hours (prolonged in elderly patients and those with hepatic insufficiency).

CONTRAINDICATIONS AND PRECAUTIONS

Contraindicated in: ♦ Hypersensitivity to the drug ♦ Pregnancy, lactation, and children under age 18 (safety has not been established) ✦ In combination with other CNS depressants.

Use Cautiously in: ✦ Elderly and debilitated patients ✦ Patients with hepatic, renal, or respiratory dysfunction ✦ Individuals with history of drug abuse/addiction ✦ Depressed/suicidal patients.

ADVERSE REACTIONS AND SIDE EFFECTS*

CNS: <u>drowsiness</u>, <u>dizziness</u>, <u>headache</u>, <u>drugged feeling</u>, depression, lethargy, abnormal dreams, amnesia, nervousness.
CV: palpitation.
Derm: rash.
GI: <u>nausea</u>, <u>vomiting</u>, <u>diarrhea</u>, constipation, dyspepsia, abdominal pain, anorexia.
GU: urinary tract infection.
MS: myalgia, arthralgia.
Resp: upper respiratory infection, sinusitis, pharyngitis, rhinitis.
Other: tolerance, physical and psychological dependence, dry mouth, flu-like symptoms.

INTERACTIONS

Drug-Drug: ✦ **Alcohol and any other drug that produces CNS depressant effects:** additive CNS depression ✦ **Flumazenil:** reversal of zolpidem's sedative-hypnotic effect.
Drug-Food: Food decreases and delays absorption of zolpidem.

ROUTE AND DOSAGE

Insomnia

✦ **PO (Adults):** 10 mg at bedtime (most effective on an empty stomach). ● An initial dose of 5 mg is recommended for elderly and debilitated patients and for patients with hepatic insufficiency.

PHARMACODYNAMICS

Route	Onset	Peak	Duration
PO	30–60 min	1.5–2 hr	7–8 hr

NURSING IMPLICATIONS

Assessment

✦ Assess sleep patterns. Keep records for adequate baseline data before the initiation of therapy.
✦ Assess for suicidal ideation (CNS depressants aggravate symptoms in depressed patients).
✦ Assess history of allergies, sensitivity to this drug.
✦ Assess date of last menses (possible pregnancy); use of contraceptives.
✦ Assess if currently breast-feeding a child.
✦ Assess current and past alcohol and drug consumption.
✦ Assess operation of automobile and/ or other dangerous machinery.
✦ Assess for presence of adverse reactions or side effects.
✦ Assess patient/family knowledge about illness and need for medication.
✦ **Lab Test Alterations:** May cause increase in AST, ALT, BUN, serum glucose, serum cholesterol, and serum lipids.
✦ **Withdrawal:** Assess for symptoms of withdrawal. May occur when drug is discontinued suddenly after being used daily for an extended time. In some cases, symptoms can occur even after only a week or two of use. Mild withdrawal symptoms might include rebound insomnia or a generalized feeling of discomfort. More severe withdrawal symptoms might include abdominal and muscle cramps, nausea and vomiting, flushing, tremors, panic attack, and seizures.
✦ **Withdrawal Management:** ● monitor vital signs ● place in quiet room with low stimuli ● institute seizure precautions.
✦ **Overdose:** Assess for symptoms of overdose: Various stages of impaired consciousness, from somnolence to light coma.

---

*<u>Underlines</u> indicate most frequent; CAPITALS indicate life-threatening.

♦ **Overdose Management:** • monitor vital signs • provide supportive care • initiate immediate gastric lavage when appropriate • intravenous fluids as needed • flumazenil may be beneficial in reversing CNS depression • medical treatment should be administered for hypotension and CNS depression if warranted • sedating drugs should not be given, even if excitation occurs • dialysis is not useful in the treatment of zolpidem overdose.

Potential Nursing Diagnoses

♦ High risk for injury related to abrupt withdrawal from long-term use; effects of drug overdose; decreased mental alertness caused by residual sedation.
♦ High risk for self-directed violence related to depressed mood aggravated by use of CNS depressants.
♦ Sleep pattern disturbance related to situational crises; physical condition; severe level of anxiety.
♦ High risk for activity intolerance related to side effects of lethargy, drowsiness, dizziness, myalgia.
♦ Knowledge deficit related to medication regimen.

Plan/Implementation

♦ Monitor vital signs before beginning therapy and at regular (bid) intervals throughout therapy.
♦ Ensure patient is protected from injury. Supervise and assist with ambulation if dizziness and myalgia are problems. Pad siderails and headboard for patient who experiences seizures (withdrawal).
♦ Administer on empty stomach for fast onset. However, drug may be given with food if nausea is a problem.
♦ Ensure capsule has been swallowed and not "cheeked" to avoid medication or hoard for later use.
♦ Raise siderails and ensure patient remains in bed following administration.
♦ Discourage smoking following administration.
♦

Store at controlled room temperatures between 15° and 30°C (59°–86°F). Protect from heat, light, and moisture.

Patient/Family Education

♦ Do not drive or operate dangerous machinery while taking zolpidem.
♦ Do not stop the drug abruptly. Doing so can produce serious withdrawal symptoms.
♦ Do not consume other CNS depressants unless prescribed by physician. Do not consume alcohol.
♦ Do not take nonprescription medication without approval from physician.
♦ Be aware of possible risks of taking zolpidem during pregnancy. Safety during pregnancy has not been established. Notify physician of desirability to discontinue drug if pregnancy is suspected or planned.
♦ Do not take zolpidem if you are breast-feeding a baby. Zolpidem is excreted in breast milk, but the effect on the infant is unknown.
♦ Be aware of potential side effects. Refer to written materials furnished by healthcare providers regarding correct method of self-administration.
♦ Carry card or piece of paper at all times stating names of medications being taken.
♦ Be aware that zolpidem is only for short-term use and that other methods for achieving sleep must be explored (e.g., relaxation exercises, soft music, warm bath before bedtime). Try to identify stressors that may be interfering with sleep and seek help if necessary for resolution.

Evaluation

♦ Patient demonstrates a subsiding/resolution of the symptoms for which zolpidem was prescribed (insomnia; sleep disturbances).
♦ Patient verbalizes understanding of side effects and regimen required for prudent self-administration of zolpidem.

APPENDIX A

Controlled Substance Categories

Drugs are categorized according to their abuse potential and regulated under the Controlled Substance Act of 1970. The following categories have been defined:

SCHEDULE I (C-I)

Drugs in this category have a high abuse potential. They have no accepted medical use, and their only legitimate purpose is investigational. Examples include heroin, marijuana, LSD.

SCHEDULE II (C-II)

These drugs have a high abuse potential that may lead to severe physical or psychological dependence. Prescriptions must be written in ink (or typewritten) and signed by the physician. They may not be renewed.

Schedule II drugs included in this drug guide:

amobarbital, p. 42	methamphetamine HCl, p. 254
amphetamine sulfate, p. 49	methylphenidate, p. 263
dextroamphetamine sulfate, p. 132	pentobarbital, p. 298
glutethimide, p. 189	phenmetrazine HCl, p. 317
methadone HCl, p. 250	secobarbital, p. 377

SCHEDULE III (C-III)

Some potential for abuse exists with drugs in this category, although less than in Schedules I and II. Low to moderate physical and/or high psychological dependence may be experienced. Up to five renewals are permitted within a 6-month period.

Schedule III drugs included in this Drug Guide:

aprobarbital, p. 54	phendimetrazine, p. 310
benzphetamine, p. 60	thiamylal sodium, p. 396
butabarbital, p. 83	thiopental sodium, p. 399
methyprylon, p. 266	

SCHEDULE IV (C-IV)

These drugs have low potential for abuse, with limited physical or psychological dependence. Up to five renewals are permitted within a 6-month period.

Schedule IV drugs included in this Drug Guide:

SCHEDULE V (C-V)

These drugs have limited abuse potential. Federal law permits limited quantities to be purchased without a prescription, subject to state and local regulations. Purchaser must be 18 years of age and all transactions are recorded by the pharmacist. Examples include small amounts of narcotics (codeine) used as antitussives or antidiarrheals.

APPENDIX B

Key to FDA Pregnancy Control Categories

The Food and Drug Administration has established five categories of potential risk from drug use during pregnancy. The potential is based on risk to the fetus balanced against the drug's potential benefits to the patient. The five categories and their interpretations are as follows:

CATEGORY A

Adequate studies in pregnant women have not demonstrated a risk to the fetus in the first trimester of pregnancy, and there is no evidence of risk in later trimesters.

CATEGORY B

Animal studies have not demonstrated a risk to the fetus, but there are no adequate studies in pregnant women. OR, animal studies have shown an adverse effect, but adequate studies in pregnant women have not demonstrated a risk to the fetus during the first trimester of pregnancy and there is no evidence of risk in later trimesters. Category B drugs included in this Drug Guide:

bupropion, p. 78
buspirone, p. 81
clozapine, p. 124
diphenhydramine, p. 144
fluoxetine, p. 178
glycopyrrolate (parenteral), p. 192

maprotiline, p. 229
methyprylon, p. 266
paroxetine, p. 291
pemoline, p. 294
sertraline, p. 381
zolpidem, p. 452

CATEGORY C

Animal studies have shown an adverse effect on the fetus, but there are no adequate studies in humans; the benefits from the use of the drug in pregnant women may be acceptable despite its potential risks. OR, there are no animal reproduction studies and no adequate studies in humans. Category C drugs included in this Drug Guide:

acetazolamide, p. 24
acetophenazine, p. 26
amantadine, p. 34
amitriptyline, p. 38
amoxapine, p. 45
amphetamine sulfate, p. 49
atropine sulfate, p. 56

benztropine, p. 63
bethanechol, p. 67
biperiden, p. 70
bromocriptine, p. 74
carbamazepine, p. 86
carbidopa/levodopa, p. 90
chloral hydrate, p. 94

CATEGORY D

There is evidence of human fetal risk, but the potential benefits from the use of the drug in pregnant women may be acceptable despite its potential risks. Category D drugs included in this Drug Guide:

prazepam, p. 340
primidone, p. 343
secobarbital, p. 377

trimethadione, p. 436
valproic acid, p. 442

CATEGORY X:

Studies in animals or humans demonstrate fetal abnormalities, or adverse reaction reports indicate evidence of fetal risk. The risk of use in a pregnant woman clearly outweighs any possible benefit. Category X drugs included in this Drug Guide:

benzphetamine, p. 60
temazepam, p. 394

triazolam, p. 419

APPENDIX C

Measurement Conversion Table*

METRIC SYSTEM EQUIVALENTS

1 gram (g) = 1000 milligrams (mg)
1000 grams = 1 kilogram (kg)
1 liter (L) = 1000 milliliters (mL)
1 milliliter = 1 cubic centimeter (cc)
1 meter = 100 centimeters (cm)
1 meter = 1000 millimeters (mm)

CONVERSION EQUIVALENTS

Volume
1 milliliter = 15 minims (M) = 15 drops (gtt)
5 milliliters = 1 fluidram (fz) = 1 teaspoon (tsp)
15 milliliters = 4 fluidrams = 1 tablespoon (T)
30 milliliters = 1 ounce (oz) = 2 tablespoons
500 milliliters = 1 pint (pt)
1000 milliliters = 1 quart (qt)

Weight
1 kilogram = 2.2 pounds (lb)
1 gram (g) = 1000 milligrams = 15 grains (gr)
0.6 gram = 600 milligrams = 10 grains
0.5 gram = 500 milligrams = 7.5 grains
0.3 gram = 300 milligrams = 5 grains
0.06 gram = 60 milligrams = 1 grain

Length
2.5 centimeters = 1 inch

CENTIGRADE-FAHRENHEIT CONVERSIONS

$C = (F - 32) \times \frac{5}{9}$
$F = (C \times \frac{9}{5}) + 32$

---

*Adapted from Deglin, J and Vallerand, A: *Davis's Drug Guide for Nurses.* FA Davis, Philadelphia, 1988.

APPENDIX D

Dietary Guidelines for Food Sources*

POTASSIUM-RICH FOODS

avocados
dried fruits
lima beans
sunflower seeds
nuts
navy beans
cantaloupe
prunes
spinach
tomatoes
rhubarb
oranges
bananas
grapefruit

SODIUM-RICH FOODS

parmesan cheese
buttermilk
butter/margarine
cured meats
canned seafood
canned soups
canned chili
macaroni and cheese
potato salad
pretzels, potato chips
canned spaghetti sauce
canned pork and beans
sauerkraut
tomato ketchup
barbecue sauce
pickles
dry soup mixes
fast-food items (hamburgers,
    french fries, pizza, fried
    chicken)

LOW-SODIUM FOODS

sherbet
egg yolk
low-calorie mayonnaise
lean meats
baked or broiled poultry
fruit
grits (except instant)
puffed wheat or rice
macaroons
red kidney or lima beans
unsalted nuts
honey
jams and jellies
fresh vegetables
potatoes
canned pumpkin
cooked turnips

CALCIUM-RICH FOODS

milk and dairy products
canned salmon/sardines
broccoli
bok choy
tofu

*Adapted from Deglin, J and Vallerand, A: *Davis's Drug Guide for Nurses,* ed 3. FA Davis, Philadelphia, 1993.

molasses
cream soups

VITAMIN K-RICH FOODS

milk
cabbage
yogurt
cheeses
spinach
asparagus
broccoli
brussels sprouts
collard greens
mustard greens
turnips

FOODS THAT ACIDIFY URINE

meats
fish
poultry
eggs
cheeses
grains (breads and cereals)
cranberries
prunes
plums

FOODS THAT ALKALINIZE URINE

all vegetables
milk
all fruits (except cranberries,
prunes, and plums)

FOODS CONTAINING TYRAMINE

red wine
beer
aged cheeses
yeasts
avocados
bananas
yogurt
sour cream
soy sauce
smoked or pickled fish
chocolate
liver
fermented sausage (bologna,
salami, pepperoni)
caffeine-containing beverages
overripe fruit
raisins

APPENDIX E

Common Street Names of Drugs by Classification

I. ANTIANXIETY AGENTS/SEDATIVE-HYPNOTICS (CNS DEPRESSANTS)

Substances

Antianxiety Agents
diazepam (Valium)
chlordiazepoxide (Librium)
oxazepam (Serax)
alprazolam (Xanex)
lorazepam (Ativan)
clorazepate (Tranxene)
prazepam (Centrax)
halazepam (Paxipam)
meprobamate (Equanil, Miltown)

Sedative-Hypnotics
aprobarbital (Alurate)
secobarbital (Seconal)
pentobarbital (Nembutal)
phenobarbital (Luminal)
amobarbital (Amytal)
butabarbital (Butisol)
thiopental (Pentothal)
methohexital (Brevital)
triazolam (Halcion)
flurazepam (Dalmane)
temazepam (Restoril)
chloral hydrate (Noctec)
ethchlorvynol (Placidyl)
glutethimide (Doriden)
methaqualone (Quaalude)
zolpidem (Ambien)

Common Street Names

- downers, goofballs, peanuts, sleepers (barbiturates and tranquilizers)
- ludes, sopers, love drug (methaqualone [Quaalude])
- dyls (ethchlorvynol [Placidyl])
- green-and-whites, libs, roaches (chlordiazepoxide [Librium])
- blues (diazepam [Valium] 10 mg)
- yellows (diazepam [Valium] 5 mg)
- red birds, red devils (secobarbital [Seconal])
- yellow jackets, nembies, yellow birds (pentobarbital [Nembutal])
- Peter, Mickey (chloral hydrate [Noctec])
- bluebirds, blue angels, blue devils (amobarbital [Amytal])
- gorilla pills, GBs, Cibas, D (glutethimide [Doriden])

II. CANNABINOLS

Substances
Marijuana, Hashish

Common Street Names

♦ joint, reefer, pot, grass, Mary Jane, MJ, roach, weed, hemp, jive, loco weed, lid, sativa, tea, Texas tea, Sweet Lucy, hash, gage, bhang, Acapulco gold, viper's weed, baby

III. CNS STIMULANTS

Substances

♦ cocaine
♦ hydrochloride cocaine
♦ amphetamine sulfate (Benzedrine)
♦ methamphetamine (Desoxyn)
♦ dextroamphetamine (Dexedrine)
♦ diethylpropion (Tenuate)
♦ methylphenidate (Ritalin)
♦ phenmetrazine (Preludin)
♦ pemoline (Cylert)
♦ mazindol (Mazanor)
♦ phentermine (Parmine, Phentrol)
♦ phendimetrazine (Plegine)
♦ fenfluramine (Pondimin)
♦ benzphetamine (Didrex)

Common Street Names

♦ coke, snow, gold dust, girl, flake, C, Carrie, Cecil, dream, happy dust, heaven dust, joy powder, nose candy, crystal (cocaine)
♦ rock, crack (hydrochloride cocaine)
♦ bennies, footballs, greenies, uppers, co-pilots, crossroads, peaches, pep pills, roses, truck drivers, wake ups, whites, black beauties, jolly beans (amphetamine sulfate [Benzedrine])
♦ Chris, Christine, crystal, meth, speed, crank (methamphetamine [Desoxyn])
♦ dexies, oranges, hearts, Christmas trees, wedges, spots (dextroamphetamine [Dexedrine])
♦ speedball (mixture of heroin and cocaine)
♦ diet pills (amphetamines, anorexigenics)

IV. HALLUCINOGENS

Substances:

♦ lysergic acid diethylamide (LSD)
♦ mescaline (peyote)
♦ phencyclidine
♦ psilocybin
♦ dimethyltryptamine
♦ dimethoxymethyl amphetamine

Common Street Names

♦ acid, cube, big D, California sunshine, blue dots, Owsley's acid, barrels, black magic, blue acid, blue heaven, brown dots, chief, chocolate chips, cupcakes, domes, flats, grape parfait, Hawaiian sunshine, micro dots, orange wedges, peace tablets, squirrels, strawberry field, twenty-five, white lightning, yellow dimples, purple haze, purple ozone (LSD)
♦ DMT, businessman's trip (dimethyltryptamine)
♦ magic mushroom (mushroom containing psilocybin)

* angel dust, PCP, hog, peace pill, rocket fuel, crystal (phencyclidine)
* TMA (combination of LSD, mescaline, and tetrahydrocannabinol)
* cactus, mesc, mescal, half moon, big chief (mescaline)
* DOM, STP ("serenity, tranquility, peace") (dimethoxymethyl amphetamine)
* pearly gates (morning glory seeds)
* product IV (combination capsules of PCP and LSD)

V. OPIATES/NARCOTICS

Substances

* heroin
* codeine
* morphine
* opium (Paregoric)
* hydromorphone (Dilaudid)
* meperidine (Demerol)
* methadone (Dolophine)
* oxycodone (Percodan)
* pentazocine (Talwin)
* propoxyphene (Darvon)

Common Street Names

* H, horse, junk, noise, pee, scag, shit, skid, smack, boy, doojee, dujie, foolish powder, hairy, Harry, TNT (heroin)
* black stuff, poppy, tar, hop, pin, yen, skee, wen shee, big O (opium)
* M, morph, morphie, morpho, white stuff, cube juice, emsel, hocus, Miss Emma, unkie, white merchandise (morphine)
* schoolboy, robo, romo, syrup (codeine)
* terp, turps (terpin hydrate cough syrup with codeine)
* spaghetti sauce (Robitussin A-C cough syrup with codeine)
* lords, little D (hydromorphine [Dilaudid])
* perkies (oxycodone [Percodan])
* PG or PO (Paregoric)
* dollies (methadone [Dolophine])
* blue velvet (a mixture of Paregoric and antihistamine)
* T's (pentazocine [Talwin])
* doctors (Demerol)

VI. DESIGNER DRUGS

Designer drugs are analogs of known pharmacological agents, synthesized by underground chemists, for sale on the street. The chemical structure of a drug is manipulated to create a totally new compound.

Substances

* 3,4-methylenedioxymethamphetamine fentanyl analogs:
  alpha-methyl-p-fluoro-3-methyl
  alpha-methyl-acetylfentanyl
* meperidine analog
  1-methyl-4-phenyl-4-propionpiperidine

Common Street Names

* MDMA, MDA, Adam, Ecstasy, XTC (3,4-methylene-dioxymethamphetamine)
* China White (fentanyl analogs)
* MPPP, synthetic heroin (meperidine analog)

Alphabetical Listing of NANDA Nursing Diagnoses*

Activity intolerance
Activity intolerance, high risk for
Adjustment, impaired
Airway clearance, ineffective
Anxiety [specify level]
Aspiration, high risk for

Body image disturbance
Body temperature, altered, high risk for
Bowel incontinence
Breastfeeding, effective
Breastfeeding, ineffective
Breastfeeding, interrupted
Breathing pattern, ineffective

Cardiac output, decreased
Caregiver role strain
Caregiver role strain, high risk for
Communication, impaired verbal
Constipation
Constipation, colonic
Constipation, perceived
Coping, defensive
Coping, family: potential for growth
Coping, ineffective family: compromised
Coping, ineffective family: disabling
Coping, ineffective individual

Decisional conflict (specify)
Denial, ineffective
Diarrhea
Disuse syndrome, high risk for
Diversional activity deficit
Dysreflexia

---

*Through 11th National Conference, March 1994.

Family processes, altered
Fatigue
Fear
Feeding pattern, infant: ineffective
Fluid volume deficit
Fluid volume deficit, high risk for
Fluid volume excess

Gas exchange, impaired
Grieving, anticipatory
Grieving, dysfunctional
Growth and development, altered

Health maintenance, altered
Health-seeking behaviors (specify)
Home maintenance management, impaired
Hopelessness
Hyperthermia
Hypothermia

Incontinence, functional
Incontinence, reflex
Incontinence, stress
Incontinence, total
Incontinence, urge
Infection, high risk for
Injury, high risk for

Knowledge deficit (specify)

Management of therapeutic regimen, ineffective
Mobility, impaired physical

Noncompliance (specify)
Nutrition, altered: less than body requirements
Nutrition, altered: more than body requirements
Nutrition, altered: high risk for more than body requirements

Oral mucous membrane, altered

Pain
Pain, chronic
Parental role conflict
Parenting, altered
Parenting, altered, potential
Peripheral neurovascular dysfunction, high risk for
Personal identity disturbance
Poisoning, high risk for
Post-trauma response

Powerlessness
Protection, altered

Rape-trauma syndrome
Rape-trauma syndrome: compound reaction
Rape-trauma syndrome: silent reaction
Relocation stress syndrome
Role performance, altered

Self-care deficit, bathing/hygiene
Self-care deficit, dressing/grooming
Self-care deficit, feeding
• Self-care deficit, toileting
Self-esteem disturbance
Self-esteem, chronic low
Self-esteem, situational low
Self-mutilation, high risk for
Sensory/perceptual alteration: visual, auditory, kinesthetic, gustatory, tactile, olfactory
Sexual dysfunction
Sexuality patterns, altered
Skin integrity, impaired
Skin integrity, impaired, high risk for
Sleep pattern disturbance
Social interaction, impaired
Social isolation
Spiritual distress
Suffocation, high risk for
Swallowing, impaired

Thermoregulation, ineffective
Thought processes, altered
Tissue integrity, impaired
Tissue perfusion, altered: renal, cerebral, cardiopulmonary, gastrointestinal, peripheral
Trauma, high risk for

Unilateral neglect
Urinary elimination, altered patterns
Urinary retention

Ventilation, spontaneous: inability to sustain
Ventilatory weaning response, dysfunctional
Violence, high risk for: self-directed or directed at others

Classification of NANDA Nursing Diagnoses by Doenges'/ Moorhouse's Diagnostic Divisions

ACTIVITY/REST

Activity Intolerance
Activity Intolerance, high risk for
Disuse Syndrome, high risk for
Diversional Activity deficit
Fatigue
Sleep Pattern disturbance

CIRCULATION

Cardiac Output, decreased
Dysreflexia
Tissue Perfusion, altered (specify): cerebral, cardiopulmonary, renal, gastrointes-
tinal, peripheral

EGO INTEGRITY

Adjustment, impaired
Anxiety [specify level]
Body Image disturbance
Coping, defensive
Coping, Individual, ineffective
Decisional Conflict (specify)
Denial, ineffective
Fear
Grieving, anticipatory
Grieving, dysfunctional
Hopelessness
Personal Identity disturbance
Post-Trauma Response
Powerlessness
Rape-Trauma Syndrome
Rape-Trauma Syndrome: compound reaction
Rape-Trauma Syndrome: silent reaction
Relocation Stress Syndrome
Self Esteem, chronic low

Self Esteem, disturbance
Self Esteem, situational low
Spiritual Distress (distress of the human spirit)

ELIMINATION

Bowel Incontinence
Constipation
Constipation, colonic
Constipation, perceived
Diarrhea
Incontinence, functional
Incontinence, reflex
Incontinence, stress
Incontinence, total
Incontinence, urge
Urinary Elimination, altered
Urinary Retention [acute/chronic]

FOOD/FLUID

Breastfeeding, effective
Breastfeeding, ineffective
Breastfeeding, interrupted
Fluid Volume deficit [active loss]
Fluid Volume deficit [regulatory failure]
Fluid Volume deficit, high risk for
Fluid Volume excess
Infant Feeding Pattern, ineffective
Nutrition, altered, less than body requirements
Nutrition, altered, more than body requirements
Nutrition, altered, high risk for more than body requirements
Oral Mucous Membrane, altered
Swallowing, impaired

HYGIENE

Self Care deficit (specify): feeding, bathing/hygiene, dressing/grooming, toileting

NEUROSENSORY

Peripheral Neurovascular dysfunction, high risk for
Sensory-Perceptual alterations (specify): visual, auditory, kinesthetic, gustatory, tactile, olfactory
Thought Processes, altered
Unilateral Neglect

PAIN/DISCOMFORT

Pain [acute]
Pain, chronic

RESPIRATION

Airway Clearance, ineffective
Aspiration, high risk for

Breathing Pattern, ineffective
Gas Exchange, impaired
Spontaneous Ventilation, inability to sustain
Ventilatory Weaning Response, dysfunctional (DVWR)

SAFETY

Body Temperature, altered, high risk for
Health Maintenance, altered
Home Maintenance Management, impaired
Hyperthermia
Hypothermia
Infection, high risk for
Injury, high risk for
Physical Mobility, impaired
Poisoning, high risk for
Protection, altered
Self-Mutilation, high risk for
Skin Integrity, impaired
Skin Integrity, impaired, high risk for
Suffocation, high risk for
Thermoregulation, ineffective
Tissue Integrity, impaired
Trauma, high risk for
Violence, high risk for, directed at self/others

SEXUALITY

Sexual dysfunction
Sexuality Patterns, altered

SOCIAL INTERACTION

Caregiver Role Strain
Caregiver Role Strain, high risk for
Communication, impaired verbal
Family Coping, ineffective: compromised
Family Coping, ineffective: disabling
Family Coping, potential for growth
Family Processes, altered
Parenteral Role Conflict
Parenting, altered
Parenting, altered, high risk for
Role Performance, altered
Social Interaction, impaired
Social Isolation

TEACHING/LEARNING

Growth and Development, altered
Health-Seeking Behaviors (specify)
Knowledge Deficit [Learning Need] (specify)
Noncompliance [Compliance, altered] (specify)
Therapeutic Regimen (Individual), ineffective management of

APPENDIX H

Classification of NANDA Nursing Diagnoses by Gordon's Functional Health Patterns*

HEALTH PERCEPTION–HEALTH MANAGEMENT PATTERN
 Altered health maintenance
 Ineffective management of therapeutic regimen (Individuals)
 Noncompliance (specify)
 Health-seeking behaviors (specify)
 High risk for infection
 High risk for injury (trauma)
 High risk for poisoning
 High risk for suffocation

NUTRITIONAL-METABOLIC PATTERN
 Altered nutrition: high risk for more than body requirements
 Altered nutrition: more than body requirements
 Altered nutrition: less than body requirements
 Ineffective breastfeeding
 Effective breastfeeding
 Interrupted breastfeeding
 Ineffective infant feeding pattern
 High risk for aspiration
 Impaired swallowing
 Altered oral mucous membrane
 High risk for fluid volume deficit
 Fluid volume deficit
 Fluid volume excess
 High risk for impaired skin integrity
 Impaired skin integrity
 Impaired tissue integrity (specify type)
 High risk for altered body temperature
 Ineffective thermoregulation
 Hyperthermia
 Hypothermia

---

*Based on Gordon, M.: Nursing Diagnosis: Process and Applications. McGraw-Hill, New York, ed. 6., 1993, with permission.

ELIMINATION PATTERN
> Constipation
> Colonic constipation
> Perceived constipation
> Diarrhea
> Bowel incontinence
> Altered urinary elimination patterns
> Functional incontinence
> Reflex incontinence
> Stress incontinence
> Urge incontinence
> Total incontinence
> Urinary retention

ACTIVITY-EXERCISE PATTERN
> High risk for activity intolerance
> Activity intolerance (specify level)
> Fatigue
> Impaired physical mobility
> High risk for disuse syndrome
> Bathing/hygiene self-care deficit
> Dressing/grooming self-care deficit
> Feeding self-care deficit
> Toileting self-care deficit
> Diversional activity deficit
> Impaired home maintenance management
> Dysfunctional Ventilatory Weaning Response (DVWR)
> Inability to sustain spontaneous ventilation
> Ineffective airway clearance
> Ineffective breathing pattern
> Impaired gas exchange
> Decreased cardiac output
> Altered tissue perfusion (specify)
> Dysreflexia
> High risk for peripheral neurovascular dysfunction
> Altered growth and development

SLEEP-REST PATTERN
> Sleep pattern disturbance

COGNITIVE-PERCEPTUAL PATTERN
> Pain
> Chronic pain
> Sensory perceptual alteration (specify)
> Unilateral neglect
> Knowledge deficit (specify)
> Altered thought process
> Decisional conflict (specify)

SELF-PERCEPTION-SELF-CONCEPT PATTERN
Fear
Anxiety
Hopelessness
Powerlessness
Self-esteem disturbance
Chronic low self-esteem
Situational low self-esteem
Body image disturbance
High risk for self-mutilation
Personal identity disturbance

ROLE-RELATIONSHIP PATTERN
Anticipatory grieving
Dysfunctional grieving
Altered role performance
Social isolation
Impaired social interaction
Relocation stress syndrome
Altered family processes
High risk for altered parenting
Altered parenting
Parental role conflict
Caregiver role strain
High risk for caregiver role strain
Impaired verbal communication
High risk for violence: self-directed or directed at others

SEXUALITY-REPRODUCTIVE PATTERN
Sexual dysfunction
Altered sexuality patterns
Rape-trauma syndrome
Rape-trauma syndrome: compound reaction
Rape-trauma syndrome: silent reaction

COPING-STRESS TOLERANCE PATTERN
Ineffective individual coping
Defensive coping
Ineffective denial
Impaired adjustment
Post-trauma response
Family coping: potential for growth
Ineffective family coping: compromised
Ineffective family coping: disabling

VALUE-BELIEF PATTERN
Spiritual distress (distress of the human spirit)

Bibliography

American Psychiatric Association: Diagnostic and Statistical Manual of Mental Disorders, ed 4. Washington, DC, 1994.

Anath, J and Lin, KM: Propranolol in psychiatry. Neuropsych 15:20, 1986.

Anthony, M and Lance, JW: Monoamine oxidase inhibition in the treatment of migraine. Arch Neurol 21:263, 1969.

August, GJ, et al: Fenfluramine treatment in infantile autism: Neurochemical, electrophysiological, and behavioral effects. J Nerv Ment Dis 172:604, 1984.

Baer, CL and Williams, BR: Clinical Pharmacology and Nursing. Springhouse, Springhouse, PA, 1988.

Baldessarini, RJ: Chemotherapy in Psychiatry: Principles and Practice, revised ed. Harvard University Press, Cambridge, MA, 1985.

Ballenger, JC and Post, RM: Carbamazepine in manic-depressive illness: A new treatment. Am J Psych 137:782, 1980.

Barton, BM and Gitlin, MJ: Verapamil in treatment-resistant mania: An open trial. J Clin Psychopharmacol 7:101, 1987.

Baum, RM: New variety of street drugs poses growing problem. Chem and Engr 9:7, 1987.

Beck, CK, et al: Mental Health-Psychiatric Nursing: A Holistic Life-Cycle Approach, ed 2. CV Mosby, St. Louis, 1988.

Bennett, G, et al (eds): Substance Abuse: Pharmacologic, Developmental and Clinical Perspectives, ed 2. Delmar Publishers, Albany, NY, 1991.

Benson, DS and Conte, RR: Nursing Meds. Appleton & Lange, 1991.

Birckhead, LM: Psychiatric/Mental Health Nursing: The Therapeutic Use of Self. JB Lippincott, Philadelphia, 1989.

Birkhimer, W, et al: Use of carbamazepine in psychiatric disorders. Clin Pharm 4:425, 1985.

Bjorkovist, SE, et al: Ambulent treatment of alcohol withdrawal symptoms with carbamazepine: A formal multicenter double-blind comparison with placebo. Acta Psychiatr Scand 53:333, 1976.

Bond, WS: Recognition and treatment of attention deficit disorder. Clin Pharm 6:617, 1987.

Bond, WS, et al: Pharmacotherapy of eating disorders: A critical review. Drug Intell Clin Pharm 20: 659, 1986.

Brotman, AW: Antidepressant therapy. J Clin Psych 45:7, 1984.

Brotman, AW, et al: Verapamil treatment of acute mania. J Clin Psych 47:136, 1986.

Brownell, LG, et al: Protriptyline in obstructive sleep apnea: A double-blind trial. N Engl J Med 307:1037, 1982.

Bryant, SG and Ereshefsky, L: Antidepressant properties of trazodone. Clin Pharm 1:406, 1982.

Bryant S, et al: Refractory bipolar illness may not respond to verapamil. J Clin Psychopharm 6:316, 1986.

Bryant, SG and Brown, C: Current concepts in clinical trials: Major affective disorders, part 2. Clin Pharm 5:385, 1986.

Burgess, AW: Psychiatric Nursing in the Hospital and the Community, ed 5. Prentice-Hall, Englewood Cliffs, NJ, 1990.

Chy, NS: Carbamazepine: Prevention of alcohol withdrawal seizures. Neurology 29:1397, 1979.

Conway, W, et al: Protriptyline therapy for upper airway sleep apnea. Am Rev Respir Dis 125 (Suppl); 102, 1982.

Cowley, G, et al: The promise of prozac. Newsweek, March 26, 1990.

Damasio, H and Lyon, L: Lithium carbonate in the treatment of cluster headaches. J Neurol 224:1, 1980.

Deglin, JH and Vallerand, AH: Davis's Drug Guide for Nurses, ed 3. FA Davis, Philadelphia, 1993.

Dhib-Jalbut, S, et al: Treatment of the neuroleptic malignant syndrome with bromocriptine. JAMA 250:484, 1983.

475

Dhib-Jalbut, S, et al: Bromocriptine treatment of neuroleptic malignant syndrome. J Clin Psych 48: 69, 1987.

Doenges, ME, et al: Psychiatric Care Plans: Guidelines for Client Care, ed 2. FA Davis, Philadelphia, 1995.

Doenges, ME and Moorhouse, MF: Nurse's Pocket Guide: Nursing Diagnoses with Interventions, ed 4. FA Davis, Philadelphia, 1993.

Dommisse, CS and DeVane, CL: Buspirone: A new type of anxiolytic. Drug Intell Clin Pharm 19: 624, 1985.

Ekbom, K: Lithium for cluster headache: Review of the literature and preliminary results of long-term treatment. Headache 21:132, 1981.

Estes, NJ, et al: Nursing Diagnosis of the Alcoholic Person. CV Mosby, St. Louis, 1980.

Estes, NJ and Hinemann, ME: Alcoholism: Development, Consequences, and Interventions, ed 2. CV Mosby, St. Louis, 1982.

Facts and Comparisons. JB Lippincott, St. Louis, 1994.

Feighner, JP: A comparative trial of fluoxetine and amitriptyline in patients with major depressive disorder. J Clin Psych 46:369, 1985.

Fischbach, F: A Manual of Laboratory Diagnostic Tests, ed 3. JB Lippincott, Philadelphia, 1988.

Gahart, BL: Intravenous Medications: A Handbook for Nurses and Other Allied Health Personnel, ed 8. CV Mosby, St. Louis, 1992.

Geller, E, et al: Preliminary observations on the effect of fenfluramine on blood serotonin and symptoms in three autistic boys. N Engl J Med 307:165, 1982.

Gelman, D: Drugs vs. the couch. Newsweek, March 26, 1990.

Gerald, MC, and O'Bannon, FV: Nursing Pharmacology and Therapeutics, ed 2. Appleton & Lange, Norwalk, CT, 1988.

Giannini, AJ, et al: Comparison of antimanic efficacy of clonidine and verapamil. J Clin Pharmacol 25:307, 1985.

Gilman, AG, et al (eds): Goodman and Gilman's The Pharmacological Basis of Therapeutics, ed 7. MacMillan, New York, 1985.

Goa, KL and Ward, A: Buspirone: A preliminary review of its pharmacological properties and therapeutic efficacy as anxiolytic. Drugs 32:114, 1986.

Govoni, LE and Hayes, JE: Drugs and Nursing Implications, ed. 7. Appleton & Lange, Norwalk, CT, 1992.

Greenwald, BS, et al: Serotoninergic treatment of screaming and banging in dementia. Lancet 2: 1464, 1986.

Haber, J, et al: Comprehensive Psychiatric Nursing, ed 4. McGraw-Hill, New York, 1992.

Hannsen, T, et al: Propranolol in schizophrenia. Arch Gen Psychiatry 37:685, 1980.

Hayes, PE and Dommisse, CS: Current concepts in clinical therapeutics: Anxiety disorders, part 1. Clin Pharm 6:140, 1987.

Hayes, PE and Dommisse, CS: Current concepts in clinical therapeutics: Anxiety disorders, part 2. Clin Pharm 6:196, 1987.

Hayes, PE and Schultz, SC: The use of beta-adrenergic blocking agents in anxiety disorders and schizophrenia. Pharmacotherapy 3:101, 1983.

Hockaday, JM, et al: Bromocriptine in migraine. Headache 16:109, 1976.

Honda, Y and Hishikawa, Y: A long-term treatment of narcolepsy and excessive daytime sleepiness with pemoline. Curr Ther Res 27:425, 1980.

Hudson, JI, et al: Treatment of anorexia nervosa with antidepressants. J Clin Psychopharm 5:17, 1985.

Jann, MW, et al: Carbamazepine for patients with affective target symptoms. Drug Intell Clin Pharm 18:81, 1984.

Janosik, EH and Davies, JL: Psychiatric/Mental Health Nursing, ed 2. Jones and Bartlett, Boston, 1989.

Jenkins, SC, and Maruta, T: Therapeutic use of propranolol for intermittent explosive disorder. Mayo Clin Proc 62:204, 1987.

Johnson, BS: Psychiatric-Mental Health Nursing: Adaptation and Growth, ed 3. JB Lippincott, Philadelphia, 1993.

Johnson, GE and Hannah, KJ: Pharmacology and the Nursing Process, ed 3. WB Saunders, Philadelphia, 1992.

Jonas, JM and Schaumburg, R: Everything You Need to Know about Prozac. Bantom Nonfiction, New York, 1991.

Kales, A, et al: Insomnia and other sleep disorders. Med Clin North Am 66:971, 1982.

Kaplan, HI and Sadock, BJ: Modern Synopsis of Comprehensive Textbook of Psychiatry, ed 4. Williams & Wilkins, Baltimore, 1985.

Karch, A and Boyd, E: Handbook of Drugs and the Nursing Process. JB Lippincott, Philadelphia, 1989.

Kastenholz, KV and Crismon, ML: Buspirone: A novel nonbenzodiazepine anxiolytic. Clin Pharm 3: 600, 1984.

Knoben, JE and Anderson, PO: Handbook of Clinical Drug Data, ed 6. Drug Intelligence, Hamilton, IL, 1988.

Kudrow, L: Lithium prophylaxis for chronic cluster headache. Headache 17:15, 1977.

Kudrow, L: Cluster Headache: Mechanisms and Management. Oxford University Press, Oxford, 1980.

Lenzi, A, et al: Use of carbamazepine in acute psychiatrics: A controlled study. J Int Med Res 14: 78, 1986.

Lickey, ME and Gordon, B: Drugs for Mental Illness: A Revolution in Psychiatry. W. H. Freeman, New York, 1983.

Love, HL, et al: The use of alternative drug therapy in nine patients with recurrent affective disorder resistant to conventional prophylaxis. Biol Psychiatry 21:1344, 1986.

Lydiard, RB and Gelenberg, AJ: Amoxapine—an antidepressant with some neuroleptic properties? Pharmacotherapy 1:163, 1981.

Markley, HG, et al: Verapamil in prophylactic therapy of migraine. Neurology 34:973, 1984.

Masters, JC and Spitler, R: Neuroleptic malignant syndrome. J Psychoscoc Nurs 24(9):11–16.

Mathewson, MK: Pharmacotherapeutics: A Nursing Process Approach, ed 2. FA Davis, Philadelphia, 1991.

McCord, MA: Relating nursing diagnoses to drug therapy. Nursing 88, October 1988.

McEvoy, GK (ed): American Hospital Formulary Service: Drug Information '88. American Society of Hospital Pharmacists, Bethesda, MD, 1988.

McHenry, LM, et al: Pharmacology in Nursing, ed 17. C. V. Mosby, St. Louis, 1989.

Meyer, JS, et al: Clinical and hemodynamic effects during treatment of vascular headaches with verapamil. Headache 24:313, 1984.

Mueller, PS, et al: Neuroleptic malignant syndrome: Successful treatment with bromocriptine. JAMA 249:386, 1983.

Murray, RB and Huelskoetter, MM: Psychiatric/Mental Health Nursing: Giving Emotional Care, ed 2. Appleton & Lange, Norwalk, CT, 1987.

Myers, DH, et al: A trial of propranolol in chronic schizophrenia. Br J Psychiatry 139:1181, 1981.

Overall, JE, et al: Broad-spectrum screening of psychotherapeutic drugs: Thiothixene as an antipsychotic and antidepressant. Clin Pharmacol Ther 10:36, 1969.

Pasquali, EA, et al: Mental Health Nursing: A Holistic Approach, ed 3. CV Mosby, St. Louis, 1989.

Physicians' Desk Reference, ed 48. Medical Economics, Oradell, NJ, 1994.

Pickar, D, et al: Clinical and biochemical effects of verapamil administration to schizophrenic patients. Arch Gen Psychiatry 44:113, 1987.

Pope, HG: Antidepressant therapy of bulimia—2 year study. J Clin Psychopharm 5:320, 1985.

Post, RM and Uhde, TW: Carbamazepine in bipolar disorder. Psychopharmacol Bull 21:10, 1985.

Poutanen, P: Experience with carbamazepine in the treatment of withdrawal symptoms in alcohol abusers. Br J Addict 74:210, 1979.

Price, WA and Giannini, AJ: Neurotoxicity caused by lithium-verapamil synergism. J Clin Pharmacol 26:717, 1986.

Raskin, NH and Appenzeller, O: Headache, Major Problems in Internal Medicine, Vol. XIX. WB Saunders, Philadelphia, 1980.

Rawls, WN: Trazodone. Drug Intell Clin Pharm 16:7, 1982.

Ritvo, ER, et al: Effects of fenfluramine on 14 outpatients with the syndrome of autism. J Am Acad Child Psych 22:549, 1983.

Ritvo, ER, et al: Study of fenfluramine in outpatients with the syndrome of autism. J Pediatr 105: 823, 1984.

Roberts, PW: The use of propranolol in treating tardive dyskinesia. Can Med Assoc J 123:1106, 1980.

Robinson, L: Psychiatric Nursing as a Human Experience, ed 3. WB Saunders, Philadelphia, 1983.

Rowbothan, MC, et al: Trazodone-oral cocaine interactions. Arch Gen Psych 1:895, 1984.

Saper, JR and Magee, KR: Freedom from Headaches. Simon and Schuster, New York, 1981.

Schatzberg, AF and Cole, JO: Manual of Clinical Psychopharmacology. American Psychiatric Press, Washington, 1986.

Scherer, JC (ed). Lippincott's Nurses' Drug Manual. JB Lippincott, Philadelphia, 1985.

Schuckit, MA: Drug and Alcohol Abuse: A Clinical Guide to Diagnosis and Treatment. Plenum Medical Book Co., New York, 1979.

Simeon, J, et al: Thiothixene in the treatment of anxiety and depression in outpatients. Curr Ther Res 12:369, 1970.

Simpson, GM, et al: Role of antidepressants and neuroleptics in the treatment of depression. Arch Gen Psych 27:337, 1972.

Skidmore-Roth, L: Mosby's Nursing Drug Reference. CV Mosby, St. Louis, 1994.

Solomon, GD, et al: Verapamil prophylaxis of migraine. JAMA 250:2500, 1983.

Sommi, RW, et al: Fluoxetine: A serotonin-specific, second-generation antidepressant. Pharmacotherapy 7:1, 1987.

Spratto, GR and Woods, AL: Nurse's Drug Reference. Delmar Publishers, Albany, NY, 1994.

Stark, P and Hardison, CD: A review of multicenter controlled studies of fluoxetine versus imipramine and placebo in outpatients with major depressive disorder. J Clin Psych 46:53, 1985.

Stimmel, GL: Antidepressants: Old and new. Clin Pharm 1:462, 1982.

Stimmel, GL and Escobar, JI: Antidepressants in chronic pain: A review of efficacy. Pharmacotherapy 6:262, 1986.

Stromgren, LS and Boller, S: Carbamazepine in treatment and prophylaxis of manic-depressive disorder. Psychiatr Dev 3:349, 1985.

Stuart, GW and Sundeen, SJ: Principles and Practice of Psychiatric Nursing, ed 4. CV Mosby, St. Louis, 1991.

Tatro, DS (ed): Drug Interaction Facts. JB Lippincott, St. Louis, 1988.

Townsend, MC: Nursing Diagnoses in Psychiatric Nursing: A Pocket Guide for Care Plan Construction, ed 3. FA Davis, Philadelphia, 1994.

Townsend, MC: Psychiatric Mental Health Nursing: Concepts of Care. FA Davis, Philadelphia, 1993.

Walsh, BT, et al: Treatment of bulimia with monoamine oxidase inhibitors. Am J Psychiatry 159:1625, 1982.

Walsh, BT, et al: Treatment of bulimia with phenelzine. Arch Gen Psych 41:1105, 1984.

Warner-Lambert Company: The first therapeutic agent for the treatment of mild to moderate Alzheimer's disease. Am J Psychiatry, January 1994.

Washton, AM and Resnick, RB: Clonidine in opiate withdrawal: Review and appraisal of clinical findings. Pharmacotherapy 1:140, 1981.

Wells, BG and Gelenberg, AJ: Chemistry, pharmacology, pharmacokinetics, adverse effects, and efficacy of the antidepressant maprotiline hydrochloride. Pharmacotherapy 1:121, 1981.

Wilbur, R and Kulik, RA: Anticonvulsant drugs in alcohol withdrawal: Use of phenytoin, primidone, carbamazepine, valproic acid, and the sedative anticonvulsants. Am J Hosp Pharm 38:1138, 1981.

Wilcock, GK, et al: Trazodone/tryptophan for aggressive behavior. Lancet 1:929, 1987.

Wilson, HS and Kneisl, CR: Psychiatric Nursing, ed 3. Addison-Wesley, Menlo Park, CA, 1988.

Yager, J: Treatment of eating disorders. J Clin Psych 49:18, 1988.

Yorkston, NJ, et al: Propranolol as an adjunct to the treatment of schizophrenia. Lancet 2:575, 1977.

Young, LY and Koda-Kimble, MA (eds): Applied Therapeutics: The Clinical Use of Drugs, ed 4. Applied Therapeutics, Vancouver, WA, 1988.

Comprehensive Index:
generic/Trade/CLASSIFICATION*

*Entries for **generic** names appear in **boldface** type, trade names appear in regular type, and CLASSIFICATIONS appear in SMALL CAPS.

479